H·C·P·C·S

Health Care Procedure Coding System

National Level II Medicare Codes

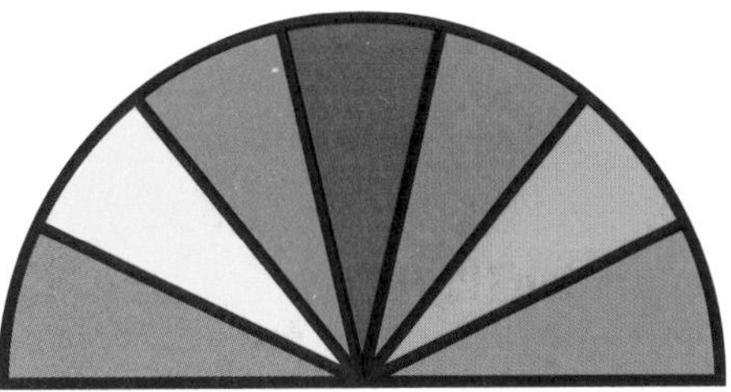

Color Coded

2017

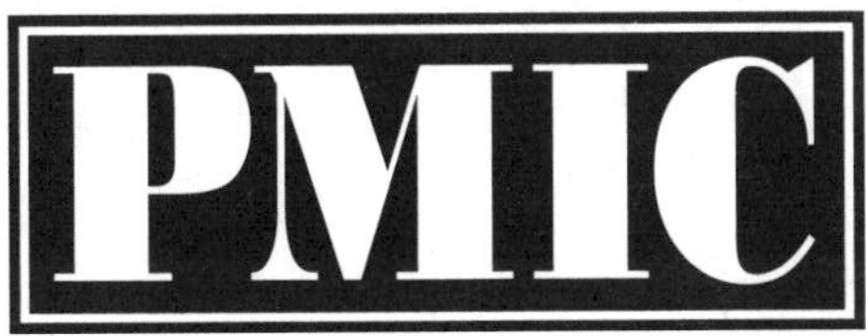

ISBN 978-1-943009-43-5 (Perfect Bound)
ISBN 978-1-943009-42-8 (Spiral Bound)
ISBN 978-1-943009-44-2 (e-book)

Practice Management Information Corporation (PMIC)
4727 Wilshire Boulevard
Los Angeles, California 90010
1-800-MED-SHOP
http://pmiconline.com

Printed in China

Additional copies of this book may be purchased from any medical book store, from PMIC by mail to the above address, by visiting our web site at http://pmiconline.com or by calling 1-800-MED-SHOP.

FOREWORD

The Health Care Procedure Coding System (HCPCS), National Level II, is a listing of codes and descriptive terminology used for reporting the provision of supplies, materials, injections and certain services and procedures to Medicare. HCPCS 2017 is the most recent revision of the HCPCS National Level II codes. The changes that appear in this revision have been prepared by our editorial staff using the HCPCS revisions released by the Center for Medicare and Medicaid Services (CMS), which is overseen by the Department of Health and Human Services (DHHS).

HCPCS 2017 codes must be used to report supplies, materials, injections and some quality measures on your Medicare claims for items and services provided from January 1, 2017 through December 31, 2017. The proper selection and reporting of HCPCS codes can improve your reimbursement and reduce your audit liability.

James B. Davis, President

DISCLAIMER

This publication is designed to offer basic information regarding coding and billing of medical services, supplies and procedures using the HCPCS coding system. The information presented is based upon material obtained from the Center for Medicare and Medicaid Services (CMS), and the experience and interpretations of the editors and publisher. Though all of the information has been carefully researched and checked for accuracy and completeness, the publisher accepts no responsibility or liability with regard to errors, omissions, misuse or misinterpretation.

CONTENTS

INTRODUCTION

HCPCS is an acronym for Health Care Procedure Coding System. This coding system was developed in 1983 by the Health Care Financing Administration (HCFA) for the purpose of standardizing the coding systems used to process Medicare claims. In 2001, HCFA changed its name to the Center for Medicare and Medicaid Services (CMS) to reflect its increased emphasis on improving Medicare and Medicaid beneficiary services and information.

The HCPCS coding system is primarily used to bill Medicare for supplies, materials and injections. It is also used to bill for certain services and procedures which are not defined in CPT. HCPCS codes must be used when billing Medicare carriers, and in some states, Medicaid carriers. Some private insurance carriers also allow or mandate the use of HCPCS codes, mostly those that are processing Medicare claims.

STRUCTURE OF HCPCS

HCPCS is a systematic method for coding supplies, materials, injections and services performed by health care professionals. Each supply, material, injection or service is identified with a five digit alphanumeric code. With the HCPCS coding system, the supplies, materials and injections can be accurately identified and properly reimbursed. There are three levels of codes within the HCPCS coding system.

LEVEL I CPT CODES

The major portion of the HCPCS coding system, referred to as Level I, is CPT. Most of the procedures and services you perform, even for Medicare patients, are billed using CPT codes. However, one of the major deficiencies of CPT is that it has limited code selections to describe supplies, materials and injections.

LEVEL II NATIONAL CODES

HCPCS National Level II codes are alphanumeric codes which start with a letter followed by four numbers. The range of HCPCS National Level II codes is from A0000 through V0000. There are also HCPCS National Level II modifiers. HCPCS National Level II codes are uniform in description throughout the United States. However, due to what is known as "carrier discretion" the processing and reimbursement of HCPCS National Level II codes is not necessarily uniform.

There are over 5,600 HCPCS National Level II codes covering supplies, materials, injections and services. A fundamental understanding of when and how to use HCPCS National Level II or Local Level III codes can have a significant impact on your Medicare reimbursement. The majority of health care professionals use codes from the Medical and Surgical Supplies section and Drugs Administered by Other Than Oral Method, commonly referred to as "A" codes and "J" codes.

HCPCS CODE OVERLAP

As may be expected, there is some overlap among the HCPCS code levels. On occasion you may have a coding situation where a specific code exists at all three levels for the same service or material. When faced with this situation, the general rule is that Local Level II codes have the highest priority, followed by CPT codes. You should consult your local Medicare carrier if you have any questions regarding HCPCS code overlap.

SECTIONS

The main body of HCPCS National Level II codes is divided into sections. The supplies, materials, injections and services are presented in alphanumeric order within each section. The sections of HCPCS National Level II are:

SECTION	CODE SERIES
Transportation Services	A0000-A0999
Medical And Surgical Supplies	A4000-A8999
Miscellaneous And Experimental	A9000-A9999
Enteral And Parenteral Therapy	B0000-B9999
Temporary Hospital Outpatient PPS	C0000-C9999
Durable Medical Equipment (DME)	E0000-E9999
Temporary Procedures & Professional Services	G0000-G9999
Rehabilitative Services	H0000-H9999
Drugs Administered Other Than Oral Method	J0000-J8999
Chemotherapy Drugs	J9000-J9999
Temporary Codes For DMERCS	K0000-K9999
Orthotic Procedures	L0000-L4999
Prosthetic Procedures	L5000-L9999
Medical Services	M0000-M9999
Pathology and Laboratory	P0000-P9999
Temporary Codes	Q0000-Q9999
Diagnostic Radiology Services	R0000-R9999
Private Payer Codes	S0000-S9999
State Medicaid Agency Codes	T0000-T9999
Vision Services	V0000-V2999
Hearing Services	V5000-V5999

INSTRUCTIONS for USE OF HCPCS NATIONAL LEVEL II CODES

A health care professional using the HCPCS National Level II codes selects the name of the material, supply, injection, service or procedure that most accurately identifies the service performed or supply delivered. Most often, HCPCS National Level II codes will be used instead of, or in addition to, CPT codes for visits, evaluation and management services, or other procedures performed at the same time or during the same visit. All services, procedures, supplies, materials and injections should be properly documented in the medical record.

The listing of a supply, material, injection or service and its code number in a specific section of HCPCS does not usually restrict its use to a specific profession or specialty group. However, there are some HCPCS National Level II codes that are by definition, profession or specialty specific.

GUIDELINES

Specific GUIDELINES are presented at the beginning of most of the sections. These GUIDELINES define items that are necessary to appropriately interpret and report the supplies, materials, injections, services and procedures listed in that section.

HCPCS MODIFIERS

A modifier provides the means by which the health care professional can indicate that a service or procedure that has been performed has been altered by some specific circumstance but not changed in its definition or code. HCPCS modifiers may be used to indicate the following:

- A service was supervised by an anesthesiologist
- A service was performed by a specific health care professional, for example, a clinical psychologist, clinical social worker, nurse practitioner, or physician assistant.
- A service was provided as part of a specific government program
- A service was provided to a specific side of the body
- Equipment was purchased or rented
- Single or multiple patients were seen during nursing home visits

It is important to note that HCPCS National Level II modifiers can be combined with CPT codes when reporting services to Medicare.

An example of the use of HCPCS National Level II modifiers is:

E1280-NR Heavy duty wheelchair; detachable arms (desk or full length) elevating leg rests - new when rented

A listing of modifiers pertinent to each section of HCPCS National Level II are located in the GUIDELINES of each section. A complete listing of HCPCS National Level II modifiers is found in APPENDIX A.

UNLISTED PROCEDURE or SERVICE

A service or procedure may be provided that is not listed in this edition of HCPCS National Level II. When reporting such a service, the appropriate "unlisted procedure" code may be used to indicate the service, identifying it by "special report" as defined below. HCPCS National Level II terminology is inconsistent in defining unlisted procedures. The procedure definition may include the term(s) "unlisted," "not otherwise classified," "unspecified," "unclassified," "other" and "miscellaneous." Prior to using these codes, try to determine if a Local Level III or CPT code is available. When an unlisted procedure code is used, the supply, material, injection, service or procedure must be described. Each of these unlisted procedure codes relates to a specific section of HCPCS National Level II and is presented in the GUIDELINES of that section.

SPECIAL REPORT

A supply, material, injection, service or procedure that is rarely provided, unusual, variable or new may require a special report for reimbursement purposes. Pertinent information should include an adequate definition or description of the nature, extent, and need for the supply, material, injection, service or procedure.

HCPCS CODE CHANGES

Each year numerous codes are added, changed or deleted. A summary of revisions to HCPCS 2017 is found in APPENDIX B. The following symbols, identical to those used in CPT, are used to indicate additions, changes and deletions in HCPCS National Level II.

ADDITIONS TO HCPCS

New HCPCS National Level II codes are identified with a small black circle placed to the left of the code number. An example of a new code in HCPCS 2017 is:

• **A4225** Supplies for external insulin infusion pump, syringe type cartridge, sterile, each

MCM: 60-14

CHANGES TO HCPCS

Changes in HCPCS National Level II code definitions are identified with a small black triangle placed to the left of the code number. An example of a changed code in HCPCS 2017 is:

▲ **E0629** Seat lift mechanism, non-electric, any type

MCM: 4107.8

DELETIONS FROM HCPCS

Deleted HCPCS National Level II codes are enclosed within parentheses, along with an italicized reference to replacement codes when available. An example of a deleted code in HCPCS 2017 is:

(**Q9981** Code deleted December 31, 2016). Use J8670.

QUALITY REVIEW SYSTEM (PQRS) INDICATOR

Ⓟ Indicates a code included in one or more PQRS measures. The specific measures may be found in Appendix E.

An example of a PQRS flagged code in HCPCS 2017 is:

Ⓟ **G8735** Elder maltreatment screen documented as positive, follow-up plan not documented, reason not specified

SPECIAL COVERAGE SYMBOLS

NOT PAYABLE BY MEDICARE

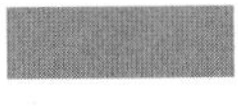

There are codes listed in HCPCS which are not payable by Medicare. These codes are identified by a red bar over the HCPCS code. These codes should not be used to report services to Medicare.

NON-COVERED BY MEDICARE

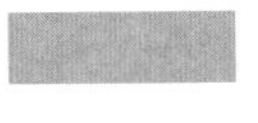

There are numerous supplies, materials, injections, services and procedures which are not covered by Medicare, either by program definition or by legislative statute. Examples of non-covered services include routine services and appliances, foot care and supportive devices for feet, custodial care, personal comfort items, and cosmetic surgery. These codes are identified by an orange bar over the HCPCS code. These codes should not be used to report services to Medicare; however, in most cases, you may bill the patient directly for non-covered services.

SPECIAL COVERAGE INSTRUCTIONS

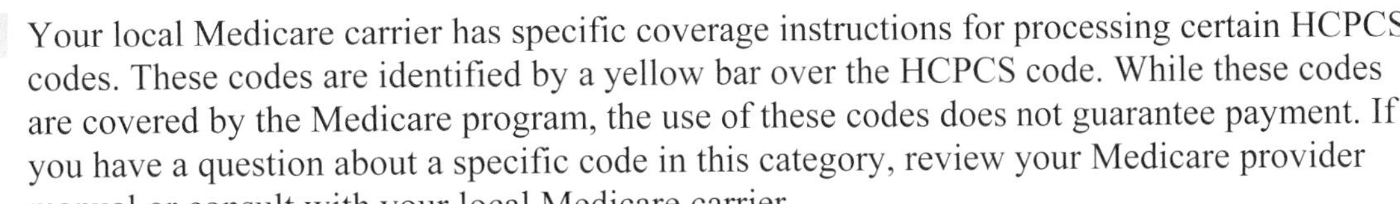

Your local Medicare carrier has specific coverage instructions for processing certain HCPCS codes. These codes are identified by a yellow bar over the HCPCS code. While these codes are covered by the Medicare program, the use of these codes does not guarantee payment. If you have a question about a specific code in this category, review your Medicare provider manual or consult with your local Medicare carrier.

CARRIER JUDGMENT

Processing and payment for these codes is done at the discretion of each insurance carrier. These codes are identified by a blue bar over the HCPCS code. For codes in this category, you should check with your Medicare carrier for proper billing instructions prior to filing an insurance claim.

DURABLE MEDICAL EQUIPMENT MEDICARE ADMINISTRATIVE CONTRACTORS (DME-MACs)

All Medicare claims for durable medical equipment (DME), prosthetics, orthotics and supplies go to one of four durable medical equipment Medicare administrative contractors, or DME-MACs (formerly known as DMERCs).

MEDICARE SUPPLIER NUMBER

Before submitting claims to DME-MACs, you must apply for a supplier number. You must use this number when submitting claims to all four carriers. To find out more information, go to the Medicare website at http://www.cms.gov.

GIONALIZATION OF CLAIM PROCESSING

Listed below are the contracted carriers and the states that they serve. The residence of the beneficiary is what determines which regional carrier processes the claim.

REGION A: CT, DE, DC, MA, MD, ME, NH, NJ, NY, PA, RI, VT

National Heritage Insurance Co
Mailing address varies depending on type of item dispensed.
866-419-9458 Check claims via an Integrated Voice Response (IVR) system.
866-590-6731 Speak to a person.
http://www.medicarenhic.com/DME/index.shtml

REGION B: IL, IN, KY, MI, MN, OH, WI

National Government Services (NGS)
Address varies depending on type of item dispensed.
877.299.7900 Check claims via an Integrated Voice Response (IVR) system.
866.590.6727 Speak to a person.
http://www.ngsMedicare.com

REGION C: AL, AR, CO, FL, GA, LA, MS, NM, NC, OK, PR, SC, TN, TX, VA, WV

CIGNA Government Services Administrators
Medicare DME MAC Operations
Address varies depending on type of item dispensed.
866.238.9650 Check claims via an Integrated Voice Response (IVR) system.
866.270.4909 Speak to a person.
http://www.cignagovernmentservices.com/jc/index.html

REGION D: AK, AZ, CA, GUAM, HI, IA, ID, KS, MO, MT, ND, NE, NV, OR, SD, UT, WA, WY

Noridian Healthcare Solutions
P.O. Box 6727
Fargo. ND 58108-6727
877.320.0390 Check claims via an Integrated Voice Response (IVR) system.
866.243.7272 Speak to a person.
http://www.noridianMedicare.com

CHANGE OF CLAIM JURISDICTION

Prior to October 1, 1993, Medicare carriers processed durable medical equipment (DME), prosthetics, and orthotics claims based on where the trasaction for the sale or rental took place. This is called the point of sale. Beginning October 1, 1993 and according to the state by state transfer schedule, regional processing of supplier claims began using beneficiary residence to determine which regional carrier had claim jurisdiction.

ELECTRONIC CLAIM FILING

The Center for Medicare and Medicaid Services is strongly encouraging electronic claims submission to DME-MACs. Suppliers submitting claims electronic must use the designated National Standard Format which meets all Medicare billing requirements and is accepted by other third-party insurance carriers. The regional carriers will assist you in converting to electronic claims submission. You can contact the Electronic Media Coordinator (EMC) at the DME-MACs listed above.

APPENDICES

APPENDIX A: Modifiers: Lists all National Level II modifiers, ambulance service, and PET scan modifiers.

APPENDIX B: Summary of Changes: Includes a summary of official additions, changes, and deletions to the current edition of HCPCS.

APPENDIX C: Table of Drugs: Includes drug names, cross references along with selected dosage, administration route, and HCPCS codes from the official HCPCS Table of Drugs.

APPENDIX D: Medicare References: Includes the complete text from all Medicare Coverage Instruction Manual (CIM) and Medicare Carriers Manual (MCM) citations in the body of the HCPCS book.

APPENDIX E: Physician Quality Review System (PQRS) measures. Includes all PQRS measures that reference HCPCS codes.

HCPCS 2017 DATA FILES

HCPCS codes are available in a data file format on CD-ROM. The HCPCS data file includes all official HCPCS codes with both short and full descriptions. The data file can be uploaded to your PC for inclusion in billing programs. For more information regarding the HCPCS data file call PMIC at 1-800-MED-SHOP or visit http://pmiconline.com.

TRANSPORTATION SERVICES

Guidelines

In addition to the information presented in the INTRODUCTION, several other items unique to this section are defined or identified here:

1. VEHICLE AND CREW REQUIREMENTS: The ambulance must be designed and equipped for transporting the sick or injured and include patient care equipment, such as a stretcher, clean linens, first aid supplies, oxygen equipment and other safety and lifesaving equipment required by state or local authorities. The ambulance crew must have two members, one of which has medical training equivalent to the standard and advanced Red Cross training. The vehicle and personnel supplier must provide a statement that describes the first-aid, safety and other patient-care items in the vehicle, the extent of first-aid training of the personnel and the supplier's agreement to notify Medicare of any changes that could affect coverage.

2. AIR AMBULANCE SERVICE: Air ambulance services are covered when the point o[illegible] up is inaccessible by land vehicle; distances or other obstacles are involved in getting the p[illegible] to the nearest hospital with appropriate facilities; and, all other conditions of coverage are met.

3. AMBULANCE SERVICE CLAIMS: Reimbursement may be made for expenses incurred for ambulance services when specific conditions have been met and the appropriate medical documentation is provided.

4. MATERIALS SUPPLIED BY AMBULANCE SERVICE: Reusable devices, such as back boards, neck boards and inflatable leg and arm splints, are considered part of general ambulance services and included in the charge for the trip. A separate reasonable charge may be recognized for non-reusable items and disposable supplies, such as oxygen, gauze and dressings, that are required for patient care during the trip.

5. UNLISTED SERVICE OR PROCEDURE: A service or procedure may be provided that is not listed in this edition of HCPCS. When reporting such a service, the appropriate "unlisted procedure" code may be used to indicate the service, identifying it by "special report" as defined below. HCPCS terminology is inconsistent in defining unlisted procedures. The procedure definition may include the term(s) "unlisted", "not otherwise classified", "unspecified", "unclassified", "other" and "miscellaneous". Prior to using these codes, try to determine if a Local Level III code or CPT code is available. The "unlisted procedures" and accompanying codes for TRANSPORTATION SERVICES are as follows:

   A0999 Unlisted ambulance service

6. SPECIAL REPORT: A service, material or supply that is rarely provided, unusual, variable or new may require a special report in determining medical appropriateness for reimbursement purposes. Pertinent information should include an adequate definition or description of the nature, extent, and need for the service, material or supply.

7. MODIFIERS: Listed services may be modified under certain circumstances. When appropriate, the modifying circumstance is identified by adding a modifier to the basic procedure code. CPT and HCPCS National Level II modifiers may be used with CPT and HCPCS National Level II procedure

codes. One digit codes are to be used in combination. The first digit should indicate the origin; the second digit should indicate the destination.

The Level II modifiers commonly used with TRANSPORTATION codes are as follows:

-GM Multiple patients on one ambulance trip

-QM Ambulance service provided under arrangement by a provider of services

-QN Ambulance services furnished directly by a provider of services

AMBULANCE SERVICE MODIFIERS

For ambulance service, one-digit modifiers are combined to form a two-digit modifier that identifies the ambulance's place of origin with the first digit, and ambulance's destination with the second digit. They are used in items 12 and 13 on the CMS Form 1491.

One digit ambulance modifiers:

-D Diagnostic or therapeutic site other than -P or -H when these are used as origin codes

-E Residential, domiciliary, custodial facility (other than an 1819 facility)

-G Hospital-based dialysis facility (hospital or hospital related)

-H Hospital

-I Site of transfer (for example, airport or helicopter pad) between types of ambulance

-J Non-hospital-based dialysis facility

-N Skilled nursing facility (SNF) (1819 facility)

-P Physician's office (includes HMO non-hospital facility, clinic, etc.)

-R Residence

-S Scene of accident or acute event

-X (Destination code only) Intermediate stop at physician's office on the way to the hospital (includes HMO non-hospital facility, clinic, etc.)

8. CPT CODE CROSS-REFERENCE: Unless specified otherwise, there is no equivalent CPT code for listings in this section.

Transportation Services Including Ambulance

A0021 Ambulance service, outside state per mile, transport (medicaid only) A0030

Ambulance Waiting Time Table			
Units	Time (Hrs)	Units	Time (Hrs)
1	1/2 to 1	6	3 to 3 ½
2	1 to 1 ½	7	3 ½ to 4
3	1 ½ to 2	8	4 to 4 ½
4	2 to 2 ½	9	4 ½ to 5
5	2 to 3	10	5 to 5 ½

A0080 Non-emergency transportation, per mile - vehicle provided by volunteer (individual or organization), with no vested interest

A0090 Non-emergency transportation, per mile - vehicle provided by individual (family member, self, neighbor) with vested interest

A0100 Non-emergency transportation; taxi

A0110 Non-emergency transportation and bus, intra or inter state carrier

A0120 Non-emergency transportation: mini-bus, mountain area transports, or other transportation systems

A0130 Non-emergency transportation: wheelchair van

A0140 Non-emergency transportation and air travel (private or commercial) intra or inter state

A0160 Non-emergency transportation: per mile - case worker or social worker

A0170 Transportation ancillary: parking fees, tolls, other

A0180 Non-emergency transportation: ancillary: lodging-recipient

A0190 Non-emergency transportation: ancillary: meals-recipient

A0200 Non-emergency transportation: ancillary: lodging escort

A0210 Non-emergency transportation: ancillary: meals-escort

A0225 Ambulance service, neonatal transport, base rate, emergency transport, one way

A0380 BLS mileage (per mile) A0425

A0382 BLS routine disposable supplies

A0384 BLS specialized service disposable supplies; defibrillation (used by ALS ambulances and BLS ambulances in jurisdictions where defibrillation is permitted in BLS ambulances)

A0390 ALS mileage (per mile) A0425

A0392 ALS specialized service disposable supplies; defibrillation (to be used only in jurisdictions where defibrillation cannot be performed in BLS ambulances)

A0394 ALS specialized service disposable supplies; iv drug therapy

A0396 ALS specialized service disposable supplies; esophageal intubation

A0398 ALS routine disposable supplies

A0420 Ambulance waiting time (ALS or BLS), one half (1/2) hour increments

A0422 Ambulance (ALS or BLS) oxygen and oxygen supplies, life sustaining situation

A0424 Extra ambulance attendant, ground (ALS or BLS) or air (fixed or rotary winged); (requires medical review)

A0425 Ground mileage, per statute mile

A0426 Ambulance service, advanced life support, non-emergency transport, level 1 (ALS 1)

A0427 Ambulance service, advanced life support, emergency transport, level 1 (ALS 1 - emergency)

A0428 Ambulance service, basic life support, non-emergency transport, (BLS)

A0429 Ambulance service, basic life support, emergency transport (BLS-emergency)

A0430 Ambulance service, conventional air services, transport, one way (fixed wing)

A0431 Ambulance service, conventional air services, transport, one way (rotary wing)

A0432 Paramedic intercept (pi), rural area, transport furnished by a volunteer ambulance company which is prohibited by state law from billing third party payers

A0433 Advanced life support, level 2 (ALS 2)

A0434 Specialty care transport (SCT)

A0435 Fixed wing air mileage, per statute mile

A0436 Rotary wing air mileage, per statute mile

A0888 Noncovered ambulance mileage, per mile (e.g., for miles traveled beyond closest appropriate facility)

MCM: 2125

A0998 Ambulance response and treatment, no transport

A0999 Unlisted ambulance service

MCM: 2120.1, 2125

MEDICAL AND SURGICAL SUPPLIES

Guidelines

In addition to the information presented in the INTRODUCTION, several other items unique to this section are defined or identified here:

1. SUBSECTION INFORMATION: Some of the listed subheadings or subsections have special needs or instructions unique to that section. Where these are indicated, special "notes" will be presented preceding or following the listings. Those subsections within the MEDICAL AND SURGICAL SUPPLIES section that have "notes" are as follows:

Subsection	Code Numbers
External urinary supplies	A4356-A4358
Tracheostomy supplies	A4622-A4626
Supplies for ESRD	A4650-A4927

2. UNLISTED SERVICE OR PROCEDURE: A service or procedure may be provided that is not listed in this edition of HCPCS. When reporting such a service, the appropriate "unlisted procedure" code may be used to indicate the service, identifying it by "special report" as defined below. HCPCS terminology is inconsistent in defining unlisted procedures. The procedure definition may include the term(s) "unlisted", "not otherwise classified", "unspecified", "unclassified", "other" and "miscellaneous". Prior to using these codes, try to determine if a Local Level III code or CPT code is available. The "unlisted procedures" and accompanying codes for MEDICAL AND SURGICAL SUPPLIES are as follows:

   A4335 Incontinence supply; miscellaneous
   A4421 Ostomy supply; miscellaneous
   A4649 Surgical supply; miscellaneous
   A4913 Miscellaneous dialysis supplies, not otherwise specified
   A6261 Wound filler, gel/paste, per fluid ounce, not elsewhere classified
   A6262 Wound filler, dry foam, per gram, not elsewhere classified

3. SPECIAL REPORT: A service, material or supply that is rarely provided, unusual, variable or new may require a special report in determining medical appropriateness for reimbursement purposes. Pertinent information should include an adequate definition or description of the nature, extent, and need for the service, material or supply.

4. MODIFIERS: Listed services may be modified under certain circumstances. When appropriate, the modifying circumstance is identified by adding a modifier to the basic procedure code. CPT and HCPCS National Level II modifiers may be used with CPT and HCPCS National Level II procedure codes. Modifiers commonly used with MEDICAL AND SURGICAL SUPPLIES are as follows:

   -CC Procedure code change (use "CC" when the procedure code submitted was changed either for administrative reasons or because an incorrect code was filed)

   -LT Left side (used to identify procedures performed on the left side of the body)

   -RT Right side (used to identify procedures performed on the right side of the body)

5. CPT CODE CROSS-REFERENCE: Unless specified otherwise, the equivalent CPT code for all listings in this section is 99070.

6. DURABLE MEDICAL EQUIPMENT REGIONAL CARRIERS (DMERCS): Effective October 1, 1993 claims for supplies must be billed to one of four regional carriers depending upon the residence of the beneficiary. The transition dates for DMERC claims is from November 1, 1993 to March 1, 1994, also depending upon the state you practice in. See the Introduction for a complete discussion of DMERCs.

Medical and Surgical Supplies

A4206 Syringe with needle, sterile, 1 cc or less, each

A4207 Syringe with needle, sterile 2 cc, each

A4208 Syringe with needle, sterile 3 cc, each

A4209 Syringe with needle, sterile 5 cc or greater, each

A4210 Needle-free injection device, each

CIM: 60-9

A4211 Supplies for self-administered injections

MCM: 2049

A4212 Non-coring needle or stylet with or without catheter

A4213 Syringe, sterile, 20 cc or greater, each

A4215 Needle, sterile, any size, each

A4216 Sterile water, saline and/or dextrose, diluent/flush, 10 ml

MCM: 2049

A4217 Sterile water/saline, 500 ml

MCM: 2049

A4218 Sterile saline or water, metered dose dispenser, 10 ml

A4220 Refill kit for implantable infusion pump

CIM: 60-14

▲ **A4221** Supplies for maintenance of non-insulin drug infusion catheter, per week (list drugs separately)

A4222 Infusion supplies for external drug infusion pump, per cassette or bag (list drugs separately)

A4223 Infusion supplies not used with external infusion pump, per cassette or bag (list drugs separately)

• **A4224** Supplies for maintenance of insulin infusion catheter, per week

• **A4225** Supplies for external insulin infusion pump, syringe type cartridge, sterile, each

MCM: 60-14

A4230 Infusion set for external insulin pump, non needle cannula type

CIM: 60-14

A4231 Infusion set for external insulin pump, needle type

CIM: 60-14

A4232 Syringe with needle for external insulin pump, sterile, 3 cc

CIM: 60-14

A4233 Replacement battery, alkaline (other than j cell), for use with medically necessary home blood glucose monitor owned by patient, each

A4234 Replacement battery, alkaline, j cell, for use with medically necessary home blood glucose monitor owned by patient, each

A4235 Replacement battery, lithium, for use with medically necessary home blood glucose monitor owned by patient, each

A4236 Replacement battery, silver oxide, for use with medically necessary home blood glucose monitor owned by patient, each

A4244 Alcohol or peroxide, per pint

A4245 Alcohol wipes, per box

A4246 Betadine or pHisoHex solution, per pint

A4247 Betadine or iodine swabs/wipes, per box

A4248 Chlorhexidine containing antiseptic, 1 ml

A4250 Urine test or reagent strips or tablets (100 tablets or strips)

MCM: 2100

A4252 Blood ketone test or reagent strip, each

Statute: 1861(n)

A4253 Blood glucose test or reagent strips for home blood glucose monitor, per 50 strips

CIM: 60-11

A4255 Platforms for home blood glucose monitor, 50 per box

CIM: 60-11

A4256 Normal, low and high calibrator solution / chips

CIM: 60-11

A4257 Replacement lens shield cartridge for use with laser skin piercing device, each

A4258 Spring-powered device for lancet, each

CIM: 60-11

A4259 Lancets, per box of 100

CIM: 60-11

A4261 Cervical cap for contraceptive use

Statute: 1862a1

A4262 Temporary, absorbable lacrimal duct implant, each

A4263 Permanent, long term, non-dissolvable lacrimal duct implant, each

MCM: 15030

A4264 Permanent implantable contraceptive intratubal occlusion device(s) and delivery system

A4265 Paraffin, per pound

CIM: 60-9

A4266 Diaphragm for contraceptive use

A4267 Contraceptive supply, condom, male, each

A4268 Contraceptive supply, condom, female, each

A4269 Contraceptive supply, spermicide (e.g., foam, gel), each

A4270 Disposable endoscope sheath, each

A4280 Adhesive skin support attachment for use with external breast prosthesis, each

A4281 Tubing for breast pump, replacement

A4282 Adapter for breast pump, replacement

A4283 Cap for breast pump bottle, replacement

A4284 Breast shield and splash protector for use with breast pump, replacement

A4285 Polycarbonate bottle for use with breast pump, replacement

A4286 Locking ring for breast pump, replacement

A4290 Sacral nerve stimulation test lead, each

Vascular Catheters

A4300 Implantable access catheter, (e.g., venous, arterial, epidural subarachnoid, or peritoneal, etc.) external access

MCM: 2130

A4301 Implantable access total catheter, port/reservoir (e.g., venous, arterial, epidural, subarachnoid, peritoneal, etc.)

A4305 Disposable drug delivery system, flow rate of 50 ml or greater per hour

A4306 Disposable drug delivery system, flow rate of less than 50 ml per hour

Incontinence Appliances and Care Supplies

A4310 Insertion tray without drainage bag and without catheter (accessories only)

MCM: 2130

A4311 Insertion tray without drainage bag with indwelling catheter, Foley type, two-way latex with coating (Teflon, silicone, silicone elastomer or hydrophilic, etc.)

MCM: 2130

A4312 Insertion tray without drainage bag with indwelling catheter, Foley type, two-way, all silicone

MCM: 2130

A4313 Insertion tray without drainage bag with indwelling catheter, Foley type, three-way, for continuous irrigation

MCM: 2130

A4314 Insertion tray with drainage bag with indwelling catheter, Foley type, two-way latex with coating (Teflon, silicone, silicone elastomer or hydrophilic, etc.)

MCM: 2130

A4315 Insertion tray with drainage bag with indwelling catheter, Foley type, two-way, all silicone

MCM: 2130

A4316 Insertion tray with drainage bag with indwelling catheter, Foley type, three-way, for continuous irrigation

MCM: 2130

A4320 Irrigation tray with bulb or piston syringe, any purpose

MCM: 2130

A4321 Therapeutic agent for urinary catheter irrigation

MCM: 2130

A4322 Irrigation syringe, bulb or piston, each

MCM: 2130

A4326 Male external catheter with integral collection chamber, any type, each

MCM: 2130

A4327 Female external urinary collection device; meatal cup, each

MCM: 2130

A4328 Female external urinary collection device; pouch, each

MCM: 2130

A4330 Perianal fecal collection pouch with adhesive, each

MCM: 2130

A4331 Extension drainage tubing, any type, any length, with connector/adaptor, for use with urinary leg bag or urostomy pouch, each

MCM: 2130

A4332 Lubricant, individual sterile packet, each

MCM: 2130

A4333 Urinary catheter anchoring device, adhesive skin attachment, each

MCM: 2130

A4334 Urinary catheter anchoring device, leg strap, each

MCM: 2130

A4335 Incontinence supply; miscellaneous

MCM: 2130

A4336 Incontinence supply, urethral insert, any type, each

A4337 Incontinence supply, rectal insert, any type, each

MCM: 2130

A4338 Indwelling catheter; Foley type, two-way latex with coating (Teflon, silicone, silicone elastomer, or hydrophilic, etc.), each

MCM: 2130

A4340 Indwelling catheter; specialty type, (e.g., coude, mushroom, wing, etc.), each

MCM: 2130

A4344 Indwelling catheter, Foley type, two-way, all silicone, each

MCM: 2130

A4346 Indwelling catheter; Foley type, three way for continuous irrigation, each

MCM: 2130

A4349 Male external catheter, with or without adhesive, disposable, each

MCM: 2130

A4351 Intermittent urinary catheter; straight tip, with or without coating (Teflon, silicone, silicone elastomer, or hydrophilic, etc.), each

MCM: 2130

A4352 Intermittent urinary catheter; coude (curved) tip, with or without coating (Teflon, silicone, silicone elastomeric, or hydrophilic, etc.), each

MCM: 2130

A4353 Intermittent urinary catheter, with insertion supplies

MCM: 2130

A4354 Insertion tray with drainage bag but without catheter

MCM: 2130

A4355 Irrigation tubing set for continuous bladder irrigation through a three-way indwelling Foley catheter, each

MCM: 2130

External Urinary Supplies

A4356 External urethral clamp or compression device (not to be used for catheter clamp), each

MCM: 2130

A4357 Bedside drainage bag, day or night, with or without anti-reflux device, with or without tube, each

MCM: 2130

A4358 Urinary drainage bag, leg or abdomen, vinyl, with or without tube, with straps, each

MCM: 2130

Ostomy Supplies

A4360 Disposable external urethral clamp or compression device, with pad and/or pouch, each

A4361 Ostomy faceplate, each

MCM: 2130

A4362 Skin barrier; solid, 4 x 4 or equivalent; each

MCM: 2130

A4363 Ostomy clamp, any type, replacement only, each

A4364 Adhesive, liquid or equal, any type, per oz

MCM: 2130

A4366 Ostomy vent, any type, each

A4367 Ostomy belt, each

MCM: 2130A

A4368 Ostomy filter, any type, each

A4369 Ostomy skin barrier, liquid (spray, brush, etc.), per oz

MCM: 2130

A4371 Ostomy skin barrier, powder, per oz

MCM: 2130

A4372 Ostomy skin barrier, solid 4 x 4 or equivalent, standard wear, with built-in convexity, each

MCM: 2130

A4373 Ostomy skin barrier, with flange (solid, flexible or accordion), with built-in convexity, any size, each

MCM: 2130

A4375 Ostomy pouch, drainable, with faceplate attached, plastic, each

MCM: 2130

A4376 Ostomy pouch, drainable, with faceplate attached, rubber, each

MCM: 2130

A4377 Ostomy pouch, drainable, for use on faceplate, plastic, each

MCM: 2130

A4378 Ostomy pouch, drainable, for use on faceplate, rubber, each

MCM: 2130

A4379 Ostomy pouch, urinary, with faceplate attached, plastic, each

MCM: 2130

A4380 Ostomy pouch, urinary, with faceplate attached, rubber, each

MCM: 2130

A4381 Ostomy pouch, urinary, for use on faceplate, plastic, each

MCM: 2130

A4382 Ostomy pouch, urinary, for use on faceplate, heavy plastic, each

MCM: 2130

A4383 Ostomy pouch, urinary, for use on faceplate, rubber, each

MCM: 2130

A4384 Ostomy faceplate equivalent, silicone ring, each

MCM: 2130

A4385 Ostomy skin barrier, solid 4 x 4 or equivalent, extended wear, without built-in convexity, each

MCM: 2130

A4387 Ostomy pouch, closed, with barrier attached, with built-in convexity (1 piece), each

MCM: 2130

A4388 Ostomy pouch, drainable, with extended wear barrier attached, (1 piece), each

MCM: 2130

A4389 Ostomy pouch, drainable, with barrier attached, with built-in convexity (1 piece), each

MCM: 2130

A4390 Ostomy pouch, drainable, with extended wear barrier attached, with built-in convexity (1 piece), each

MCM: 2130

A4391 Ostomy pouch, urinary, with extended wear barrier attached (1 piece), each

MCM: 2130

A4392 Ostomy pouch, urinary, with standard wear barrier attached, with built-in convexity (1 piece), each

MCM: 2130

A4393 Ostomy pouch, urinary, with extended wear barrier attached, with built-in convexity (1 piece), each

MCM: 2130

A4394 Ostomy deodorant, with or without lubricant, for use in ostomy pouch, per fluid ounce

MCM: 2130

A4395 Ostomy deodorant for use in ostomy pouch, solid, per tablet

MCM: 2130

A4396 Ostomy belt with peristomal hernia support

MCM: 2130

A4397 Irrigation supply; sleeve, each

MCM: 2130

A4398 Ostomy irrigation supply; bag, each

MCM: 2130

A4399 Ostomy irrigation supply; cone/catheter, with or without brush

MCM: 2130

A4400 Ostomy irrigation set

MCM: 2130

A4402 Lubricant, per ounce

MCM: 2130

A4404 Ostomy ring, each

MCM: 2130

A4405 Ostomy skin barrier, non-pectin based, paste, per ounce

MCM: 2130

A4406 Ostomy skin barrier, pectin-based, paste, per ounce

MCM: 2130

A4407 Ostomy skin barrier, with flange (solid, flexible, or accordion), extended wear, with built-in convexity, 4 x 4 inches or smaller, each

MCM: 2130

A4408 Ostomy skin barrier, with flange (solid, flexible or accordion), extended wear, with built-in convexity, larger than 4 x 4 inches, each

MCM: 2130

A4409 Ostomy skin barrier, with flange (solid, flexible or accordion), extended wear, without built-in convexity, 4 x 4 inches or smaller, each

MCM: 2130

A4410 Ostomy skin barrier, with flange (solid, flexible or accordion), extended wear, without built-in convexity, larger than 4 x 4 inches, each

MCM: 2130

A4411 Ostomy skin barrier, solid 4 x 4 or equivalent, extended wear, with built-in convexity, each

A4412 Ostomy pouch, drainable, high output, for use on a barrier with flange (2 piece system), without filter, each

MCM: 2130

A4413 Ostomy pouch, drainable, high output, for use on a barrier with flange (2 piece system), with filter, each

MCM: 2130

A4414 Ostomy skin barrier, with flange (solid, flexible or accordion), without built-in convexity, 4 x 4 inches or smaller, each

MCM: 2130

A4415 Ostomy skin barrier, with flange (solid, flexible or accordion), without built-in convexity, larger than 4 x 4 inches, each

MCM: 2130

A4416 Ostomy pouch, closed, with barrier attached, with filter (1 piece), each

A4417 Ostomy pouch, closed, with barrier attached, with built-in convexity, with filter (1 piece), each

A4418 Ostomy pouch, closed; without barrier attached, with filter (1 piece), each

A4419 Ostomy pouch, closed; for use on barrier with non-locking flange, with filter (2 piece), each

A4420 Ostomy pouch, closed; for use on barrier with locking flange (2 piece), each

A4421 Ostomy supply; miscellaneous

A4422 Ostomy absorbent material (sheet/pad/crystal packet) for use in ostomy pouch to thicken liquid stomal output, each

MCM: 2130

A4423 Ostomy pouch, closed; for use on barrier with locking flange, with filter (2 piece), each

A4424 Ostomy pouch, drainable, with barrier attached, with filter (1 piece), each

A4425 Ostomy pouch, drainable; for use on barrier with non-locking flange, with filter (2 piece system), each

A4426 Ostomy pouch, drainable; for use on barrier with locking flange (2 piece system), each

A4427 Ostomy pouch, drainable; for use on barrier with locking flange, with filter (2 piece system), each

A4428 Ostomy pouch, urinary, with extended wear barrier attached, with faucet-type tap with valve (1 piece), each

A4429 Ostomy pouch, urinary, with barrier attached, with built-in convexity, with faucet-type tap with valve (1 piece), each

A4430 Ostomy pouch, urinary, with extended wear barrier attached, with built-in convexity, with faucet-type tap with valve (1 piece), each

A4431 Ostomy pouch, urinary; with barrier attached, with faucet-type tap with valve (1 piece), each

A4432 Ostomy pouch, urinary; for use on barrier with non-locking flange, with faucet-type tap with valve (2 piece), each

A4433 Ostomy pouch, urinary; for use on barrier with locking flange (2 piece), each

A4434 Ostomy pouch, urinary; for use on barrier with locking flange, with faucet-type tap with valve (2 piece), each

A4435 Ostomy pouch, drainable, high output, with extended wear barrier (one-piece system), with or without filter, each

Supplies

A4450 Tape, non-waterproof, per 18 square inches

MCM: 2130

A4452 Tape, waterproof, per 18 square inches

MCM: 2130

A4455 Adhesive remover or solvent (for tape, cement or other adhesive), per ounce

MCM: 2130

A4456 Adhesive remover, wipes, any type, each

MCM: 2130

A4458 Enema bag with tubing, reusable

A4459 Manual pump-operated enema system, includes balloon, catheter and all accessories, reusable, any type

A4461 Surgical dressing holder, non-reusable, each

A4463 Surgical dressing holder, reusable, each

A4465 Non-elastic binder for extremity

(**A4466** Code deleted December 31, 2016). Use A4467.

• **A4467** Belt, strap, sleeve, garment, or covering, any type

A4470 Gravlee jet washer

CIM: 50-4

MCM: 2320

A4480 Vabra aspirator

CIM: 50-10

MCM: 2320

A4481 Tracheostoma filter, any type, any size, each

MCM: 2130

A4483 Moisture exchanger, disposable, for use with invasive mechanical ventilation

MCM: 2130

A4490 Surgical stockings above knee length, each

CIM: 60-9

MCM: 2079, 2100

A4495 Surgical stockings thigh length, each

CIM: 60-9

MCM: 2079, 2100

A4500 Surgical stockings below knee length, each

CIM: 60-9

MCM: 2079, 2100

A4510 Surgical stockings full length, each

CIM: 60-9

MCM: 2079, 2100

A4520 Incontinence garment, any type, (e.g., brief, diaper), each

CIM: 60-9

A4550 Surgical trays

MCM: 15030

• **A4553** Non-disposable underpads, all sizes

A4554 Disposable underpads, all sizes

CIM: 60-9

A4555 Electrode/transducer for use with electrical stimulation device used for cancer treatment, replacement only

A4556 Electrodes, (e.g., apnea monitor), per pair

A4557 Lead wires, (e.g., apnea monitor), per pair

A4558 Conductive gel or paste, for use with electrical device (e.g., tens, NMES), per O

A4559 Coupling gel or paste, for use with ultrasound device, per oz

A4561 Pessary, rubber, any type

A4562 Pessary, non rubber, any type

A4565 Slings

A4566 Shoulder sling or vest design, abduction restrainer, with or without swathe control, prefabricated, includes fitting and adjustment

A4570 Splint

MCM: 2079

A4575 Topical hyperbaric oxygen chamber, disposable

CIM: 35-10

A4580 Cast supplies (e.g., plaster)

MCM: 2079

A4590 Special casting material (e.g., fiberglass)

MCM: 2079

A4595 Electrical stimulator supplies, 2 lead, per month, (e.g., tens, NMES)

CIM: 45-25

Supplies for Oxygen and Related Respiratory Equipment

A4600 Sleeve for intermittent limb compression device, replacement only, each

A4601 Lithium ion battery, rechargeable, for non-prosthetic use, replacement

A4602 Replacement battery for external infusion pump owned by patient, lithium, 1.5 volt, each

A4604 Tubing with integrated heating element for use with positive airway pressure device

A4605 Tracheal suction catheter, closed system, each

A4606 Oxygen probe for use with oximeter device, replacement

A4608 Transtracheal oxygen catheter, each

A4611 Battery, heavy duty; replacement for patient owned ventilator

Statute: 1834a3A

A4612 Battery cables; replacement for patient-owned ventilator

Statute: 1834a3A

A4613 Battery charger; replacement for patient-owned ventilator

Statute: 1834a3A

A4614 Peak expiratory flow rate meter, hand held

A4615 Cannula, nasal

CIM: 60-4

MCM: 3312

A4616 Tubing (oxygen), per foot

CIM: 60-4

MCM: 3312

A4617 Mouth piece

CIM: 60-4

MCM: 3312

A4618 Breathing circuits

CIM: 60-4

MCM: 3312

A4619 Face tent

CIM: 60-4

MCM: 3312

A4620 Variable concentration mask

CIM: 60-4

MCM: 3312

A4623 Tracheostomy, inner cannula

CIM: 65-16

MCM: 2130

A4624 Tracheal suction catheter, any type other than closed system, each

A4625 Tracheostomy care kit for new tracheostomy

MCM: 2130

A4626 Tracheostomy cleaning brush, each

MCM: 2130

A4627 Spacer, bag or reservoir, with or without mask, for use with metered dose inhaler

MCM: 2100

A4628 Oropharyngeal suction catheter, each

A4629 Tracheostomy care kit for established tracheostomy

MCM: 2130

Supplies for Other Durable Medical Equipment

A4630 Replacement batteries, medically necessary, transcutaneous electrical stimulator, owned by patient

CIM: 65-8

A4633 Replacement bulb/lamp for ultraviolet light therapy system, each

A4634 Replacement bulb for therapeutic light box, tabletop model

A4635 Underarm pad, crutch, replacement, each

CIM: 60-9

A4636 Replacement, handgrip, cane, crutch, or walker, each

CIM: 60-9

A4637 Replacement, tip, cane, crutch, walker, each.

CIM: 60-9

A4638 Replacement battery for patient-owned ear pulse generator, each

A4639 Replacement pad for infrared heating pad system, each

A4640 Replacement pad for use with medically necessary alternating pressure pad owned by patient

CIM: 60-9

MCM: 4107.6

Supplies for Radiological Procedures

A4641 Radiopharmaceutical, diagnostic, not otherwise classified

A4642 Indium in-111 satumomab pendetide, diagnostic, per study dose, up to 6 millicuries

A4648 Tissue marker, implantable, any type, each

A4649 Surgical supply; miscellaneous

Supplies for ESRD

A4650 Implantable radiation dosimeter, each

A4651 Calibrated microcapillary tube, each

MCM: 4270

A4652 Microcapillary tube sealant

MCM: 4270

A4653 Peritoneal dialysis catheter anchoring device, belt, each

A4657 Syringe, with or without needle, each

MCM: 4270

A4660 Sphygmomanometer/blood pressure apparatus with cuff and stethoscope

MCM: 4270

A4663 Blood pressure cuff only

MCM: 4270

A4670 Automatic blood pressure monitor

CIM: 50-42

MCM: 4270

A4671 Disposable cycler set used with cycler dialysis machine, each

MCM: 4270

A4672 Drainage extension line, sterile, for dialysis, each

MCM: 4270

A4673 Extension line with easy lock connectors, used with dialysis

MCM: 4270

A4674 Chemicals/antiseptics solution used to clean/sterilize dialysis equipment, per 8 oz

MCM: 4270

A4680 Activated carbon filter for hemodialysis, each

CIM: 55-1

MCM: 4270

A4690 Dialyzer (artificial kidneys), all types, all sizes, for hemodialysis, each

MCM: 4270

A4706 Bicarbonate concentrate, solution, for hemodialysis, per gallon

MCM: 4270

A4707 Bicarbonate concentrate, powder, for hemodialysis, per packet

MCM: 4270

A4708 Acetate concentrate solution, for hemodialysis, per gallon

MCM: 4270

A4709 Acid concentrate, solution, for hemodialysis, per gallon

MCM: 4270

A4714 Treated water (deionized, distilled, or reverse osmosis) for peritoneal dialysis, per gallon

CIM: 55-1

MCM: 4270

A4719 "y set" tubing for peritoneal dialysis

MCM: 4270

A4720 Dialysate solution, any concentration of dextrose, fluid volume greater than 249cc, but less than or equal to 999 cc, for peritoneal dialysis

MCM: 4270

A4721 Dialysate solution, any concentration of dextrose, fluid volume greater than 999 cc but less than or equal to 1999 cc, for peritoneal dialysis

MCM: 4270

A4722 Dialysate solution, any concentration of dextrose, fluid volume greater than 1999 cc but less than or equal to 2999 cc, for peritoneal dialysis

MCM: 4270

A4723 Dialysate solution, any concentration of dextrose, fluid volume greater than 2999 cc but less than or equal to 3999 cc, for peritoneal dialysis

MCM: 4270

A4724 Dialysate solution, any concentration of dextrose, fluid volume greater than 3999 cc but less than or equal to 4999 cc, for peritoneal dialysis

MCM: 4270

A4725 Dialysate solution, any concentration of dextrose, fluid volume greater than 4999 cc but less than or equal to 5999 cc, for peritoneal dialysis

MCM: 4270

A4726 Dialysate solution, any concentration of dextrose, fluid volume greater than 5999 cc, for peritoneal dialysis

MCM: 4270

A4728 Dialysate solution, non-dextrose containing, 500 ml

A4730 Fistula cannulation set for hemodialysis, each

MCM: 4270

A4736 Topical anesthetic, for dialysis, per gram

MCM: 4270

A4737 Injectable anesthetic, for dialysis, per 10 ml

MCM: 4270

A4740 Shunt accessory, for hemodialysis, any type, each

MCM: 4270

A4750 Blood tubing, arterial or venous, for hemodialysis, each

MCM: 4270

A4755 Blood tubing, arterial and venous combined, for hemodialysis, each

MCM: 4270

A4760 Dialysate solution test kit, for peritoneal dialysis, any type, each

MCM: 4270

A4765 Dialysate concentrate, powder, additive for peritoneal dialysis, per packet

MCM: 4270

A4766 Dialysate concentrate, solution, additive for peritoneal dialysis, per 10 ml

MCM: 4270

A4770 Blood collection tube, vacuum, for dialysis, per 50

MCM: 4270

A4771 Serum clotting time tube, for dialysis, per 50

MCM: 4270

A4772 Blood glucose test strips, for dialysis, per 50

MCM: 4270

A4773 Occult blood test strips, for dialysis, per 50

MCM: 4270

A4774 Ammonia test strips, for dialysis, per 50

MCM: 4270

A4802 Protamine sulfate, for hemodialysis, per 50 mg

MCM: 4270

A4860 Disposable catheter tips for peritoneal dialysis, per 10

MCM: 4270

A4870 Plumbing and/or electrical work for home hemodialysis equipment

MCM: 4270

A4890 Contracts, repair and maintenance, for hemodialysis equipment

MCM: 2100.4

A4911 Drain bag/bottle, for dialysis, each

A4913 Miscellaneous dialysis supplies, not otherwise specified

A4918 Venous pressure clamp, for hemodialysis, each

A4927 Gloves, non-sterile, per 100

A4928 Surgical mask, per 20

A4929 Tourniquet for dialysis, each

A4930 Gloves, sterile, per pair

A4931 Oral thermometer, reusable, any type, each

A4932 Rectal thermometer, reusable, any type, each

Additional Ostomy Supplies

A5051 Ostomy pouch, closed; with barrier attached (1 piece), each

MCM: 2130

A5052 Ostomy pouch, closed; without barrier attached (1 piece), each

MCM: 2130

A5053 Ostomy pouch, closed; for use on faceplate, each

MCM: 2130

A5054 Ostomy pouch, closed; for use on barrier with flange (2 piece), each

MCM: 2130

A5055 Stoma cap

MCM: 2130

A5056 Ostomy pouch, drainable, with extended wear barrier attached, with filter, (1 piece), each

MCM: 2130

A5057 Ostomy pouch, drainable, with extended wear barrier attached, with built in convexity, with filter, (1 piece), each

MCM: 2130

A5061 Ostomy pouch, drainable; with barrier attached, (1 piece), each

A5062 Ostomy pouch, drainable; without barrier attached (1 piece), each

MCM: 2130

A5063 Ostomy pouch, drainable; for use on barrier with flange (2 piece system), each

MCM: 2130

A5071 Ostomy pouch, urinary; with barrier attached (1 piece), each

MCM: 2130

A5072 Ostomy pouch, urinary; without barrier attached (1 piece), each

MCM: 2130

A5073 Ostomy pouch, urinary; for use on barrier with flange (2 piece), each

MCM: 2130

A5081 Stoma plug or seal, any type

MCM: 2130

A5082 Continent device; catheter for continent stoma

MCM: 2130

A5083 Continent device, stoma absorptive cover for continent stoma

A5093 Ostomy accessory; convex insert

MCM: 2130

Additional Incontinence Appliances/Supplies

A5102 Bedside drainage bottle with or without tubing, rigid or expandable, each

MCM: 2130

A5105 Urinary suspensory with leg bag, with or without tube, each

MCM: 2130

A5112 Urinary drainage bag, leg or abdomen, latex, with or without tube, with straps, each

MCM: 2130

A5113 Leg strap; latex, replacement only, per set

MCM: 2130

A5114 Leg strap; foam or fabric, replacement only, per set

MCM: 2130

Supplies for Either Incontinence or Ostomy Appliances

A5120 Skin barrier, wipes or swabs, each

MCM: 2130

A5121 Skin barrier; solid, 6 x 6 or equivalent, each

MCM: 2130

A5122 Skin barrier; solid, 8 x 8 or equivalent, each

MCM: 2130

A5126 Adhesive or non-adhesive; disk or foam pad

MCM: 2130

A5131 Appliance cleaner, incontinence and ostomy appliances, per 16 oz.

MCM: 2130

A5200 Percutaneous catheter/tube anchoring device, adhesive skin attachment

MCM: 2130

Shoe Supplies for Diabetics

A5500 For diabetics only, fitting (including follow-up), custom preparation and supply of off-the-shelf depth-inlay shoe manufactured to accommodate multi-density insert(s), per shoe

MCM: 2134

A5501 For diabetics only, fitting (including follow-up), custom preparation and supply of shoe molded from cast(s) of patient's foot (custom molded shoe), per shoe

MCM: 2134

A5503 For diabetics only, modification (including fitting) of off-the-shelf depth-inlay shoe or custom-molded shoe with roller or rigid rocker bottom, per shoe

MCM: 2134

A5504 For diabetics only, modification (including fitting) of off-the-shelf depth-inlay shoe or custom-molded shoe with wedge(s), per shoe

MCM: 2134

A5505 For diabetics only, modification (including fitting) of off-the-shelf depth-inlay shoe or custom-molded shoe with metatarsal bar, per shoe

MCM: 2134

A5506 For diabetics only, modification (including fitting) of off-the-shelf depth-inlay shoe or custom-molded shoe with off-set heel(s), per shoe

MCM: 2134

A5507 For diabetics only, not otherwise specified modification (including fitting) of off-the-shelf depth-inlay shoe or custom-molded shoe, per shoe

MCM: 2134

A5508 For diabetics only, deluxe feature of off-the-shelf depth-inlay shoe or custom-molded shoe, per shoe

MCM: 2134

A5510 For diabetics only, direct formed, compression molded to patient's foot without external heat source, multiple-density insert(s) prefabricated, per shoe

MCM: 2134

A5512 For diabetics only, multiple density insert, direct formed, molded to foot after external heat source of 230 degrees Fahrenheit or higher, total contact with patient's foot, including arch, base layer minimum of 1/4 inch material of shore a 35 durometer or 3/16 inch material of shore a 40 durometer (or higher), prefabricated, each

A5513 For diabetics only, multiple density insert, custom molded from model of patient's foot, total contact with patient's foot, including arch, base layer minimum of 3/16 inch material of shore a 35 durometer or higher), includes arch filler and other shaping material, custom fabricated, each

Wound Dressings

A6000 Non-contact wound warming wound cover for use with the non-contact wound warming device and warming card

MCM: 2303

A6010 Collagen based wound filler, dry form, sterile, per gram of collagen

MCM: 2079

A6011 Collagen based wound filler, gel/paste, per gram of collagen

MCM: 2079

A6021 Collagen dressing, sterile, size 16 sq. in. or less, each

MCM: 2079

A6022 Collagen dressing, sterile, size more than 16 sq. in. but less than or equal to 48 sq. in., each

MCM: 2079

A6023 Collagen dressing, sterile, size more than 48 sq. in., each

MCM: 2079

A6024 Collagen dressing wound filler, sterile, per 6 inches

MCM: 2079

A6025 Gel sheet for dermal or epidermal application, (e.g., silicone, hydrogel, other), each

A6154 Wound pouch, each

MCM: 2079

A6196 Alginate or other fiber gelling dressing, wound cover, sterile, pad size 16 sq. in. or less, each dressing

MCM: 2079

A6197 Alginate or other fiber gelling dressing, wound cover, sterile, pad size more than 16 sq. in. but less than or equal to 48 sq. in., each dressing

MCM: 2079

A6198 Alginate or other fiber gelling dressing, wound cover, sterile, pad size more than 48 sq. in., each dressing

MCM: 2079

A6199 Alginate or other fiber gelling dressing, wound filler, sterile, per 6 inches

MCM: 2079

A6203 Composite dressing, sterile, pad size 16 sq. in. or less, with any size adhesive border, each dressing

MCM: 2079

A6204 Composite dressing, sterile, pad size more than 16 sq. in. but less than or equal to 48 sq. in., with any size adhesive border, each dressing

MCM: 2079

A6205 Composite dressing, sterile, pad size more than 48 sq. in., with any size adhesive border, each dressing

MCM: 2079

A6206 Contact layer, sterile, 16 sq. in. or less, each dressing

MCM: 2079

A6207 Contact layer, sterile, more than 16 sq. in. but less than or equal to 48 sq. in., each dressing

MCM: 2079

A6208 Contact layer, sterile, more than 48 sq. in., each dressing

MCM: 2079

A6209 Foam dressing, wound cover, sterile, pad size 16 sq. in. or less, without adhesive border, each dressing

MCM: 2079

A6210 Foam dressing, wound cover, sterile, pad size more than 16 sq. in. but less than or equal to 48 sq. in., without adhesive border, each dressing

MCM: 2079

A6211 Foam dressing, wound cover, sterile, pad size more than 48 sq. in., without adhesive border, each dressing

MCM: 2079

A6212 Foam dressing, wound cover, sterile, pad size 16 sq. in. or less, with any size adhesive border, each dressing

MCM: 2079

A6213 Foam dressing, wound cover, sterile, pad size more than 16 sq. in. but less than or equal to 48 sq. in., with any size adhesive border, each dressing

MCM: 2079

A6214 Foam dressing, wound cover, sterile, pad size more than 48 sq. in., with any size adhesive border, each dressing

MCM: 2079

A6215 Foam dressing, wound filler, sterile, per gram

MCM: 2079

A6216 Gauze, non-impregnated, non-sterile, pad size 16 sq. in. or less, without adhesive border, each dressing

MCM: 2079

A6217 Gauze, non-impregnated, non-sterile, pad size more than 16 sq. in. but less than or equal to 48 sq. in., without adhesive border, each dressing

MCM: 2079

A6218 Gauze, non-impregnated, non-sterile, pad size more than 48 sq. in., without adhesive border, each dressing

MCM: 2079

A6219 Gauze, non-impregnated, sterile, pad size 16 sq. in. or less, with any size adhesive border, each dressing

MCM: 2079

A6220 Gauze, non-impregnated, sterile, pad size more than 16 sq. in. but less than or equal to 48 sq. in., with any size adhesive border, each dressing

MCM: 2079

A6221 Gauze, non-impregnated, sterile, pad size more than 48 sq. in., with any size adhesive border, each dressing

MCM: 2079

A6222 Gauze, impregnated with other than water, normal saline, or hydrogel, sterile, pad size 16 sq. in. or less, without adhesive border, each dressing

MCM: 2079

A6223 Gauze, impregnated with other than water, normal saline, or hydrogel, sterile, pad size more than 16 sq. in., but less than or equal to 48 sq. in., without adhesive border, each dressing

MCM: 2079

A6224 Gauze, impregnated with other than water, normal saline, or hydrogel, sterile, pad size more than 48 sq. in., without adhesive border, each dressing

MCM: 2079

A6228 Gauze, impregnated, water or normal saline, sterile, pad size 16 sq. in. or less, without adhesive border, each dressing

MCM: 2079

A6229 Gauze, impregnated, water or normal saline, sterile, pad size more than 16 sq. in. but less than or equal to 48 sq. in., without adhesive border, each dressing

MCM: 2079

A6230 Gauze, impregnated, water or normal saline, sterile, pad size more than 48 sq. in., without adhesive border, each dressing

MCM: 2079

A6231 Gauze, impregnated, hydrogel, for direct wound contact, sterile, pad size 16 sq. in. or less, each dressing

MCM: 2079

A6232 Gauze, impregnated, hydrogel, for direct wound contact, sterile, pad size greater than 16 sq. in., but less than or equal to 48 sq. in., each dressing

MCM: 2079

A6233 Gauze, impregnated, hydrogel, for direct wound contact, sterile, pad size more than 48 sq. in., each dressing

MCM: 2079

A6234 Hydrocolloid dressing, wound cover, sterile, pad size 16 sq. in. or less, without adhesive border, each dressing

MCM: 2079

A6235 Hydrocolloid dressing, wound cover, sterile, pad size more than 16 sq. in. but less than or equal to 48 sq. in., without adhesive border, each dressing

MCM: 2079

A6236 Hydrocolloid dressing, wound cover, sterile, pad size more than 48 sq. in., without adhesive border, each dressing

MCM: 2079

A6237 Hydrocolloid dressing, wound cover, sterile, pad size 16 sq. in. or less, with any size adhesive border, each dressing

MCM: 2079

A6238 Hydrocolloid dressing, wound cover, sterile, pad size more than 16 sq. in. but less than or equal to 48 sq. in., with any size adhesive border, each dressing

MCM: 2079

A6239 Hydrocolloid dressing, wound cover, sterile, pad size more than 48 sq. in., with any size adhesive border, each dressing

MCM: 2079

A6240 Hydrocolloid dressing, wound filler, paste, sterile, per ounce

MCM: 2079

A6241 Hydrocolloid dressing, wound filler, dry form, sterile, per gram

MCM: 2079

A6242 Hydrogel dressing, wound cover, sterile, pad size 16 sq. in. or less, without adhesive border, each dressing

MCM: 2079

A6243 Hydrogel dressing, wound cover, sterile, pad size more than 16 sq. in. but less than or equal to 48 sq. in., without adhesive border, each dressing

MCM: 2079

A6244 Hydrogel dressing, wound cover, sterile, pad size more than 48 sq. in., without adhesive border, each dressing

MCM: 2079

A6245 Hydrogel dressing, wound cover, sterile, pad size 16 sq. in. or less, with any size adhesive border, each dressing

MCM: 2079

A6246 Hydrogel dressing, wound cover, sterile, pad size more than 16 sq. in. but less than or equal to 48 sq. in., with any size adhesive border, each dressing

MCM: 2079

A6247 Hydrogel dressing, wound cover, sterile, pad size more than 48 sq. in., with any size adhesive border, each dressing

MCM: 2079

A6248 Hydrogel dressing, wound filler, gel, per fluid ounce

MCM: 2079

A6250 Skin sealants, protectants, moisturizers, ointments, any type, any size

MCM: 2079

A6251 Specialty absorptive dressing, wound cover, sterile, pad size 16 sq. in. or less, without adhesive border, each dressing

MCM: 2079

A6252 Specialty absorptive dressing, wound cover, sterile, pad size more than 16 sq. in. but less than or equal to 48 sq. in., without adhesive border, each dressing

MCM: 2079

A6253 Specialty absorptive dressing, wound cover, sterile, pad size more than 48 sq. in., without adhesive border, each dressing

MCM: 2079

A6254 Specialty absorptive dressing, wound cover, sterile, pad size 16 sq. in. or less, with any size adhesive border, each dressing

MCM: 2079

A6255 Specialty absorptive dressing, wound cover, sterile, pad size more than 16 sq. in. but less than or equal to 48 sq. in., with any size adhesive border, each dressing

MCM: 2079

A6256 Specialty absorptive dressing, wound cover, sterile, pad size more than 48 sq. in., with any size adhesive border, each dressing

MCM: 2079

A6257 Transparent film, sterile, 16 sq. in. or less, each dressing

MCM: 2079

A6258 Transparent film, sterile, more than 16 sq. in. but less than or equal to 48 sq. in., each dressing

MCM: 2079

A6259 Transparent film, sterile, more than 48 sq. in., each dressing

MCM: 2079

A6260 Wound cleansers, any type, any size

MCM: 2079

A6261 Wound filler, gel/paste, per fluid ounce, not otherwise specified

MCM: 2079

A6262 Wound filler, dry form, per gram, not otherwise specified

MCM: 2079

A6266 Gauze, impregnated, other than water, normal saline, or zinc paste, sterile, any width, per linear yard

MCM: 2079

A6402 Gauze, non-impregnated, sterile, pad size 16 sq. in. or less, without adhesive border, each dressing

MCM: 2079

A6403 Gauze, non-impregnated, sterile, pad size more than 16 sq. in. less than or equal to 48 sq. in., without adhesive border, each dressing

MCM: 2079

A6404 Gauze, non-impregnated, sterile, pad size more than 48 sq. in., without adhesive border, each dressing

MCM: 2079

A6407 Packing strips, non-impregnated, sterile, up to 2 inches in width, per linear yard

A6410 Eye pad, sterile, each

MCM: 2079

A6411 Eye pad, non-sterile, each

MCM: 2079

A6412 Eye patch, occlusive, each

A6413 Adhesive bandage, first-aid type, any size, each

Statute: 1861(s)(5)

A6441 Padding bandage, non-elastic, non-woven/non-knitted, width greater than or equal to three inches and less than five inches, per yard

A6442 Conforming bandage, non-elastic, knitted/woven, non-sterile, width less than three inches, per yard

A6443 Conforming bandage, non-elastic, knitted/woven, non-sterile, width greater than or equal to three inches and less than five inches, per yard

A6444 Conforming bandage, non-elastic, knitted/woven, non-sterile, width greater than or equal to 5 inches, per yard

A6445 Conforming bandage, non-elastic, knitted/woven, sterile, width less than three inches, per yard

A6446 Conforming bandage, non-elastic, knitted/woven, sterile, width greater than or equal to three inches and less than five inches, per yard

A6447 Conforming bandage, non-elastic, knitted/woven, sterile, width greater than or equal to five inches, per yard

A6448 Light compression bandage, elastic, knitted/woven, width less than three inches, per yard

A6449 Light compression bandage, elastic, knitted/woven, width greater than or equal to three inches and less than five inches, per yard

A6450 Light compression bandage, elastic, knitted/woven, width greater than or equal to five inches, per yard

A6451 Moderate compression bandage, elastic, knitted/woven, load resistance of 1.25 to 1.34 foot pounds at 50% maximum stretch, width greater than or equal to three inches and less than five inches, per yard

A6452 High compression bandage, elastic, knitted/woven, load resistance greater than or equal to 1.35 foot pounds at 50% maximum stretch, width greater than or equal to three inches and less than five inches, per yard

A6453 Self-adherent bandage, elastic, non-knitted/non-woven, width less than three inches, per yard

A6454 Self-adherent bandage, elastic, non-knitted/non-woven, width greater than or equal to three inches and less than five inches, per yard

A6455 Self-adherent bandage, elastic, non-knitted/non-woven, width greater than or equal to five inches, per yard

A6456 Zinc paste impregnated bandage, non-elastic, knitted/woven, width greater than or equal to three inches and less than five inches, per yard

A6457 Tubular dressing with or without elastic, any width, per linear yard

A6501 Compression burn garment, bodysuit (head to foot), custom fabricated

MCM: 2079

A6502 Compression burn garment, chin strap, custom fabricated

MCM: 2079

A6503 Compression burn garment, facial hood, custom fabricated

MCM: 2079

A6504 Compression burn garment, glove to wrist, custom fabricated

MCM: 2079

A6505 Compression burn garment, glove to elbow, custom fabricated

MCM: 2079

A6506 Compression burn garment, glove to axilla, custom fabricated

MCM: 2079

A6507 Compression burn garment, foot to knee length, custom fabricated

MCM: 2079

A6508 Compression burn garment, foot to thigh length, custom fabricated

MCM: 2079

A6509 Compression burn garment, upper trunk to waist including arm openings (vest), custom fabricated

MCM: 2079

A6510 Compression burn garment, trunk, including arms down to leg openings (leotard), custom fabricated

MCM: 2079

A6511 Compression burn garment, lower trunk including leg openings (panty), custom fabricated

MCM: 2079

A6512 Compression burn garment, not otherwise classified

MCM: 2079

A6513 Compression burn mask, face and/or neck, plastic or equal, custom fabricated

A6530 Gradient compression stocking, below knee, 18-30 mmhg, each

CIM: 60-9

A6531 Gradient compression stocking, below knee, 30-40 mmhg, each

MCM: 2079

A6532 Gradient compression stocking, below knee, 40-50 mmhg, each

MCM: 2079

A6533 Gradient compression stocking, thigh length, 18-30 mmhg, each

CIM: 60-9

MCM: 2133

A6534 Gradient compression stocking, thigh length, 30-40 mmhg, each

CIM: 60-9

MCM: 2133

A6535 Gradient compression stocking, thigh length, 40-50 mmhg, each

CIM: 60-9

MCM: 2133

A6536 Gradient compression stocking, full length/chap style, 18-30 mmhg, each

CIM: 60-9

MCM: 2133

A6537 Gradient compression stocking, full length/chap style, 30-40 mmhg, each

CIM: 60-9

MCM: 2133

A6538 Gradient compression stocking, full length/chap style, 40-50 mmhg, each

CIM: 60-9

MCM: 2133

A6539 Gradient compression stocking, waist length, 18-30 mmhg, each

CIM: 60-9

MCM: 2133

A6540 Gradient compression stocking, waist length, 30-40 mmhg, each

CIM: 60-9

MCM: 2133

A6541 Gradient compression stocking, waist length, 40-50 mmhg, each

CIM: 60-9

MCM: 2133

A6544 Gradient compression stocking, garter belt

CIM: 60-9

MCM: 2133

A6545 Gradient compression wrap, non-elastic, below knee, 30-50 mm hg, each

MCM: 2079

A6549 Gradient compression stocking/sleeve, not otherwise specified

CIM: 60-9

MCM: 2133

A6550 Wound care set, for negative pressure wound therapy electrical pump, includes all supplies and accessories

A7000 Canister, disposable, used with suction pump, each

A7001 Canister, non-disposable, used with suction pump, each

A7002 Tubing, used with suction pump, each

A7003 Administration set, with small volume nonfiltered pneumatic nebulizer, disposable

A7004 Small volume nonfiltered pneumatic nebulizer, disposable

A7005 Administration set, with small volume nonfiltered pneumatic nebulizer, non-disposable

A7006 Administration set, with small volume filtered pneumatic nebulizer

A7007 Large volume nebulizer, disposable, unfilled, used with aerosol compressor

A7008 Large volume nebulizer, disposable, prefilled, used with aerosol compressor

A7009 Reservoir bottle, non-disposable, used with large volume ultrasonic nebulizer

A7010 Corrugated tubing, disposable, used with large volume nebulizer, 100 feet

(**A7011** Code deleted December 31, 2015.)

A7012 Water collection device, used with large volume nebulizer

A7013 Filter, disposable, used with aerosol compressor or ultrasonic generator

A7014 Filter, nondisposable, used with aerosol compressor or ultrasonic generator

A7015 Aerosol mask, used with DME nebulizer

A7016 Dome and mouthpiece, used with small volume ultrasonic nebulizer

A7017 Nebulizer, durable, glass or autoclavable plastic, bottle type, not used with oxygen

CIM: 60-9

A7018 Water, distilled, used with large volume nebulizer, 1000 ml

A7020 Interface for cough stimulating device, includes all components, replacement only

A7025 High frequency chest wall oscillation system vest, replacement for use with patient owned equipment, each

A7026 High frequency chest wall oscillation system hose, replacement for use with patient owned equipment, each

A7027 Combination oral/nasal mask, used with continuous positive airway pressure device, each

A7028 Oral cushion for combination oral/nasal mask, replacement only, each

A7029 Nasal pillows for combination oral/nasal mask, replacement only, pair

A7030 Full face mask used with positive airway pressure device, each

A7031 Face mask interface, replacement for full face mask, each

A7032 Cushion for use on nasal mask interface, replacement only, each

A7033 Pillow for use on nasal cannula type interface, replacement only, pair

A7034 Nasal interface (mask or cannula type) used with positive airway pressure device, with or without head strap

A7035 Headgear used with positive airway pressure device

A7036 Chinstrap used with positive airway pressure device

A7037 Tubing used with positive airway pressure device

A7038 Filter, disposable, used with positive airway pressure device

A7039 Filter, non disposable, used with positive airway pressure device

A7040 One way chest drain valve

A7041 Water seal drainage container and tubing for use with implanted chest tube

A7044 Oral interface used with positive airway pressure device, each

A7045 Exhalation port with or without swivel used with accessories for positive airway devices, replacement only

CIM: 60-17

A7046 Water chamber for humidifier, used with positive airway pressure device, replacement, each

CIM: 60-17

A7047 Oral interface used with respiratory suction pump, each

A7048 Vacuum drainage collection unit and tubing kit, including all supplies needed for collection unit change, for use with implanted catheter, each

A7501 Tracheostoma valve, including diaphragm, each

MCM: 2130

A7502 Replacement diaphragm/faceplate for tracheostoma valve, each

MCM: 2130

A7503 Filter holder or filter cap, reusable, for use in a tracheostoma heat and moisture exchange system, each

MCM: 2130

A7504 Filter for use in a tracheostoma heat and moisture exchange system, each

MCM: 2130

A7505 Housing, reusable without adhesive, for use in a heat and moisture exchange system and/or with a tracheostoma valve, each

MCM: 2130

A7506 Adhesive disc for use in a heat and moisture exchange system and/or with tracheostoma valve, any type each

MCM: 2130

A7507 Filter holder and integrated filter without adhesive, for use in a tracheostoma heat and moisture exchange system, each

MCM: 2130

A7508 Housing and integrated adhesive, for use in a tracheostoma heat and moisture exchange system and/or with a tracheostoma valve, each

MCM: 2130

A7509 Filter holder and integrated filter housing, and adhesive, for use as a tracheostoma heat and moisture exchange system, each

MCM: 2130

A7520 Tracheostomy/laryngectomy tube, non-cuffed, polyvinylchloride (pvc), silicone or equal, each

A7521 Tracheostomy/laryngectomy tube, cuffed, polyvinylchloride (pvc), silicone or equal, each

A7522 Tracheostomy/laryngectomy tube, stainless steel or equal (sterilizable and reusable), each

A7523 Tracheostomy shower protector, each

A7524 Tracheostoma stent/stud/button, each

A7525 Tracheostomy mask, each

A7526 Tracheostomy tube collar/holder, each

A7527 Tracheostomy/laryngectomy tube plug/stop, each

A8000 Helmet, protective, soft, prefabricated, includes all components and accessories

A8001 Helmet, protective, hard, prefabricated, includes all components and accessories

A8002 Helmet, protective, soft, custom fabricated, includes all components and accessories

A8003 Helmet, protective, hard, custom fabricated, includes all components and accessories

A8004 Soft interface for helmet, replacement only

ADMINISTRATIVE, MISCELLANEOUS AND INVESTIGATIONAL

NOTE: The following codes do not imply that codes in other sections are necessarily covered.

Guidelines

In addition to the information presented in the INTRODUCTION, several other items unique to this section are defined or identified here:

1. SPECIAL REPORT: A service, material or supply that is rarely provided, unusual, variable or new may require a special report in determining medical appropriateness for reimbursement purposes. Pertinent information should include an adequate definition or description of the nature, extent, and need for the service, material or supply.

2. CPT CODE CROSS-REFERENCE: Unless specified otherwise, there is no equivalent CPT code for listings in this section.

Miscellaneous and Experimental

A9150 Non-prescription drugs

MCM: 2050.5

A9152 Single vitamin/mineral/trace element, oral, per dose, not otherwise specified

A9153 Multiple vitamins, with or without minerals and trace elements, oral, per dose, not otherwise specified

A9155 Artificial saliva, 30 ml

A9180 Pediculosis (lice infestation) treatment, topical, for administration by patient/caretaker

A9270 Non-covered item or service

MCM: 2303

A9272 Wound suction, disposable, includes dressing, all accessories and components, any type, each

Statute: 1861(n)

A9273 Hot water bottle, ice cap or collar, heat and/or cold wrap, any type

A9274 External ambulatory insulin delivery system, disposable, each, includes all supplies and accessories

Statute: 1861(n)

A9275 Home glucose disposable monitor, includes test strips

A9276 Sensor; invasive (e.g., subcutaneous), disposable, for use with interstitial continuous glucose monitoring system, one unit = 1 day supply

Statute: 1861(n)

A9277 Transmitter; external, for use with interstitial continuous glucose monitoring system

Statute: 1861(n)

A9278 Receiver (monitor); external, for use with interstitial continuous glucose monitoring system

Statute: 1861(n)

A9279 Monitoring feature/device, stand-alone or integrated, any type, includes all accessories, components and electronics, not otherwise classified

Statute: 1861(n)

A9280 Alert or alarm device, not otherwise classified

Statute: 1861

A9281 Reaching/grabbing device, any type, any length, each

Statute: 1862 SSA

A9282 Wig, any type, each

Statute: 1861SSA

A9283 Foot pressure off loading/supportive device, any type, each

Statute: 1862a(i)13

A9284 Spirometer, non-electronic, includes all accessories

• **A9285** Inversion/eversion correction device

• **A9286** Hygienic item or device, disposable or non-disposable, any type, each

Statute: 1834

A9300 Exercise equipment

CIM: 60-9

MCM: 2100.1

A9500 Technetium tc-99m sestamibi, diagnostic, per study dose

A9501 Technetium tc-99m teboroxime, diagnostic, per study dose

A9502 Technetium tc-99m tetrofosmin, diagnostic, per study dose

A9503 Technetium tc-99m medronate, diagnostic, per study dose, up to 30 millicuries

A9504 Technetium tc-99m apcitide, diagnostic, per study dose, up to 20 millicuries

A9505 Thallium tl-201 thallous chloride, diagnostic, per millicurie

A9507 Indium in-111 capromab pendetide, diagnostic, per study dose, up to 10 millicuries

A9508 Iodine i-131 iobenguane sulfate, diagnostic, per 0.5 millicurie

A9509 Iodine i-123 sodium iodide, diagnostic, per millicurie

A9510 Technetium tc-99m disofenin, diagnostic, per study dose, up to 15 millicuries

A9512 Technetium tc-99m pertechnetate, diagnostic, per millicurie

• **A9515** Choline c-11, diagnostic, per study dose up to 20 millicuries

A9516 Iodine i-123 sodium iodide, diagnostic, per 100 microcuries, up to 999 microcuries

A9517 Iodine i-131 sodium iodide capsule(s), therapeutic, per millicurie

A9520 Technetium tc-99m tilmanocept, diagnostic, up to 0.5 millicuries

A9521 Technetium tc-99m exametazime, diagnostic, per study dose, up to 25 millicuries

A9524 Iodine i-131 iodinated serum albumin, diagnostic, per 5 microcuries

A9526 Nitrogen n-13 ammonia, diagnostic, per study dose, up to 40 millicuries

A9527 Iodine i-125, sodium iodide solution, therapeutic, per millicurie

A9528 Iodine i-131 sodium iodide capsule(s), diagnostic, per millicurie

A9529 Iodine i-131 sodium iodide solution, diagnostic, per millicurie

A9530 Iodine i-131 sodium iodide solution, therapeutic, per millicurie

A9531 Iodine i-131 sodium iodide, diagnostic, per microcurie (up to 100 microcuries)

A9532 Iodine i-125 serum albumin, diagnostic, per 5 microcuries

A9536 Technetium tc-99m depreotide, diagnostic, per study dose, up to 35 millicuries

A9537 Technetium tc-99m mebrofenin, diagnostic, per study dose, up to 15 millicuries

A9538 Technetium tc-99m pyrophosphate, diagnostic, per study dose, up to 25 millicuries

A9539 Technetium tc-99m pentetate, diagnostic, per study dose, up to 25 millicuries

A9540 Technetium tc-99m macroaggregated albumin, diagnostic, per study dose, up to 10 millicuries

A9541 Technetium tc-99m sulfur colloid, diagnostic, per study dose, up to 20 millicuries

A9542 Indium in-111 ibritumomab tiuxetan, diagnostic, per study dose, up to 5 millicuries

A9543 Yttrium y-90 ibritumomab tiuxetan, therapeutic, per treatment dose, up to 40 millicuries

(**A9544** Code deleted December 31, 2016).

(**A9545** Code deleted December 31, 2016).

A9546 Cobalt co-57/58, cyanocobalamin, diagnostic, per study dose, up to 1 microcurie

A9547 Indium in-111 oxyquinoline, diagnostic, per 0.5 millicurie

A9548 Indium in-111 pentetate, diagnostic, per 0.5 millicurie

A9550 Technetium tc-99m sodium gluceptate, diagnostic, per study dose, up to 25 millicurie

A9551 Technetium tc-99m succimer, diagnostic, per study dose, up to 10 millicuries

A9552 Fluorodeoxyglucose f-18 fdg, diagnostic, per study dose, up to 45 millicuries

A9553 Chromium cr-51 sodium chromate, diagnostic, per study dose, up to 250 microcuries

A9554 Iodine i-125 sodium iothalamate, diagnostic, per study dose, up to 10 microcuries

A9555 Rubidium rb-82, diagnostic, per study dose, up to 60 millicuries

A9556 Gallium ga-67 citrate, diagnostic, per millicurie

A9557 Technetium tc-99m bicisate, diagnostic, per study dose, up to 25 millicuries

A9558 Xenon xe-133 gas, diagnostic, per 10 millicuries

A9559 Cobalt co-57 cyanocobalamin, oral, diagnostic, per study dose, up to 1 microcurie

A9560 Technetium tc-99m labeled red blood cells, diagnostic, per study dose, up to 30 millicuries

A9561 Technetium tc-99m oxidronate, diagnostic, per study dose, up to 30 millicuries

A9562 Technetium tc-99m mertiatide, diagnostic, per study dose, up to 15 millicuries

A9563 Sodium phosphate p-32, therapeutic, per millicurie

A9564 Chromic phosphate p-32 suspension, therapeutic, per millicurie

A9566 Technetium tc-99m fanolesomab, diagnostic, per study dose, up to 25 millicuries

A9567 Technetium tc-99m pentetate, diagnostic, aerosol, per study dose, up to 75 millicuries

A9568 Technetium tc-99m arcitumomab, diagnostic, per study dose, up to 45 millicuries

A9569 Technetium tc-99m exametazime labeled autologous white blood cells, diagnostic, per study dose

A9570 Indium in-111 labeled autologous white blood cells, diagnostic, per study dose

A9571 Indium in-111 labeled autologous platelets, diagnostic, per study dose

A9572 Indium in-111 pentetreotide, diagnostic, per study dose, up to 6 millicuries

A9575 Injection, gadoterate meglumine, 0.1 ml

A9576 Injection, gadoteridol, (ProHance multipack), per ml

A9577 Injection, gadobenate dimeglumine (MultiHance), per ml

A9578 Injection, gadobenate dimeglumine (MultiHance multipack), per ml

A9579 Injection, gadolinium-based magnetic resonance contrast agent, not otherwise specified (nos), per ml

A9580 Sodium fluoride f-18, diagnostic, per study dose, up to 30 millicuries

A9581 Injection, gadoxetate disodium, 1 ml

A9582 Iodine i-123 iobenguane, diagnostic, per study dose, up to 15 millicuries

A9583 Injection, gadofosveset trisodium, 1 ml

A9584 Iodine 1-123 ioflupane, diagnostic, per study dose, up to 5 millicuries

A9585 Injection, gadobutrol, 0.1 ml

A9586 Florbetapir f18, diagnostic, per study dose, up to 10 millicuries

• **A9587** Gallium ga-68, dotatate, diagnostic, 0.1 millicurie

• **A9588** Fluciclovine f-18, diagnostic, 1 millicurie

• **A9597** Positron emission tomography radiopharmaceutical, diagnostic, for tumor identification, not otherwise classified

• **A9598** Positron emission tomography radiopharmaceutical, diagnostic, for non-tumor identification, not otherwise classified

▲ **A9599** Radiopharmaceutical, diagnostic, for beta-amyloid positron emission tomography (pet) imaging, per study dose, not otherwise specified

A9600 Strontium sr-89 chloride, therapeutic, per millicurie

A9604 Samarium sm-153 lexidronam, therapeutic, per treatment dose, up to 150 millicuries

A9606 Radium ra-223 dichloride, therapeutic, per microcurie

A9698 Non-radioactive contrast imaging material, not otherwise classified, per study

MCM: 15022

A9699 Radiopharmaceutical, therapeutic, not otherwise classified

A9700 Supply of injectable contrast material for use in echocardiography, per study

MCM: 15360

A9900 Miscellaneous DME supply, accessory, and/or service component of another HCPCS code

A9901 DME delivery, set up, and/or dispensing service component of another HCPCS code

A9999 Miscellaneous DME supply or accessory, not otherwise specified

ENTERAL AND PARENTERAL THERAPY

Guidelines

In addition to the information presented in the INTRODUCTION, several other items unique to this section are defined or identified here:

1. SUBSECTION INFORMATION: Some of the listed subheadings or subsections have special needs or instructions unique to that section. Where these are indicated, special "notes" will be presented preceding or following the listings. Those subsections within the ENTERAL AND PARENTERAL THERAPY section that have "notes" are as follows:

SUBSECTION	CODE SERIES
Enteral formulae and enteral medical supplies	B4034-B5200

2. UNLISTED SERVICE OR PROCEDURE: A service or procedure may be provided that is not listed in this edition of HCPCS. When reporting such a service, the appropriate "unlisted procedure" code may be used to indicate the service, identifying it by "special report" as defined below. HCPCS terminology is inconsistent in defining unlisted procedures. The procedure definition may include the term(s) "unlisted", "not otherwise classified", "unspecified", "unclassified", "other" and "miscellaneous". Prior to using these codes, try to determine if a Local Level III code or CPT code is available. The "unlisted procedures" and accompanying codes for ENTERAL AND PARENTERAL THERAPY are as follows:

   B9998 NOC for enteral supplies
   B9999 NOC for parenteral supplies

3. SPECIAL REPORT: A service, material or supply that is rarely provided, unusual, variable or new may require a special report in determining medical appropriateness for reimbursement purposes. Pertinent information should include an adequate definition or description of the nature, extent, and need for the service, material or supply.

4. MODIFIERS: Listed services may be modified under certain circumstances. When appropriate, the modifying circumstance is identified by adding a modifier to the basic procedure code. CPT and HCPCS National Level II modifiers may be used with CPT and HCPCS National Level II procedure codes. Modifiers commonly used with ENTERAL AND PARENTERAL THERAPY are as follows:

   -CC Procedure code change (used when the procedure code submitted was changed either for administrative reasons or because an incorrect code was filed)

5. CPT CODE CROSS-REFERENCE: Unless specified otherwise, the equivalent CPT code for all listings in this section is 99070.

Enteral Formulae and Enteral Medical Supplies

B4034 Enteral feeding supply kit; syringe fed, per day, includes but not limited to feeding/flushing syringe, administration set tubing, dressings, tape

CIM: 65-10

MCM: 2130, 4450

B4035 Enteral feeding supply kit; pump fed, per day, includes but not limited to feeding/flushing syringe, administration set tubing, dressings, tape

CIM: 65-10

MCM: 2130, 4450

B4036 Enteral feeding supply kit; gravity fed, per day, includes but not limited to feeding/flushing syringe, administration set tubing, dressings, tape

CIM: 65-10

MCM: 2130, 4450

B4081 Nasogastric tubing with stylet

CIM: 65-10

MCM: 2130, 4450

B4082 Nasogastric tubing without stylet

CIM: 65-10

MCM: 2130, 4450

B4083 Stomach tube - Levine type

CIM: 65-10

MCM: 2130, 4450

B4087 Gastrostomy/jejunostomy tube, standard, any material, any type, each

B4088 Gastrostomy/jejunostomy tube, low-profile, any material, any type, each

B4100 Food thickener, administered orally, per ounce

CIM: 60-9

B4102 Enteral formula, for adults, used to replace fluids and electrolytes (e.g., clear liquids), 500 ml = 1 unit

CIM: 65-10

B4103 Enteral formula, for pediatrics, used to replace fluids and electrolytes (e.g., clear liquids), 500 ml = 1 unit

CIM: 65-10

B4104 Additive for enteral formula (e.g., fiber)

CIM: 65-10

B4149 Enteral formula, manufactured blenderized natural foods with intact nutrients, includes proteins, fats, carbohydrates, vitamins and minerals, may include fiber, administered through an enteral feeding tube, 100 calories = 1 unit

CIM: 65-10

MCM: 2130, 4450

B4150 Enteral formula, nutritionally complete with intact nutrients, includes proteins, fats, carbohydrates, vitamins and minerals, may include fiber, administered through an enteral feeding tube, 100 calories = 1 unit

CIM: 65-10

MCM: 2130, 4450

B4152 Enteral formula, nutritionally complete, calorically dense (equal to or greater than 1.5 kcal/ml) with intact nutrients, includes proteins, fats, carbohydrates, vitamins and minerals, may include fiber, administered through an enteral feeding tube, 100 calories = 1 unit

CIM: 65-10

MCM: 2130, 4450

B4153 Enteral formula, nutritionally complete, hydrolyzed proteins (amino acids and peptide chain), includes fats, carbohydrates, vitamins and minerals, may include fiber, administered through an enteral feeding tube, 100 calories = 1 unit

CIM: 65-10

MCM: 2130, 4450

B4154 Enteral formula, nutritionally complete, for special metabolic needs, excludes inherited disease of metabolism, includes altered composition of proteins, fats, carbohydrates, vitamins and/or minerals, may include fiber, administered through an enteral feeding tube, 100 calories = 1 unit

CIM: 65-10

MCM: 2130, 4450

B4155 Enteral formula, nutritionally incomplete/modular nutrients, includes specific nutrients, carbohydrates (e.g., glucose polymers), proteins/amino acids (e.g., glutamine, arginine), fat (e.g., medium chain triglycerides) or combination, administered through an enteral feeding tube, 100 calories = 1 unit

CIM: 65-10

MCM: 2130, 4450

B4157 Enteral formula, nutritionally complete, for special metabolic needs for inherited disease of metabolism, includes proteins, fats, carbohydrates, vitamins and minerals, may include fiber, administered through an enteral feeding tube, 100 calories = 1 unit

CIM: 65-10

B4158 Enteral formula, for pediatrics, nutritionally complete with intact nutrients, includes proteins, fats, carbohydrates, vitamins and minerals, may include fiber and/or iron, administered through an enteral feeding tube, 100 calories = 1 unit

CIM: 65-10

B4159 Enteral formula, for pediatrics, nutritionally complete soy based with intact nutrients, includes proteins, fats, carbohydrates, vitamins and minerals, may include fiber and/or iron, administered through an enteral feeding tube, 100 calories = 1 unit

CIM: 65-10

B4160 Enteral formula, for pediatrics, nutritionally complete calorically dense (equal to or greater than 0.7 kcal/ml) with intact nutrients, includes proteins, fats, carbohydrates, vitamins and minerals, may include fiber, administered through an enteral feeding tube, 100 calories = 1 unit

CIM: 65-10

B4161 Enteral formula, for pediatrics, hydrolyzed/amino acids and peptide chain proteins, includes fats, carbohydrates, vitamins and minerals, may include fiber, administered through an enteral feeding tube, 100 calories = 1 unit

CIM: 65-10

B4162 Enteral formula, for pediatrics, special metabolic needs for inherited disease of metabolism, includes proteins, fats, carbohydrates, vitamins and minerals, may include fiber, administered through an enteral feeding tube, 100 calories = 1 unit

CIM: 65-10

Parenteral Nutrition

B4164 Parenteral nutrition solution: carbohydrates (dextrose), 50% or less (500 ml = 1 unit) - home mix

CIM: 65-10

MCM: 2130, 4450

B4168 Parenteral nutrition solution; amino acid, 3.5%, (500 ml = 1 unit) - home mix

CIM: 65-10

MCM: 2130, 4450

B4172 Parenteral nutrition solution; amino acid, 5.5% through 7%, (500 ml = 1 unit) - home mix

CIM: 65-10

MCM: 2130, 4450

B4176 Parenteral nutrition solution; amino acid, 7% through 8.5%, (500 ml = 1 unit) - home mix

CIM: 65-10

MCM: 2130, 4450

B4178 Parenteral nutrition solution: amino acid, greater than 8.5% (500 ml = 1 unit) - home mix

CIM: 65-10

MCM: 2130, 4450

B4180 Parenteral nutrition solution; carbohydrates (dextrose), greater than 50% (500 ml = 1 unit) - home mix

CIM: 65-10

MCM: 2130, 4450

B4185 Parenteral nutrition solution, per 10 grams lipids

B4189 Parenteral nutrition solution; compounded amino acid and carbohydrates with electrolytes, trace elements, and vitamins, including preparation, any strength, 10 to 51 grams of protein - premix

CIM: 65-10

MCM: 2130, 4450

B4193 Parenteral nutrition solution; compounded amino acid and carbohydrates with electrolytes, trace elements, and vitamins, including preparation, any strength, 52 to 73 grams of protein - premix

CIM: 65-10

MCM: 2130, 4450

B4197 Parenteral nutrition solution; compounded amino acid and carbohydrates with electrolytes, trace elements and vitamins, including preparation, any strength, 74 to 100 grams of protein - premix

CIM: 65-10

MCM: 2130, 4450

B4199 Parenteral nutrition solution; compounded amino acid and carbohydrates with electrolytes, trace elements and vitamins, including preparation, any strength, over 100 grams of protein - premix

CIM: 65-10

MCM: 2130, 4450

B4216 Parenteral nutrition; additives (vitamins, trace elements, heparin, electrolytes), home mix, per day

CIM: 65-10

MCM: 2130, 4450

B4220 Parenteral nutrition supply kit; premix, per day

CIM: 65-10

MCM: 2130, 4450

B4222 Parenteral nutrition supply kit; home mix, per day

CIM: 65-10

MCM: 2130, 4450

B4224 Parenteral nutrition administration kit, per day

CIM: 65-10

MCM: 2130, 4450

B5000 Parenteral nutrition solution compounded amino acid and carbohydrates with electrolytes, trace elements, and vitamins, including preparation, any strength, renal-Aminosyn-rf, NephrAmine, renamine-premix

CIM: 65-10

MCM: 2130, 4450

B5100 Parenteral nutrition solution compounded amino acid and carbohydrates with electrolytes, trace elements, and vitamins, including preparation, any strength, hepatic, HepatAmine-premix

CIM: 65-10

MCM: 2130, 4450

B5200 Parenteral nutrition solution compounded amino acid and carbohydrates with electrolytes, trace elements, and vitamins, including preparation, any strength, stress-branch chain amino acids-FreAmine-HBc-premix

CIM: 65-10

MCM: 2130, 4450

Enteral and Parenteral Pumps

(**B9000** Code deleted December 31, 2016).

▲ **B9002** Enteral nutrition infusion pump, any type

CIM: 65-10

MCM: 2130, 4450

B9004 Parenteral nutrition infusion pump, portable

CIM: 65-10

MCM: 2130, 4450

B9006 Parenteral nutrition infusion pump, stationary

CIM: 65-10

MCM: 2130, 4450

B9998 NOC for enteral supplies

CIM: 65-10

MCM: 2130, 4450

B9999 NOC for parenteral supplies

CIM: 65-10

MCM: 2130, 4450

HOSPITAL OUTPATIENT PPS CODES

Guidelines

The "C" codes are unique temporary codes established by CMS for use under the Hospital Outpatient Prospective Payment System (OPPS). Non-OPPS use of these codes for Medicare is not valid.

The purpose of the "C" codes is to provide hospitals with a list of codes and long descriptors for drugs, biologicals and devices eligible for transitional pass-through payments, and for items classified in "new technology" ambulatory payment classifications (APCs) under the new Hospital Outpatient Prospective Payment System (OPPS).

The listing of HCPCS codes in this section does not assure coverage of the specific item or service in a given case. To be eligible for pass-through and new technology payments, the items reported with "C" codes must be considered reasonable and necessary.

All of the "C" codes are used exclusively for services paid under the Hospital Outpatient Prospective Payment System and may not be used to bill for services paid under other Medicare payment systems.

In addition to the information presented above, several other items unique to this section are defined here:

1. SPECIAL REPORT: A service, material or supply that is rarely provided, unusual, variable or new may require a special report in determining medical appropriateness for reimbursement purposes. Pertinent information should include an adequate definition or description of the nature, extent, and need for the service, material or supply.

2. MODIFIERS: Listed services may be modified under certain circumstances. When appropriate, the modifying circumstance is identified by adding a modifier to the basic procedure code. CPT and HCPCS National Level II modifiers may be used with CPT and HCPCS National Level II procedure codes.

Hospital Outpatient PPS Codes

C1713 Anchor/screw for opposing bone-to-bone or soft tissue-to-bone (implantable)

Statute: 1833(T)

C1714 Catheter, transluminal atherectomy, directional

Statute: 1833(T)

C1715 Brachytherapy needle

Statute: 1833(T)

C1716 Brachytherapy source, non-stranded, gold-198, per source

Statute: 1833(T)

C1717 Brachytherapy source, non-stranded, high dose rate iridium-192, per source

Statute: 1833(T)

C1719 Brachytherapy source, non-stranded, non-high dose rate iridium-192, per source

Statute: 1833(T)

C1721 Cardioverter-defibrillator, dual chamber (implantable)

Statute: 1833(T)

C1722 Cardioverter-defibrillator, single chamber (implantable)

Statute: 1833(T)

C1724 Catheter, transluminal atherectomy, rotational

Statute: 1833(T)

C1725 Catheter, transluminal angioplasty, non-laser (may include guidance, infusion/perfusion capability)

Statute: 1833(T)

C1726 Catheter, balloon dilatation, non-vascular

Statute: 1833(T)

C1727 Catheter, balloon tissue dissector, non-vascular (insertable)

Statute: 1833(T)

C1728 Catheter, brachytherapy seed administration

Statute: 1833(T)

C1729 Catheter, drainage

Statute: 1833(T)

C1730 Catheter, electrophysiology, diagnostic, other than 3d mapping (19 or fewer electrodes)

Statute: 1833(T)

C1731 Catheter, electrophysiology, diagnostic, other than 3d mapping (20 or more electrodes)

Statute: 1833(T)

C1732 Catheter, electrophysiology, diagnostic/ablation, 3d or vector mapping

Statute: 1833(T)

C1733 Catheter, electrophysiology, diagnostic/ablation, other than 3d or vector mapping, other than cool-tip

Statute: 1833(T)

C1749 Endoscope, retrograde imaging/illumination colonoscope device (implantable)

Statute: 1833(t)

C1750 Catheter, hemodialysis/peritoneal, long-term

Statute: 1833(T)

C1751 Catheter, infusion, inserted peripherally, centrally or midline (other than hemodialysis)

Statute: 1833(T)

C1752 Catheter, hemodialysis/peritoneal, short-term

Statute: 1833(T)

C1753 Catheter, intravascular ultrasound

Statute: 1833(T)

C1754 Catheter, intradiscal

Statute: 1833(T)

C1755 Catheter, intraspinal

Statute: 1833(T)

C1756 Catheter, pacing, transesophageal

Statute: 1833(T)

C1757 Catheter, thrombectomy/embolectomy

Statute: 1833(T)

C1758 Catheter, ureteral

Statute: 1833(T)

C1759 Catheter, intracardiac echocardiography

Statute: 1833(T)

C1760 Closure device, vascular (implantable/insertable)

Statute: 1833(T)

C1762 Connective tissue, human (includes fascia lata)

Statute: 1833(T)

C1763 Connective tissue, non-human (includes synthetic)

Statute: 1833(T)

C1764 Event recorder, cardiac (implantable)

Statute: 1833(T)

C1765 Adhesion barrier

Statute: 1833(T)

C1766 Introducer/sheath, guiding, intracardiac electrophysiological, steerable, other than peel-away

Statute: 1833(T)

C1767 Generator, neurostimulator (implantable), non-rechargeable

Statute: 1833(T)

C1768 Graft, vascular

Statute: 1833(T)

C1769 Guide wire

Statute: 1833(T)

C1770 Imaging coil, magnetic resonance (insertable)

Statute: 1833(T)

C1771 Repair device, urinary, incontinence, with sling graft

Statute: 1833(T)

C1772 Infusion pump, programmable (implantable)

Statute: 1833(T)

C1773 Retrieval device, insertable (used to retrieve fractured medical devices)

Statute: 1833(T)

C1776 Joint device (implantable)

Statute: 1833(T)

C1777 Lead, cardioverter-defibrillator, endocardial single coil (implantable)

Statute: 1833(T)

C1778 Lead, neurostimulator (implantable)

Statute: 1833(T)

C1779 Lead, pacemaker, transvenous VDD single pass

Statute: 1833(T)

C1780 Lens, intraocular (new technology)

Statute: 1833(T)

C1781 Mesh (implantable)

Statute: 1833(T)

C1782 Morcellator

Statute: 1833(T)

C1783 Ocular implant, aqueous drainage assist device

Statute: 1833(T)

C1784 Ocular device, intraoperative, detached retina

Statute: 1833(T)

C1785 Pacemaker, dual chamber, rate-responsive (implantable)

Statute: 1833(T)

C1786 Pacemaker, single chamber, rate-responsive (implantable)

Statute: 1833(T)

C1787 Patient programmer, neurostimulator

Statute: 1833(T)

C1788 Port, indwelling (implantable)

Statute: 1833(T)

C1789 Prosthesis, breast (implantable)

Statute: 1833(T)

C1813 Prosthesis, penile, inflatable

Statute: 1833(T)

C1814 Retinal tamponade device, silicone oil

Statute: 1833t

C1815 Prosthesis, urinary sphincter (implantable)

Statute: 1833(T)

C1816 Receiver and/or transmitter, neurostimulator (implantable)

Statute: 1833(T)

C1817 Septal defect implant system, intracardiac

Statute: 1833(T)

C1818 Integrated keratoprosthesis

Statute: 1833T

C1819 Surgical tissue localization and excision device (implantable)

Statute: 1833T

C1820 Generator, neurostimulator (implantable), non high-frequency with rechargeable battery and charging system

Statute: 1833(T)

C1821 Interspinous process distraction device (implantable)

Statute: 1833(T)

C1822 Generator, neurostimulator (implantable), high frequency, with rechargeable battery and charging system

Statute: 1833(T)

C1830 Powered bone marrow biopsy needle

Statute: 1833(t)

C1840 Lens, intraocular (telescopic)

Statute: 1833(t)

C1841 Retinal prosthesis, includes all internal and external components

Statute: 1833(t)

C1874 Stent, coated/covered, with delivery system

Statute: 1833(T)

C1875 Stent, coated/covered, without delivery system

Statute: 1833(T)

C1876 Stent, non-coated/non-covered, with delivery system

Statute: 1833(T)

C1877 Stent, non-coated/non-covered, without delivery system

Statute: 1833(T)

C1878 Material for vocal cord medialization, synthetic (implantable)

Statute: 1833(T)

C1880 Vena cava filter

Statute: 1833(T)

C1881 Dialysis access system (implantable)

Statute: 1833(T)

C1882 Cardioverter-defibrillator, other than single or dual chamber (implantable)

Statute: 1833(T)

C1883 Adapter/extension, pacing lead or neurostimulator lead (implantable)

Statute: 1833(T)

C1884 Embolization protective system

Statute: 1833T

C1885 Catheter, transluminal angioplasty, laser

Statute: 1833(T)

C1886 Catheter, extravascular tissue ablation, any modality (insertable)

Statute: 1833(t)

C1887 Catheter, guiding (may include infusion/perfusion capability)

Statute: 1833(T)

C1888 Catheter, ablation, non-cardiac, endovascular (implantable)

Statute: 1833(T)

• **C1889** Implantable/insertable device for device intensive procedure, not otherwise classified

Statute: 1833(T)

C1891 Infusion pump, non-programmable, permanent (implantable)

Statute: 1833(T)

C1892 Introducer/sheath, guiding, intracardiac electrophysiological, fixed-curve, peel-away

Statute: 1833(T)

C1893 Introducer/sheath, guiding, intracardiac electrophysiological, fixed-curve, other than peel-away

Statute: 1833(T)

C1894 Introducer/sheath, other than guiding, other than intracardiac electrophysiological, non-laser

Statute: 1833(T)

C1895 Lead, cardioverter-defibrillator, endocardial dual coil (implantable)

Statute: 1833(T)

C1896 Lead, cardioverter-defibrillator, other than endocardial single or dual coil (implantable)

Statute: 1833(T)

C1897 Lead, neurostimulator test kit (implantable)

Statute: 1833(T)

C1898 Lead, pacemaker, other than transvenous VDD single pass

Statute: 1833(T)

C1899 Lead, pacemaker/cardioverter-defibrillator combination (implantable)

Statute: 1833(T)

C1900 Lead, left ventricular coronary venous system

Statute: 1833(T)

C2613 Lung biopsy plug with delivery system

Statute: 1833(t)

C2614 Probe, percutaneous lumbar discectomy

Statute: 1833(T)

C2615 Sealant, pulmonary, liquid

Statute: 1833(T)

C2616 Brachytherapy source, non-stranded, yttrium-90, per source

Statute: 1833(T)

C2617 Stent, non-coronary, temporary, without delivery system

Statute: 1833(T)

C2618 Probe/needle, cryoablation

Statute: 1833(T)

C2619 Pacemaker, dual chamber, non rate-responsive (implantable)

Statute: 1833(T)

C2620 Pacemaker, single chamber, non rate-responsive (implantable)

Statute: 1833(T)

C2621 Pacemaker, other than single or dual chamber (implantable)

Statute: 1833(T)

C2622 Prosthesis, penile, non-inflatable

Statute: 1833(T)

C2623 Catheter, transluminal angioplasty, drug-coated, non-laser

Statute: 1833(t)

C2624 Implantable wireless pulmonary artery pressure sensor with delivery catheter, including all system components

Statute: 1833(t)

C2625 Stent, non-coronary, temporary, with delivery system

Statute: 1833(T)

C2626 Infusion pump, non-programmable, temporary (implantable)

Statute: 1833(T)

C2627 Catheter, suprapubic/cystoscopic

Statute: 1833(T)

C2628 Catheter, occlusion

Statute: 1833(T)

C2629 Introducer/sheath, other than guiding, other than intracardiac electrophysiological, laser

Statute: 1833(T)

C2630 Catheter, electrophysiology, diagnostic/ablation, other than 3d or vector mapping, cool-tip

Statute: 1833(T)

C2631 Repair device, urinary, incontinence, without sling graft

Statute: 1833(T)

C2634 Brachytherapy source, non-stranded, high activity, iodine-125, greater than 1.01 mCi (nist), per source

Statute: 1833(T)

C2635 Brachytherapy source, non-stranded, high activity, palladium-103, greater than 2.2 mCi (nist), per source

Statute: 1833(T)

C2636 Brachytherapy linear source, non-stranded, palladium-103, per 1 mm

Statute: 1833(T)

C2637 Brachytherapy source, non-stranded, ytterbium-169, per source

Statute: 1833(T)

C2638 Brachytherapy source, stranded, iodine-125, per source

Statute: 1833(t)(2)

C2639 Brachytherapy source, non-stranded, iodine-125, per source

Statute: 1833(t)(2)

C2640 Brachytherapy source, stranded, palladium-103, per source

Statute: 1833(t)(2)

C2641 Brachytherapy source, non-stranded, palladium-103, per source

Statute: 1833(t)(2)

C2642 Brachytherapy source, stranded, cesium-131, per source

Statute: 1833(t)(2)

C2643 Brachytherapy source, non-stranded, cesium-131, per source

Statute: 1833(t)(2)

C2644 Brachytherapy source, cesium-131 chloride solution, per millicurie

Statute: 1833(t)

C2645 Brachytherapy planar source, palladium-103, per square millimeter

Statute: 1833(T)

C2698 Brachytherapy source, stranded, not otherwise specified, per source

Statute: 1833(t)(2)

C2699 Brachytherapy source, non-stranded, not otherwise specified, per source

Statute: 1833(t)(2)

C5271 Application of low cost skin substitute graft to trunk, arms, legs, total wound surface area up to 100 sq cm; first 25 sq cm or less wound surface area

Statute: 1833(t)

C5272 Application of low cost skin substitute graft to trunk, arms, legs, total wound surface area up to 100 sq cm; each additional 25 sq cm wound surface area, or part thereof (list separately in addition to code for primary procedure)

Statute: 1833(t)

C5273 Application of low cost skin substitute graft to trunk, arms, legs, total wound surface area greater than or equal to 100 sq cm; first 100 sq cm wound surface area, or 1% of body area of infants and children

Statute: 1833(t)

C5274 Application of low cost skin substitute graft to trunk, arms, legs, total wound surface area greater than or equal to 100 sq cm; each additional 100 sq cm wound surface area, or part thereof, or each additional 1% of body area of infants and children, or part thereof (list separately in addition to code for primary procedure)

Statute: 1833(t)

C5275 Application of low cost skin substitute graft to face, scalp, eyelids, mouth, neck, ears, orbits, genitalia, hands, feet, and/or multiple digits, total wound surface area up to 100 sq cm; first 25 sq cm or less wound surface area

Statute: 1833(t)

C5276 Application of low cost skin substitute graft to face, scalp, eyelids, mouth, neck, ears, orbits, genitalia, hands, feet, and/or multiple digits, total wound surface area up to 100 sq cm; each additional 25 sq cm wound surface area, or part thereof (list separately in addition to code for primary procedure)

Statute: 1833(t)

C5277 Application of low cost skin substitute graft to face, scalp, eyelids, mouth, neck, ears, orbits, genitalia, hands, feet, and/or multiple digits, total wound surface area greater than or equal to 100 sq cm; first 100 sq cm wound surface area, or 1% of body area of infants and children

Statute: 1833(t)

C5278 Application of low cost skin substitute graft to face, scalp, eyelids, mouth, neck, ears, orbits, genitalia, hands, feet, and/or multiple digits, total wound surface area greater than or equal to 100 sq cm; each additional 100 sq cm wound surface area, or part thereof, or each additional 1% of body area of infants and children, or part thereof (list separately in addition to code for primary procedure)

Statute: 1833(t)

C8900 Magnetic resonance angiography with contrast, abdomen

Statute: 1833(t)(2)

C8901 Magnetic resonance angiography without contrast, abdomen

Statute: 1833(t)(2)

C8902 Magnetic resonance angiography without contrast followed by with contrast, abdomen

Statute: 1833(t)(2)

C8903 Magnetic resonance imaging with contrast, breast; unilateral

Statute: 1833(t)(2)

C8904 Magnetic resonance imaging without contrast, breast; unilateral

Statute: 1833(t)(2)

C8905 Magnetic resonance imaging without contrast followed by with contrast, breast; unilateral

Statute: 1833(t)(2)

C8906 Magnetic resonance imaging with contrast, breast; bilateral

Statute: 1833(t)(2)

C8907 Magnetic resonance imaging without contrast, breast; bilateral

Statute: 1833(t)(2)

C8908 Magnetic resonance imaging without contrast followed by with contrast, breast; bilateral

Statute: 1833(t)(2)

C8909 Magnetic resonance angiography with contrast, chest (excluding myocardium)

Statute: 1833(t)(2)

C8910 Magnetic resonance angiography without contrast, chest (excluding myocardium)

Statute: 1833(t)(2)

C8911 Magnetic resonance angiography without contrast followed by with contrast, chest (excluding myocardium)

Statute: 1833(t)(2)

C8912 Magnetic resonance angiography with contrast, lower extremity

Statute: 1833(t)(2)

C8913 Magnetic resonance angiography without contrast, lower extremity

Statute: 1833(t)(2)

C8914 Magnetic resonance angiography without contrast followed by with contrast, lower extremity

Statute: 1833(t)(2)

C8918 Magnetic resonance angiography with contrast, pelvis

Statute: 430 BIPA

C8919 Magnetic resonance angiography without contrast, pelvis

Statute: 430 BIPA

C8920 Magnetic resonance angiography without contrast followed by with contrast, pelvis

Statute: 430 BIPA

C8921 Transthoracic echocardiography with contrast, or without contrast followed by with contrast, for congenital cardiac anomalies; complete

Statute: 1833(t)(2)

C8922 Transthoracic echocardiography with contrast, or without contrast followed by with contrast, for congenital cardiac anomalies; follow-up or limited study

Statute: 1833(t)(2)

C8923 Transthoracic echocardiography with contrast, or without contrast followed by with contrast, real-time with image documentation (2d), includes m-mode recording, when performed, complete, without spectral or color Doppler echocardiography

Statute: 1833(t)(2)

C8924 Transthoracic echocardiography with contrast, or without contrast followed by with contrast, real-time with image documentation (2d), includes m-mode recording, when performed, follow-up or limited study

Statute: 1833(t)(2)

C8925 Transesophageal echocardiography (tee) with contrast, or without contrast followed by with contrast, real time with image documentation (2d) (with or without m-mode recording); including probe placement, image acquisition, interpretation and report

Statute: 1833(t)(2)

C8926 Transesophageal echocardiography (tee) with contrast, or without contrast followed by with contrast, for congenital cardiac anomalies; including probe placement, image acquisition, interpretation and report

Statute: 1833(t)(2)

C8927 Transesophageal echocardiography (tee) with contrast, or without contrast followed by with contrast, for monitoring purposes, including probe placement, real time 2-dimensional image acquisition and interpretation leading to ongoing (continuous)

assessment of (dynamically changing) cardiac pumping function and to therapeutic measures on an immediate time basis

Statute: 1833(t)(2)

C8928 Transthoracic echocardiography with contrast, or without contrast followed by with contrast, real-time with image documentation (2d), includes m-mode recording, when performed, during rest and cardiovascular stress test using treadmill, bicycle exercise and/or pharmacologically induced stress, with interpretation and report

Statute: 1833(t)(2)

C8929 Transthoracic echocardiography with contrast, or without contrast followed by with contrast, real-time with image documentation (2d), includes m-mode recording, when performed, complete, with spectral Doppler echocardiography, and with color flow Doppler echocardiography

Statute: 1833(t)(2)

C8930 Transthoracic echocardiography, with contrast, or without contrast followed by with contrast, real-time with image documentation (2d), includes m-mode recording, when performed, during rest and cardiovascular stress test using treadmill, bicycle exercise and/or pharmacologically induced stress, with interpretation and report; including performance of continuous electrocardiographic monitoring, with physician supervision

Statute: 1833(t)(2)

C8931 Magnetic resonance angiography with contrast, spinal canal and contents

Statute: 1833(t)

C8932 Magnetic resonance angiography without contrast, spinal canal and contents

Statute: 1833(t)

C8933 Magnetic resonance angiography without contrast followed by with contrast, spinal canal and contents

Statute: 1833(t)

C8934 Magnetic resonance angiography with contrast, upper extremity

Statute: 1833(t)

C8935 Magnetic resonance angiography without contrast, upper extremity

Statute: 1833(t)

C8936 Magnetic resonance angiography without contrast followed by with contrast, upper extremity

Statute: 1833(t)

C8957 Intravenous infusion for therapy/diagnosis; initiation of prolonged infusion (more than 8 hours), requiring use of portable or implantable pump

Statute: 1833(t)

(**C9025** Code deleted December 31, 2015.) Use J9308.

(**C9026** Code deleted December 31, 2015.) Use J3380.

(**C9027** Code deleted December 31, 2015.) Use J9271.

C9113 Injection, pantoprazole sodium, per vial

Statute: 1833(T)

(**C9121** Code deleted December 31, 2016). Use J0883.

C9132 Prothrombin complex concentrate (human), Kcentra, per i.u. of factor ix activity

Statute: 1833(t)

(**C9136** Code deleted December 31, 2015.) Use Q9975.

(**C9137** Code deleted December 31, 2016). Use J7207.

(**C9138** Code deleted December 31, 2016). Use J7209.

(**C9139** Code deleted December 31, 2016). Use J7202.

C9248 Injection, clevidipine butyrate, 1 mg

Statute: 1833(t)

C9250 Human plasma fibrin sealant, vapor-heated, solvent-detergent (Artiss), 2 ml

Statute: 621MMA

C9254 Injection, lacosamide, 1 mg

Statute: 621MMA

C9257 Injection, bevacizumab, 0.25 mg

Statute: 1833(t)

C9275 Injection, hexaminolevulinate hydrochloride, 100 mg, per study dose

Statute: 1833(t)

C9285 Lidocaine 70 mg/tetracaine 70 mg, per patch

Statute: 1833(t)

C9290 Injection, bupivacaine liposome, 1 mg

Statute: 1833(t)

C9293 Injection, glucarpidase, 10 units

Statute: 1833(t)

(**C9349** Code deleted December 31, 2016). Use Q4172.

C9352 Microporous collagen implantable tube (NeuraGen nerve guide), per centimeter length

Statute: 621MMA

C9353 Microporous collagen implantable slit tube (neurawrap nerve protector), per centimeter length

Statute: 621MMA

C9354 Acellular pericardial tissue matrix of non-human origin (veritas), per square centimeter

Statute: 621MMA

C9355 Collagen nerve cuff (neuromatrix), per 0.5 centimeter length

Statute: 621MMA

C9356 Tendon, porous matrix of cross-linked collagen and glycosaminoglycan matrix (TenoGlide tendon protector sheet), per square centimeter

Statute: 621 MMA

C9358 Dermal substitute, native, non-denatured collagen, fetal bovine origin (Surgimend collagen matrix), per 0.5 square centimeters

Statute: 621 MMA

C9359 Porous purified collagen matrix bone void filler (Integra Mozaik osteoconductive scaffold putty, Integra os osteoconductive scaffold putty), per 0.5 cc

Statute: 1833(T)

C9360 Dermal substitute, native, non-denatured collagen, neonatal bovine origin (Surgimend collagen matrix), per 0.5 square centimeters

Statute: 621MMA

C9361 Collagen matrix nerve wrap (neuromend collagen nerve wrap), per 0.5 centimeter length

Statute: 621MMA

C9362 Porous purified collagen matrix bone void filler (Integra Mozaik osteoconductive scaffold strip), per 0.5 cc

Statute: 621MMA

C9363 Skin substitute, Integra meshed bilayer wound matrix, per square centimeter

Statute: 621MMA

C9364 Porcine implant, Permacol, per square centimeter

Statute: 621MMA

C9399 Unclassified drugs or biologicals

Statute: 621MMA

(**C9442** Code deleted December 31, 2015.) Use J9032.

(**C9443** Code deleted December 31, 2015.) Use J0875.

(**C9444** Code deleted December 31, 2015.) Use J2407.

(**C9445** Code deleted December 31, 2015.) Use J0596.

(**C9446** Code deleted December 31, 2015.) Use J3090.

C9447 Injection, phenylephrine and ketorolac, 4 ml vial

Statute: 1833(t)

(**C9448** Code deleted December 31, 2015.) Use Q9978.

(**C9449** Code deleted December 31, 2015.) Use J9039.

(**C9450** Code deleted December 31, 2015.) Use J7313.

(**C9451** Code deleted December 31, 2015.) Use J2547.

(**C9452** Code deleted December 31, 2015.) Use J0695.

(**C9453** Code deleted December 31, 2015.) Use J9299.

(**C9454** Code deleted December 31, 2015.) Use J2502.

(**C9455** Code deleted December 31, 2015.) Use J2860.

(**C9456** Code deleted December 31, 2015.) Use J1833.

(**C9457** Code deleted December 31, 2015.) Use Q9950.

(**C9458** Code deleted June 30, 2016.) Use Q9983.

(**C9459** Code deleted June 30, 2016.) Use Q9982.

C9460 Injection, cangrelor, 1 mg

Statute: 1833(t)

(**C9461** Code deleted December 31, 2016). Use A9515.

(**C9461** Code deleted December 31, 2016). Use A9515.

(**C9470** Code deleted December 31, 2016). Use J1942.

(**C9471** Code deleted December 31, 2016). Use J7322.

(**C9472** Code deleted December 31, 2016). Use J9325.

(**C9473** Code deleted December 31, 2016). Use J2182.

(**C9474** Code deleted December 31, 2016). Use J9205.

(**C9475** Code deleted December 31, 2016). Use J9295.

(**C9476** Code deleted December 31, 2016). Use J9145.

(**C9477** Code deleted December 31, 2016). Use J9176.

(**C9478** Code deleted December 31, 2016). Use J2840.

(**C9479** Code deleted December 31, 2016). Use J7342.

(**C9480** Code deleted December 31, 2016). Use J9352.

• **C9482** Injection, sotalol hydrochloride, 1 mg

Statute: 1833(t)

• **C9483** Injection, atezolizumab, 10 mg

Statute: 1833(t)

C9497 Loxapine, inhalation powder, 10 mg

Statute: 1833(t)

C9600 Percutaneous transcatheter placement of drug eluting intracoronary stent(s), with coronary angioplasty when performed; single major coronary artery or branch

Statute: 1833(t)

C9601 Percutaneous transcatheter placement of drug-eluting intracoronary stent(s), with coronary angioplasty when performed; each additional branch of a major coronary artery (list separately in addition to code for primary procedure)

Statute: 1833(t)

C9602 Percutaneous transluminal coronary atherectomy, with drug eluting intracoronary stent, with coronary angioplasty when performed; single major coronary artery or branch

Statute: 1833(t)

C9603 Percutaneous transluminal coronary atherectomy, with drug-eluting intracoronary stent, with coronary angioplasty when performed; each additional branch of a major coronary artery (list separately in addition to code for primary procedure)

Statute: 1833(t)

C9604 Percutaneous transluminal revascularization of or through coronary artery bypass graft (internal mammary, free arterial, venous), any combination of drug-eluting intracoronary stent, atherectomy and angioplasty, including distal protection when performed; single vessel

Statute: 1833(t)

C9605 Percutaneous transluminal revascularization of or through coronary artery bypass graft (internal mammary, free arterial, venous), any combination of drug-eluting intracoronary stent, atherectomy and angioplasty, including distal protection when performed; each additional branch subtended by the bypass graft (list separately in addition to code for primary procedure)

Statute: 1833(t)

C9606 Percutaneous transluminal revascularization of acute total/subtotal occlusion during acute myocardial infarction, coronary artery or coronary artery bypass graft, any combination of drug-eluting intracoronary stent, atherectomy and angioplasty, including aspiration thrombectomy when performed, single vessel

Statute: 1833(t)

C9607 Percutaneous transluminal revascularization of chronic total occlusion, coronary artery, coronary artery branch, or coronary artery bypass graft, any combination of drug-eluting intracoronary stent, atherectomy and angioplasty; single vessel

Statute: 1833(t)

C9608 Percutaneous transluminal revascularization of chronic total occlusion, coronary artery, coronary artery branch, or coronary artery bypass graft, any combination of drug-eluting intracoronary stent, atherectomy and angioplasty; each additional coronary artery, coronary artery branch, or bypass graft (list separately in addition to code for primary procedure)

Statute: 1833(t)

(**C9724** Code deleted December 31, 2015.) Use 43210.

C9725 Placement of endorectal intracavitary applicator for high intensity brachytherapy

Statute: 1833(T)

C9726 Placement and removal (if performed) of applicator into breast for intraoperative radiation therapy, add-on to primary breast procedure

Statute: 1833(T)

C9727 Insertion of implants into the soft palate; minimum of three implants

Statute: 1833(T)

C9728 Placement of interstitial device(s) for radiation therapy/surgery guidance (e.g., fiducial markers, dosimeter), for other than the following sites (any approach): abdomen, pelvis, prostate, retroperitoneum, thorax, single or multiple

Statute: 1833(T)

C9733 Non-ophthalmic fluorescent vascular angiography

Statute: 1833(t)

C9734 Focused ultrasound ablation/therapeutic intervention, other than uterine leiomyomata, with magnetic resonance (mr) guidance

Statute: 1833(t)

(**C9737** Code deleted December 31, 2015.) Use 0392T.

C9739 Cystourethroscopy, with insertion of transprostatic implant; 1 to 3 implants

Statute: 1833(t)

C9740 Cystourethroscopy, with insertion of transprostatic implant; 4 or more implants

Statute: 1833(t)

C9741 Right heart catheterization with implantation of wireless pressure sensor in the pulmonary artery, including any type of measurement, angiography, imaging supervision, interpretation, and report

Statute: 1833(t)

(**C9742** Code deleted December 31, 2016). Use 31573, 31574.

(**C9743** Code deleted June 30, 2016). Use 0438T.

• **C9744** Ultrasound, abdominal, with contrast

Statute: 1833(t)

(**C9800** Code deleted December 31, 2016). Use G0429.

C9898 Radiolabeled product provided during a hospital inpatient stay

C9899 Implanted prosthetic device, payable only for inpatients who do not have inpatient coverage

Statute: 1833(t)

DURABLE MEDICAL EQUIPMENT

Guidelines

In addition to the information presented in the INTRODUCTION, several other items unique to this section are defined or identified here:

1. DEFINITION OF DURABLE MEDICAL EQUIPMENT: Durable medical equipment (DME) can withstand repeated use and is used primarily to serve a medical purpose. It generally is not useful in the absence of an illness or injury, and is appropriate for use in the home. Expendable medical supplies, such as incontinent pads, lamb's wool pads, catheters, ace bandages, elastic stockings, surgical face masks, irrigating kits, sheets and bags, are not considered to be DME.

2. REASONABLE AND NECESSARY: DME may not be covered in every instance. The equipment must be reasonable and necessary for the illness or injury being treated or for improving the functioning of a malformed body part. A physician's prescription is normally sufficient to establish that the equipment is necessary. To determine reasonableness, the following conditions must be met: the expense must be proportionate to the therapeutic benefits of using the equipment; the cost must not substantially exceed a medically appropriate care plan; and, the item must not serve the same purpose as equipment already available to the patient. Claims for items that are not reasonable will be denied except when it is determined that no alternative plan of care is available for which payment could be made.

3. SUBSECTION INFORMATION: Some of the listed subheadings or subsections have special needs or instructions unique to that section. Where these are indicated, special "notes" will be presented preceding or following the listings. Those subsections within the DURABLE MEDICAL EQUIPMENT section that have "notes" are as follows:

SUBSECTION	CODE SERIES
Artificial kidney machines and accessories	E1510-E1699

4. UNLISTED SERVICE OR PROCEDURE: A service or procedure may be provided that is not listed in this edition of HCPCS. When reporting such a service, the appropriate "unlisted procedure" code may be used to indicate the service, identifying it by "special report" as defined below. HCPCS terminology is inconsistent in defining unlisted procedures. The procedure definition may include the term(s) "unlisted", "not otherwise classified", "unspecified", "unclassified", "other" and "miscellaneous". Prior to using these codes, try to determine if a Local Level III code or CPT code is available. The "unlisted procedures" and accompanying codes for DURABLE MEDICAL EQUIPMENT are as follows:

   E1399 Durable medical equipment, miscellaneous
   E1699 Dialysis equipment, not otherwise specified

5. SPECIAL REPORT: A service, material or supply that is rarely provided, unusual, variable or new may require a special report in determining medical appropriateness for reimbursement purposes. Pertinent information should include an adequate definition or description of the nature, extent, and need for the service, material or supply.

E CODES

6. MODIFIERS: Listed services may be modified under certain circumstances. When appropriate, the modifying circumstance is identified by adding a modifier to the basic procedure code. CPT and HCPCS National Level II modifiers may be used with CPT and HCPCS National Level II procedure codes. Modifiers commonly used with DURABLE MEDICAL EQUIPMENT are as follows:

   -CC Procedure code change (use "CC" when the procedure code submitted was changed either for administrative reasons or because an incorrect code was filed)

   -LL Lease/rental (used the "LL" modifier when DME rental is to be applied against the purchase price)

   -LT Left side (used to identify procedures performed on the left side of the body)

   -MS Six-month maintenance and servicing fee for reasonable and necessary parts and labor which are not covered under any manufacturer or supplier warranty

   -NR New when rented (use the "NR" modifier when DME which was new at the time of rental is subsequently purchased)

   -NU New equipment

   -QE Prescribed amount of oxygen is less than 1 liter per minute (LPM)

   -QF Prescribed amount of oxygen exceeds 4 liters per minute (LPM) and portable oxygen is prescribed

   -QG Prescribed amount of oxygen is greater than 4 liters per minute (LPM)

   -QH Oxygen conserving device is being used with an oxygen delivery system

   -QT Recording and storage on tape by an analog tape recorder

   -RP Replacement and repair (may be used to indicate replacement of DME, orthotic and prosthetic devices which have been in use for some time. The claim shows the code for the part, followed by the "RP" modifier and the charge for the part.)

   -RR Rental (used when DME is to be rented)

   -RT Right side (used to identify procedures performed on the right side of the body)

   -TC Technical component. Under certain circumstances, a charge may be made for the technical component alone. Under those circumstances, the technical component charge is identified by adding modifier -TC to the usual procedure code. Technical component charges are institutional charges and are not billed separately by physicians. However, portable x-ray suppliers bill only for technical component and should utilize modifier -TC. The charge data from portable x-ray suppliers will then be used to build customary and prevailing profiles.

   -UE Used durable medical equipment

7. CPT CODE CROSS-REFERENCE: Unless otherwise specified, the equivalent CPT code for all listings in this section is 99070.

8. DURABLE MEDICAL EQUIPMENT REGIONAL CARRIERS (DMERCS): Effective October 1, 1993 claims for durable medical equipment (DME) must be billed to one of four regional carriers depending upon the residence of the beneficiary. The transition dates for DMERC claims is from November 1, 1993 to March 1, 1994 depending upon the state you practice in. See the Introduction for a complete discussion of DMERCs.

Durable Medical Equipment Canes

E0100 Cane, includes canes of all materials, adjustable or fixed, with tip

CIM: 60-3, 60-9

MCM: 2100.1

E0105 Cane, quad or three prong, includes canes of all materials, adjustable or fixed, with tips

CIM: 60-15, 60-9

MCM: 2100.1

Crutches

E0110 Crutches, forearm, includes crutches of various materials, adjustable or fixed, pair, complete with tips and handgrips

CIM: 60-9

MCM: 2100.1

E0111 Crutch forearm, includes crutches of various materials, adjustable or fixed, each, with tip and handgrips

CIM: 60-9

MCM: 2100.1

E0112 Crutches underarm, wood, adjustable or fixed, pair, with pads, tips and handgrips

CIM: 60-9

MCM: 2100.1

E0113 Crutch underarm, wood, adjustable or fixed, each, with pad, tip and handgrip

CIM: 60-9

MCM: 2100.1

E0114 Crutches underarm, other than wood, adjustable or fixed, pair, with pads, tips and handgrips

CIM: 60-9

MCM: 2100.1

E0116 Crutch, underarm, other than wood, adjustable or fixed, with pad, tip, handgrip, with or without shock absorber, each

CIM: 60-9

MCM: 2100.1

E0117 Crutch, underarm, articulating, spring assisted, each

MCM: 2100.1

E0118 Crutch substitute, lower leg platform, with or without wheels, each

Walkers

E0130 Walker, rigid (pickup), adjustable or fixed height

CIM: 60-9

MCM: 2100.1

E0135 Walker, folding (pickup), adjustable or fixed height

CIM: 60-9

MCM: 2100.1

E0140 Walker, with trunk support, adjustable or fixed height, any type

CIM: 60-9

MCM: 2100.1

E0141 Walker, rigid, wheeled, adjustable or fixed height

CIM: 60-9

MCM: 2100.1

E0143 Walker, folding, wheeled, adjustable or fixed height

CIM: 60-9

MCM: 2100.1

E0144 Walker, enclosed, four sided framed, rigid or folding, wheeled with posterior seat

CIM: 60-9

MCM: 2100.1

E0147 Walker, heavy duty, multiple braking system, variable wheel resistance

CIM: 60-15

MCM: 2100.1

E0148 Walker, heavy duty, without wheels, rigid or folding, any type, each

E0149 Walker, heavy duty, wheeled, rigid or folding, any type

Attachments

E0153 Platform attachment, forearm crutch, each

E0154 Platform attachment, walker, each

E0155 Wheel attachment, rigid pick-up walker, per pair

E0156 Seat attachment, walker

E0157 Crutch attachment, walker, each

E0158 Leg extensions for walker, per set of four (4)

E0159 Brake attachment for wheeled walker, replacement, each

Commodes

E0160 Sitz type bath or equipment, portable, used with or without commode

CIM: 60-9

E0161 Sitz type bath or equipment, portable, used with or without commode, with faucet attachment/s

CIM: 60-9

E0162 Sitz bath chair

CIM: 60-9

E0163 Commode chair, mobile or stationary, with fixed arms

CIM: 60-9

MCM: 2100.1

E0165 Commode chair, mobile or stationary, with detachable arms

CIM: 60-9

MCM: 2100.1

E0167 Pail or pan for use with commode chair, replacement only

CIM: 60-9

E0168 Commode chair, extra wide and/or heavy duty, stationary or mobile, with or without arms, any type, each

E0170 Commode chair with integrated seat lift mechanism, electric, any type

E0171 Commode chair with integrated seat lift mechanism, non-electric, any type

E0172 Seat lift mechanism placed over or on top of toilet, any type

Statute: 1861SSA

E0175 Foot rest, for use with commode chair, each

Decubitus Care Equipment

E0181 Powered pressure reducing mattress overlay/pad, alternating, with pump, includes heavy duty

CIM: 60-9

MCM: 4107.6

E0182 Pump for alternating pressure pad, for replacement only

CIM: 60-9

MCM: 4107.6

E0184 Dry pressure mattress

CIM: 60-9

MCM: 4107.6

E0185 Gel or gel-like pressure pad for mattress, standard mattress length and width

CIM: 60-9

MCM: 4107.6

E0186 Air pressure mattress

CIM: 60-9

E0187 Water pressure mattress

CIM: 60-9

E0188 Synthetic sheepskin pad

CIM: 60-9

MCM: 4107.6

E0189 Lambs wool sheepskin pad, any size

CIM: 60-9

MCM: 4107.6

E0190 Positioning cushion/pillow/wedge, any shape or size, includes all components and accessories

MCM: 2100.1

E0191 Heel or elbow protector, each

E0193 Powered air flotation bed (low air loss therapy)

E0194 Air fluidized bed

CIM: 60-19

E0196 Gel pressure mattress

CIM: 60-9

E0197 Air pressure pad for mattress, standard mattress length and width

CIM: 60-9

E0198 Water pressure pad for mattress, standard mattress length and width

CIM: 60-9

E0199 Dry pressure pad for mattress, standard mattress length and width

CIM: 60-9

Heat/Cold Application

E0200 Heat lamp, without stand (table model), includes bulb, or infrared element

CIM: 60-9

MCM: 2100.1

E0202 Phototherapy (bilirubin) light with photometer

E0203 Therapeutic light box, minimum 10,000 lux, table top model

CIM: 60-9

E0205 Heat lamp, with stand, includes bulb, or infrared element

CIM: 60-9

MCM: 2100.1

E0210 Electric heat pad, standard

CIM: 60-9

E0215 Electric heat pad, moist

CIM: 60-9

E0217 Water circulating heat pad with pump

CIM: 60-9

E0218 Water circulating cold pad with pump

CIM: 60-9

E0221 Infrared heating pad system

E0225 Hydrocollator unit, includes pads

CIM: 60-9

MCM: 2210.3

E0231 Non-contact wound warming device (temperature control unit, ac adapter and power cord) for use with warming card and wound cover

MCM: 2303

E0232 Warming card for use with the non contact wound warming device and non contact wound warming wound cover

MCM: 2303

E0235 Paraffin bath unit, portable (see medical supply code a4265 for paraffin)

CIM: 60-9

MCM: 2210.3

E0236 Pump for water circulating pad

CIM: 60-9

E0239 Hydrocollator unit, portable

CIM: 60-9

MCM: 2210.3

Bath and Toilet Aids

E0240 Bath/shower chair, with or without wheels, any size

CIM: 60-9

E0241 Bath tub wall rail, each

CIM: 60-9

MCM: 2100.1

E0242 Bath tub rail, floor base

CIM: 60-9

MCM: 2100.1

E0243 Toilet rail, each

CIM: 60-9

MCM: 2100.1

E0244 Raised toilet seat

CIM: 60-9

E0245 Tub stool or bench

CIM: 60-9

E0246 Transfer tub rail attachment

E0247 Transfer bench for tub or toilet with or without commode opening

CIM: 60-9

E0248 Transfer bench, heavy duty, for tub or toilet with or without commode opening

CIM: 60-9

E0249 Pad for water circulating heat unit, for replacement only

CIM: 60-9

Hospital Beds and Accessories

E0250 Hospital bed, fixed height, with any type side rails, with mattress

CIM: 60-18

MCM: 2100.1

E0251 Hospital bed, fixed height, with any type side rails, without mattress

CIM: 60-18

MCM: 2100.1

E0255 Hospital bed, variable height, hi-lo, with any type side rails, with mattress

CIM: 60-18

MCM: 2100.1

E0256 Hospital bed, variable height, hi-lo, with any type side rails, without mattress

CIM: 60-18

MCM: 2100.1

E0260 Hospital bed, semi-electric (head and foot adjustment), with any type side rails, with mattress

CIM: 60-18

MCM: 2100.1

E0261 Hospital bed, semi-electric (head and foot adjustment), with any type side rails, without mattress

CIM: 60-18

MCM: 2100.1

E0265 Hospital bed, total electric (head, foot and height adjustments), with any type side rails, with mattress

CIM: 60-18

MCM: 2100.1

E0266 Hospital bed, total electric (head, foot and height adjustments), with any type side rails, without mattress

CIM: 60-18

MCM: 2100.1

E0270 Hospital bed, institutional type includes: oscillating, circulating and Stryker frame, with mattress

CIM: 60-9

E0271 Mattress, innerspring

CIM: 60-18, 60-9

E0272 Mattress, foam rubber

CIM: 60-18, 60-9

E0273 Bed board

CIM: 60-9

E0274 Over-bed table

CIM: 60-9

E0275 Bed pan, standard, metal or plastic

CIM: 60-9

E0276 Bed pan, fracture, metal or plastic

CIM: 60-9

E0277 Powered pressure-reducing air mattress

CIM: 60-9

E0280 Bed cradle, any type

E0290 Hospital bed, fixed height, without side rails, with mattress

CIM: 60-18

MCM: 2100.1

E0291 Hospital bed, fixed height, without side rails, without mattress

CIM: 60-18

MCM: 2100.1

E0292 Hospital bed, variable height, hi-lo, without side rails, with mattress

CIM: 60-18

MCM: 2100.1

E0293 Hospital bed, variable height, hi-lo, without side rails, without mattress

CIM: 60-18

MCM: 2100.1

E0294 Hospital bed, semi-electric (head and foot adjustment), without side rails, with mattress

CIM: 60-18

MCM: 2100.1

E0295 Hospital bed, semi-electric (head and foot adjustment), without side rails, without mattress

CIM: 60-18

MCM: 2100.1

E0296 Hospital bed, total electric (head, foot and height adjustments). without side rails, with mattress

CIM: 60-18

MCM: 2100.1

E0297 Hospital bed, total electric (head, foot and height adjustments), without side rails, without mattress

CIM: 60-18

MCM: 2100.1

E0300 Pediatric crib, hospital grade, fully enclosed, with or without top enclosure

E0301 Hospital bed, heavy duty, extra wide, with weight capacity greater than 350 pounds, but less than or equal to 600 pounds, with any type side rails, without mattress

CIM: 60-18

E0302 Hospital bed, extra heavy duty, extra wide, with weight capacity greater than 600 pounds, with any type side rails, without mattress

CIM: 60-18

E0303 Hospital bed, heavy duty, extra wide, with weight capacity greater than 350 pounds, but less than or equal to 600 pounds, with any type side rails, with mattress

CIM: 60-18

E0304 Hospital bed, extra heavy duty, extra wide, with weight capacity greater than 600 pounds, with any type side rails, with mattress

CIM: 60-18

E0305 Bed side rails, half length

CIM: 60-18

E0310 Bed side rails, full length

CIM: 60-18

E0315 Bed accessory: board, table, or support device, any type

CIM: 60-9

E0316 Safety enclosure frame/canopy for use with hospital bed, any type

E0325 Urinal; male, jug-type, any material

CIM: 60-9

E0326 Urinal; female, jug-type, any material

CIM: 60-9

E0328 Hospital bed, pediatric, manual, 360 degree side enclosures, top of headboard, footboard and side rails up to 24 inches above the spring, includes mattress

E0329 Hospital bed, pediatric, electric or semi-electric, 360 degree side enclosures, top of headboard, footboard and side rails up to 24 inches above the spring, includes mattress

E0350 Control unit for electronic bowel irrigation/evacuation system

E0352 Disposable pack (water reservoir bag, speculum, valving mechanism and collection bag/box) for use with the electronic bowel irrigation/evacuation system

E0370 Air pressure elevator for heel

E0371 Nonpowered advanced pressure reducing overlay for mattress, standard mattress length and width

E0372 Powered air overlay for mattress, standard mattress length and width

E0373 Nonpowered advanced pressure reducing mattress

Oxygen and Related Respiratory Equipment

E0424 Stationary compressed gaseous oxygen system, rental; includes container, contents, regulator, flowmeter, humidifier, nebulizer, cannula or mask, and tubing

CIM: 60-4

MCM: 4107.9

E0425 Stationary compressed gas system, purchase; includes regulator, flowmeter, humidifier, nebulizer, cannula or mask, and tubing

CIM: 60-4

MCM: 4107.9

E0430 Portable gaseous oxygen system, purchase; includes regulator, flowmeter, humidifier, cannula or mask, and tubing

CIM: 60-4

MCM: 4107.9

E0431 Portable gaseous oxygen system, rental; includes portable container, regulator, flowmeter, humidifier, cannula or mask, and tubing

CIM: 60-4

MCM: 4107.9

E0433 Portable liquid oxygen system, rental; home liquefier used to fill portable liquid oxygen containers, includes portable containers, regulator, flowmeter, humidifier, cannula or mask and tubing, with or without supply reservoir and contents gauge

E0434 Portable liquid oxygen system, rental; includes portable container, supply reservoir, humidifier, flowmeter, refill adaptor, contents gauge, cannula or mask, and tubing

CIM: 60-4

MCM: 4107.9

E0435 Portable liquid oxygen system, purchase; includes portable container, supply reservoir, flowmeter, humidifier, contents gauge, cannula or mask, tubing and refill adaptor

CIM: 60-4

MCM: 4107.9

E0439 Stationary liquid oxygen system, rental; includes container, contents, regulator, flowmeter, humidifier, nebulizer, cannula or mask, & tubing

CIM: 60-4

MCM: 4107.9

E0440 Stationary liquid oxygen system, purchase; includes use of reservoir, contents indicator, regulator, flowmeter, humidifier, nebulizer, cannula or mask, and tubing

CIM: 60-4

MCM: 4107.9

E0441 Stationary oxygen contents, gaseous, 1 month's supply = 1 unit

CIM: 60-4

MCM: 4107.9

E0442 Stationary oxygen contents, liquid, 1 month's supply = 1 unit

CIM: 60-4

MCM: 4107.9

E0443 Portable oxygen contents, gaseous, 1 month's supply = 1 unit

CIM: 60-4

MCM: 4107.9

E0444 Portable oxygen contents, liquid, 1 month's supply = 1 unit

CIM: 60-4

MCM: 4107.9

E0445 Oximeter device for measuring blood oxygen levels non-invasively

E0446 Topical oxygen delivery system, not otherwise specified, includes all supplies and accessories

(**E0450** Code deleted December 31, 2015.)

E0455 Oxygen tent, excluding croup or pediatric tents

CIM: 60-4

MCM: 4107.9

E0457 Chest shell (cuirass)

E0459 Chest wrap

(**E0460** Code deleted December 31, 2015.)

(**E0461** Code deleted December 31, 2015.)

E0462 Rocking bed with or without side rails

(**E0463** Code deleted December 31, 2015.)

(**E0464** Code deleted December 31, 2015.)

E0465 Home ventilator, any type, used with invasive interface, (e.g., tracheostomy tube)

MCM: 60-9

E0466 Home ventilator, any type, used with non-invasive interface, (e.g., mask, chest shell)

MCM: 60-9

E0470 Respiratory assist device, bi-level pressure capability, without backup rate feature, used with noninvasive interface, e.g., nasal or facial mask (intermittent assist device with continuous positive airway pressure device)

CIM: 60-9

E0471 Respiratory assist device, bi-level pressure capability, with back-up rate feature, used with noninvasive interface, e.g., nasal or facial mask (intermittent assist device with continuous positive airway pressure device)

CIM: 60-9

E0472 Respiratory assist device, bi-level pressure capability, with backup rate feature, used with invasive interface, e.g., tracheostomy tube (intermittent assist device with continuous positive airway pressure device)

CIM: 60-9

E0480 Percussor, electric or pneumatic, home model

CIM: 60-9

E0481 Intrapulmonary percussive ventilation system and related accessories

CIM: 60-21

E0482 Cough stimulating device, alternating positive and negative airway pressure

E0483 High frequency chest wall oscillation air-pulse generator system, (includes hoses and vest), each

E0484 Oscillatory positive expiratory pressure device, non-electric, any type, each

E0485 Oral device/appliance used to reduce upper airway collapsibility, adjustable or non-adjustable, prefabricated, includes fitting and adjustment

E0486 Oral device/appliance used to reduce upper airway collapsibility, adjustable or non-adjustable, custom fabricated, includes fitting and adjustment

E0487 Spirometer, electronic, includes all accessories

IPPB Machines

E0500 IPPB machine, all types, with built-in nebulization; manual or automatic valves; internal or external power source

CIM: 60-9

Humidifiers/Nebulizers for Use With Oxygen IPPB Equipment

E0550 Humidifier, durable for extensive supplemental humidification during IPPB treatments or oxygen delivery

CIM: 60-9

E0555 Humidifier, durable, glass or autoclavable plastic bottle type, for use with regulator or flowmeter

CIM: 60-9

MCM: 4107.9

E0560 Humidifier, durable for supplemental humidification during IPPB treatment or oxygen delivery

CIM: 60-9

E0561 Humidifier, non-heated, used with positive airway pressure device

E0562 Humidifier, heated, used with positive airway pressure device

E0565 Compressor, air power source for equipment which is not self-contained or cylinder driven

E0570 Nebulizer, with compressor

CIM: 60-9

MCM: 4107.9

E0572 Aerosol compressor, adjustable pressure, light duty for intermittent use

E0574 Ultrasonic/electronic aerosol generator with small volume nebulizer

E0575 Nebulizer, ultrasonic, large volume

CIM: 60-9

E0580 Nebulizer, durable, glass or autoclavable plastic, bottle type, for use with regulator or flowmeter

CIM: 60-9

MCM: 4107.9

E0585 Nebulizer, with compressor and heater

CIM: 60-9

MCM: 4107.9

Suction Pump/Room Vaporizers

E0600 Respiratory suction pump, home model, portable or stationary, electric

CIM: 60-9

E0601 Continuous positive airway pressure (CPAP) device

CIM: 60-17

E0602 Breast pump, manual, any type

E0603 Breast pump, electric (ac and/or dc), any type

E0604 Breast pump, hospital grade, electric (ac and / or dc), any type

E0605 Vaporizer, room type

CIM: 60-9

E0606 Postural drainage board

CIM: 60-9

Monitoring Equipment

E0607 Home blood glucose monitor

CIM: 60-11

Pacemaker Monitor

E0610 Pacemaker monitor, self-contained, (checks battery depletion, includes audible and visible check systems)

CIM: 60-7, 50-1

E0615 Pacemaker monitor, self contained, checks battery depletion and other pacemaker components, includes digital/visible check systems

CIM: 60-7, 50-1

E0616 Implantable cardiac event recorder with memory, activator and programmer

E0617 External defibrillator with integrated electrocardiogram analysis

E0618 Apnea monitor, without recording feature

E0619 Apnea monitor, with recording feature

E0620 Skin piercing device for collection of capillary blood, laser, each

Patient Lifts

E0621 Sling or seat, patient lift, canvas or nylon

CIM: 60-9

E0625 Patient lift, bathroom or toilet, not otherwise classified

CIM: 60-9

▲ **E0627** Seat lift mechanism, electric, any type

CIM: 60-8

MCM: 4107.8

(**E0628** Code deleted December 31, 2016). Use Q0078.

▲ **E0629** Seat lift mechanism, non-electric, any type

MCM: 4107.8

E0630 Patient lift, hydraulic or mechanical, includes any seat, sling, strap(s) or pad(s)

CIM: 60-9

E0635 Patient lift, electric with seat or sling

CIM: 60-9

E0636 Multipositional patient support system, with integrated lift, patient accessible controls

E0637 Combination sit to stand frame/table system, any size including pediatric, with seat lift feature, with or without wheels

CIM: 60-9

E0638 Standing frame/table system, one position (e.g., upright, supine or prone stander), any size including pediatric, with or without wheels

CIM: 60-9

E0639 Patient lift, moveable from room to room with disassembly and reassembly, includes all components/accessories

E0640 Patient lift, fixed system, includes all components/accessories

E0641 Standing frame/table system, multi-position (e.g., three-way stander), any size including pediatric, with or without wheels

CIM: 60-9

E0642 Standing frame/table system, mobile (dynamic stander), any size including pediatric

CIM: 60-9

Pneumatic Compressor and Appliances (Lymphedema Pump)

E0650 Pneumatic compressor, non-segmental home model

CIM: 60-16

E0651 Pneumatic compressor, segmental home model without calibrated gradient pressure

CIM: 60-16

E0652 Pneumatic compressor, segmental home model with calibrated gradient pressure

CIM: 60-16

E0655 Non-segmental pneumatic appliance for use with pneumatic compressor, half arm

CIM: 60-16

E0656 Segmental pneumatic appliance for use with pneumatic compressor, trunk

E0657 Segmental pneumatic appliance for use with pneumatic compressor, chest

E0660 Non-segmental pneumatic appliance for use with pneumatic compressor, full leg

CIM: 60-16

E0665 Non-segmental pneumatic appliance for use with pneumatic compressor, full arm

CIM: 60-16

E0666 Non-segmental pneumatic appliance for use with pneumatic compressor, half leg

CIM: 60-16

E0667 Segmental pneumatic appliance for use with pneumatic compressor, full leg

CIM: 60-16

E0668 Segmental pneumatic appliance for use with pneumatic compressor, full arm

CIM: 60-16

E0669 Segmental pneumatic appliance for use with pneumatic compressor, half leg

CIM: 60-16

E0670 Segmental pneumatic appliance for use with pneumatic compressor, integrated, 2 full legs and trunk

CIM: 60-16

E0671 Segmental gradient pressure pneumatic appliance, full leg

CIM: 60-16

E0672 Segmental gradient pressure pneumatic appliance, full arm

CIM: 60-16

E0673 Segmental gradient pressure pneumatic appliance, half leg

CIM: 60-16

E0675 Pneumatic compression device, high pressure, rapid inflation/deflation cycle, for arterial insufficiency (unilateral or bilateral system)

E0676 Intermittent limb compression device (includes all accessories), not otherwise specified

Ultraviolet Cabinet

E0691 Ultraviolet light therapy system, includes bulbs/lamps, timer and eye protection; treatment area 2 square feet or less

E0692 Ultraviolet light therapy system panel, includes bulbs/lamps, timer and eye protection, 4 foot panel

E0693 Ultraviolet light therapy system panel, includes bulbs/lamps, timer and eye protection, 6 foot panel

E0694 Ultraviolet multidirectional light therapy system in 6 foot cabinet, includes bulbs/lamps, timer and eye protection

Safety Equipment

E0700 Safety equipment, device or accessory, any type

Restraints

E0705 Transfer device, any type, each

E0710 Restraints, any type (body, chest, wrist or ankle)

Transcutaneous And/Or Neuromuscular Electrical Nerve Stimulators - TENS

E0720 Transcutaneous electrical nerve stimulation (tens) device, two lead, localized stimulation

CIM: 35-20, 35-46

MCM: 4107.6

E0730 Transcutaneous electrical nerve stimulation (tens) device, four or more leads, for multiple nerve stimulation

CIM: 35-20, 35-46

MCM: 4107.6

E0731 Form fitting conductive garment for delivery of tens or NMES (with conductive fibers separated from the patient's skin by layers of fabric)

CIM: 45-25

▲ **E0740** Non-implanted pelvic floor electrical stimulator, complete system

CIM: 60.24

E0744 Neuromuscular stimulator for scoliosis

E0745 Neuromuscular stimulator, electronic shock unit

CIM: 35-77

E0746 Electromyography (EMG), biofeedback device

CIM: 35-27

E0747 Osteogenesis stimulator, electrical, non-invasive, other than spinal applications

CIM: 35-48

E0748 Osteogenesis stimulator, electrical, non-invasive, spinal applications

CIM: 35-48

E0749 Osteogenesis stimulator, electrical, surgically implanted

CIM: 35-48

E0755 Electronic salivary reflex stimulator (intra-oral/non-invasive)

E0760 Osteogenesis stimulator, low intensity ultrasound, non-invasive

MCM: 35-48

E0761 Non-thermal pulsed high frequency radio waves, high peak power electromagnetic energy treatment device

CIM: 35-102

E0762 Transcutaneous electrical joint stimulation device system, includes all accessories

E0764 Functional neuromuscular stimulation, transcutaneous stimulation of sequential muscle groups of ambulation with computer control, used for walking by spinal cord injured, entire system, after completion of training program

CIM: 35-77

E0765 FDA approved nerve stimulator, with replaceable batteries, for treatment of nausea and vomiting

E0766 Electrical stimulation device used for cancer treatment, includes all accessories, any type

E0769 Electrical stimulation or electromagnetic wound treatment device, not otherwise classified

CIM: 35-102

E0770 Functional electrical stimulator, transcutaneous stimulation of nerve and/or muscle groups, any type, complete system, not otherwise specified

Infusion Pumps

E0776 IV pole

E0779 Ambulatory infusion pump, mechanical, reusable, for infusion 8 hours or greater

E0780 Ambulatory infusion pump, mechanical, reusable, for infusion less than 8 hours

E0781 Ambulatory infusion pump, single or multiple channels, electric or battery operated, with administrative equipment, worn by patient

CIM: 60-14

E0782 Infusion pump, implantable, non-programmable (includes all components, e.g., pump, catheter, connectors, etc.)

CIM: 60-14

E0783 Infusion pump system, implantable, programmable (includes all components, e.g., pump, catheter, connectors, etc.)

CIM: 60-14

E0784 External ambulatory infusion pump, insulin

CIM: 60-14

E0785 Implantable intraspinal (epidural/intrathecal) catheter used with implantable infusion pump, replacement

MCM: 60-14

E0786 Implantable programmable infusion pump, replacement (excludes implantable intraspinal catheter)

CIM: 60-14

E0791 Parenteral infusion pump, stationary, single or multi-channel

CIM: 65-10

MCM: 2130, 4450

Traction Equipment

E0830 Ambulatory traction device, all types, each

CIM: 60-9

E0840 Traction frame, attached to headboard, cervical traction

CIM: 60-9

E0849 Traction equipment, cervical, free-standing stand/frame, pneumatic, applying traction force to other than mandible

E0850 Traction stand, free standing, cervical traction

CIM: 60-9

E0855 Cervical traction equipment not requiring additional stand or frame

E0856 Cervical traction device, with inflatable air bladder(s)

E0860 Traction equipment, overdoor, cervical

CIM: 60-9

E0870 Traction frame, attached to footboard, extremity traction, (e.g., buck's)

CIM: 60-9

E0880 Traction stand, free standing, extremity traction, (e.g., buck's)

CIM: 60-9

E0890 Traction frame, attached to footboard, pelvic traction

CIM: 60-9

E0900 Traction stand, free standing, pelvic traction, (e.g., buck's)

CIM: 60-9

Trapeze Equipment, Fracture Frame, and Other Orthopedic Devices

E0910 Trapeze bars, a/k/a patient helper, attached to bed, with grab bar

CIM: 60-9

E0911 Trapeze bar, heavy duty, for patient weight capacity greater than 250 pounds, attached to bed, with grab bar

CIM: 60-9

E0912 Trapeze bar, heavy duty, for patient weight capacity greater than 250 pounds, free standing, complete with grab bar

CIM: 60-9

E0920 Fracture frame, attached to bed, includes weights

CIM: 60-9

E0930 Fracture frame, free standing, includes weights

CIM: 60-9

E0935 Continuous passive motion exercise device for use on knee only

CIM: 60-9

E0936 Continuous passive motion exercise device for use other than knee

E0940 Trapeze bar, free standing, complete with grab bar

CIM: 60-9

E0941 Gravity assisted traction device, any type

CIM: 60-9

E0942 Cervical head harness/halter

E0944 Pelvic belt/harness/boot

E0945 Extremity belt/harness

E0946 Fracture, frame, dual with cross bars, attached to bed, (e.g., Balken, 4 poster)

CIM: 60-9

E0947 Fracture frame, attachments for complex pelvic traction

CIM: 60-9

E0948 Fracture frame, attachments for complex cervical traction

CIM: 60-9

Wheelchair Accessories

E0950 Wheelchair accessory, tray, each

CIM: 60-9

E0951 Heel loop/holder, any type, with or without ankle strap, each

E0952 Toe loop/holder, any type, each

CIM: 60-9

E0955 Wheelchair accessory, headrest, cushioned, any type, including fixed mounting hardware, each

E0956 Wheelchair accessory, lateral trunk or hip support, any type, including fixed mounting hardware, each

E0957 Wheelchair accessory, medial thigh support, any type, including fixed mounting hardware, each

E0958 Manual wheelchair accessory, one-arm drive attachment, each

CIM: 60-9

E0959 Manual wheelchair accessory, adapter for amputee, each

CIM: 60-9

E0960 Wheelchair accessory, shoulder harness/straps or chest strap, including any type mounting hardware

E0961 Manual wheelchair accessory, wheel lock brake extension (handle), each

CIM: 60-9

E0966 Manual wheelchair accessory, headrest extension, each

CIM: 60-9

▲ **E0967** Manual wheelchair accessory, hand rim with projections, any type, replacement only, each

CIM: 60-9

E0968 Commode seat, wheelchair

CIM: 60-9

E0969 Narrowing device, wheelchair

CIM: 60-9

E0970 No. 2 footplates, except for elevating leg rest

CIM: 60-9

E0971 Manual wheelchair accessory, anti-tipping device, each

CIM: 60-9 K0021

E0973 Wheelchair accessory, adjustable height, detachable armrest, complete assembly, each

CIM: 60-9

E0974 Manual wheelchair accessory, anti-rollback device, each

CIM: 60-9

E0978 Wheelchair accessory, positioning belt/safety belt/pelvic strap, each

E0980 Safety vest, wheelchair

E0981 Wheelchair accessory, seat upholstery, replacement only, each

E0982 Wheelchair accessory, back upholstery, replacement only, each

E0983 Manual wheelchair accessory, power add-on to convert manual wheelchair to motorized wheelchair, joystick control

E0984 Manual wheelchair accessory, power add-on to convert manual wheelchair to motorized wheelchair, tiller control

E0985 Wheelchair accessory, seat lift mechanism

E0986 Manual wheelchair accessory, push-rim activated power assist system

E0988 Manual wheelchair accessory, lever-activated, wheel drive, pair

E0990 Wheelchair accessory, elevating leg rest, complete assembly, each

CIM: 60-9

E0992 Manual wheelchair accessory, solid seat insert

E0994 Arm rest, each

CIM: 60-9

▲ **E0995** Wheelchair accessory, calf rest/pad, replacement only, each

CIM: 60-9

E1002 Wheelchair accessory, power seating system, tilt only

E1003 Wheelchair accessory, power seating system, recline only, without shear reduction

E1004 Wheelchair accessory, power seating system, recline only, with mechanical shear reduction

E1005 Wheelchair accessory, power seating system, recline only, with power shear reduction

E1006 Wheelchair accessory, power seating system, combination tilt and recline, without shear reduction

E1007 Wheelchair accessory, power seating system, combination tilt and recline, with mechanical shear reduction

E1008 Wheelchair accessory, power seating system, combination tilt and recline, with power shear reduction

E1009 Wheelchair accessory, addition to power seating system, mechanically linked leg elevation system, including pushrod and leg rest, each

E1010 Wheelchair accessory, addition to power seating system, power leg elevation system, including leg rest, pair

E1011 Modification to pediatric size wheelchair, width adjustment package (not to be dispensed with initial chair)

CIM: 60-9

E1012 Wheelchair accessory, addition to power seating system, center mount power elevating leg rest/platform, complete system, any type, each

E1014 Reclining back, addition to pediatric size wheelchair

CIM: 60-9

E1015 Shock absorber for manual wheelchair, each

MCM: 60.9

E1016 Shock absorber for power wheelchair, each

MCM: 60.9

E1017 Heavy duty shock absorber for heavy duty or extra heavy duty manual wheelchair, each

MCM: 60.9

E1018 Heavy duty shock absorber for heavy duty or extra heavy duty power wheelchair, each

MCM: 60.9

E1020 Residual limb support system for wheelchair, any type

MCM: 60-6

E1028 Wheelchair accessory, manual Swing-Away, retractable or removable mounting hardware for joystick, other control interface or positioning accessory

E1029 Wheelchair accessory, ventilator tray, fixed

E1030 Wheelchair accessory, ventilator tray, gimbaled

Rollabout Chair

E1031 Rollabout chair, any and all types with casters 5" or greater

CIM: 60-9

E1035 Multi-positional patient transfer system, with integrated seat, operated by care giver, patient weight capacity up to and including 300 lbs

MCM: 2100

E1036 Multi-positional patient transfer system, extra-wide, with integrated seat, operated by caregiver, patient weight capacity greater than 300 lbs

E1037 Transport chair, pediatric size

CIM: 60-9

E1038 Transport chair, adult size, patient weight capacity up to and including 300 pounds

CIM: 60-9

E1039 Transport chair, adult size, heavy duty, patient weight capacity greater than 300 pounds

Wheelchairs; Fully-Reclining, Semi-Reclining, Standard, Amputee, and Special Size

E1050 Fully-reclining wheelchair, fixed full length arms, swing away detachable elevating leg rests

CIM: 60-9

E1060 Fully-reclining wheelchair, detachable arms, desk or full length, swing away detachable elevating leg rests

CIM: 60-9

E1070 Fully-reclining wheelchair, detachable arms (desk or full length) swing away detachable footrest

CIM: 60-9

E1083 Hemi-wheelchair, fixed full length arms, swing away detachable elevating leg rest

CIM: 60-9

E1084 Hemi-wheelchair, detachable arms desk or full length arms, swing away detachable elevating leg rests

CIM: 60-9

E1085 Hemi-wheelchair, fixed full length arms, swing away detachable foot rests

CIM: 60-9 K0002

E1086 Hemi-wheelchair detachable arms desk or full length, swing away detachable footrests

CIM: 60-9 K0002

E1087 High strength lightweight wheelchair, fixed full length arms, swing away detachable elevating leg rests

CIM: 60-9

E1088 High strength lightweight wheelchair, detachable arms desk or full length, swing away detachable elevating leg rests

CIM: 60-9

E1089 High strength lightweight wheelchair, fixed length arms, swing away detachable footrest

CIM: 60-9 K0004

E1090 High strength lightweight wheelchair, detachable arms desk or full length, swing away detachable foot rests

CIM: 60-9 K0004

E1092 Wide heavy duty wheel chair, detachable arms (desk or full length), swing away detachable elevating leg rests

CIM: 60-9

E1093 Wide heavy duty wheelchair, detachable arms desk or full length arms, swing away detachable footrests

CIM: 60-9

E1100 Semi-reclining wheelchair, fixed full length arms, swing away detachable elevating leg rests

CIM: 60-9

E1110 Semi-reclining wheelchair, detachable arms (desk or full length) elevating leg rest

CIM: 60-9

E1130 Standard wheelchair, fixed full length arms, fixed or swing away detachable footrests

CIM: 60-9 K0001

E1140 Wheelchair, detachable arms, desk or full length, swing away detachable footrests

CIM: 60-9 K0001

E1150 Wheelchair, detachable arms, desk or full length swing away detachable elevating leg rests

CIM: 60-9

E1160 Wheelchair, fixed full length arms, swing away detachable elevating leg rests

CIM: 60-9

E1161 Manual adult size wheelchair, includes tilt in space

E1170 Amputee wheelchair, fixed full length arms, swing away detachable elevating leg rests

CIM: 60-9

E1171 Amputee wheelchair, fixed full length arms, without footrests or leg rest

CIM: 60-9

E1172 Amputee wheelchair, detachable arms (desk or full length) without footrests or leg rest

CIM: 60-9

E1180 Amputee wheelchair, detachable arms (desk or full length) swing away detachable footrests

CIM: 60-9

E1190 Amputee wheelchair, detachable arms (desk or full length) swing away detachable elevating leg rests

CIM: 60-9

E1195 Heavy duty wheelchair, fixed full length arms, swing away detachable elevating leg rests

CIM: 60-9

E1200 Amputee wheelchair, fixed full length arms, swing away detachable footrest

CIM: 60-9

E1220 Wheelchair; specially sized or constructed, (indicate brand name, model number, if any) and justification

CIM: 60-6

E1221 Wheelchair with fixed arm, footrests

CIM: 60-6

E1222 Wheelchair with fixed arm, elevating leg rests

CIM: 60-6

E1223 Wheelchair with detachable arms, footrests

CIM: 60-6

E1224 Wheelchair with detachable arms, elevating leg rests

CIM: 60-6

E1225 Wheelchair accessory, manual semi-reclining back, (recline greater than 15 degrees, but less than 80 degrees), each

CIM: 60-6

E1226 Wheelchair accessory, manual fully reclining back, (recline greater than 80 degrees), each

CIM: 60-9

E1227 Special height arms for wheelchair

CIM: 60-6

E1228 Special back height for wheelchair

CIM: 60-6

E1229 Wheelchair, pediatric size, not otherwise specified

Power Operated Vehicle

E1230 Power operated vehicle (three or four wheel non highway) specify brand name and model number

CIM: 60-5

MCM: 4107.6

Wheelchairs; Lightweight and Heavy Duty

E1231 Wheelchair, pediatric size, tilt-in-space, rigid, adjustable, with seating system

CIM: 60-9

E1232 Wheelchair, pediatric size, tilt-in-space, folding, adjustable, with seating system

CIM: 60-9

E1233 Wheelchair, pediatric size, tilt-in-space, rigid, adjustable, without seating system

CIM: 60-9

E1234 Wheelchair, pediatric size, tilt-in-space, folding, adjustable, without seating system

CIM: 60-9

E1235 Wheelchair, pediatric size, rigid, adjustable, with seating system

CIM: 60-9

E1236 Wheelchair, pediatric size, folding, adjustable, with seating system

CIM: 60-9

E1237 Wheelchair, pediatric size, rigid, adjustable, without seating system

CIM: 60-9

E1238 Wheelchair, pediatric size, folding, adjustable, without seating system

CIM: 60-9

E1239 Power wheelchair, pediatric size, not otherwise specified

E1240 Lightweight wheelchair, detachable arms, (desk or full length) swing away detachable, elevating leg rest

CIM: 60-9

E1250 Lightweight wheelchair, fixed full length arms, swing away detachable footrest

CIM: 60-9 K0003

E1260 Lightweight wheelchair, detachable arms (desk or full length) swing away detachable footrest

CIM: 60-9 K0003

E1270 Lightweight wheelchair, fixed full length arms, swing away detachable elevating leg rests

CIM: 60-9

E1280 Heavy duty wheelchair, detachable arms (desk or full length) elevating leg rests

CIM: 60-9

E1285 Heavy duty wheelchair, fixed full length arms, swing away detachable footrest

CIM: 60-9 K0006

E1290 Heavy duty wheelchair, detachable arms (desk or full length) swing away detachable footrest

CIM: 60-9 K0006

E1295 Heavy duty wheelchair, fixed full length arms, elevating leg rest

CIM: 60-9

E1296 Special wheelchair seat height from floor

CIM: 60-6

E1297 Special wheelchair seat depth, by upholstery

CIM: 60-6

E1298 Special wheelchair seat depth and/or width, by construction

CIM: 60-6

Whirlpool Equipment

E1300 Whirlpool, portable (over tub type)

CIM: 60-9

E1310 Whirlpool, non-portable (built-in type)

CIM: 60-9

Additional Oxygen Related Supplies and Equipment

E1352 Oxygen accessory, flow regulator capable of positive inspiratory pressure

E1353 Regulator

CIM: 60-4

MCM: 4107.9

E1354 Oxygen accessory, wheeled cart for portable cylinder or portable concentrator, any type, replacement only, each

E1355 Stand/rack

CIM: 60-4

E1356 Oxygen accessory, battery pack/cartridge for portable concentrator, any type, replacement only, each

E1357 Oxygen accessory, battery charger for portable concentrator, any type, replacement only, each

E1358 Oxygen accessory, dc power adapter for portable concentrator, any type, replacement only, each

E1372 Immersion external heater for nebulizer

CIM: 60-4

E1390 Oxygen concentrator, single delivery port, capable of delivering 85 percent or greater oxygen concentration at the prescribed flow rate

CIM: 60-4

E1391 Oxygen concentrator, dual delivery port, capable of delivering 85 percent or greater oxygen concentration at the prescribed flow rate, each

CIM: 60-4

E1392 Portable oxygen concentrator, rental

CIM: 60-4

E1399 Durable medical equipment, miscellaneous

E1405 Oxygen and water vapor enriching system with heated delivery

CIM: 60-4

MCM: 4107

E1406 Oxygen and water vapor enriching system without heated delivery

CIM: 60-4

MCM: 4107

Artificial Kidney Machines and Accessories

E1500 Centrifuge, for dialysis

E1510 Kidney, dialysate delivery syst kidney machine, pump recirculating, air removal syst, flowrate meter, power off, heater and temperature control with alarm, i.v. poles, pressure gauge, concentrate container

E1520 Heparin infusion pump for hemodialysis

E1530 Air bubble detector for hemodialysis, each, replacement

E1540 Pressure alarm for hemodialysis, each, replacement

E1550 Bath conductivity meter for hemodialysis, each

E1560 Blood leak detector for hemodialysis, each, replacement

E1570 Adjustable chair, for ESRD patients

E1575 Transducer protectors/fluid barriers, for hemodialysis, any size, per 10

E1580 Unipuncture control system for hemodialysis

E1590 Hemodialysis machine

E1592 Automatic intermittent peritoneal dialysis system

E1594 Cycler dialysis machine for peritoneal dialysis

E1600 Delivery and/or installation charges for hemodialysis equipment

E1610 Reverse osmosis water purification system, for hemodialysis

CIM: 55-1A

E1615 Deionizer water purification system, for hemodialysis

CIM: 55-1A

E1620 Blood pump for hemodialysis, replacement

E1625 Water softening system, for hemodialysis

CIM: 55-1B

E1630 Reciprocating peritoneal dialysis system

E1632 Wearable artificial kidney, each

E1634 Peritoneal dialysis clamps, each

MCM: 4270

E1635 Compact (portable) travel hemodialyzer system

E1636 Sorbent cartridges, for hemodialysis, per 10

E1637 Hemostats, each

E1639 Scale, each

E1699 Dialysis equipment, not otherwise specified

Extension/Flexion Devices

E1700 Jaw motion rehabilitation system

E1701 Replacement cushions for jaw motion rehabilitation system, pkg. of 6

E1702 Replacement measuring scales for jaw motion rehabilitation system, pkg. of 200

E1800 Dynamic adjustable elbow extension/flexion device, includes soft interface material

E1801 Static progressive stretch elbow device, extension and/or flexion, with or without range of motion adjustment, includes all components and accessories

E1802 Dynamic adjustable forearm pronation/supination device, includes soft interface material

E1805 Dynamic adjustable wrist extension / flexion device, includes soft interface material

E1806 Static progressive stretch wrist device, flexion and/or extension, with or without range of motion adjustment, includes all components and accessories

E1810 Dynamic adjustable knee extension / flexion device, includes soft interface material

E1811 Static progressive stretch knee device, extension and/or flexion, with or without range of motion adjustment, includes all components and accessories

E1812 Dynamic knee, extension/flexion device with active resistance control

E1815 Dynamic adjustable ankle extension/flexion device, includes soft interface material

E1816 Static progressive stretch ankle device, flexion and/or extension, with or without range of motion adjustment, includes all components and accessories

E1818 Static progressive stretch forearm pronation / supination device, with or without range of motion adjustment, includes all components and accessories

E1820 Replacement soft interface material, dynamic adjustable extension/flexion device

E1821 Replacement soft interface material/cuffs for bi-directional static progressive stretch device

E1825 Dynamic adjustable finger extension/flexion device, includes soft interface material

E1830 Dynamic adjustable toe extension/flexion device, includes soft interface material

E1831 Static progressive stretch toe device, extension and/or flexion, with or without range of motion adjustment, includes all components and accessories

E1840 Dynamic adjustable shoulder flexion / abduction / rotation device, includes soft interface material

E1841 Static progressive stretch shoulder device, with or without range of motion adjustment, includes all components and accessories

E1902 Communication board, non-electronic augmentative or alternative communication device

E2000 Gastric suction pump, home model, portable or stationary, electric

E2100 Blood glucose monitor with integrated voice synthesizer

CIM: 60-11

E2101 Blood glucose monitor with integrated lancing/blood sample

CIM: 60-11

E2120 Pulse generator system for tympanic treatment of inner ear endolymphatic fluid

Manual Wheelchair Accessories

E2201 Manual wheelchair accessory, nonstandard seat frame, width greater than or equal to 20

Not payable by Medicare | Non-covered by Medicare | Special coverage instructions | Carrier judgement inches and less than 24 inches

E2202 Manual wheelchair accessory, nonstandard seat frame width, 24-27 inches

E2203 Manual wheelchair accessory, nonstandard seat frame depth, 20 to less than 22 inches

E2204 Manual wheelchair accessory, nonstandard seat frame depth, 22 to 25 inches

E2205 Manual wheelchair accessory, hand rim without projections (includes ergonomic or contoured), any type, replacement only, each

▲ **E2206** Manual wheelchair accessory, wheel lock assembly, complete, replacement only, each

E2207 Wheelchair accessory, crutch and cane holder, each

E2208 Wheelchair accessory, cylinder tank carrier, each

E2209 Accessory, arm trough, with or without hand support, each

E2210 Wheelchair accessory, bearings, any type, replacement only, each

E2211 Manual wheelchair accessory, pneumatic propulsion tire, any size, each

E2212 Manual wheelchair accessory, tube for pneumatic propulsion tire, any size, each

E2213 Manual wheelchair accessory, insert for pneumatic propulsion tire (removable), any type, any size, each

E2214 Manual wheelchair accessory, pneumatic caster tire, any size, each

E2215 Manual wheelchair accessory, tube for pneumatic caster tire, any size, each

E2216 Manual wheelchair accessory, foam filled propulsion tire, any size, each

E2217 Manual wheelchair accessory, foam filled caster tire, any size, each

E2218 Manual wheelchair accessory, foam propulsion tire, any size, each

E2219 Manual wheelchair accessory, foam caster tire, any size, each

▲ **E2220** Manual wheelchair accessory, solid (rubber/plastic) propulsion tire, any size, replacement only, each

▲ **E2221** Manual wheelchair accessory, solid (rubber/plastic) caster tire (removable), any size, replacement only, each

▲ **E2222** Manual wheelchair accessory, solid (rubber/plastic) caster tire with integrated wheel, any size, replacement only, each

▲ **E2224** Manual wheelchair accessory, propulsion wheel excludes tire, any size, replacement only, each

E2225 Manual wheelchair accessory, caster wheel excludes tire, any size, replacement only, each

E2226 Manual wheelchair accessory, caster fork, any size, replacement only, each

E2227 Manual wheelchair accessory, gear reduction drive wheel, each

E2228 Manual wheelchair accessory, wheel braking system and lock, complete, each

E2230 Manual wheelchair accessory, manual standing system

E2231 Manual wheelchair accessory, solid seat support base (replaces sling seat), includes any type mounting hardware

E2291 Back, planar, for pediatric size wheelchair including fixed attaching hardware

E2292 Seat, planar, for pediatric size wheelchair including fixed attaching hardware

E2293 Back, contoured, for pediatric size wheelchair including fixed attaching hardware

E2294 Seat, contoured, for pediatric size wheelchair including fixed attaching hardware

E2295 Manual wheelchair accessory, for pediatric size wheelchair, dynamic seating frame, allows coordinated movement of multiple positioning features

E2300 Wheelchair accessory, power seat elevation system, any type

E2301 Wheelchair accessory, power standing system, any type

Power Wheelchair Accessories

E2310 Power wheelchair accessory, electronic connection between wheelchair controller and one power seating system motor, including all related electronics, indicator feature, mechanical function selection switch, and fixed mounting hardware

E2311 Power wheelchair accessory, electronic connection between wheelchair controller and two or more power seating system motors, including all related electronics, indicator feature, mechanical function selection switch, and fixed mounting hardware

E2312 Power wheelchair accessory, hand or chin control interface, mini-proportional remote joystick, proportional, including fixed mounting hardware

E2313 Power wheelchair accessory, harness for upgrade to expandable controller, including all fasteners, connectors and mounting hardware, each

E2321 Power wheelchair accessory, hand control interface, remote joystick, nonproportional, including all related electronics, mechanical stop switch, and fixed mounting hardware

E2322 Power wheelchair accessory, hand control interface, multiple mechanical switches, nonproportional, including all related electronics, mechanical stop switch, and fixed mounting hardware

E2323 Power wheelchair accessory, specialty joystick handle for hand control interface, prefabricated

E2324 Power wheelchair accessory, chin cup for chin control interface

E2325 Power wheelchair accessory, sip and puff interface, nonproportional, including all related electronics, mechanical stop switch, and manual Swing-Away mounting hardware

E2326 Power wheelchair accessory, breath tube kit for sip and puff interface

E2327 Power wheelchair accessory, head control interface, mechanical, proportional, including all related electronics, mechanical direction change switch, and fixed mounting hardware

E2328 Power wheelchair accessory, head control or extremity control interface, electronic, proportional, including all related electronics and fixed mounting hardware

E2329 Power wheelchair accessory, head control interface, contact switch mechanism, nonproportional, including all related electronics, mechanical stop switch, mechanical direction change switch, head array, and fixed mounting hardware

E2330 Power wheelchair accessory, head control interface, proximity switch mechanism, nonproportional, including all related electronics, mechanical stop switch, mechanical direction change switch, head array, and fixed mounting hardware

E2331 Power wheelchair accessory, attendant control, proportional, including all related electronics and fixed mounting hardware

E2340 Power wheelchair accessory, nonstandard seat frame width, 20-23 inches

E2341 Power wheelchair accessory, nonstandard seat frame width, 24-27 inches

E2342 Power wheelchair accessory, nonstandard seat frame depth, 20 or 21 inches

E2343 Power wheelchair accessory, nonstandard seat frame depth, 22-25 inches

E2351 Power wheelchair accessory, electronic interface to operate speech generating device using power wheelchair control interface

E2358 Power wheelchair accessory, group 34 non-sealed lead acid battery, each

E2359 Power wheelchair accessory, group 34 sealed lead acid battery, each (e.g., gel cell, absorbed glassmat)

E2360 Power wheelchair accessory, 22nf non-sealed lead acid battery, each

E2361 Power wheelchair accessory, 22nf sealed lead acid battery, each, (e.g., gel cell, absorbed glassmat)

E2362 Power wheelchair accessory, group 24 non-sealed lead acid battery, each

E2363 Power wheelchair accessory, group 24 sealed lead acid battery, each (e.g., gel cell, absorbed glassmat)

E2364 Power wheelchair accessory, u-1 non-sealed lead acid battery, each

E2365 Power wheelchair accessory, u-1 sealed lead acid battery, each (e.g., gel cell, absorbed glassmat)

E2366 Power wheelchair accessory, battery charger, single mode, for use with only one battery type, sealed or non-sealed, each

E2367 Power wheelchair accessory, battery charger, dual mode, for use with either battery type, sealed or non-sealed, each

E2368 Power wheelchair component, drive wheel motor, replacement only

E2369 Power wheelchair component, drive wheel gear box, replacement only

E2370 Power wheelchair component, integrated drive wheel motor and gear box combination, replacement only

E2371 Power wheelchair accessory, group 27 sealed lead acid battery, (e.g., gel cell, absorbed glassmat), each

E2372 Power wheelchair accessory, group 27 non-sealed lead acid battery, each

E2373 Power wheelchair accessory, hand or chin control interface, compact remote joystick, proportional, including fixed mounting hardware

E2374 Power wheelchair accessory, hand or chin control interface, standard remote joystick (not including controller), proportional, including all related electronics and fixed mounting hardware, replacement only

E2375 Power wheelchair accessory, non-expandable controller, including all related electronics and mounting hardware, replacement only

E2376 Power wheelchair accessory, expandable controller, including all related electronics and mounting hardware, replacement only

E2377 Power wheelchair accessory, expandable controller, including all related electronics and mounting hardware, upgrade provided at initial issue

E2378 Power wheelchair component, actuator, replacement only

E2381 Power wheelchair accessory, pneumatic drive wheel tire, any size, replacement only, each

E2382 Power wheelchair accessory, tube for pneumatic drive wheel tire, any size, replacement only, each

E2383 Power wheelchair accessory, insert for pneumatic drive wheel tire (removable), any type, any size, replacement only, each

E2384 Power wheelchair accessory, pneumatic caster tire, any size, replacement only, each

E2385 Power wheelchair accessory, tube for pneumatic caster tire, any size, replacement only, each

E2386 Power wheelchair accessory, foam filled drive wheel tire, any size, replacement only, each

E2387 Power wheelchair accessory, foam filled caster tire, any size, replacement only, each

E2388 Power wheelchair accessory, foam drive wheel tire, any size, replacement only, each

E2389 Power wheelchair accessory, foam caster tire, any size, replacement only, each

E2390 Power wheelchair accessory, solid (rubber/plastic) drive wheel tire, any size, replacement only, each

E2391 Power wheelchair accessory, solid (rubber/plastic) caster tire (removable), any size, replacement only, each

E2392 Power wheelchair accessory, solid (rubber/plastic) caster tire with integrated wheel, any size, replacement only, each

E2394 Power wheelchair accessory, drive wheel excludes tire, any size, replacement only, each

E2395 Power wheelchair accessory, caster wheel excludes tire, any size, replacement only, each

E2396 Power wheelchair accessory, caster fork, any size, replacement only, each

E2397 Power wheelchair accessory, lithium-based battery, each

E2402 Negative pressure wound therapy electrical pump, stationary or portable

Speech Generating Device and Accessories

E2500 Speech generating device, digitized speech, using pre-recorded messages, less than or equal to 8 minutes recording time

CIM: 60-23

E2502 Speech generating device, digitized speech, using pre-recorded messages, greater than 8 minutes but less than or equal to 20 minutes recording time

CIM: 60-23

E2504 Speech generating device, digitized speech, using pre-recorded messages, greater than 20 minutes but less than or equal to 40 minutes recording time

CIM: 60-23

E2506 Speech generating device, digitized speech, using pre-recorded messages, greater than 40 minutes recording time

CIM: 60-23

E2508 Speech generating device, synthesized speech, requiring message formulation by spelling and access by physical contact with the device

CIM: 60-23

E2510 Speech generating device, synthesized speech, permitting multiple methods of message formulation and multiple methods of device access

CIM: 60-23

E2511 Speech generating software program, for personal computer or personal digital assistant

CIM: 60-23

E2512 Accessory for speech generating device, mounting system

CIM: 60-23

E2599 Accessory for speech generating device, not otherwise classified

CIM: 60-23

Wheelchair Cushions and Support Devices

E2601 General use wheelchair seat cushion, width less than 22 inches, any depth

E2602 General use wheelchair seat cushion, width 22 inches or greater, any depth

E2603 Skin protection wheelchair seat cushion, width less than 22 inches, any depth

E2604 Skin protection wheelchair seat cushion, width 22 inches or greater, any depth

E2605 Positioning wheelchair seat cushion, width less than 22 inches, any depth

E2606 Positioning wheelchair seat cushion, width 22 inches or greater, any depth

E2607 Skin protection and positioning wheelchair seat cushion, width less than 22 inches, any depth

E2608 Skin protection and positioning wheelchair seat cushion, width 22 inches or greater, any depth

E2609 Custom fabricated wheelchair seat cushion, any size

E2610 Wheelchair seat cushion, powered

E2611 General use wheelchair back cushion, width less than 22 inches, any height, including any type mounting hardware

E2612 General use wheelchair back cushion, width 22 inches or greater, any height, including any type mounting hardware

E2613 Positioning wheelchair back cushion, posterior, width less than 22 inches, any height, including any type mounting hardware

E2614 Positioning wheelchair back cushion, posterior, width 22 inches or greater, any height, including any type mounting hardware

E2615 Positioning wheelchair back cushion, posterior-lateral, width less than 22 inches, any height, including any type mounting hardware

E2616 Positioning wheelchair back cushion, posterior-lateral, width 22 inches or greater, any height, including any type mounting hardware

E2617 Custom fabricated wheelchair back cushion, any size, including any type mounting hardware

E2619 Replacement cover for wheelchair seat cushion or back cushion, each

E2620 Positioning wheelchair back cushion, planar back with lateral supports, width less than 22 inches, any height, including any type mounting hardware

E2621 Positioning wheelchair back cushion, planar back with lateral supports, width 22 inches or greater, any height, including any type mounting hardware

E2622 Skin protection wheelchair seat cushion, adjustable, width less than 22 inches, any depth

E2623 Skin protection wheelchair seat cushion, adjustable, width 22 inches or greater, any depth

E2624 Skin protection and positioning wheelchair seat cushion, adjustable, width less than 22 inches, any depth

E2625 Skin protection and positioning wheelchair seat cushion, adjustable, width 22 inches or greater, any depth

E2626 Wheelchair accessory, shoulder elbow, mobile arm support attached to wheelchair, balanced, adjustable

E2627 Wheelchair accessory, shoulder elbow, mobile arm support attached to wheelchair, balanced, adjustable rancho type

E2628 Wheelchair accessory, shoulder elbow, mobile arm support attached to wheelchair, balanced, reclining

E2629 Wheelchair accessory, shoulder elbow, mobile arm support attached to wheelchair, balanced, friction arm support (friction dampening to proximal and distal joints)

E2630 Wheelchair accessory, shoulder elbow, mobile arm support, monosuspension arm and hand support, overhead elbow forearm hand sling support, yoke type suspension support

E2631 Wheelchair accessory, addition to mobile arm support, elevating proximal arm

E2632 Wheelchair accessory, addition to mobile arm support, offset or lateral rocker arm with elastic balance control

E2633 Wheelchair accessory, addition to mobile arm support, supinator

Gait Trainer

E8000 Gait trainer, pediatric size, posterior support, includes all accessories and components

E8001 Gait trainer, pediatric size, upright support, includes all accessories and components

E8002 Gait trainer, pediatric size, anterior support, includes all accessories and components

PROCEDURES AND PROFESSIONAL SERVICES

Guidelines

In addition to the information presented in the INTRODUCTION, several other items unique to this section are defined or identified here:

1. TEMPORARY CODES: The codes listed in this section are assigned by CMS on a temporary basis to identify procedures/services.

Procedures/Professional Services

G0008 Administration of influenza virus vaccine

G0009 Administration of pneumococcal vaccine

G0010 Administration of hepatitis b vaccine

G0027 Semen analysis; presence and/or motility of sperm excluding Huhner

Ⓟ **G0101** Cervical or vaginal cancer screening; pelvic and clinical breast examination

G0102 Prostate cancer screening; digital rectal examination

CIM: 50-55

MCM: 4182

G0103 Prostate cancer screening; prostate specific antigen test (PSA)

CIM: 50-55

MCM: 4182

G0104 Colorectal cancer screening; flexible sigmoidoscopy

Ⓟ **G0105** Colorectal cancer screening; colonoscopy on individual at high risk

Ⓟ **G0106** Colorectal cancer screening; alternative to g0104, screening sigmoidoscopy, barium enema

Ⓟ **G0108** Diabetes outpatient self-management training services, individual, per 30 minutes

G0109 Diabetes outpatient self-management training services, group session (2 or more), per 30 minutes

G0117 Glaucoma screening for high risk patients furnished by an optometrist or ophthalmologist

G0118 Glaucoma screening for high risk patient furnished under the direct supervision of an optometrist or ophthalmologist

Ⓟ **G0120** Colorectal cancer screening; alternative to g0105, screening colonoscopy, barium enema.

Ⓟ **G0121** Colorectal cancer screening; colonoscopy on individual not meeting criteria for high risk

Ⓟ **G0122** Colorectal cancer screening; barium enema

G0123 Screening cytopathology, cervical or vaginal (any reporting system), collected in preservative fluid, automated thin layer preparation, screening by cytotechnologist under physician supervision

CIM: 50-20

G0124 Screening cytopathology, cervical or vaginal (any reporting system), collected in preservative fluid, automated thin layer preparation, requiring interpretation by physician

CIM: 50-20

G0127 Trimming of dystrophic nails, any number

MCM: 2323

G0128 Direct (face-to-face with patient) skilled nursing services of a registered nurse provided in a comprehensive outpatient rehabilitation facility, each 10 minutes beyond the first 5 minutes

Statute: 1833(a)

G0129 Occupational therapy services requiring the skills of a qualified occupational therapist, furnished as a component of a partial hospitalization treatment program, per session (45 minutes or more)

G0130 Single energy x-ray absorptiometry (sexa) bone density study, one or more sites; appendicular skeleton (peripheral) (e.g., radius, wrist, heel)

CIM: 50-44

G0141 Screening cytopathology smears, cervical or vaginal, performed by automated system, with manual rescreening, requiring interpretation by physician

G0143 Screening cytopathology, cervical or vaginal (any reporting system), collected in preservative fluid, automated thin layer preparation, with manual screening and rescreening by cytotechnologist under physician supervision

G0144 Screening cytopathology, cervical or vaginal (any reporting system), collected in preservative fluid, automated thin layer preparation, with screening by automated system, under physician supervision

G0145 Screening cytopathology, cervical or vaginal (any reporting system), collected in preservative fluid, automated thin layer preparation, with screening by automated system and manual rescreening under physician supervision

G0147 Screening cytopathology smears, cervical or vaginal, performed by automated system under physician supervision

G0148 Screening cytopathology smears, cervical or vaginal, performed by automated system with manual rescreening

G0151 Services performed by a qualified physical therapist in the home health or hospice setting, each 15 minutes

G0152 Services performed by a qualified occupational therapist in the home health or hospice setting, each 15 minutes

G0153 Services performed by a qualified speech-language pathologist in the home health or hospice setting, each 15 minutes

(**G0154** Code deleted February 29, 2016).

Ⓟ **G0155** Services of clinical social worker in home health or hospice settings, each 15 minutes

G0156 Services of home health/hospice aide in home health or hospice settings, each 15 minutes

G0157 Services performed by a qualified physical therapist assistant in the home health or hospice setting, each 15 minutes

G0158 Services performed by a qualified occupational therapist assistant in the home health or hospice setting, each 15 minutes

G0159 Services performed by a qualified physical therapist, in the home health setting, in the establishment or delivery of a safe and effective physical therapy maintenance program, each 15 minutes

G0160 Services performed by a qualified occupational therapist, in the home health setting, in the establishment or delivery of a safe and effective occupational therapy maintenance program, each 15 minutes

G0161 Services performed by a qualified speech-language pathologist, in the home health setting, in the establishment or delivery of a safe and effective speech-language pathology maintenance program, each 15 minutes

G0162 Skilled services by a registered nurse (RN) for management and evaluation of the plan of care; each 15 minutes (the patient's underlying condition or complication requires an RN to ensure that essential non-skilled care achieves its purpose in the home health or hospice setting)

(**G0163** Code deleted December 31, 2016).

(**G0164** Code deleted December 31, 2016).

G0166 External counterpulsation, per treatment session

CIM: 35-74

G0168 Wound closure utilizing tissue adhesive(s) only

G0175 Scheduled interdisciplinary team conference (minimum of three exclusive of patient care nursing staff) with patient present

Ⓟ **G0176** Activity therapy, such as music, dance, art or play therapies not for recreation, related to the care and treatment of patient's disabling mental health problems, per session (45 minutes or more)

Ⓟ **G0177** Training and educational services related to the care and treatment of patient's disabling mental health problems per session (45 minutes or more)

G0179 Physician re-certification for medicare-covered home health services under a home health plan of care (patient not present), including contacts with home health agency and review of reports of patient status required by physicians to affirm the initial implementation of the plan of care that meets patient's needs, per re-certification period

G0180 Physician certification for medicare-covered home health services under a home health plan of care (patient not present), including contacts with home health agency and review of reports of patient status required by physicians to affirm the initial implementation of the plan of care that meets patient's needs, per certification period

G0181 Physician supervision of a patient receiving medicare-covered services provided by a participating home health agency (patient not present) requiring complex and multidisciplinary care modalities involving regular physician development and/or revision of care plans, review of subsequent reports of patient status, review of laboratory and other studies, communication (including telephone calls) with other health care professionals involved in the patient's care, integration of new information into the medical treatment plan and/or adjustment of medical therapy, within a calendar month, 30 minutes or more

G0182 Physician supervision of a patient under a medicare-approved hospice (patient not present) requiring complex and multidisciplinary care modalities involving regular physician development and/or revision of care plans, review of subsequent reports of patient status, review of laboratory and other studies, communication (including telephone calls) with other health care professionals involved in the patient's care, integration of new information into the medical treatment plan and/or adjustment of medical therapy, within a calendar month, 30 minutes or more

G0186 Destruction of localized lesion of choroid (for example, choroidal neovascularization); photocoagulation, feeder vessel technique (one or more sessions)

▲Ⓟ **G0202** Screening mammography, bilateral (2-view study of each breast), including computer-aided detection (cad) when performed

▲ **G0204** Diagnostic mammography, including computer-aided detection (cad) when performed; bilateral

▲ **G0206** Diagnostic mammography, including computer-aided detection (cad) when performed; unilateral

G0219 Pet imaging whole body; melanoma for non-covered indications

CIM: 50-36

MCM: 4173

G0235 Pet imaging, any site, not otherwise specified

CIM: 50-36

G0237 Therapeutic procedures to increase strength or endurance of respiratory muscles, face to face, one on one, each 15 minutes (includes monitoring)

G0238 Therapeutic procedures to improve respiratory function, other than described by g0237, one on one, face to face, per 15 minutes (includes monitoring)

G0239 Therapeutic procedures to improve respiratory function or increase strength or endurance of respiratory muscles, two or more individuals (includes monitoring)

G0245 Initial physician evaluation and management of a diabetic patient with diabetic sensory neuropathy resulting in a loss of protective sensation (lops) which must include: (1) the diagnosis of lops, (2) a patient history, (3) a physical examination that consists of at least the following elements: (a) visual inspection of the forefoot, hindfoot and toe web spaces, (b) evaluation of a protective sensation, (c) evaluation of foot structure and biomechanics, (d) evaluation of vascular status and skin integrity, and (e) evaluation and recommendation of footwear and (4) patient education

CIM: 50.81

G0246 Follow-up physician evaluation and management of a diabetic patient with diabetic sensory neuropathy resulting in a loss of protective sensation (lops) to include at least the following: (1) a patient history, (2) a physical examination that includes: (a) visual inspection of the forefoot, hindfoot and toe web spaces, (b) evaluation of protective sensation, (c) evaluation of foot structure and biomechanics, (d) evaluation of vascular status and skin integrity, and (e) evaluation and recommendation of footwear, and (3) patient education

CIM: 50.81

G0247 Routine foot care by a physician of a diabetic patient with diabetic sensory neuropathy resulting in a loss of protective sensation (lops) to include, the local care of superficial wounds (i.e. superficial to muscle and fascia) and at least the following if present: (1) local care of superficial wounds, (2) debridement of corns and calluses, and (3) trimming and debridement of nails

CIM: 50.81

G0248 Demonstration, prior to initiation of home INR monitoring, for patient with either mechanical heart valve(s), chronic atrial fibrillation, or venous thromboembolism who meets Medicare coverage criteria, under the direction of a physician; includes: face-to-face demonstration of use and care of the INR monitor, obtaining at least one blood sample, provision of instructions for reporting home INR test results, and documentation of patient's ability to perform testing and report results

CIM: 50.55

G0249 Provision of test materials and equipment for home INR monitoring of patient with either mechanical heart valve(s), chronic atrial fibrillation, or venous thromboembolism who meets Medicare coverage criteria; includes: provision of materials for use in the home and reporting of test results to physician; testing not occurring more frequently than once a week; testing materials, billing units of service include 4 tests

CIM: 50.55

G0250 Physician review, interpretation, and patient management of home INR testing for patient with either mechanical heart valve(s), chronic atrial fibrillation, or venous thromboembolism who meets Medicare coverage criteria; testing not occurring more frequently than once a week; billing units of service include 4 tests

CIM: 50.55

G0252 Pet imaging, full and partial-ring pet scanners only, for initial diagnosis of breast cancer and/or surgical planning for breast cancer (e.g., initial staging of axillary lymph nodes)

CIM: 50-36

G0255 Current perception threshold/sensory nerve conduction test, (sNCT) per limb, any nerve

CIM: 50-57

G0257 Unscheduled or emergency dialysis treatment for an ESRD patient in a hospital outpatient department that is not certified as an ESRD facility

G0259 Injection procedure for sacroiliac joint; arthrography

G0260 Injection procedure for sacroiliac joint; provision of anesthetic, steroid and/or other therapeutic agent, with or without arthrography

G0268 Removal of impacted cerumen (one or both ears) by physician on same date of service as audiologic function testing

G0269 Placement of occlusive device into either a venous or arterial access site, post surgical or interventional procedure (e.g., Angio-Seal plug, vascular plug)

Ⓟ **G0270** Medical nutrition therapy; reassessment and subsequent intervention(s) following second referral in same year for change in diagnosis, medical condition or treatment regimen (including additional hours needed for renal disease), individual, face to face with the patient, each 15 minutes

Ⓟ **G0271** Medical nutrition therapy, reassessment and subsequent intervention(s) following second referral in same year for change in diagnosis, medical condition, or treatment regimen (including additional hours needed for renal disease), group (2 or more individuals), each 30 minutes

G0276 Blinded procedure for lumbar stenosis, percutaneous image-guided lumbar decompression (pild) or placebo-control, performed in an approved coverage with evidence development (CED) clinical trial

G0277 Hyperbaric oxygen under pressure, full body chamber, per 30 minute interval

CIM: 35-10

Ⓟ **G0278** Iliac and/or femoral artery angiography, non-selective, bilateral or ipsilateral to catheter insertion, performed at the same time as cardiac catheterization and/or coronary angiography, includes positioning or placement of the catheter in the distal aorta or ipsilateral femoral or iliac artery, injection of dye, production of permanent images, and radiologic supervision and interpretation (list separately in addition to primary procedure)

G0279 Diagnostic digital breast tomosynthesis, unilateral or bilateral (list separately in addition to G0204 or G0206)

G0281 Electrical stimulation, (unattended), to one or more areas, for chronic stage iii and stage iv pressure ulcers, arterial ulcers, diabetic ulcers, and venous stasis ulcers not demonstrating measurable signs of healing after 30 days of conventional care, as part of a therapy plan of care

G0282 Electrical stimulation, (unattended), to one or more areas, for wound care other than described in g0281

MCM: 35-98

G0283 Electrical stimulation (unattended), to one or more areas for indication(s) other than wound care, as part of a therapy plan of care

G0288 Reconstruction, computed tomographic angiography of aorta for surgical planning for vascular surgery

G0289 Arthroscopy, knee, surgical, for removal of loose body, foreign body, debridement/shaving of articular cartilage (chondroplasty) at the time of other surgical knee arthroscopy in a different compartment of the same knee

G0293 Noncovered surgical procedure(s) using conscious sedation, regional, general or spinal anesthesia in a Medicare qualifying clinical trial, per day

G0294 Noncovered procedure(s) using either no anesthesia or local anesthesia only, in a Medicare qualifying clinical trial, per day

G0295 Electromagnetic therapy, to one or more areas, for wound care other than described in G0329 or for other uses

CIM: 35-98

G0296 Counseling visit to discuss need for lung cancer screening (ldct) using low dose ct scan (service is for eligibility determination and shared decision making)

G0297 Low dose ct scan (ldct) for lung cancer screening

G0298 HIV antigen/antibody, combination assay, screening

G0299 Direct skilled nursing services of a registered nurse (RN) in the home health or hospice setting, each 15 minutes

G0300 Direct skilled nursing services of a license practical nurse (LPN) in the home health or hospice setting, each 15 minutes

G0302 Pre-operative pulmonary surgery services for preparation for LVRS, complete course of services, to include a minimum of 16 days of services

G0303 Pre-operative pulmonary surgery services for preparation for LVRS, 10 to 15 days of services

G0304 Pre-operative pulmonary surgery services for preparation for LVRS, 1 to 9 days of services

G0305 Post-discharge pulmonary surgery services after LVRS, minimum of 6 days of services

G0306 Complete CBC, automated (hgb, hCT, rbc, wbc, without platelet count) and automated wbc differential count

G0307 Complete (CBC), automated (hgb, hCT, rbc, wbc; without platelet count)

G0328 Colorectal cancer screening; fecal occult blood test, immunoassay, 1-3 simultaneous

G0329 Electromagnetic therapy, to one or more areas for chronic stage iii and stage iv pressure ulcers, arterial ulcers, diabetic ulcers and venous stasis ulcers not demonstrating measurable signs of healing after 30 days of conventional care as part of a therapy plan of care

G0333 Pharmacy dispensing fee for inhalation drug(s); initial 30-day supply as a beneficiary

G0337 Hospice evaluation and counseling services, pre-election

G0339 Image-guided robotic linear accelerator-based stereotactic radiosurgery, complete course of therapy in one session or first session of fractionated treatment

G0340 Image-guided robotic linear accelerator-based stereotactic radiosurgery, delivery including collimator changes and custom plugging, fractionated treatment, all lesions, per session, second through fifth sessions, maximum five sessions per course of treatment

G0341 Percutaneous islet cell transplant, includes portal vein catheterization and infusion

CIM: 260.3

G0342 Laparoscopy for islet cell transplant, includes portal vein catheterization and infusion

CIM: 35-82

G0343 Laparotomy for islet cell transplant, includes portal vein catheterization and infusion

CIM: 35-82

G0364 Bone marrow aspiration performed with bone marrow biopsy through the same incision on the same date of service

G0365 Vessel mapping of vessels for hemodialysis access (services for preoperative vessel mapping prior to creation of hemodialysis access using an autogenous hemodialysis conduit, including arterial inflow and venous outflow)

G0372 Physician service required to establish and document the need for a power mobility device

G0378 Hospital observation service, per hour

G0379 Direct admission of patient for hospital observation care

G0380 Level 1 hospital emergency department visit provided in a type b emergency department; (the ed must meet at least one of the following requirements: (1) it is licensed by the state in which it is located under applicable state law as an emergency room or emergency department; (2) it is held out to the public (by name, posted signs, advertising, or other means) as a place that provides care for emergency medical conditions on an urgent basis without requiring a previously scheduled appointment; or (3) during the calendar year immediately preceding the calendar year in which a determination under 42 cfr 489.24 is being made, based on a representative sample of patient visits that occurred during that calendar year, it provides at least one-third of all of its outpatient visits for the treatment of emergency medical conditions on an urgent basis without requiring a previously scheduled appointment)

G0381 Level 2 hospital emergency department visit provided in a type b emergency department; (the ed must meet at least one of the following requirements: (1) it is licensed by the state in which it is located under applicable state law as an emergency room or emergency department; (2) it is held out to the public (by name, posted signs, advertising, or other means) as a place that provides care for emergency medical conditions on an urgent basis without requiring a previously scheduled appointment; or (3) during the calendar year immediately preceding the calendar year in which a determination under 42 cfr 489.24 is being made, based on a representative sample of patient visits that occurred during that calendar year, it provides at least one-third of all of its outpatient visits for the treatment of emergency medical conditions on an urgent basis without requiring a previously scheduled appointment)

G0382 Level 3 hospital emergency department visit provided in a type b emergency department; (the ed must meet at least one of the following requirements: (1) it is licensed by the state in which it is located under applicable state law as an emergency room or emergency department; (2) it is held out to the public (by name, posted signs, advertising, or other means) as a place that provides care for emergency medical conditions on an urgent basis without requiring a previously scheduled appointment; or (3) during the calendar year immediately preceding the calendar year in which a determination under 42 cfr 489.24 is being made, based on a representative sample of patient visits that occurred during that calendar year, it provides at least one-third of all of its outpatient visits for the treatment of emergency medical conditions on an urgent basis without requiring a previously scheduled appointment)

G0383 Level 4 hospital emergency department visit provided in a type b emergency department; (the ed must meet at least one of the following requirements: (1) it is licensed by the state in which it is located under applicable state law as an emergency room or emergency department; (2) it is held out to the public (by name, posted signs, advertising, or other means) as a place that provides care for emergency medical conditions on an urgent basis without requiring a previously scheduled appointment; or (3) during the calendar year immediately preceding the calendar year in which a determination under 42 cfr 489.24 is being made, based on a representative sample of patient visits that occurred during that calendar year, it provides at least one-third of all of its outpatient visits for the treatment of emergency medical conditions on an urgent basis without requiring a previously scheduled appointment)

G0384 Level 5 hospital emergency department visit provided in a type b emergency department; (the ed must meet at least one of the following requirements: (1) it is licensed by the state in which it is located under applicable state law as an emergency room or emergency department; (2) it is held out to the public (by name, posted signs, advertising, or other means) as a place that provides care for emergency medical conditions on an urgent basis without requiring a previously scheduled appointment; or (3) during the calendar year immediately preceding the calendar year in which a determination under 42 cfr 489.24 is being made, based on a representative sample of patient visits that occurred during that calendar year, it provides at least one-third of all of its outpatient visits for the treatment of emergency medical conditions on an urgent basis without requiring a previously scheduled appointment)

(**G0389** Code deleted December 31, 2016).

G0390 Trauma response team associated with hospital critical care service

G0396 Alcohol and/or substance (other than tobacco) abuse structured assessment (e.g., audit, DAST), and brief intervention 15 to 30 minutes

G0397 Alcohol and/or substance (other than tobacco) abuse structured assessment (e.g., audit, DAST), and intervention, greater than 30 minutes

G0398 Home sleep study test (hst) with type ii portable monitor, unattended; minimum of 7 channels: eeg, eog, EMG, ECG/heart rate, airflow, respiratory effort and oxygen saturation

G0399 Home sleep test (hst) with type iii portable monitor, unattended; minimum of 4 channels: 2 respiratory movement/airflow, 1 ECG/heart rate and 1 oxygen saturation

G0400 Home sleep test (hst) with type iv portable monitor, unattended; minimum of 3 channels

Ⓟ **G0402** Initial preventive physical examination; face-to-face visit, services limited to new beneficiary during the first 12 months of Medicare enrollment

G0403 Electrocardiogram, routine ECG with 12 leads; performed as a screening for the initial preventive physical examination with interpretation and report

G0404 Electrocardiogram, routine ECG with 12 leads; tracing only, without interpretation and report, performed as a screening for the initial preventive physical examination

G0405 Electrocardiogram, routine ECG with 12 leads; interpretation and report only, performed as a screening for the initial preventive physical examination

G0406 Follow-up inpatient consultation, limited, physicians typically spend 15 minutes communicating with the patient via telehealth

G0407 Follow-up inpatient consultation, intermediate, physicians typically spend 25 minutes communicating with the patient via telehealth

G0408 Follow-up inpatient consultation, complex, physicians typically spend 35 minutes communicating with the patient via telehealth

Ⓟ **G0409** Social work and psychological services, directly relating to and/or furthering the patient's rehabilitation goals, each 15 minutes, face-to-face; individual (services provided by a corf-qualified social worker or psychologist in a corf)

Ⓟ **G0410** Group psychotherapy other than of a multiple-family group, in a partial hospitalization setting, approximately 45 to 50 minutes

Ⓟ **G0411** Interactive group psychotherapy, in a partial hospitalization setting, approximately 45 to 50 minutes

G0412 Open treatment of iliac spine(s), tuberosity avulsion, or iliac wing fracture(s), unilateral or bilateral for pelvic bone fracture patterns which do not disrupt the pelvic ring includes internal fixation, when performed

G0413 Percutaneous skeletal fixation of posterior pelvic bone fracture and/or dislocation, for fracture patterns which disrupt the pelvic ring, unilateral or bilateral, (includes ilium, sacroiliac joint and/or sacrum)

G0414 Open treatment of anterior pelvic bone fracture and/or dislocation for fracture patterns which disrupt the pelvic ring, unilateral or bilateral, includes internal fixation when performed (includes pubic symphysis and/or superior/inferior rami)

G0415 Open treatment of posterior pelvic bone fracture and/or dislocation, for fracture patterns which disrupt the pelvic ring, unilateral or bilateral, includes internal fixation, when performed (includes ilium, sacroiliac joint and/or sacrum)

G0416 Surgical pathology, gross and microscopic examinations, for prostate needle biopsy, any method

G0420 Face-to-face educational services related to the care of chronic kidney disease;

individual, per session, per one hour

G0421 Face-to-face educational services related to the care of chronic kidney disease; group, per session, per one hour

G0422 Intensive cardiac rehabilitation; with or without continuous ECG monitoring with exercise, per session

G0423 Intensive cardiac rehabilitation; with or without continuous ECG monitoring; without exercise, per session

G0424 Pulmonary rehabilitation, including exercise (includes monitoring), one hour, per session, up to two sessions per day

G0425 Telehealth consultation, emergency department or initial inpatient, typically 30 minutes communicating with the patient via telehealth

G0426 Telehealth consultation, emergency department or initial inpatient, typically 50 minutes communicating with the patient via telehealth

G0427 Telehealth consultation, emergency department or initial inpatient, typically 70 minutes or more communicating with the patient via telehealth

G0428 Collagen meniscus implant procedure for filling meniscal defects (e.g., CMI, collagen scaffold, menaflex)

G0429 Dermal filler injection(s) for the treatment of facial lipodystrophy syndrome (lds) (e.g., as a result of highly active antiretroviral therapy)

(**G0431** Code deleted December 31, 2015.)

G0432 Infectious agent antibody detection by enzyme immunoassay (EIA) technique, hiv-1 and/or hiv-2, screening

G0433 Infectious agent antibody detection by enzyme-linked immunosorbent assay (ELISA) technique, hiv-1 and/or hiv-2, screening

(**G0434** Code deleted December 31, 2015.)

G0435 Infectious agent antibody detection by rapid antibody test, hiv-1 and/or hiv-2, screening

(**G0436** Code deleted 09/30/16). Use 99406, 99407.

(**G0437** Code deleted 09/30/16). Use 99406, 99407.

Ⓟ **G0438** Annual wellness visit; includes a personalized prevention plan of service (pps), initial visit

Ⓟ **G0439** Annual wellness visit, includes a personalized prevention plan of service (pps), subsequent visit

G0442 Annual alcohol misuse screening, 15 minutes

G0443 Brief face-to-face behavioral counseling for alcohol misuse, 15 minutes

Ⓟ **G0444** Annual depression screening, 15 minutes

G0445 High intensity behavioral counseling to prevent sexually transmitted infection; face-to-face, individual, includes: education, skills training and guidance on how to change sexual behavior; performed semi-annually, 30 minutes

G0446 Annual, face-to-face intensive behavioral therapy for cardiovascular disease, individual, 15 minutes

Ⓟ **G0447** Face-to-face behavioral counseling for obesity, 15 minutes

G0448 Insertion or replacement of a permanent pacing cardioverter-defibrillator system with transvenous lead(s), single or dual chamber with insertion of pacing electrode, cardiac venous system, for left ventricular pacing

G0451 Development testing, with interpretation and report, per standardized instrument form

G0452 Molecular pathology procedure; physician interpretation and report

G0453 Continuous intraoperative neurophysiology monitoring, from outside the operating room (remote or nearby), per patient, (attention directed exclusively to one patient) each 15 minutes (list in addition to primary procedure)

G0454 Physician documentation of face-to-face visit for durable medical equipment determination performed by nurse practitioner, physician assistant or clinical nurse specialist

G0455 Preparation with instillation of fecal microbiota by any method, including assessment of donor specimen

G0458 Low dose rate (LDR) prostate brachytherapy services, composite rate

G0459 Inpatient telehealth pharmacologic management, including prescription, use, and review of medication with no more than minimal medical psychotherapy

G0460 Autologous platelet rich plasma for chronic wounds/ulcers, including phlebotomy, centrifugation, and all other preparatory procedures, administration and dressings, per treatment

Ⓟ **G0463** Hospital outpatient clinic visit for assessment and management of a patient

G0464 Colorectal cancer screening; stool-based DNA and fecal occult hemoglobin (e.g., KRAS, ndrg4 and bmp3)

G0466 Federally qualified health center (fqhc) visit, new patient; a medically-necessary, face-to-face encounter (one-on-one) between a new patient and a fqhc practitioner during which time one or more fqhc services are rendered and includes a typical bundle of medicare-covered services that would be furnished per diem to a patient receiving a fqhc visit

G0467 Federally qualified health center (fqhc) visit, established patient; a medically-necessary, face-to-face encounter (one-on-one) between an established patient and a fqhc practitioner during which time one or more fqhc services are rendered and includes a typical bundle of medicare-covered services that would be furnished per diem to a patient receiving a fqhc visit

G0468 Federally qualified health center (fqhc) visit, IPPE or AWV; a fqhc visit that includes an initial preventive physical examination (IPPE) or annual wellness visit (AWV) and includes a typical bundle of medicare-covered services that would be furnished per diem to a patient receiving an IPPE or AWV

G0469 Federally qualified health center (fqhc) visit, mental health, new patient; a medically-necessary, face-to-face mental health encounter (one-on-one) between a new patient and a fqhc practitioner during which time one or more fqhc services are rendered and includes a typical bundle of medicare-covered services that would be furnished per diem to a patient receiving a mental health visit

G0470 Federally qualified health center (fqhc) visit, mental health, established patient; a medically-necessary, face-to-face mental health encounter (one-on-one) between an established patient and a fqhc practitioner during which time one or more fqhc services are rendered and includes a typical bundle of medicare-covered services that would be furnished per diem to a patient receiving a mental health visit

G0471 Collection of venous blood by venipuncture or urine sample by catheterization from an individual in a skilled nursing facility (snf) or by a laboratory on behalf of a home health agency (HHA)

G0472 Hepatitis c antibody screening, for individual at high risk and other covered indication(s)

Statute: 1861SSA

G0473 Face-to-face behavioral counseling for obesity, group (2-10), 30 minutes

G0475 HIV antigen/antibody, combination assay, screening

G0476 Infectious agent detection by nucleic acid (DNA or rna); human papillomavirus (HPV), high-risk types (eg, 16, 18, 31, 33, 35, 39, 45, 51, 52, 56, 58, 59, 68) for cervical cancer screening, must be performed in addition to pap test

• **G0490** Face-to-face home health nursing visit by a rural health clinic (RHC) or federally qualified health center (fqhc) in an area with a shortage of home health agencies; (services limited to RN or LPN only)

• **G0491** Dialysis procedure at a Medicare certified ESRD facility for acute kidney injury without ESRD

• **G0492** Dialysis procedure with single evaluation by a physician or other qualified health care professional for acute kidney injury without ESRD

• **G0493** Skilled services of a registered nurse (RN) for the observation and assessment of the patient's condition, each 15 minutes (the change in the patient's condition requires skilled nursing personnel to identify and evaluate the patient's need for possible modification of treatment in the home health or hospice setting)

• **G0494** Skilled services of a licensed practical nurse (LPN) for the observation and assessment of the patient's condition, each 15 minutes (the change in the patient's condition requires skilled nursing personnel to identify and evaluate the patient's need for possible modification of treatment in the home health or hospice setting)

• **G0495** Skilled services of a registered nurse (RN), in the training and/or education of a patient or family member, in the home health or hospice setting, each 15 minutes

• **G0496** Skilled services of a licensed practical nurse (LPN), in the training and/or education of a patient or family member, in the home health or hospice setting, each 15 minutes

• **G0498** Chemotherapy administration, intravenous infusion technique; initiation of infusion in the office/clinic setting using office/clinic pump/supplies, with continuation of the infusion in the community setting (e.g., home, domiciliary, rest home or assisted living) using a portable pump provided by the office/clinic, includes follow up office/clinic visit at the conclusion of the infusion

• **G0499** Hepatitis b screening in non-pregnant, high risk individual includes hepatitis b surface antigen (HBsAg) followed by a neutralizing confirmatory test for initially reactive results, and antibodies to HBsAg (anti-HBs) and hepatitis b core antigen (anti-HBc)

• **G0500** Moderate sedation services provided by the same physician or other qualified health care professional performing a gastrointestinal endoscopic service that sedation supports, requiring the presence of an independent trained observer to assist in the monitoring of the patient's level of consciousness and physiological status; initial 15 minutes of intra-service time; patient age 5 years or older (additional time may be reported with 99153, as appropriate)

• **G0501** Resource-intensive services for patients for whom the use of specialized mobility-assistive technology (such as adjustable height chairs or tables, patient lift, and adjustable padded leg supports) is medically necessary and used during the provision of an office/outpatient, evaluation and management visit (list separately in addition to primary service)

• **G0502** Initial psychiatric collaborative care management, first 70 minutes in the first calendar month of behavioral health care manager activities, in consultation with a psychiatric consultant, and directed by the treating physician or other qualified health care professional, with the following required elements: outreach to and engagement in treatment of a patient directed by the treating physician or other qualified health care professional; initial assessment of the patient, including administration of validated rating scales, with the development of an individualized treatment plan; review by the psychiatric consultant with modifications of the plan if recommended; entering patient in a registry and tracking patient follow-up and progress using the registry, with appropriate documentation, and participation in weekly caseload consultation with the psychiatric consultant; and provision of brief interventions using evidence-based techniques such as behavioral activation, motivational interviewing, and other focused treatment strategies

• **G0503** Subsequent psychiatric collaborative care management, first 60 minutes in a subsequent month of behavioral health care manager activities, in consultation with a psychiatric consultant, and directed by the treating physician or other qualified health care professional, with the following required elements: tracking patient follow-up and progress using the registry, with appropriate documentation; participation in weekly caseload consultation with the psychiatric consultant; ongoing collaboration with and coordination of the patient's mental health care with the treating physician or other qualified health care professional and any other treating mental health providers; additional review of progress and recommendations for changes in treatment, as indicated, including medications, based on recommendations provided by the psychiatric consultant; provision of brief interventions using evidence-based techniques such as behavioral activation, motivational interviewing, and other focused treatment strategies; monitoring of patient outcomes using validated rating scales; and relapse prevention planning with patients as they achieve remission of symptoms and/or other treatment goals and are prepared for discharge from active treatment

• **G0504** Initial or subsequent psychiatric collaborative care management, each additional 30 minutes in a calendar month of behavioral health care manager activities, in consultation with a psychiatric consultant, and directed by the treating physician or other qualified health care professional (list separately in addition to code for primary procedure); (use G0504 in conjunction with G0502, G0503)

• **G0505** Cognition and functional assessment using standardized instruments with development of recorded care plan for the patient with cognitive impairment, history obtained from patient and/or caregiver, in office or other outpatient setting or home or domiciliary or rest home

• **G0506** Comprehensive assessment of and care planning for patients requiring chronic care management services (list separately in addition to primary monthly care management service)

• **G0507** Care management services for behavioral health conditions, at least 20 minutes of clinical staff time, directed by a physician or other qualified health care professional, per calendar month, with the following required elements: initial assessment or follow-up monitoring, including the use of applicable validated rating scales; behavioral health care planning in relation to behavioral/psychiatric health problems, including revision for patients who are not progressing or whose status changes; facilitating and coordinating treatment such as psychotherapy, pharmacotherapy, counseling and/or psychiatric consultation; and continuity of care with a designated member of the care team

• **G0508** Telehealth consultation, critical care, initial , physicians typically spend 60 minutes communicating with the patient and providers via telehealth

• **G0509** Telehealth consultation, critical care, subsequent, physicians typically spend 50 minutes communicating with the patient and providers via telehealth

Ⓟ **G0913** Improvement in visual function achieved within 90 days following cataract surgery

Ⓟ **G0914** Patient care survey was not completed by patient

Ⓟ **G0915** Improvement in visual function not achieved within 90 days following cataract surgery

Ⓟ **G0916** Satisfaction with care achieved within 90 days following cataract surgery

Ⓟ **G0917** Patient satisfaction survey was not completed by patient

Ⓟ **G0918** Satisfaction with care not achieved within 90 days following cataract surgery

(**G3001** Code deleted December 31, 2016).

G6001 Ultrasonic guidance for placement of radiation therapy fields

CIM: 50-7

G6002 Stereoscopic x-ray guidance for localization of target volume for the delivery of radiation therapy

G6003 Radiation treatment delivery, single treatment area, single port or parallel opposed ports, simple blocks or no blocks: up to 5 mev

G6004 Radiation treatment delivery, single treatment area, single port or parallel opposed ports, simple blocks or no blocks: 6-10 mev

G6005 Radiation treatment delivery, single treatment area, single port or parallel opposed ports, simple blocks or no blocks: 11-19 mev

G6006 Radiation treatment delivery, single treatment area, single port or parallel opposed ports, simple blocks or no blocks: 20 mev or greater

G6007 Radiation treatment delivery, 2 separate treatment areas, 3 or more ports on a single treatment area, use of multiple blocks: up to 5 mev

G6008 Radiation treatment delivery, 2 separate treatment areas, 3 or more ports on a single treatment area, use of multiple blocks: 6-10 mev

G6009 Radiation treatment delivery, 2 separate treatment areas, 3 or more ports on a single treatment area, use of multiple blocks: 11-19 mev

G6010 Radiation treatment delivery, 2 separate treatment areas, 3 or more ports on a single treatment area, use of multiple blocks: 20 mev or greater

G6011 Radiation treatment delivery,3 or more separate treatment areas, custom blocking, tangential ports, wedges, rotational beam, compensators, electron beam; up to 5 mev

G6012 Radiation treatment delivery,3 or more separate treatment areas, custom blocking, tangential ports, wedges, rotational beam, compensators, electron beam; 6-10 mev

G6013 Radiation treatment delivery,3 or more separate treatment areas, custom blocking, tangential ports, wedges, rotational beam, compensators, electron beam; 11-19 mev

G6014 Radiation treatment delivery,3 or more separate treatment areas, custom blocking, tangential ports, wedges, rotational beam, compensators, electron beam; 20 mev or greater

G6015 Intensity modulated treatment delivery, single or multiple fields/arcs, via narrow spatially and temporally modulated beams, binary, dynamic mlc, per treatment session

G6016 Compensator-based beam modulation treatment delivery of inverse planned treatment using 3 or more high resolution (milled or cast) compensator, convergent beam modulated fields, per treatment session

G6017 Intra-fraction localization and tracking of target or patient motion during delivery of radiation therapy (eg,3d positional tracking, gating, 3d surface tracking), each fraction of treatment

(**G6018** Code deleted December 31, 2015.)

(**G6019** Code deleted December 31, 2015.)

(**G6020** Code deleted December 31, 2015.)

(**G6021** Code deleted December 31, 2015.)

(**G6022** Code deleted December 31, 2015.)

(**G6023** Code deleted December 31, 2015.)

(**G6024** Code deleted December 31, 2015.)

(**G6025** Code deleted December 31, 2015.)

(**G6027** Code deleted December 31, 2015.)

(**G6028** Code deleted December 31, 2015.)

G6030 Amitriptyline

G6031 Benzodiazepines

G6032 Desipramine

G6034 Doxepin

G6035 Gold

G6036 Assay of imipramine

G6037 Nortriptyline

G6038 Salicylate

G6039 Acetaminophen

G6040 Alcohol (ethanol); any specimen except breath

G6041 Alkaloids, urine, quantitative

G6042 Amphetamine or methamphetamine

G6043 Barbiturates, not elsewhere specified

G6044 Cocaine or metabolite

G6045 Dihydrocodeinone

G6046 Dihydromorphinone

G6047 Dihydrotestosterone

G6048 Dimethadione

G6049 Epiandrosterone

G6050 Ethchlorvynol

G6051 Flurazepam

G6052 Meprobamate

G6053 Methadone

G6054 Methsuximide

G6055 Nicotine

G6056 Opiate(s), drug and metabolites, each procedure

G6057 Phenothiazine

G6058 Drug confirmation, each procedure

Physician's Voluntary Reporting Program Codes

These HCPCS codes are to be used for the physician's voluntary reporting program in which CMS seeks to analyze the quality of care provided to Medicare beneficiaries. Reporting of these codes is
voluntary. Physicians should not charge for these codes. Unless otherwise indicated, report these codes in addition to office visit, home visit, nursing facility and domiciliary evaluation and management codes.

G8395 Left ventricular ejection fraction (LVEF) >= 40% or documentation as normal or mildly depressed left ventricular systolic function

G8396 Left ventricular ejection fraction (LVEF) not performed or documented

Ⓟ **G8397** Dilated macular or fundus exam performed, including documentation of the presence or absence of macular edema and level of severity of retinopathy

Ⓟ **G8398** Dilated macular or fundus exam not performed

Ⓟ **G8399** Patient with documented results of a central dual-energy x-ray absorptiometry (DXA) ever being performed

Ⓟ **G8400** Patient with central dual-energy x-ray absorptiometry (DXA) results not documented, reason not given

(**G8401** Code deleted December 31, 2016).

Ⓟ **G8404** Lower extremity neurological exam performed and documented

Ⓟ **G8405** Lower extremity neurological exam not performed

Ⓟ **G8410** Footwear evaluation performed and documented

Ⓟ **G8415** Footwear evaluation was not performed

Ⓟ **G8416** Clinician documented that patient was not an eligible candidate for footwear evaluation measure

Ⓟ **G8417** BMI is documented above normal parameters and a follow-up plan is documented

Ⓟ **G8418** BMI is documented below normal parameters and a follow-up plan is documented

Ⓟ **G8419** BMI documented outside normal parameters, no follow-up plan documented, no reason given

Ⓟ **G8420** BMI is documented within normal parameters and no follow-up plan is required

Ⓟ **G8421** BMI not documented and no reason is given

Ⓟ **G8422** BMI not documented, documentation the patient is not eligible for BMI calculation

▲Ⓟ **G8427** Eligible clinician attests to documenting in the medical record they obtained, updated, or reviewed the patient's current medications

▲Ⓟ **G8428** Current list of medications not documented as obtained, updated, or reviewed by the eligible clinician, reason not given

▲Ⓟ **G8430** Eligible clinician attests to documenting in the medical record the patient is not eligible for a current list of medications being obtained, updated, or reviewed by the eligible clinician

▲Ⓟ **G8431** Screening for depression is documented as being positive and a follow-up plan is documented

▲Ⓟ **G8432** Depression screening not documented, reason not given

▲Ⓟ **G8433** Screening for depression not completed, documented reason

Ⓟ **G8442** Pain assessment not documented as being performed, documentation the patient is not eligible for a pain assessment using a standardized tool

Ⓟ **G8450** Beta-blocker therapy prescribed

Ⓟ **G8451** Beta-blocker therapy for LVEF < 40% not prescribed for reasons documented by the clinician (e.g., low blood pressure, fluid overload, asthma, patients recently treated with an intravenous positive inotropic agent, allergy, intolerance, other medical reasons, patient declined, other patient reasons, or other reasons attributable to the healthcare system)

Ⓟ **G8452** Beta-blocker therapy not prescribed

(**G8458** Code deleted December 31, 2016).

(**G8460** Code deleted December 31, 2016).

(**G8461** Code deleted December 31, 2016).

Ⓟ **G8465** High or very high risk of recurrence of prostate cancer

Ⓟ **G8473** Angiotensin converting enzyme (ace) inhibitor or angiotensin receptor blocker (arb) therapy prescribed

Ⓟ **G8474** Angiotensin converting enzyme (ace) inhibitor or angiotensin receptor blocker (arb) therapy not prescribed for reasons documented by the clinician (e.g., allergy, intolerance, pregnancy, renal failure due to ace inhibitor, diseases of the aortic or mitral valve, other medical reasons) or (e.g., patient declined, other patient reasons) or (e.g., lack of drug availability, other reasons attributable to the health care system)

Ⓟ **G8475** Angiotensin converting enzyme (ace) inhibitor or angiotensin receptor blocker (arb) therapy not prescribed, reason not given

Ⓟ **G8476** Most recent blood pressure has a systolic measurement of < 140 mmhg and a diastolic measurement of < 90 mmhg

Ⓟ **G8477** Most recent blood pressure has a systolic measurement of >= 140 mmhg and/or a diastolic measurement of >= 90 mmhg

Ⓟ **G8478** Blood pressure measurement not performed or documented, reason not given

Ⓟ **G8482** Influenza immunization administered or previously received

Ⓟ **G8483** Influenza immunization was not administered for reasons documented by clinician (e.g., patient allergy or other medical reasons, patient declined or other patient reasons, vaccine not available or other system reasons)

Ⓟ **G8484** Influenza immunization was not administered, reason not given

(**G8485** Code deleted December 31, 2016).

(**G8486** Code deleted December 31, 2016).

(**G8487** Code deleted December 31, 2016).

(**G8489** Code deleted December 31, 2016).

(**G8490** Code deleted December 31, 2016).

(**G8491** Code deleted December 31, 2016).

(**G8494** Code deleted December 31, 2016).

(**G8495** Code deleted December 31, 2016).

(**G8496** Code deleted December 31, 2016).

(**G8497** Code deleted December 31, 2016).

(**G8498** Code deleted December 31, 2016).

(**G8499** Code deleted December 31, 2016).

(**G8500** Code deleted December 31, 2016).

Ⓟ **G8506** Patient receiving angiotensin converting enzyme (ace) inhibitor or angiotensin receptor blocker (arb) therapy

Ⓟ **G8509** Pain assessment documented as positive using a standardized tool, follow-up plan not documented, reason not given

▲Ⓟ **G8510** Screening for depression is documented as negative, a follow-up plan is not required

▲Ⓟ **G8511** Screening for depression documented as positive, follow-up plan not documented, reason not given

(**G8530** Code deleted December 31, 2015.)

(**G8531** Code deleted December 31, 2015.)

(**G8532** Code deleted December 31, 2015.)

Ⓟ **G8535** Elder maltreatment screen not documented; documentation that patient not eligible for the elder maltreatment screen

Ⓟ **G8536** No documentation of an elder maltreatment screen, reason not given

Ⓟ **G8539** Functional outcome assessment documented as positive using a standardized tool and a care plan based on identified deficiencies on the date of functional outcome assessment, is documented

Ⓟ **G8540** Functional outcome assessment not documented as being performed, documentation the patient is not eligible for a functional outcome assessment using a standardized tool

Ⓟ **G8541** Functional outcome assessment using a standardized tool not documented, reason not given

Ⓟ **G8542** Functional outcome assessment using a standardized tool is documented; no functional deficiencies identified, care plan not required

Ⓟ **G8543** Documentation of a positive functional outcome assessment using a standardized tool; care plan not documented, reason not given

(**G8544** Code deleted December 31, 2016).

(**G8545** Code deleted December 31, 2016).

(**G8548** Code deleted December 31, 2016).

(**G8549** Code deleted December 31, 2016).

(**G8551** Code deleted December 31, 2016).

G8559 Patient referred to a physician (preferably a physician with training in disorders of the ear) for an otologic evaluation

G8560 Patient has a history of active drainage from the ear within the previous 90 days

G8561 Patient is not eligible for the referral for otologic evaluation for patients with a history of active drainage measure

G8562 Patient does not have a history of active drainage from the ear within the previous 90 days

G8563 Patient not referred to a physician (preferably a physician with training in disorders of the ear) for an otologic evaluation, reason not given

G8564 Patient was referred to a physician (preferably a physician with training in disorders of the ear) for an otologic evaluation, reason not specified)

G8565 Verification and documentation of sudden or rapidly progressive hearing loss

G8566 Patient is not eligible for the "referral for otologic evaluation for sudden or rapidly progressive hearing loss" measure

G8567 Patient does not have verification and documentation of sudden or rapidly progressive hearing loss

G8568 Patient was not referred to a physician (preferably a physician with training in disorders of the ear) for an otologic evaluation, reason not given

Ⓟ **G8569** Prolonged postoperative intubation (> 24 hrs) required

Ⓟ **G8570** Prolonged postoperative intubation (> 24 hrs) not required

G8571 Development of deep sternal wound infection/mediastinitis within 30 days postoperatively

G8572 No deep sternal wound infection/mediastinitis

G8573 Stroke following isolated CABG surgery

G8574 No stroke following isolated CABG surgery

G8575 Developed postoperative renal failure or required dialysis

G8576 No postoperative renal failure/dialysis not required

G8577 Re-exploration required due to mediastinal bleeding with or without tamponade, graft occlusion, valve dysfunction or other cardiac reason

	G8578	Re-exploration not required due to mediastinal bleeding with or without tamponade, graft occlusion, valve dysfunction or other cardiac reason
▲Ⓟ	G8598	Aspirin or another antiplatelet therapy used
▲Ⓟ	G8599	Aspirin or another antiplatelet therapy not used, reason not given
Ⓟ	G8600	IV t-pa initiated within three hours (<= 180 minutes) of time last known well
Ⓟ	G8601	IV t-pa not initiated within three hours (<= 180 minutes) of time last known well for reasons documented by clinician
Ⓟ	G8602	IV t-pa not initiated within three hours (<= 180 minutes) of time last known well, reason not given
Ⓟ	G8627	Surgical procedure performed within 30 days following cataract surgery for major complications (e.g., retained nuclear fragments, endophthalmitis, dislocated or wrong power IOL, retinal detachment, or wound dehiscence)
Ⓟ	G8628	Surgical procedure not performed within 30 days following cataract surgery for major complications (e.g., retained nuclear fragments, endophthalmitis, dislocated or wrong power IOL, retinal detachment, or wound dehiscence)
Ⓟ	G8633	Pharmacologic therapy (other than minerals/vitamins) for osteoporosis prescribed
(	G8634	Code deleted December 31, 2016).
Ⓟ	G8635	Pharmacologic therapy for osteoporosis was not prescribed, reason not given
(	G8645	Code deleted December 31, 2016).
(	G8646	Code deleted December 31, 2016).
Ⓟ	G8647	Risk-adjusted functional status change residual score for the knee successfully calculated and the score was equal to zero (0) or greater than zero (>0)
Ⓟ	G8648	Risk-adjusted functional status change residual score for the knee successfully calculated and the score was less than zero (<0)
▲Ⓟ	G8649	Risk-adjusted functional status change residual scores for the knee not measured because the patient did not complete foto's status survey near discharge, not appropriate
Ⓟ	G8650	Risk-adjusted functional status change residual scores for the knee not measured because the patient did not complete foto's functional intake on admission and/or follow up status survey near discharge, reason not given
Ⓟ	G8651	Risk-adjusted functional status change residual score for the hip successfully calculated and the score was equal to zero (0) or greater than zero (>0)
Ⓟ	G8652	Risk-adjusted functional status change residual score for the hip successfully calculated and the score was less than zero (<0)
▲Ⓟ	G8653	Risk-adjusted functional status change residual scores for the hip not measured because the patient did not complete follow up status survey near discharge, patient not appropriate
Ⓟ	G8654	Risk-adjusted functional status change residual scores for the hip not measured

because the patient did not complete foto's functional intake on admission and/or follow up status survey near discharge, reason not given

▲Ⓟ **G8655** Risk-adjusted functional status change residual score for the foot or ankle successfully calculated and the score was equal to zero (0) or greater than zero (> 0)

▲Ⓟ **G8656** Risk-adjusted functional status change residual score for the foot or ankle successfully calculated and the score was less than zero (< 0)

▲Ⓟ **G8657** Risk-adjusted functional status change residual scores for the foot or ankle not measured because the patient did not complete foto's status survey near discharge, patient not appropriate

▲Ⓟ **G8658** Risk-adjusted functional status change residual scores for the foot or ankle not measured because the patient did not complete foto's functional intake on admission and/or follow up status survey near discharge, reason not given

▲Ⓟ **G8659** Risk-adjusted functional status change residual score for the lumbar impairment successfully calculated and the score was equal to zero (0) or greater than zero (> 0)

▲Ⓟ **G8660** Risk-adjusted functional status change residual score for the lumbar impairment successfully calculated and the score was less than zero (< 0)

▲Ⓟ **G8661** Risk-adjusted functional status change residual scores for the lumbar impairment not measured because the patient did not complete foto's status survey near discharge, patient not appropriate

▲Ⓟ **G8662** Risk-adjusted functional status change residual scores for the lumbar impairment not measured because the patient did not complete foto's functional intake on admission and/or follow up status survey near discharge, reason not given

Ⓟ **G8663** Risk-adjusted functional status change residual score for the shoulder successfully calculated and the score was equal to zero (0) or greater than zero (>0)

Ⓟ **G8664** Risk-adjusted functional status change residual score for the shoulder successfully calculated and the score was less than zero (<0)

▲Ⓟ **G8665** Risk-adjusted functional status change residual scores for the shoulder not measured because the patient did not complete foto's functional status survey near discharge, patient not appropriate

Ⓟ **G8666** Risk-adjusted functional status change residual scores for the shoulder not measured because the patient did not complete foto's functional intake on admission and/or follow up status survey near discharge, reason not given

Ⓟ **G8667** Risk-adjusted functional status change residual score for the elbow, wrist or hand successfully calculated and the score was equal to zero (0) or greater than zero (>0)

Ⓟ **G8668** Risk-adjusted functional status change residual score for the elbow, wrist or hand successfully calculated and the score was less than zero (<0)

▲Ⓟ **G8669** Risk-adjusted functional status change residual scores for the elbow, wrist or hand not measured because the patient did not complete foto's functional follow up status survey near discharge, patient not appropriate

Ⓟ **G8670** Risk-adjusted functional status change residual scores for the elbow, wrist or hand not measured because the patient did not complete foto's functional intake on admission and/or follow up status survey near discharge, reason not given

▲Ⓟ **G8671** Risk-adjusted functional status change residual score for the neck, cranium, mandible, thoracic spine, ribs, or other general orthopaedic impairment successfully calculated and the score was equal to zero (0) or greater than zero (> 0)

▲Ⓟ **G8672** Risk-adjusted functional status change residual score for the neck, cranium, mandible, thoracic spine, ribs, or other general orthopedic impairment successfully calculated and the score was less than zero (<0)

▲Ⓟ **G8673** Risk-adjusted functional status change residual scores for the neck, cranium, mandible, thoracic spine, ribs, or other general orthopaedic impairment not measured because the patient did not complete foto's functional follow up status survey near discharge, patient not appropriate

▲Ⓟ **G8674** Risk-adjusted functional status change residual scores for the neck, cranium, mandible, thoracic spine, ribs, or other general orthopaedic impairment not measured because the patient did not complete foto's functional intake on admission and/or follow up status survey near discharge, reason not given

Ⓟ **G8694** Left ventricular ejection fraction (LVEF) < 40%

Ⓟ **G8696** Antithrombotic therapy prescribed at discharge

▲Ⓟ **G8697** Antithrombotic therapy not prescribed for documented reasons (e.g., patient had stroke during hospital stay, patient expired during inpatient stay, other medical reason(s)); (e.g., patient left against medical advice, other patient reason(s))

Ⓟ **G8698** Antithrombotic therapy was not prescribed at discharge, reason not given

Ⓟ **G8708** Patient not prescribed or dispensed antibiotic

Ⓟ **G8709** Patient prescribed or dispensed antibiotic for documented medical reason(s) (e.g., intestinal infection, pertussis, bacterial infection, lyme disease, otitis media, acute sinusitis, acute pharyngitis, acute tonsillitis, chronic sinusitis, infection of the pharynx/larynx/tonsils/adenoids, prostatitis, cellulitis, mastoiditis, or bone infections, acute lymphadenitis, impetigo, skin staph infections, pneumonia/gonococcal infections, venereal disease (syphilis, chlamydia, inflammatory diseases (female reproductive organs)), infections of the kidney, cystitis or UTI, and acne)

Ⓟ **G8710** Patient prescribed or dispensed antibiotic

Ⓟ **G8711** Prescribed or dispensed antibiotic

G8712 Antibiotic not prescribed or dispensed

(**G8713** Code deleted December 31, 2015.)

(**G8714** Code deleted December 31, 2015.)

(**G8717** Code deleted December 31, 2015.)

(**G8718** Code deleted December 31, 2015.)

(**G8720** Code deleted December 31, 2015.)

Ⓟ **G8721** Pt category (primary tumor), pn category (regional lymph nodes), and histologic grade were documented in pathology report

Ⓟ **G8722** Documentation of medical reason(s) for not including the pt category, the pn category or the histologic grade in the pathology report (e.g., re-excision without residual tumor; non-carcinomas anal canal)

Ⓟ **G8723** Specimen site is other than anatomic location of primary tumor

Ⓟ **G8724** Pt category, pn category and histologic grade were not documented in the pathology report, reason not given

(**G8725** Code deleted December 31, 2016).

(**G8726** Code deleted December 31, 2016).

(**G8728** Code deleted December 31, 2016).

Ⓟ **G8730** Pain assessment documented as positive using a standardized tool and a follow-up plan is documented

Ⓟ **G8731** Pain assessment using a standardized tool is documented as negative, no follow-up plan required

Ⓟ **G8732** No documentation of pain assessment, reason not given

Ⓟ **G8733** Elder maltreatment screen documented as positive and a follow-up plan is documented

Ⓟ **G8734** Elder maltreatment screen documented as negative, no follow-up required

Ⓟ **G8735** Elder maltreatment screen documented as positive, follow-up plan not documented, reason not given

Ⓟ **G8749** Absence of signs of melanoma (cough, dyspnea, tenderness, localized neurologic signs such as weakness, jaundice or any other sign suggesting systemic spread) or absence of

symptoms of melanoma (pain, paresthesia, or any other symptom suggesting the possibility of systemic spread of melanoma)

Ⓟ **G8752** Most recent systolic blood pressure < 140 mmhg

Ⓟ **G8753** Most recent systolic blood pressure >= 140 mmhg

Ⓟ **G8754** Most recent diastolic blood pressure < 90 mmhg

Ⓟ **G8755** Most recent diastolic blood pressure >= 90 mmhg

Ⓟ **G8756** No documentation of blood pressure measurement, reason not given

(**G8757** Code deleted December 31, 2016).

(**G8758** Code deleted December 31, 2016).

(**G8759** Code deleted December 31, 2016).

(**G8761** Code deleted December 31, 2016).

(**G8762** Code deleted December 31, 2016).

(**G8765** Code deleted December 31, 2016).

ⓟ	**G8783**	Normal blood pressure reading documented, follow-up not required
(	**G8784**	Code deleted December 31, 2016).
ⓟ	**G8785**	Blood pressure reading not documented, reason not given
ⓟ	**G8797**	Specimen site other than anatomic location of esophagus
ⓟ	**G8798**	Specimen site other than anatomic location of prostate
ⓟ	**G8806**	Performance of trans-abdominal or trans-vaginal ultrasound
ⓟ	**G8807**	Trans-abdominal or trans-vaginal ultrasound not performed for reasons documented by clinician (e.g., patient has visited the ed multiple times within 72 hours, patient has a documented intrauterine pregnancy [IUP])
ⓟ	**G8808**	Performance of trans-abdominal or trans-vaginal ultrasound not ordered, reason not given (e.g., patient has visited the ed multiple times with no documentation of a trans-abdominal or trans-vaginal ultrasound within ed or from referring eligible professional)
ⓟ	**G8809**	Rh-immunoglobulin (RhoGAM) ordered
ⓟ	**G8810**	Rh-immunoglobulin (RhoGAM) not ordered for reasons documented by clinician (e.g., patient had prior documented receipt of RhoGAM within 12 weeks, patient refusal)
ⓟ	**G8811**	Documentation Rh-immunoglobulin (RhoGAM) was not ordered, reason not given
▲ⓟ	**G8815**	Documented reason in the medical records for why the statin therapy was not prescribed (i.e., lower extremity bypass was for a patient with non-atherosclerotic disease)
ⓟ	**G8816**	Statin medication prescribed at discharge
ⓟ	**G8817**	Statin therapy not prescribed at discharge, reason not given
ⓟ	**G8818**	Patient discharge to home no later than post-operative day #7
ⓟ	**G8825**	Patient not discharged to home by post-operative day #7
ⓟ	**G8826**	Patient discharge to home no later than post-operative day #2 following EVAR
ⓟ	**G8833**	Patient not discharged to home by post-operative day #2 following EVAR
ⓟ	**G8834**	Patient discharged to home no later than post-operative day #2 following CEA
ⓟ	**G8838**	Patient not discharged to home by post-operative day #2 following CEA
	G8839	Sleep apnea symptoms assessed, including presence or absence of snoring and daytime sleepiness
	G8840	Documentation of reason(s) for not documenting an assessment of sleep symptoms (e.g., patient didn't have initial daytime sleepiness, patient visited between initial testing and initiation of therapy)
	G8841	Sleep apnea symptoms not assessed, reason not given

G8842 Apnea hypopnea index (AHI) or respiratory disturbance index (RDI) measured at the time of initial diagnosis

G8843 Documentation of reason(s) for not measuring an apnea hypopnea index (AHI) or a respiratory disturbance index (RDI) at the time of initial diagnosis (e.g., psychiatric disease, dementia, patient declined, financial, insurance coverage, test ordered but not yet completed)

G8844 Apnea hypopnea index (AHI) or respiratory disturbance index (RDI) not measured at the time of initial diagnosis, reason not given

G8845 Positive airway pressure therapy prescribed

G8846 Moderate or severe obstructive sleep apnea (apnea hypopnea index (AHI) or respiratory disturbance index (RDI) of 15 or greater)

(**G8848** Code deleted December 31, 2016).

G8849 Documentation of reason(s) for not prescribing positive airway pressure therapy (e.g., patient unable to tolerate, alternative therapies use, patient declined, financial, insurance coverage)

G8850 Positive airway pressure therapy not prescribed, reason not given

G8851 Objective measurement of adherence to positive airway pressure therapy, documented

G8852 Positive airway pressure therapy prescribed

(**G8853** Code deleted December 31, 2016).

G8854 Documentation of reason(s) for not objectively measuring adherence to positive airway pressure therapy (e.g., patient didn't bring data from continuous positive airway pressure [CPAP], therapy not yet initiated, not available on machine)

G8855 Objective measurement of adherence to positive airway pressure therapy not performed, reason not given

Ⓟ **G8856** Referral to a physician for an otologic evaluation performed

Ⓟ **G8857** Patient is not eligible for the referral for otologic evaluation measure (e.g., patients who are already under the care of a physician for acute or chronic dizziness)

Ⓟ **G8858** Referral to a physician for an otologic evaluation not performed, reason not given

Ⓟ **G8861** Within the past 2 years, central dual-energy x-ray absorptiometry (DXA) ordered and documented, review of systems and medication history or pharmacologic therapy (other than minerals/vitamins) for osteoporosis prescribed

G8863 Patients not assessed for risk of bone loss, reason not given

G8864 Pneumococcal vaccine administered or previously received

G8865 Documentation of medical reason(s) for not administering or previously receiving pneumococcal vaccine (e.g., patient allergic reaction, potential adverse drug reaction)

G8866 Documentation of patient reason(s) for not administering or previously receiving pneumococcal vaccine (e.g., patient refusal)

G8867 Pneumococcal vaccine not administered or previously received, reason not given

(**G8868** Code deleted December 31, 2016).

Ⓟ **G8869** Patient has documented immunity to hepatitis b and is receiving a first course of anti-TNF therapy

(**G8870** Code deleted December 31, 2015.)

(**G8871** Code deleted December 31, 2015.)

Ⓟ **G8872** Excised tissue evaluated by imaging intraoperatively to confirm successful inclusion of targeted lesion

Ⓟ **G8873** Patients with needle localization specimens which are not amenable to intraoperative imaging such as MRI needle wire localization, or targets which are tentatively identified on mammogram or ultrasound which do not contain a biopsy marker but which can be verified on intraoperative inspection or pathology (e.g., needle biopsy site where the biopsy marker is remote from the actual biopsy site)

Ⓟ **G8874** Excised tissue not evaluated by imaging intraoperatively to confirm successful inclusion of targeted lesion

Ⓟ **G8875** Clinician diagnosed breast cancer preoperatively by a minimally invasive biopsy method

Ⓟ **G8876** Documentation of reason(s) for not performing minimally invasive biopsy to diagnose breast cancer preoperatively (e.g., lesion too close to skin, implant, chest wall, etc., lesion could not be adequately visualized for needle biopsy, patient condition prevents needle biopsy [weight, breast thickness, etc.], duct excision without imaging abnormality, prophylactic mastectomy, reduction mammoplasty, excisional biopsy performed by another physician)

Ⓟ **G8877** Clinician did not attempt to achieve the diagnosis of breast cancer preoperatively by a minimally invasive biopsy method, reason not given

Ⓟ **G8878** Sentinel lymph node biopsy procedure performed

Ⓟ **G8879** Clinically node negative (t1n0m0 or t2n0m0) invasive breast cancer

Ⓟ **G8880** Documentation of reason(s) sentinel lymph node biopsy not performed (e.g., reasons could include but not limited to; non-invasive cancer, incidental discovery of breast cancer on prophylactic mastectomy, incidental discovery of breast cancer on reduction mammoplasty, pre-operative biopsy proven lymph node (ln) metastases, inflammatory carcinoma, stage 3 locally advanced cancer, recurrent invasive breast cancer, patient refusal after informed consent)

G8881 Stage of breast cancer is greater than t1n0m0 or t2n0m0

Ⓟ **G8882** Sentinel lymph node biopsy procedure not performed, reason not given

Ⓟ **G8883** Biopsy results reviewed, communicated, tracked and documented

Ⓟ **G8884** Clinician documented reason that patient's biopsy results were not reviewed

Ⓟ **G8885** Biopsy results not reviewed, communicated, tracked or documented

(**G8898** Code deleted December 31, 2016).

(**G8899** Code deleted December 31, 2016).

(**G8900** Code deleted December 31, 2016).

(**G8902** Code deleted December 31, 2016).

(**G8903** Code deleted December 31, 2016).

(**G8906** Code deleted December 31, 2016).

G8907 Patient documented not to have experienced any of the following events: a burn prior to discharge; a fall within the facility; wrong site/side/patient/procedure/implant event; or a hospital transfer or hospital admission upon discharge from the facility

G8908 Patient documented to have received a burn prior to discharge

G8909 Patient documented not to have received a burn prior to discharge

G8910 Patient documented to have experienced a fall within asc

G8911 Patient documented not to have experienced a fall within ambulatory surgical center

G8912 Patient documented to have experienced a wrong site, wrong side, wrong patient, wrong procedure or wrong implant event

G8913 Patient documented not to have experienced a wrong site, wrong side, wrong patient, wrong procedure or wrong implant event

G8914 Patient documented to have experienced a hospital transfer or hospital admission upon discharge from asc

G8915 Patient documented not to have experienced a hospital transfer or hospital admission upon discharge from asc

G8916 Patient with preoperative order for iv antibiotic surgical site infection (ssi) prophylaxis, antibiotic initiated on time

G8917 Patient with preoperative order for iv antibiotic surgical site infection (ssi) prophylaxis, antibiotic not initiated on time

G8918 Patient without preoperative order for iv antibiotic surgical site infection (ssi) prophylaxis

Ⓟ **G8923** Left ventricular ejection fraction (LVEF) < 40% or documentation of moderately or severely depressed left ventricular systolic function

▲Ⓟ **G8924** Spirometry test results demonstrate fev1/fvc < 70%, fev < 60% predicted and patient has COPD symptoms (e.g., dyspnea, cough/sputum, wheezing)

▲Ⓟ **G8925** Spirometry test results demonstrate fev1 >= 60% fev1/fvc >= 70%, predicted or patient does not have COPD symptoms

Ⓟ **G8926** Spirometry test not performed or documented, reason not given

(**G8927** Code deleted December 31, 2016).

(**G8928** Code deleted December 31, 2016).

(**G8929** Code deleted December 31, 2016).

Ⓟ **G8934** Left ventricular ejection fraction (LVEF) <40% or documentation of moderately or severely depressed left ventricular systolic function

Ⓟ **G8935** Clinician prescribed angiotensin converting enzyme (ace) inhibitor or angiotensin receptor blocker (arb) therapy

Ⓟ **G8936** Clinician documented that patient was not an eligible candidate for angiotensin converting enzyme (ace) inhibitor or angiotensin receptor blocker (arb) therapy (eg, allergy, intolerance, pregnancy, renal failure due to ace inhibitor, diseases of the aortic or mitral valve, other medical reasons) or (eg, patient declined, other patient reasons) or (eg, lack of drug availability, other reasons attributable to the health care system)

Ⓟ **G8937** Clinician did not prescribe angiotensin converting enzyme (ace) inhibitor or angiotensin receptor blocker (arb) therapy, reason not given

Ⓟ **G8938** BMI is documented as being outside of normal limits, follow-up plan is not documented, documentation the patient is not eligible

Ⓟ **G8939** Pain assessment documented as positive, follow-up plan not documented, documentation the patient is not eligible

(**G8940** Code deleted December 31, 2016).

Ⓟ **G8941** Elder maltreatment screen documented as positive, follow-up plan not documented, documentation the patient is not eligible

Ⓟ **G8942** Functional outcomes assessment using a standardized tool is documented within the previous 30 days and care plan, based on identified deficiencies on the date of the functional outcome assessment, is documented

Ⓟ **G8944** AJCC melanoma cancer stage 0 through iic melanoma

Ⓟ **G8946** Minimally invasive biopsy method attempted but not diagnostic of breast cancer (e.g., high risk lesion of breast such as atypical ductal hyperplasia, lobular neoplasia, atypical lobular hyperplasia, lobular carcinoma in situ, atypical columnar hyperplastica, flat epithelial atypia, radial scar, complex sclerosing lesion, papillary lesion, or any lesion with spindle cells)

G8947 One or more neuropsychiatric symptoms

(**G8948** Code deleted December 31, 2016).

Ⓟ **G8950** Pre-hypertensive or hypertensive blood pressure reading documented, and the indicated follow-up is documented

(**G8951** Code deleted December 31, 2015.)

Ⓟ **G8952** Pre-hypertensive or hypertensive blood pressure reading documented, indicated follow-up not documented, reason not given

(**G8953** Code deleted December 31, 2016).

Ⓟ **G8955** Most recent assessment of adequacy of volume management documented

Ⓟ **G8956** Patient receiving maintenance hemodialysis in an outpatient dialysis facility

Ⓟ **G8958** Assessment of adequacy of volume management not documented, reason not given

Ⓟ **G8959** Clinician treating major depressive disorder communicates to clinician treating comorbid condition

Ⓟ **G8960** Clinician treating major depressive disorder did not communicate to clinician treating comorbid condition, reason not given

Ⓟ **G8961** Cardiac stress imaging test primarily performed on low-risk surgery patient for preoperative evaluation within 30 days preceding this surgery

Ⓟ **G8962** Cardiac stress imaging test performed on patient for any reason including those who did not have low risk surgery or test that was performed more than 30 days preceding low risk surgery

Ⓟ **G8963** Cardiac stress imaging performed primarily for monitoring of asymptomatic patient who had pci within 2 years

Ⓟ **G8964** Cardiac stress imaging test performed primarily for any other reason than monitoring of asymptomatic patient who had pci within 2 years (e.g., symptomatic patient, patient greater than 2 years since pci, initial evaluation, etc)

Ⓟ **G8965** Cardiac stress imaging test primarily performed on low CHD risk patient for initial detection and risk assessment

Ⓟ **G8966** Cardiac stress imaging test performed on symptomatic or higher than low CHD risk patient or for any reason other than initial detection and risk assessment

Ⓟ **G8967** Warfarin or another oral anticoagulant that is FDA approved prescribed

▲Ⓟ **G8968** Documentation of medical reason(s) for not prescribing warfarin or another oral anticoagulant that is FDA approved for the prevention of thromboembolism (e.g., allergy, risk of bleeding, other medical reasons)

Ⓟ **G8969** Documentation of patient reason(s) for not prescribing warfarin or another oral anticoagulant that is approved (e.g., economic, social, and/or religious impediments, noncompliance patient refusal, other patient reasons)

Ⓟ **G8970** No risk factors or one moderate risk factor for thromboembolism

Ⓟ **G8971** Warfarin or another oral anticoagulant that is approved not prescribed, reason not given

Ⓟ **G8972** One or more high risk factors for thromboembolism or more than one moderate risk factor for thromboembolism

Ⓟ **G8973** Most recent hemoglobin (hgb) level < 10 g/dl

Ⓟ **G8974** Hemoglobin level measurement not documented, reason not given

Ⓟ **G8975** Documentation of medical reason(s) for patient having a hemoglobin level < 10 g/dl (e.g., patients who have non-renal etiologies of anemia [e.g., sickle cell anemia or other hemoglobinopathies, hypersplenism, primary bone marrow disease, anemia related to chemotherapy for diagnosis of malignancy, postoperative bleeding, active bloodstream or peritoneal infection], other medical reasons)

Ⓟ **G8976** Most recent hemoglobin (hgb) level >= 10 g/dl

(**G8977** Code deleted December 31, 2016).

G8978 Mobility: walking & moving around functional limitation, current status, at therapy episode outset and at reporting intervals

	G8979	Mobility: walking & moving around functional limitation, projected goal status, at therapy episode outset, at reporting intervals, and at discharge or to end reporting
Ⓟ	**G8980**	Mobility: walking & moving around functional limitation, discharge status, at discharge from therapy or to end reporting
	G8981	Changing & maintaining body position functional limitation, current status, at therapy episode outset and at reporting intervals
	G8982	Changing & maintaining body position functional limitation, projected goal status, at therapy episode outset, at reporting intervals, and at discharge or to end reporting
Ⓟ	**G8983**	Changing & maintaining body position functional limitation, discharge status, at discharge from therapy or to end reporting
	G8984	Carrying, moving & handling objects functional limitation, current status, at therapy episode outset and at reporting intervals
	G8985	Carrying, moving and handling objects, projected goal status, at therapy episode outset, at reporting intervals, and at discharge or to end reporting
Ⓟ	**G8986**	Carrying, moving & handling objects functional limitation, discharge status, at discharge from therapy or to end reporting
	G8987	Self care functional limitation, current status, at therapy episode outset and at reporting intervals
	G8988	Self care functional limitation, projected goal status, at therapy episode outset, at reporting intervals, and at discharge or to end reporting
Ⓟ	**G8989**	Self care functional limitation, discharge status, at discharge from therapy or to end reporting
	G8990	Other physical or occupational therapy primary functional limitation, current status, at therapy episode outset and at reporting intervals
	G8991	Other physical or occupational therapy primary functional limitation, projected goal status, at therapy episode outset, at reporting intervals, and at discharge or to end reporting
Ⓟ	**G8992**	Other physical or occupational therapy primary functional limitation, discharge status, at discharge from therapy or to end reporting
	G8993	Other physical or occupational therapy subsequent functional limitation, current status, at therapy episode outset and at reporting intervals
	G8994	Other physical or occupational therapy subsequent functional limitation, projected goal status, at therapy episode outset, at reporting intervals, and at discharge or to end reporting
Ⓟ	**G8995**	Other physical or occupational therapy subsequent functional limitation, discharge status, at discharge from therapy or to end reporting
	G8996	Swallowing functional limitation, current status at therapy episode outset and at reporting intervals
	G8997	Swallowing functional limitation, projected goal status, at therapy episode outset, at

reporting intervals, and at discharge or to end reporting

G8998 Swallowing functional limitation, discharge status, at discharge from therapy or to end reporting

G8999 Motor speech functional limitation, current status at therapy episode outset and at reporting intervals

G9001 Coordinated care fee, initial rate

G9002 Coordinated care fee, maintenance rate

G9003 Coordinated care fee, risk adjusted high, initial

G9004 Coordinated care fee, risk adjusted low, initial

G9005 Coordinated care fee, risk adjusted maintenance

G9006 Coordinated care fee, home monitoring

G9007 Coordinated care fee, scheduled team conference

G9008 Coordinated care fee, physician coordinated care oversight services

G9009 Coordinated care fee, risk adjusted maintenance, level 3

G9010 Coordinated care fee, risk adjusted maintenance, level 4

G9011 Coordinated care fee, risk adjusted maintenance, level 5

G9012 Other specified case management service not elsewhere classified

G9013 Esrd demo basic bundle level i

G9014 Esrd demo expanded bundle including venous access and related services

G9016 Smoking cessation counseling, individual, in the absence of or in addition to any other evaluation and management service, per session (6-10 minutes) [demo project code only]

G9017 Amantadine hydrochloride, oral, per 100 mg (for use in a medicare-approved demonstration project)

G9018 Zanamivir, inhalation powder, administered through inhaler, per 10 mg (for use in a medicare-approved demonstration project)

G9019 Oseltamivir phosphate, oral, per 75 mg (for use in a medicare-approved demonstration project)

G9020 Rimantadine hydrochloride, oral, per 100 mg (for use in a medicare-approved demonstration project)

G9033 Amantadine hydrochloride, oral brand, per 100 mg (for use in a medicare-approved demonstration project)

G9034 Zanamivir, inhalation powder, administered through inhaler, brand, per 10 mg (for use in a medicare-approved demonstration project)

G9035 Oseltamivir phosphate, oral, brand, per 75 mg (for use in a medicare-approved demonstration project)

G9036 Rimantadine hydrochloride, oral, brand, per 100 mg (for use in a medicare-approved demonstration project)

Oncology

G9050 Oncology; primary focus of visit; work-up, evaluation, or staging at the time of cancer diagnosis or recurrence (for use in a medicare-approved demonstration project)

G9051 Oncology; primary focus of visit; treatment decision-making after disease is staged or restaged, discussion of treatment options, supervising/coordinating active cancer directed therapy or managing consequences of cancer directed therapy (for use in a medicare-approved demonstration project)

G9052 Oncology; primary focus of visit; surveillance for disease recurrence for patient who has completed definitive cancer-directed therapy and currently lacks evidence of recurrent disease; cancer directed therapy might be considered in the future (for use in a medicare-approved demonstration project)

G9053 Oncology; primary focus of visit; expectant management of patient with evidence of cancer for whom no cancer directed therapy is being administered or arranged at present; cancer directed therapy might be considered in the future (for use in a medicare-approved demonstration project)

G9054 Oncology; primary focus of visit; supervising, coordinating or managing care of patient with terminal cancer or for whom other medical illness prevents further cancer treatment; includes symptom management, end-of-life care planning, management of palliative therapies (for use in a medicare-approved demonstration project)

G9055 Oncology; primary focus of visit; other, unspecified service not otherwise listed (for use in a medicare-approved demonstration project)

G9056 Oncology; practice guidelines; management adheres to guidelines (for use in a medicare-approved demonstration project)

G9057 Oncology; practice guidelines; management differs from guidelines as a result of patient enrollment in an institutional review board approved clinical trial (for use in a medicare-approved demonstration project)

G9058 Oncology; practice guidelines; management differs from guidelines because the treating physician disagrees with guideline recommendations (for use in a medicare-approved demonstration project)

G9059 Oncology; practice guidelines; management differs from guidelines because the patient, after being offered treatment consistent with guidelines, has opted for

alternative treatment or management, including no treatment (for use in a medicare-approved demonstration project)

G9060 Oncology; practice guidelines; management differs from guidelines for reason(s) associated with patient comorbid illness or performance status not factored into guidelines (for use in a medicare-approved demonstration project)

G9061 Oncology; practice guidelines; patient's condition not addressed by available guidelines (for use in a medicare-approved demonstration project)

G9062 Oncology; practice guidelines; management differs from guidelines for other reason(s) not listed (for use in a medicare-approved demonstration project)

G9063 Oncology; disease status; limited to non-small cell lung cancer; extent of disease initially established as stage i (prior to neo-adjuvant therapy, if any) with no evidence of disease progression, recurrence, or metastases (for use in a medicare-approved demonstration project)

G9064 Oncology; disease status; limited to non-small cell lung cancer; extent of disease initially established as stage ii (prior to neo-adjuvant therapy, if any) with no evidence of disease progression, recurrence, or metastases (for use in a medicare-approved demonstration project)

G9065 Oncology; disease status; limited to non-small cell lung cancer; extent of disease initially established as stage iii a (prior to neo-adjuvant therapy, if any) with no evidence of disease progression, recurrence, or metastases (for use in a medicare-approved demonstration project)

G9066 Oncology; disease status; limited to non-small cell lung cancer; stage iii b- iv at diagnosis, metastatic, locally recurrent, or progressive (for use in a medicare-approved demonstration project)

G9067 Oncology; disease status; limited to non-small cell lung cancer; extent of disease unknown, staging in progress, or not listed (for use in a medicare-approved demonstration project)

G9068 Oncology; disease status; limited to small cell and combined small cell/non-small cell; extent of disease initially established as limited with no evidence of disease progression, recurrence, or metastases (for use in a medicare-approved demonstration project)

G9069 Oncology; disease status; small cell lung cancer, limited to small cell and combined small cell/non-small cell; extensive stage at diagnosis, metastatic, locally recurrent, or progressive (for use in a medicare-approved demonstration project)

G9070 Oncology; disease status; small cell lung cancer, limited to small cell and combined small cell/non-small; extent of disease unknown, staging in progress, or not listed (for use in a medicare-approved demonstration project)

G9071 Oncology; disease status; invasive female breast cancer (does not include ductal carcinoma in situ); adenocarcinoma as predominant cell type; stage i or stage iia-iib; or t3, n1, m0; and er and/or pr positive; with no evidence of disease progression, recurrence, or metastases (for use in a medicare-approved demonstration project)

G9072 Oncology; disease status; invasive female breast cancer (does not include ductal carcinoma in situ); adenocarcinoma as predominant cell type; stage i, or stage iia-iib; or t3, n1, m0; and er and pr negative; with no evidence of disease progression, recurrence, or metastases (for use in a medicare-approved demonstration project)

G9073 Oncology; disease status; invasive female breast cancer (does not include ductal carcinoma in situ); adenocarcinoma as predominant cell type; stage IIIa-IIIb; and not t3, n1, m0; and er and/or pr positive; with no evidence of disease progression, recurrence, or metastases (for use in a medicare-approved demonstration project)

G9074 Oncology; disease status; invasive female breast cancer (does not include ductal carcinoma in situ); adenocarcinoma as predominant cell type; stage IIIa-IIIb; and not

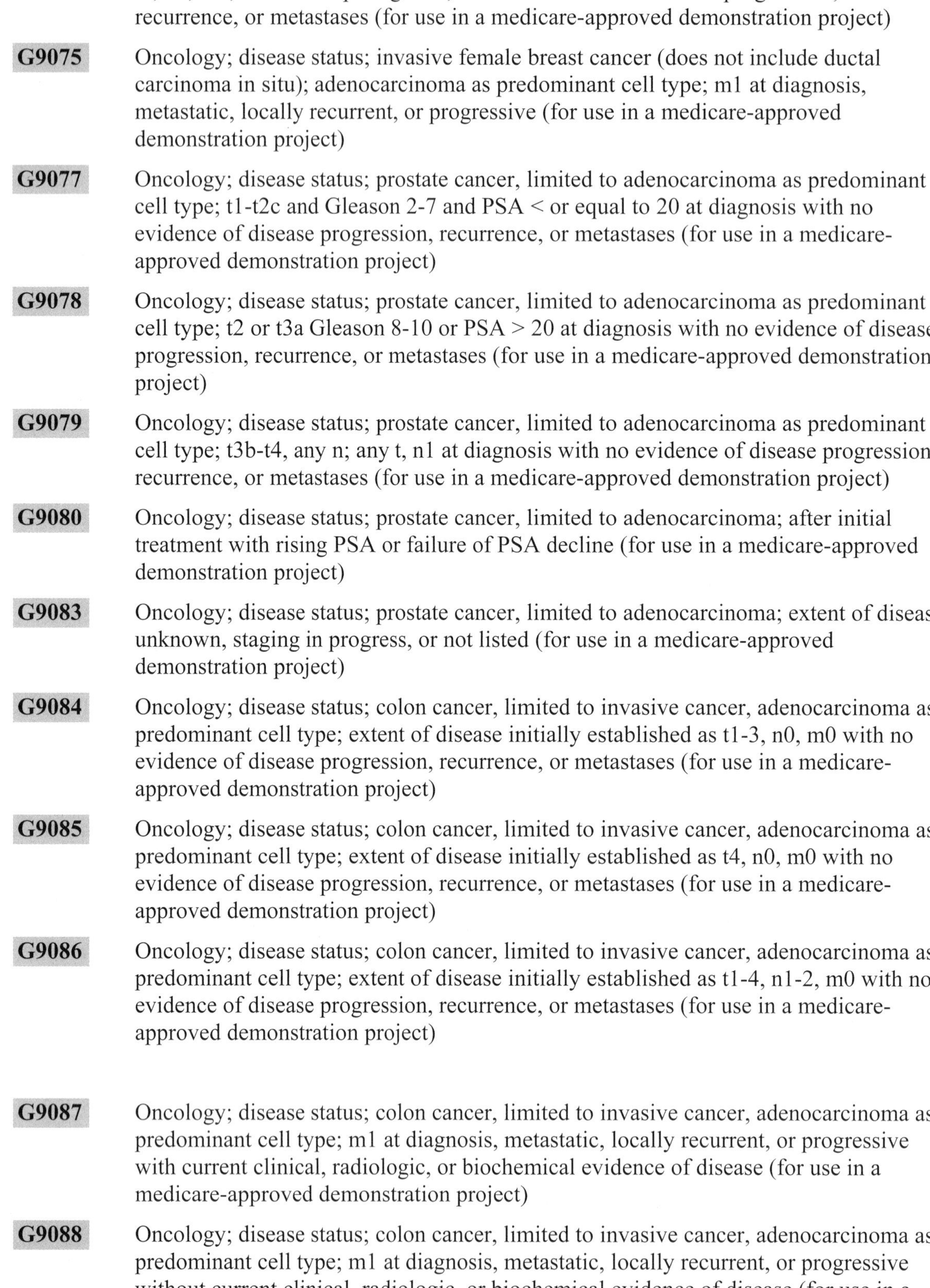

t3, n1, m0; and er and pr negative; with no evidence of disease progression, recurrence, or metastases (for use in a medicare-approved demonstration project)

G9075 Oncology; disease status; invasive female breast cancer (does not include ductal carcinoma in situ); adenocarcinoma as predominant cell type; m1 at diagnosis, metastatic, locally recurrent, or progressive (for use in a medicare-approved demonstration project)

G9077 Oncology; disease status; prostate cancer, limited to adenocarcinoma as predominant cell type; t1-t2c and Gleason 2-7 and PSA < or equal to 20 at diagnosis with no evidence of disease progression, recurrence, or metastases (for use in a medicare-approved demonstration project)

G9078 Oncology; disease status; prostate cancer, limited to adenocarcinoma as predominant cell type; t2 or t3a Gleason 8-10 or PSA > 20 at diagnosis with no evidence of disease progression, recurrence, or metastases (for use in a medicare-approved demonstration project)

G9079 Oncology; disease status; prostate cancer, limited to adenocarcinoma as predominant cell type; t3b-t4, any n; any t, n1 at diagnosis with no evidence of disease progression, recurrence, or metastases (for use in a medicare-approved demonstration project)

G9080 Oncology; disease status; prostate cancer, limited to adenocarcinoma; after initial treatment with rising PSA or failure of PSA decline (for use in a medicare-approved demonstration project)

G9083 Oncology; disease status; prostate cancer, limited to adenocarcinoma; extent of disease unknown, staging in progress, or not listed (for use in a medicare-approved demonstration project)

G9084 Oncology; disease status; colon cancer, limited to invasive cancer, adenocarcinoma as predominant cell type; extent of disease initially established as t1-3, n0, m0 with no evidence of disease progression, recurrence, or metastases (for use in a medicare-approved demonstration project)

G9085 Oncology; disease status; colon cancer, limited to invasive cancer, adenocarcinoma as predominant cell type; extent of disease initially established as t4, n0, m0 with no evidence of disease progression, recurrence, or metastases (for use in a medicare-approved demonstration project)

G9086 Oncology; disease status; colon cancer, limited to invasive cancer, adenocarcinoma as predominant cell type; extent of disease initially established as t1-4, n1-2, m0 with no evidence of disease progression, recurrence, or metastases (for use in a medicare-approved demonstration project)

G9087 Oncology; disease status; colon cancer, limited to invasive cancer, adenocarcinoma as predominant cell type; m1 at diagnosis, metastatic, locally recurrent, or progressive with current clinical, radiologic, or biochemical evidence of disease (for use in a medicare-approved demonstration project)

G9088 Oncology; disease status; colon cancer, limited to invasive cancer, adenocarcinoma as predominant cell type; m1 at diagnosis, metastatic, locally recurrent, or progressive without current clinical, radiologic, or biochemical evidence of disease (for use in a medicare-approved demonstration project)

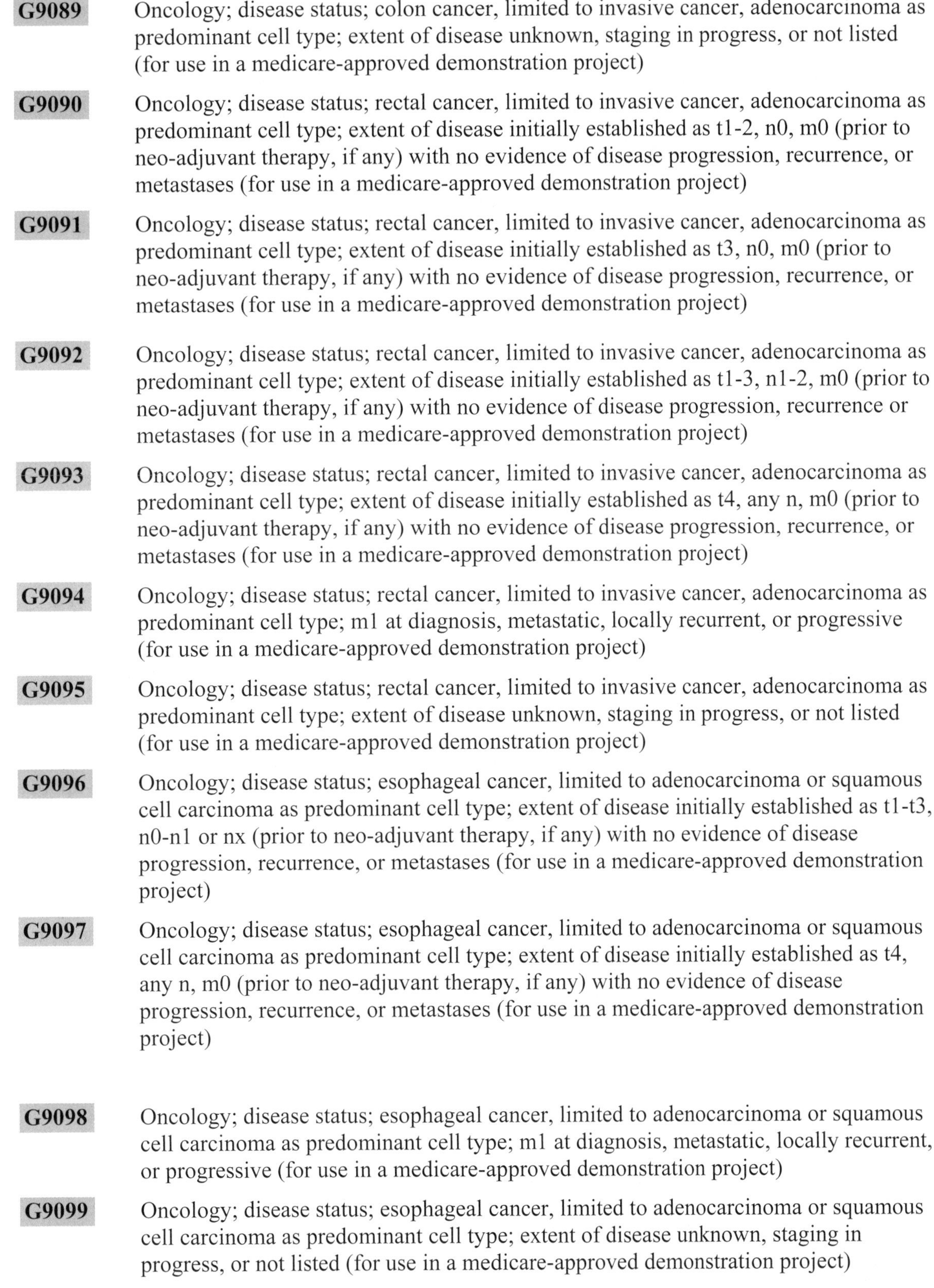

G9089 Oncology; disease status; colon cancer, limited to invasive cancer, adenocarcinoma as predominant cell type; extent of disease unknown, staging in progress, or not listed (for use in a medicare-approved demonstration project)

G9090 Oncology; disease status; rectal cancer, limited to invasive cancer, adenocarcinoma as predominant cell type; extent of disease initially established as t1-2, n0, m0 (prior to neo-adjuvant therapy, if any) with no evidence of disease progression, recurrence, or metastases (for use in a medicare-approved demonstration project)

G9091 Oncology; disease status; rectal cancer, limited to invasive cancer, adenocarcinoma as predominant cell type; extent of disease initially established as t3, n0, m0 (prior to neo-adjuvant therapy, if any) with no evidence of disease progression, recurrence, or metastases (for use in a medicare-approved demonstration project)

G9092 Oncology; disease status; rectal cancer, limited to invasive cancer, adenocarcinoma as predominant cell type; extent of disease initially established as t1-3, n1-2, m0 (prior to neo-adjuvant therapy, if any) with no evidence of disease progression, recurrence or metastases (for use in a medicare-approved demonstration project)

G9093 Oncology; disease status; rectal cancer, limited to invasive cancer, adenocarcinoma as predominant cell type; extent of disease initially established as t4, any n, m0 (prior to neo-adjuvant therapy, if any) with no evidence of disease progression, recurrence, or metastases (for use in a medicare-approved demonstration project)

G9094 Oncology; disease status; rectal cancer, limited to invasive cancer, adenocarcinoma as predominant cell type; m1 at diagnosis, metastatic, locally recurrent, or progressive (for use in a medicare-approved demonstration project)

G9095 Oncology; disease status; rectal cancer, limited to invasive cancer, adenocarcinoma as predominant cell type; extent of disease unknown, staging in progress, or not listed (for use in a medicare-approved demonstration project)

G9096 Oncology; disease status; esophageal cancer, limited to adenocarcinoma or squamous cell carcinoma as predominant cell type; extent of disease initially established as t1-t3, n0-n1 or nx (prior to neo-adjuvant therapy, if any) with no evidence of disease progression, recurrence, or metastases (for use in a medicare-approved demonstration project)

G9097 Oncology; disease status; esophageal cancer, limited to adenocarcinoma or squamous cell carcinoma as predominant cell type; extent of disease initially established as t4, any n, m0 (prior to neo-adjuvant therapy, if any) with no evidence of disease progression, recurrence, or metastases (for use in a medicare-approved demonstration project)

G9098 Oncology; disease status; esophageal cancer, limited to adenocarcinoma or squamous cell carcinoma as predominant cell type; m1 at diagnosis, metastatic, locally recurrent, or progressive (for use in a medicare-approved demonstration project)

G9099 Oncology; disease status; esophageal cancer, limited to adenocarcinoma or squamous cell carcinoma as predominant cell type; extent of disease unknown, staging in progress, or not listed (for use in a medicare-approved demonstration project)

G9100 Oncology; disease status; gastric cancer, limited to adenocarcinoma as predominant cell type; post r0 resection (with or without neoadjuvant therapy) with no evidence of disease recurrence, progression, or metastases (for use in a medicare-approved demonstration project)

G9101 Oncology; disease status; gastric cancer, limited to adenocarcinoma as predominant cell type; post r1 or r2 resection (with or without neoadjuvant therapy) with no evidence of disease progression, or metastases (for use in a medicare-approved demonstration project)

G9102 Oncology; disease status; gastric cancer, limited to adenocarcinoma as predominant cell type; clinical or pathologic m0, unresectable with no evidence of disease progression, or metastases (for use in a medicare-approved demonstration project)

G9103 Oncology; disease status; gastric cancer, limited to adenocarcinoma as predominant cell type; clinical or pathologic m1 at diagnosis, metastatic, locally recurrent, or progressive (for use in a medicare-approved demonstration project)

G9104 Oncology; disease status; gastric cancer, limited to adenocarcinoma as predominant cell type; extent of disease unknown, staging in progress, or not listed (for use in a medicare-approved demonstration project)

G9105 Oncology; disease status; pancreatic cancer, limited to adenocarcinoma as predominant cell type; post r0 resection without evidence of disease progression, recurrence, or metastases (for use in a medicare-approved demonstration project)

G9106 Oncology; disease status; pancreatic cancer, limited to adenocarcinoma; post r1 or r2 resection with no evidence of disease progression, or metastases (for use in a medicare-approved demonstration project)

G9107 Oncology; disease status; pancreatic cancer, limited to adenocarcinoma; unresectable at diagnosis, m1 at diagnosis, metastatic, locally recurrent, or progressive (for use in a medicare-approved demonstration project)

G9108 Oncology; disease status; pancreatic cancer, limited to adenocarcinoma; extent of disease unknown, staging in progress, or not listed (for use in a medicare-approved demonstration project)

G9109 Oncology; disease status; head and neck cancer, limited to cancers of oral cavity, pharynx and larynx with squamous cell as predominant cell type; extent of disease initially established as t1-t2 and n0, m0 (prior to neo-adjuvant therapy, if any) with no evidence of disease progression, recurrence, or metastases (for use in a medicare-approved demonstration project)

G9110 Oncology; disease status; head and neck cancer, limited to cancers of oral cavity, pharynx and larynx with squamous cell as predominant cell type; extent of disease initially established as t3-4 and/or n1-3, m0 (prior to neo-adjuvant therapy, if any) with no evidence of disease progression, recurrence, or metastases (for use in a medicare-approved demonstration project)

G9111 Oncology; disease status; head and neck cancer, limited to cancers of oral cavity, pharynx and larynx with squamous cell as predominant cell type; m1 at diagnosis, metastatic, locally recurrent, or progressive (for use in a medicare-approved demonstration project)

G9112 Oncology; disease status; head and neck cancer, limited to cancers of oral cavity, pharynx and larynx with squamous cell as predominant cell type; extent of disease unknown, staging in progress, or not listed (for use in a medicare-approved demonstration project)

G9113 Oncology; disease status; ovarian cancer, limited to epithelial cancer; pathologic stage ia-b (grade 1) without evidence of disease progression, recurrence, or metastases (for use in a medicare-approved demonstration project)

G9114 Oncology; disease status; ovarian cancer, limited to epithelial cancer; pathologic stage ia-b (grade 2-3); or stage ic (all grades); or stage ii; without evidence of disease progression, recurrence, or metastases (for use in a medicare-approved demonstration project)

G9115 Oncology; disease status; ovarian cancer, limited to epithelial cancer; pathologic stage iii-iv; without evidence of progression, recurrence, or metastases (for use in a medicare-approved demonstration project)

G9116 Oncology; disease status; ovarian cancer, limited to epithelial cancer; evidence of disease progression, or recurrence, and/or platinum resistance (for use in a medicare-approved demonstration project)

G9117 Oncology; disease status; ovarian cancer, limited to epithelial cancer; extent of disease unknown, staging in progress, or not listed (for use in a medicare-approved demonstration project)

G9123 Oncology; disease status; chronic myelogenous leukemia, limited to Philadelphia chromosome positive and/or bcr-abl positive; chronic phase not in hematologic, cytogenetic, or molecular remission (for use in a medicare-approved demonstration project)

G9124 Oncology; disease status; chronic myelogenous leukemia, limited to Philadelphia chromosome positive and/or bcr-abl positive; accelerated phase not in hematologic cytogenetic, or molecular remission (for use in a medicare-approved demonstration project)

G9125 Oncology; disease status; chronic myelogenous leukemia, limited to Philadelphia chromosome positive and/or bcr-abl positive; blast phase not in hematologic, cytogenetic, or molecular remission (for use in a medicare-approved demonstration project)

G9126 Oncology; disease status; chronic myelogenous leukemia, limited to Philadelphia chromosome positive and/or bcr-abl positive; in hematologic, cytogenetic, or molecular remission (for use in a medicare-approved demonstration project)

G9128 Oncology; disease status; limited to multiple myeloma, systemic disease; smoldering, stage i (for use in a medicare-approved demonstration project)

G9129 Oncology; disease status; limited to multiple myeloma, systemic disease; stage ii or higher (for use in a medicare-approved demonstration project)

G9130 Oncology; disease status; limited to multiple myeloma, systemic disease; extent of disease unknown, staging in progress, or not listed (for use in a medicare-approved demonstration project)

G9131 Oncology; disease status; invasive female breast cancer (does not include ductal carcinoma in situ); adenocarcinoma as predominant cell type; extent of disease unknown, staging in progress, or not listed (for use in a medicare-approved demonstration project)

G9132 Oncology; disease status; prostate cancer, limited to adenocarcinoma; hormone-refractory/androgen-independent (e.g., rising PSA on anti-androgen therapy or post-orchiectomy); clinical metastases (for use in a medicare-approved demonstration project)

G9133 Oncology; disease status; prostate cancer, limited to adenocarcinoma; hormone-responsive; clinical metastases or m1 at diagnosis (for use in a medicare-approved demonstration project)

G9134 Oncology; disease status; non-Hodgkin's lymphoma, any cellular classification; stage i, ii at diagnosis, not relapsed, not refractory (for use in a medicare-approved demonstration project)

G9135 Oncology; disease status; non-Hodgkin's lymphoma, any cellular classification; stage iii, iv, not relapsed, not refractory (for use in a medicare-approved demonstration project)

G9136 Oncology; disease status; non-Hodgkin's lymphoma, transformed from original cellular diagnosis to a second cellular classification (for use in a medicare-approved demonstration project)

G9137 Oncology; disease status; non-Hodgkin's lymphoma, any cellular classification; relapsed/refractory (for use in a medicare-approved demonstration project)

G9138 Oncology; disease status; non-Hodgkin's lymphoma, any cellular classification; diagnostic evaluation, stage not determined, evaluation of possible relapse or non-response to therapy, or not listed (for use in a medicare-approved demonstration project)

G9139 Oncology; disease status; chronic myelogenous leukemia, limited to Philadelphia chromosome positive and/or bcr-abl positive; extent of disease unknown, staging in progress, not listed (for use in a medicare-approved demonstration project)

G9140 Frontier extended stay clinic demonstration; for a patient stay in a clinic approved for the CMS demonstration project; the following measures should be present: the stay must be equal to or greater than 4 hours; weather or other conditions must prevent transfer or the case falls into a category of monitoring and observation cases that are permitted by the rules of the demonstration; there is a maximum frontier extended stay clinic (FESC) visit of 48 hours, except in the case when weather or other conditions prevent transfer; payment is made on each period up to 4 hours, after the first 4 hours

G9143 Warfarin responsiveness testing by genetic technique using any method, any number of specimen(s)

G9147 Outpatient intravenous insulin treatment (OIVIT) either pulsatile or continuous, by any means, guided by the results of measurements for: respiratory quotient; and/or, urine

urea nitrogen (UUN); and/or, arterial, venous or capillary glucose; and/or potassium concentration

G9148 National committee for quality assurance - level 1 medical home

G9149 National committee for quality assurance - level 2 medical home

G9150 National committee for quality assurance - level 3 medical home

G9151 Mapcp demonstration - state provided services

G9152 Mapcp demonstration - community health teams

G9153 Mapcp demonstration - physician incentive pool

G9156 Evaluation for wheelchair requiring face to face visit with physician

G9157 Transesophageal Doppler measurement of cardiac output (including probe placement, image acquisition, and interpretation per course of treatment) for monitoring purposes

Documentation and Reporting

G9158 Motor speech functional limitation, discharge status, at discharge from therapy or to end reporting

G9159 Spoken language comprehension functional limitation, current status at therapy episode outset and at reporting intervals

G9160 Spoken language comprehension functional limitation, projected goal status at therapy episode outset, at reporting intervals, and at discharge or to end reporting

G9161 Spoken language comprehension functional limitation, discharge status, at discharge from therapy or to end reporting

G9162 Spoken language expression functional limitation, current status at therapy episode outset and at reporting intervals

G9163 Spoken language expression functional limitation, projected goal status at therapy episode outset, at reporting intervals, and at discharge or to end reporting

G9164 Spoken language expression functional limitation, discharge status at discharge from therapy or to end reporting

G9165 Attention functional limitation, current status at therapy episode outset and at reporting intervals

G9166 Attention functional limitation, projected goal status at therapy episode outset, at reporting intervals, and at discharge or to end reporting

G9167 Attention functional limitation, discharge status at discharge from therapy or to end reporting

G9168 Memory functional limitation, current status at therapy episode outset and at reporting intervals

G9169 Memory functional limitation, projected goal status at therapy episode outset, at reporting intervals, and at discharge or to end reporting

G9170 Memory functional limitation, discharge status at discharge from therapy or to end reporting

G9171 Voice functional limitation, current status at therapy episode outset and at reporting intervals

G9172 Voice functional limitation, projected goal status at therapy episode outset, at reporting intervals, and at discharge or to end reporting

G9173 Voice functional limitation, discharge status at discharge from therapy or to end reporting

G9174 Other speech language pathology functional limitation, current status at therapy episode outset and at reporting intervals

G9175 Other speech language pathology functional limitation, projected goal status at therapy episode outset, at reporting intervals, and at discharge or to end reporting

G9176 Other speech language pathology functional limitation, discharge status at discharge from therapy or to end reporting

G9186 Motor speech functional limitation, projected goal status at therapy episode outset, at reporting intervals, and at discharge or to end reporting

G9187 Bundled payments for care improvement initiative home visit for patient assessment performed by a qualified health care professional for individuals not considered homebound including, but not limited to, assessment of safety, falls, clinical status, fluid status, medication reconciliation/management, patient compliance with orders/plan of care, performance of activities of daily living, appropriateness of care setting; (for use only in the Medicare-approved bundled payments for care improvement initiative); may not be billed for a 30-day period covered by a transitional care management code

Ⓟ **G9188** Beta-blocker therapy not prescribed, reason not given

Ⓟ **G9189** Beta-blocker therapy prescribed or currently being taken

Ⓟ **G9190** Documentation of medical reason(s) for not prescribing beta-blocker therapy (eg, allergy, intolerance, other medical reasons)

Ⓟ **G9191** Documentation of patient reason(s) for not prescribing beta-blocker therapy (eg, patient declined, other patient reasons)

Ⓟ **G9192** Documentation of system reason(s) for not prescribing beta-blocker therapy (eg, other reasons attributable to the health care system)

Ⓟ **G9196** Documentation of medical reason(s) for not ordering a first or second generation cephalosporin for antimicrobial prophylaxis (e.g., patients enrolled in clinical trials, patients with documented infection prior to surgical procedure of interest, patients who were receiving antibiotics more than 24 hours prior to surgery [except colon surgery patients taking oral prophylactic antibiotics], patients who were receiving antibiotics within 24 hours prior to arrival [except colon surgery patients taking oral prophylactic antibiotics], other medical reason(s))

Ⓟ **G9197** Documentation of order for first or second generation cephalosporin for antimicrobial prophylaxis

Ⓟ **G9198** Order for first or second generation cephalosporin for antimicrobial prophylaxis was not documented, reason not given

(**G9203** Code deleted December 31, 2016).

(**G9204** Code deleted December 31, 2016).

(**G9205** Code deleted December 31, 2016).

(**G9206** Code deleted December 31, 2016).

(**G9207** Code deleted December 31, 2016).

(**G9208** Code deleted December 31, 2016).

(**G9209** Code deleted December 31, 2016).

(**G9210** Code deleted December 31, 2016).

(**G9211** Code deleted December 31, 2016).

G9212 DSM-IV criteria for major depressive disorder documented at the initial evaluation

G9213 DSM-IV-tr criteria for major depressive disorder not documented at the initial evaluation, reason not otherwise specified

(**G9217** Code deleted December 31, 2016).

(**G9219** Code deleted December 31, 2016).

(**G9222** Code deleted December 31, 2016).

G9223 Pneumocystis jiroveci pneumonia prophylaxis prescribed within 3 months of low cd4+ cell count below 500 cells/mm3 or a cd4 percentage below 15%

G9225 Foot exam was not performed, reason not given

G9226 Foot examination performed (includes examination through visual inspection, sensory exam with 10-g monofilament plus testing any one of the following: vibration using 128-hz tuning fork, pinprick sensation, ankle reflexes, or vibration perception threshold, and pulse exam ? report when all of the 3 components are completed)

Ⓟ **G9227** Functional outcome assessment documented, care plan not documented, documentation the patient is not eligible for a care plan

Ⓟ **G9228** Chlamydia, gonorrhea and syphilis screening results documented (report when results are present for all of the 3 screenings)

▲Ⓟ **G9229** Chlamydia, gonorrhea, and syphilis screening results not documented (patient refusal is the only allowed exception)

Ⓟ **G9230** Chlamydia, gonorrhea, and syphilis not screened, reason not given

▲Ⓟ **G9231** Documentation of end stage renal disease (ESRD), dialysis, renal transplant before or during the measurement period or pregnancy during the measurement period

▲Ⓟ **G9232** Clinician treating major depressive disorder did not communicate to clinician treating comorbid condition for specified patient reason (e.g., patient is unable to communicate the diagnosis of a comorbid condition; the patient is unwilling to communicate the diagnosis of a comorbid condition; or the patient is unaware of the comorbid condition, or any other specified patient reason)

(**G9233** Code deleted December 31, 2016).

(**G9234** Code deleted December 31, 2016).

(**G9235** Code deleted December 31, 2016).

(**G9236** Code deleted December 31, 2016).

(**G9237** Code deleted December 31, 2016).

(**G9238** Code deleted December 31, 2016).

▲Ⓟ **G9239** Documentation of reasons for patient initiating maintenance hemodialysis with a catheter as the mode of vascular access (e.g., patient has a maturing AVF/avg, time-limited trial of hemodialysis, other medical reasons, patient declined AVF/avg, other patient reasons, patient followed by reporting nephrologist for fewer than 90 days, other system reasons)

Ⓟ **G9240** Patient whose mode of vascular access is a catheter at the time maintenance hemodialysis is initiated

Ⓟ **G9241** Patient whose mode of vascular access is not a catheter at the time maintenance hemodialysis is initiated

G9242 Documentation of viral load equal to or greater than 200 copies/ml or viral load not performed

(**G9244** Code deleted December 31, 2016).

(**G9245** Code deleted December 31, 2016).

G9245 Antiretroviral therapy prescribed

G9246 Patient did not have at least one medical visit in each 6 month period of the 24 month measurement period, with a minimum of 60 days between medical visits

G9247 Patient had at least one medical visit in each 6 month period of the 24 month measurement period, with a minimum of 60 days between medical visits

Ⓟ **G9250** Documentation of patient pain brought to a comfortable level within 48 hours from initial assessment

Ⓟ **G9251** Documentation of patient with pain not brought to a comfortable level within 48 hours from initial assessment

Ⓟ **G9254** Documentation of patient discharged to home later than post-operative day 2 following CAS

Ⓟ **G9255** Documentation of patient discharged to home no later than post operative day 2 following CAS

Ⓟ **G9256** Documentation of patient death following CAS

Ⓟ **G9257** Documentation of patient stroke following CAS

Ⓟ **G9258** Documentation of patient stroke following CEA

Ⓟ **G9259** Documentation of patient survival and absence of stroke following CAS

Ⓟ **G9260** Documentation of patient death following CEA

Ⓟ **G9261** Documentation of patient survival and absence of stroke following CEA

Ⓟ **G9262** Documentation of patient death in the hospital following endovascular aaa repair

Ⓟ **G9263** Documentation of patient survival in the hospital following endovascular aaa repair

Ⓟ **G9264** Documentation of patient receiving maintenance hemodialysis for greater than or equal to 90 days with a catheter for documented reasons (e.g., other medical reasons, patient declined AVF/avg, other patient reasons)

Ⓟ **G9265** Patient receiving maintenance hemodialysis for greater than or equal to 90 days with a catheter as the mode of vascular access

Ⓟ **G9266** Patient receiving maintenance hemodialysis for greater than or equal to 90 days without a catheter as the mode of vascular access

Ⓟ **G9267** Documentation of patient with one or more complications or mortality within 30 days

Ⓟ **G9268** Documentation of patient with one or more complications within 90 days

Ⓟ **G9269** Documentation of patient without one or more complications and without mortality within 30 days

Ⓟ **G9270** Documentation of patient without one or more complications within 90 days

G9273 Blood pressure has a systolic value of < 140 and a diastolic value of < 90

G9274 Blood pressure has a systolic value of =140 and a diastolic value of = 90 or systolic value < 140 and diastolic value = 90 or systolic value = 140 and diastolic value < 90

G9275 Documentation that patient is a current non-tobacco user

G9276 Documentation that patient is a current tobacco user

G9277 Documentation that the patient is on daily aspirin or anti-platelet or has documentation of a valid contraindication or exception to aspirin/anti-platelet; contraindications/exceptions include anti-coagulant use, allergy to aspirin or anti-platelets, history of gastrointestinal bleed and bleeding disorder; additionally, the following exceptions documented by the physician as a reason for not taking daily aspirin or anti-platelet are acceptable (use of non-steroidal anti-inflammatory agents, documented risk for drug interaction, uncontrolled hypertension defined as >180 systolic or >110 diastolic or gastroesophageal reflux)

G9278 Documentation that the patient is not on daily aspirin or anti-platelet regimen

G9279 Pneumococcal screening performed and documentation of vaccination received prior to discharge

G9280 Pneumococcal vaccination not administered prior to discharge, reason not specified

G9281 Screening performed and documentation that vaccination not indicated/patient refusal

G9282 Documentation of medical reason(s) for not reporting the histological type or NSCLC-nos classification with an explanation (e.g., biopsy taken for other purposes in a patient with a history of non-small cell lung cancer or other documented medical reasons)

G9283 Non small cell lung cancer biopsy and cytology specimen report documents classification into specific histologic type or classified as NSCLC-nos with an explanation

G9284 Non small cell lung cancer biopsy and cytology specimen report does not document classification into specific histologic type or classified as NSCLC-nos with an explanation

G9285 Specimen site other than anatomic location of lung or is not classified as non small cell lung cancer

Ⓟ **G9286** Antibiotic regimen prescribed within10 days after onset of symptoms

Ⓟ **G9287** Antibiotic regimen not prescribed within 10 days after onset of symptoms

G9288 Documentation of medical reason(s) for not reporting the histological type or NSCLC-nos classification with an explanation (e.g., a solitary fibrous tumor in a person with a history of non-small cell carcinoma or other documented medical reasons)

G9289 Non small cell lung cancer biopsy and cytology specimen report documents classification into specific histologic type or classified as NSCLC-nos with an explanation

G9290 Non small cell lung cancer biopsy and cytology specimen report does not document classification into specific histologic type or classified as NSCLC-nos with an explanation

G9291 Specimen site other than anatomic location of lung, is not classified as non small cell lung cancer or classified as NSCLC-nos

G9292 Documentation of medical reason(s) for not reporting pt category and a statement on thickness and ulceration and for pt1, mitotic rate (e.g., negative skin biopsies in a patient with a history of melanoma or other documented medical reasons)

G9293 Pathology report does not include the pt category and a statement on thickness and ulceration and for pt1, mitotic rate

G9294 Pathology report includes the pt category and a statement on thickness and ulceration and for pt1, mitotic rate

G9295 Specimen site other than anatomic cutaneous location

G9296 Patients with documented shared decision-making including discussion of conservative (non-surgical) therapy (e.g., NSAIDs, analgesics, weight loss, exercise, injections) prior to the procedure

G9297 Shared decision-making including discussion of conservative (non-surgical) therapy (e.g., NSAIDs, analgesics, weight loss, exercise, injections) prior to the procedure, not documented, reason not given

G9298 Patients who are evaluated for venous thromboembolic and cardiovascular risk factors within 30 days prior to the procedure (e.g. history of DVT, pe, mi, arrhythmia and stroke)

G9299 Patients who are not evaluated for venous thromboembolic and cardiovascular risk factors within 30 days prior to the procedure including (e.g., history of DVT, pe, mi, arrhythmia and stroke, reason not given)

G9300 Documentation of medical reason(s) for not completely infusing the prophylactic antibiotic prior to the inflation of the proximal tourniquet (e.g., a tourniquet was not used)

G9301 Patients who had the prophylactic antibiotic completely infused prior to the inflation of the proximal tourniquet

G9302 Prophylactic antibiotic not completely infused prior to the inflation of the proximal tourniquet, reason not given

G9303 Operative report does not identify the prosthetic implant specifications including the prosthetic implant manufacturer, the brand name of the prosthetic implant and the size of each prosthetic implant, reason not given

G9304 Operative report identifies the prosthetic implant specifications including the prosthetic implant manufacturer, the brand name of the prosthetic implant and the size of each prosthetic implant

G9305 Intervention for presence of leak of endoluminal contents through an anastomosis not required

G9306 Intervention for presence of leak of endoluminal contents through an anastomosis required

▲ **G9307** No return to the operating room for a surgical procedure, for complications of the principal operative procedure, within 30 days of the principal operative procedure

▲ **G9308** Unplanned return to the operating room for a surgical procedure, for complications of the principal operative procedure, within 30 days of the principal operative procedure

G9309 No unplanned hospital readmission within 30 days of principal procedure

G9310 Unplanned hospital readmission within 30 days of principal procedure

G9311 No surgical site infection

G9312 Surgical site infection

Ⓟ **G9313** Amoxicillin, with or without clavulanate, not prescribed as first line antibiotic at the time of diagnosis for documented reason (eg, cystic fibrosis, immotile cilia disorders, ciliary dyskinesia, immune deficiency, prior history of sinus surgery within the past 12 months, and anatomic abnormalities, such as deviated nasal septum, resistant organisms, allergy to medication, recurrent sinusitis, chronic sinusitis, or other reasons)

Ⓟ **G9314** Amoxicillin, with or without clavulanate, not prescribed as first line antibiotic at the time of diagnosis, reason not given

Ⓟ **G9315** Documentation amoxicillin, with or without clavulanate, prescribed as a first line antibiotic at the time of diagnosis

Ⓟ **G9316** Documentation of patient-specific risk assessment with a risk calculator based on multi-institutional clinical data, the specific risk calculator used, and communication of risk assessment from risk calculator with the patient or family

Ⓟ **G9317** Documentation of patient-specific risk assessment with a risk calculator based on multi-institutional clinical data, the specific risk calculator used, and communication of risk assessment from risk calculator with the patient or family not completed

G9318 Imaging study named according to standardized nomenclature

G9319 Imaging study not named according to standardized nomenclature, reason not given

(G9320 Code deleted December 31, 2015.)

G9321 Count of previous ct (any type of ct) and cardiac nuclear medicine (myocardial perfusion) studies documented in the 12-month period prior to the current study

G9322 Count of previous ct and cardiac nuclear medicine (myocardial perfusion) studies not documented in the 12-month period prior to the current study, reason not given

(G9323 Code deleted December 31, 2015.)

(G9324 Code deleted December 31, 2016).

(G9325 Code deleted December 31, 2015.)

▲ G9326 Ct studies performed not reported to a radiation dose index registry that is capable of collecting at a minimum all necessary data elements, reason not given

▲ G9327 Ct studies performed reported to a radiation dose index registry with all necessary data elements

(G9328 Code deleted December 31, 2015.)

G9329 DICOM format image data available to non-affiliated external healthcare facilities or entities on a secure, media free, reciprocally searchable basis with patient authorization for at least a 12-month period after the study not documented in final report, reason not given

G9340 Final report documented that DICOM format image data available to non-affiliated external healthcare facilities or entities on a secure, media free, reciprocally searchable basis with patient authorization for at least a 12-month period after the study

G9341 Search conducted for prior patient ct studies completed at non-affiliated external healthcare facilities or entities within the past 12-months and are available through a secure, authorized, media-free, shared archive prior to an imaging study being performed

G9342 Search not conducted prior to an imaging study being performed for prior patient ct studies completed at non-affiliated external healthcare facilities or entities within the past 12-months and are available through a secure, authorized, media-free, shared archive, reason not given

(G9343 Code deleted December 31, 2015.)

G9344 Due to system reasons search not conducted for DICOM format images for prior patient ct imaging studies completed at non-affiliated external healthcare facilities or entities within the past 12 months that are available through a secure, authorized, media-free, shared archive (e.g., non-affiliated external healthcare facilities or entities does not have archival abilities through a shared archival system)

G9345 Follow-up recommendations documented according to recommended guidelines for incidentally detected pulmonary nodules (e.g., follow-up ct imaging studies needed or that no follow-up is needed) based at a minimum on nodule size and patient risk factors

(G9346 Code deleted December 31, 2015.)

G9347 Follow-up recommendations not documented according to recommended guidelines for incidentally detected pulmonary nodules, reason not given

Ⓟ **G9348** Ct scan of the paranasal sinuses ordered at the time of diagnosis for documented reasons (eg, persons with sinusitis symptoms lasting at least 7 to 10 days, antibiotic resistance, immunocompromised, recurrent sinusitis, acute frontal sinusitis, acute sphenoid sinusitis, periorbital cellulitis, or other medical)

Ⓟ **G9349** Documentation of a ct scan of the paranasal sinuses ordered at the time of diagnosis or received within 28 days after date of diagnosis

Ⓟ **G9350** Ct scan of the paranasal sinuses not ordered at the time of diagnosis or received within 28 days after date of diagnosis

G9351 More than one ct scan of the paranasal sinuses ordered or received within 90 days after diagnosis

Ⓟ **G9352** More than one ct scan of the paranasal sinuses ordered or received within 90 days after the date of diagnosis, reason not given

Ⓟ **G9353** More than one ct scan of the paranasal sinuses ordered or received within 90 days after the date of diagnosis for documented reasons (eg, patients with complications, second ct obtained prior to surgery, other medical reasons)

Ⓟ **G9354** One ct scan or no ct scan of the paranasal sinuses ordered within 90 days after the date of diagnosis

Ⓟ **G9355** Elective delivery or early induction not performed

Ⓟ **G9356** Elective delivery or early induction performed

Ⓟ **G9357** Post-partum screenings, evaluations and education performed

Ⓟ **G9358** Post-partum screenings, evaluations and education not performed

▲Ⓟ **G9359** Documentation of negative or managed positive tb screen with further evidence that tb is not active within one year of patient visit

Ⓟ **G9360** No documentation of negative or managed positive tb screen

▲Ⓟ **G9361** Medical indication for induction [documentation of reason(s) for elective delivery (c-section) or early induction (e.g., hemorrhage and placental complications, hypertension, preeclampsia and eclampsia, rupture of membranes-premature or prolonged, maternal conditions complicating pregnancy/delivery, fetal conditions complicating pregnancy/ delivery, late pregnancy, prior uterine surgery, or participation in clinical trial)]

(**G9362** Code deleted December 31, 2015.)

(**G9363** Code deleted December 31, 2015.)

Ⓟ **G9364** Sinusitis caused by, or presumed to be caused by, bacterial infection

Ⓟ **G9365** One high-risk medication ordered

Ⓟ **G9366** One high-risk medication not ordered

Ⓟ **G9367** At least two different high-risk medications ordered

Ⓟ **G9368** At least two different high-risk medications not ordered

(**G9369** Code deleted December 31, 2015.)

(**G9370** Code deleted December 31, 2015.)

(**G9376** Code deleted December 31, 2015.)

(**G9377** Code deleted December 31, 2015.)

(**G9378** Code deleted December 31, 2015.)

(**G9379** Code deleted December 31, 2015.)

Ⓟ **G9380** Patient offered assistance with end of life issues during the measurement period

▲Ⓟ **G9381** Documentation of medical reason(s) for not offering assistance with end of life issues (e.g., patient in hospice care, patient in terminal phase) during the measurement period

Ⓟ **G9382** Patient not offered assistance with end of life issues during the measurement period

Ⓟ **G9383** Patient received screening for HCV infection within the 12 month reporting period

Ⓟ **G9384** Documentation of medical reason(s) for not receiving annual screening for HCV infection (e.g., decompensated cirrhosis indicating advanced disease [i.e., ascites, esophageal variceal bleeding, hepatic encephalopathy], hepatocellular carcinoma, waitlist for organ transplant, limited life expectancy, other medical reasons)

Ⓟ **G9385** Documentation of patient reason(s) for not receiving annual screening for HCV infection (e.g., patient declined, other patient reasons)

Ⓟ **G9386** Screening for HCV infection not received within the 12 month reporting period, reason not given

Ⓟ **G9389** Unplanned rupture of the posterior capsule requiring vitrectomy during cataract surgery

Ⓟ **G9390** No unplanned rupture of the posterior capsule requiring vitrectomy during cataract surgery

(**G9391** Code deleted December 31, 2015.)

(**G9392** Code deleted December 31, 2015.)

G9393 Patient with an initial phq-9 score greater than nine who achieves remission at twelve months as demonstrated by a twelve month (+/- 30 days) phq-9 score of less than five

G9394 Patient who had a diagnosis of bipolar disorder or personality disorder, death, permanent nursing home resident or receiving hospice or palliative care any time during the measurement or assessment period

G9395 Patient with an initial phq-9 score greater than nine who did not achieve remission at twelve months as demonstrated by a twelve month (+/- 30 days) phq-9 score greater than or equal to five

G9396 Patient with an initial phq-9 score greater than nine who was not assessed for remission at twelve months (+/- 30 days)

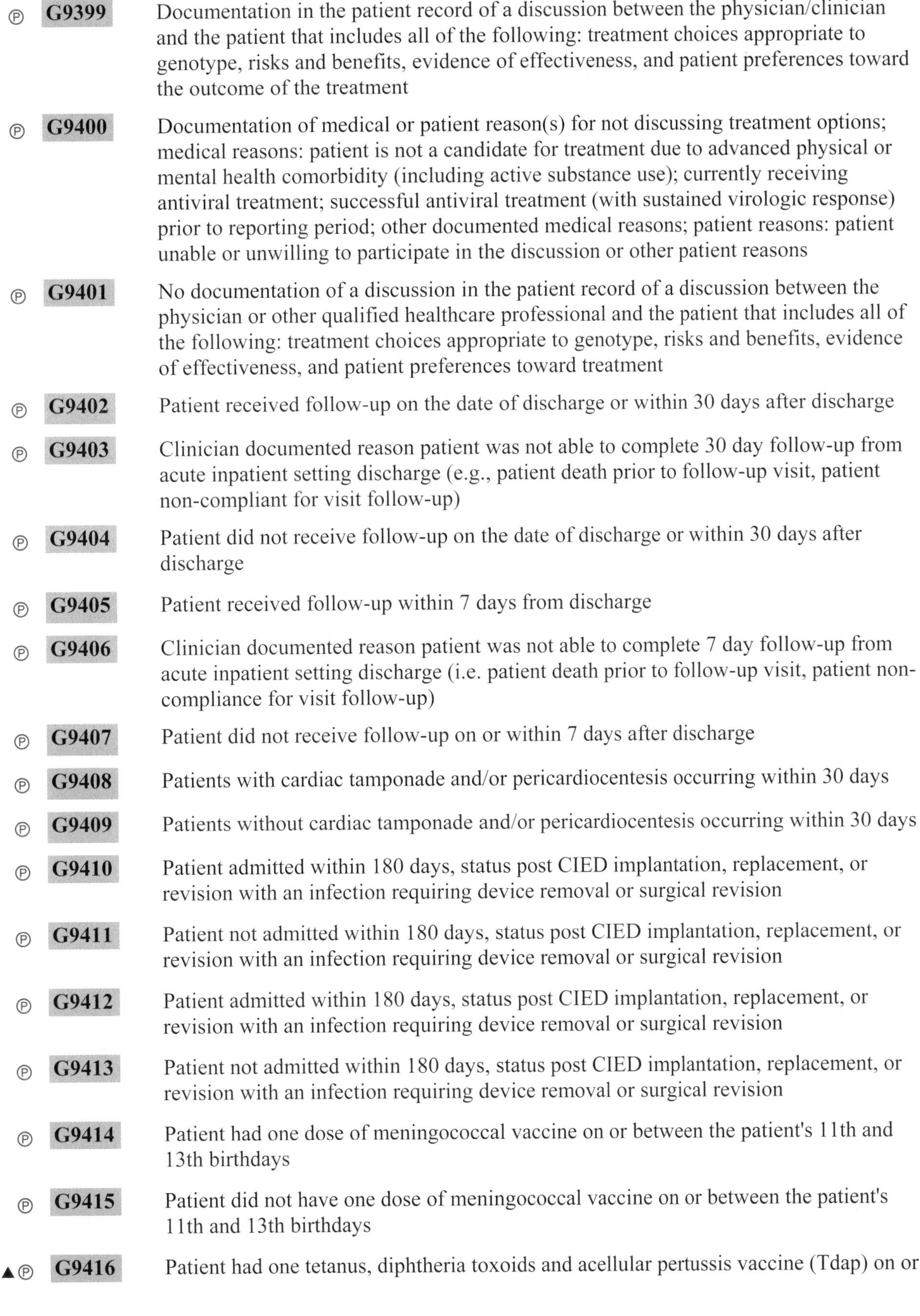

Ⓟ **G9399** Documentation in the patient record of a discussion between the physician/clinician and the patient that includes all of the following: treatment choices appropriate to genotype, risks and benefits, evidence of effectiveness, and patient preferences toward the outcome of the treatment

Ⓟ **G9400** Documentation of medical or patient reason(s) for not discussing treatment options; medical reasons: patient is not a candidate for treatment due to advanced physical or mental health comorbidity (including active substance use); currently receiving antiviral treatment; successful antiviral treatment (with sustained virologic response) prior to reporting period; other documented medical reasons; patient reasons: patient unable or unwilling to participate in the discussion or other patient reasons

Ⓟ **G9401** No documentation of a discussion in the patient record of a discussion between the physician or other qualified healthcare professional and the patient that includes all of the following: treatment choices appropriate to genotype, risks and benefits, evidence of effectiveness, and patient preferences toward treatment

Ⓟ **G9402** Patient received follow-up on the date of discharge or within 30 days after discharge

Ⓟ **G9403** Clinician documented reason patient was not able to complete 30 day follow-up from acute inpatient setting discharge (e.g., patient death prior to follow-up visit, patient non-compliant for visit follow-up)

Ⓟ **G9404** Patient did not receive follow-up on the date of discharge or within 30 days after discharge

Ⓟ **G9405** Patient received follow-up within 7 days from discharge

Ⓟ **G9406** Clinician documented reason patient was not able to complete 7 day follow-up from acute inpatient setting discharge (i.e. patient death prior to follow-up visit, patient non-compliance for visit follow-up)

Ⓟ **G9407** Patient did not receive follow-up on or within 7 days after discharge

Ⓟ **G9408** Patients with cardiac tamponade and/or pericardiocentesis occurring within 30 days

Ⓟ **G9409** Patients without cardiac tamponade and/or pericardiocentesis occurring within 30 days

Ⓟ **G9410** Patient admitted within 180 days, status post CIED implantation, replacement, or revision with an infection requiring device removal or surgical revision

Ⓟ **G9411** Patient not admitted within 180 days, status post CIED implantation, replacement, or revision with an infection requiring device removal or surgical revision

Ⓟ **G9412** Patient admitted within 180 days, status post CIED implantation, replacement, or revision with an infection requiring device removal or surgical revision

Ⓟ **G9413** Patient not admitted within 180 days, status post CIED implantation, replacement, or revision with an infection requiring device removal or surgical revision

Ⓟ **G9414** Patient had one dose of meningococcal vaccine on or between the patient's 11th and 13th birthdays

Ⓟ **G9415** Patient did not have one dose of meningococcal vaccine on or between the patient's 11th and 13th birthdays

▲Ⓟ **G9416** Patient had one tetanus, diphtheria toxoids and acellular pertussis vaccine (Tdap) on or between the patient's 10th and 13th birthdays

Ⓟ **G9417** Patient did not have one tetanus, diphtheria toxoids and acellular pertussis vaccine (Tdap) on or between the patient's 10th and 13th birthdays

Ⓟ **G9418** Primary non-small cell lung cancer biopsy and cytology specimen report documents classification into specific histologic type or classified as NSCLC-nos with an explanation
Ⓟ

Ⓟ **G9419** Documentation of medical reason(s) for not including the histological type or NSCLC-nos classification with an explanation (e.g., biopsy taken for other purposes in a patient with a history of primary non-small cell lung cancer or other documented medical reasons)

Ⓟ **G9420** Specimen site other than anatomic location of lung or is not classified as primary non-small cell lung cancer

Ⓟ **G9421** Primary non-small cell lung cancer biopsy and cytology specimen report does not document classification into specific histologic type or classified as NSCLC-nos with an explanation

Ⓟ **G9422** Primary lung carcinoma resection report documents pt category, pn category and for non-small cell lung cancer, histologic type (squamous cell carcinoma, adenocarcinoma and not NSCLC-nos)

Ⓟ **G9423** Documentation of medical reason for not including pt category, pn category and histologic type (for patient with appropriate exclusion criteria (e.g. metastatic disease, benign tumors, malignant tumors other than carcinomas, inadequate surgical specimens)

Ⓟ **G9424** Specimen site other than anatomic location of lung or classified as NSCLC-nos

Ⓟ **G9425** Primary lung carcinoma resection report does not document pt category, pn category and for non-small cell lung cancer, histologic type (squamous cell carcinoma, adenocarcinoma)

G9426 Improvement in median time from ed arrival to initial ed oral or parenteral pain medication administration performed for ed admitted patients

G9427 Improvement in median time from ed arrival to initial ed oral or parenteral pain medication administration not performed for ed admitted patients

G9428 Pathology report includes the pt category and a statement on thickness and ulceration and for pt1, mitotic rate

Ⓟ **G9429** Documentation of medical reason(s) for not including pt category and a statement on thickness and ulceration and for pt1, mitotic rate (e.g., negative skin biopsies in a patient with a history of melanoma or other documented medical reasons)

Ⓟ **G9430** Specimen site other than anatomic cutaneous location

Ⓟ **G9431** Pathology report does not include the pt category and a statement on thickness and ulceration and for pt1, mitotic rate

Ⓟ **G9432** Asthma well-controlled based on the act, c-act, acq, or ataq score and results documented

(**G9433** Code deleted December 31, 2015.)

Ⓟ **G9434** Asthma not well-controlled based on the act, c-act, acq, or ataq score, or specified asthma control tool not used, reason not given

(**G9435** Code deleted December 31, 2016).

(**G9436** Code deleted December 31, 2016).

(**G9437** Code deleted December 31, 2016).

(**G9438** Code deleted December 31, 2016).

(**G9439** Code deleted December 31, 2016).

(**G9440** Code deleted December 31, 2016).

(**G9441** Code deleted December 31, 2016).

(**G9442** Code deleted December 31, 2016).

(**G9443** Code deleted December 31, 2016).

Ⓟ **G9448** Patients who were born in the years 1945-1965

Ⓟ **G9449** History of receiving blood transfusions prior to 1992

Ⓟ **G9450** History of injection drug use

Ⓟ **G9451** Patient received one-time screening for HCV infection

Ⓟ **G9452** Documentation of medical reason(s) for not receiving one-time screening for HCV infection (e.g., decompensated cirrhosis indicating advanced disease [ie, ascites, esophageal variceal bleeding, hepatic encephalopathy], hepatocellular carcinoma, waitlist for organ transplant, limited life expectancy, other medical reasons)

Ⓟ **G9453** Documentation of patient reason(s) for not receiving one-time screening for HCV infection (e.g., patient declined, other patient reasons)

Ⓟ **G9454** One-time screening for HCV infection not received within 12 month reporting period and no documentation of prior screening for HCV infection, reason not given

Ⓟ **G9455** Patient underwent abdominal imaging with ultrasound, contrast enhanced ct or contrast MRI for hcc

Ⓟ **G9456** Documentation of medical or patient reason(s) for not ordering or performing screening for hcc. medical reason: comorbid medical conditions with expected survival < 5 years, hepatic decompensation and not a candidate for liver transplantation, or other medical reasons; patient reasons: patient declined or other patient reasons (e.g., cost of tests, time related to accessing testing equipment)

Ⓟ **G9457** Patient did not undergo abdominal imaging and did not have a documented reason for not undergoing abdominal imaging in the reporting period

Ⓟ **G9458** Patient documented as tobacco user and received tobacco cessation intervention (must include at least one of the following: advice given to quit smoking or tobacco use, counseling on the benefits of quitting smoking or tobacco use, assistance with or referral to external smoking or tobacco cessation support programs, or current enrollment in smoking or tobacco use cessation program) if identified as a tobacco user

Ⓟ **G9459** Currently a tobacco non-user

Ⓟ **G9460** Tobacco assessment or tobacco cessation intervention not performed, reason not given

(**G9463** Code deleted December 31, 2016).

(**G9464** Code deleted December 31, 2016).

(**G9465** Code deleted December 31, 2016).

(**G9466** Code deleted December 31, 2016).

(**G9467** Code deleted December 31, 2016).

G9468 Patient not receiving corticosteroids greater than or equal to 10 mg/day of prednisone equivalents for 60 or greater consecutive days or a single prescription equating to 600 mg prednisone or greater for all fills

Ⓟ **G9469** Patients who have received or are receiving corticosteroids greater than or equal to 10 mg/day of prednisone equivalents for 60 or greater consecutive days or a single prescription equating to 600 mg prednisone or greater for all fills

G9470 Patients not receiving corticosteroids greater than or equal to 10 mg/day of prednisone equivalents for 60 or greater consecutive days or a single prescription equating to 600 mg prednisone or greater for all fills

G9471 Within the past 2 years, central dual-energy x-ray absorptiometry (DXA) not ordered or documented

Ⓟ **G9472** Within the past 2 years, central dual-energy x-ray absorptiometry (DXA) not ordered and documented, no review of systems and no medication history or pharmacologic therapy (other than minerals/vitamins) for osteoporosis prescribed

G9473 Services performed by chaplain in the hospice setting, each 15 minutes

G9474 Services performed by dietary counselor in the hospice setting, each 15 minutes

G9475 Services performed by other counselor in the hospice setting, each 15 minutes

G9476 Services performed by volunteer in the hospice setting, each 15 minutes

G9477 Services performed by care coordinator in the hospice setting, each 15 minutes

G9478 Services performed by other qualified therapist in the hospice setting, each 15 minutes

G9479 Services performed by qualified pharmacist in the hospice setting, each 15 minutes

G9480 Admission to Medicare care choice model program (MCCM)

• **G9481** Remote in-home visit for the evaluation and management of a new patient for use only in the Medicare-approved comprehensive care for joint replacement model, which requires these 3 key components:

- a problem focused history;
- a problem focused examination; and
- straightforward medical decision making, furnished in real time using interactive

audio and video technology.

Counseling and coordination of care with other physicians, other qualified health care professionals or agencies are provided consistent with the nature of the problem(s) and the needs of the patient or the family or both. usually, the presenting problem(s) are self limited or minor. Typically, 10 minutes are spent with the patient or family or both via real time, audio and video intercommunications technology

• **G9482** Remote in-home visit for the evaluation and management of a new patient for use only in the Medicare-approved comprehensive care for joint replacement model, which requires these 3 key components:

- an expanded problem focused history;
- an expanded problem focused examination;
- straightforward medical decision making, furnished in real time using interactive audio and video technology.

Counseling and coordination of care with other physicians, other qualified health care professionals or agencies are provided consistent with the nature of the problem(s) and the needs of the patient or the family or both. usually, the presenting problem(s) are of low to moderate severity. Typically, 20 minutes are spent with the patient or family or both via real time, audio and video intercommunications technology

• **G9483** Remote in-home visit for the evaluation and management of a new patient for use only in the Medicare-approved comprehensive care for joint replacement model, which requires these 3 key components:

- a detailed history;
- a detailed examination;
- medical decision making of low complexity, furnished in real time using interactive audio and video technology.

Counseling and coordination of care with other physicians, other qualified health care professionals or agencies are provided consistent with the nature of the problem(s) and the needs of the patient or the family or both. usually, the presenting problem(s) are of moderate severity. Typically, 30 minutes are spent with the patient or family or both via real time, audio and video intercommunications technology

• **G9484** Remote in-home visit for the evaluation and management of a new patient for use only in the Medicare-approved comprehensive care for joint replacement model, which requires these 3 key components:

- a comprehensive history;
- a comprehensive examination;
- medical decision making of moderate complexity, furnished in real time using interactive audio and video technology.

Counseling and coordination of care with other physicians, other qualified health care professionals or agencies are provided consistent with the nature of the problem(s) and the needs of the patient or the family or both. usually, the presenting problem(s) are of moderate to high severity. Typically, 45 minutes are spent with the patient or family or both via real time, audio and video intercommunications technology

G9485 Remote in-home visit for the evaluation and management of a new patient for use only in the Medicare-approved comprehensive care for joint replacement model, which requires these 3 key components:

- a comprehensive history;
- a comprehensive examination;

- medical decision making of high complexity, furnished in real time using interactive audio and video technology.

Counseling and coordination of care with other physicians, other qualified health care professionals or agencies are provided consistent with the nature of the problem(s) and the needs of the patient or the family or both. usually, the presenting problem(s) are of moderate to high severity. Typically, 60 minutes are spent with the patient or family or both via real time, audio and video intercommunications technology

• **G9486** Remote in-home visit for the evaluation and management of an established patient for use only in the Medicare-approved comprehensive care for joint replacement model, which requires at least 2 of the following 3 key components:

- a problem focused history;
- a problem focused examination;
- straightforward medical decision making, furnished in real time using interactive audio and video technology.

Counseling and coordination of care with other physicians, other qualified health care professionals or agencies are provided consistent with the nature of the problem(s) and the needs of the patient or the family or both. usually, the presenting problem(s) are self limited or minor. Typically, 10 minutes are spent with the patient or family or both via real time, audio and video intercommunications technology

• **G9487** Remote in-home visit for the evaluation and management of an established patient for use only in the Medicare-approved comprehensive care for joint replacement model, which requires at least 2 of the following 3 key components:

- an expanded problem focused history;
- an expanded problem focused examination;
- medical decision making of low complexity, furnished in real time using interactive audio and video technology.

Counseling and coordination of care with other physicians, other qualified health care professionals or agencies are provided consistent with the nature of the problem(s) and the needs of the patient or the family or both. usually, the presenting problem(s) are of low to moderate severity. Typically, 15 minutes are spent with the patient or family or both via real time, audio and video intercommunications technology

• **G9488** Remote in-home visit for the evaluation and management of an established patient for use only in the Medicare-approved comprehensive care for joint replacement model, which requires at least 2 of the following 3 key components:

- a detailed history;
- a detailed examination;
- medical decision making of moderate complexity, furnished in real time using interactive audio and video technology.

Counseling and coordination of care with other physicians, other qualified health care professionals or agencies are provided consistent with the nature of the problem(s) and the needs of the patient or the family or both. usually, the presenting problem(s) are of moderate to high severity. Typically, 25 minutes are spent with the patient or family or both via real time, audio and video intercommunications technology

● **G9489** Remote in-home visit for the evaluation and management of an established patient for use only in the Medicare-approved comprehensive care for joint replacement model, which requires at least 2 of the following 3 key components:

- a comprehensive history;
- a comprehensive examination;
- medical decision making of high complexity, furnished in real time using interactive audio and video technology.

Counseling and coordination of care with other physicians, other qualified health care professionals or agencies are provided consistent with the nature of the problem(s) and the needs of the patient or the family or both. usually, the presenting problem(s) are of moderate to high severity. Typically, 40 minutes are spent with the patient or family or both via real time, audio and video intercommunications technology

● **G9490** Comprehensive Care for Joint Replacement model, home visit for patient assessment performed by clinical staff for an individual not considered homebound, including, but not necessarily limited to patient assessment of clinical status, safety/fall prevention, functional status/ambulation, medication reconciliation/management, compliance with orders/plan of care, performance of activities of daily living, and ensuring beneficiary connections to community and other services. (for use only in the Medicare-approved Comprehensive Care for Joint Replacement model); may not be billed for a 30 day period covered by a transitional care management code.

G9496 Documentation of reason for not detecting adenoma(s) or other neoplasm. (e.g., neoplasm detected is only diagnosed as traditional serrated adenoma, sessile serrated polyp, or sessile serrated adenoma

▲Ⓟ **G9497** Received instruction from the anesthesiologist or proxy prior to the day of surgery to abstain from smoking on the day of surgery

Ⓟ **G9498** Antibiotic regimen prescribed

(**G9499** Code deleted December 31, 2016).

▲ **G9500** Radiation exposure indices, or exposure time and number of fluorographic images in final report for procedures using fluoroscopy, documented

▲ **G9501** Radiation exposure indices, or exposure time and number of fluorographic images not documented in final report for procedure using fluoroscopy, reason not given

G9502 Documentation of medical reason for not performing foot exam (i.e., patients who have had either a bilateral amputation above or below the knee, or both a left and right amputation above or below the knee before or during the measurement period)

Ⓟ **G9503** Patient taking tamsulosin hydrochloride

Ⓟ **G9504** Documented reason for not assessing hepatitis b virus (HBV) status (e.g. patient not receiving a first course of anti-TNF therapy, patient declined) within one year prior to first course of anti-TNF therapy

Ⓟ **G9505** Antibiotic regimen prescribed within 10 days after onset of symptoms for documented medical reason

Ⓟ **G9506** Biologic immune response modifier prescribed

G9507 Documentation that the patient is on a statin medication or has documentation of a valid contraindication or exception to statin medications; contraindications/exceptions that can be defined by diagnosis codes include pregnancy during the measurement period, active liver disease, rhabdomyolysis, end stage renal disease on dialysis and heart failure; provider documented contraindications/exceptions include breastfeeding during the measurement period, woman of child-bearing age not actively taking birth control, allergy to statin, drug interaction (hiv protease inhibitors, nefazodone, cyclosporine, gemfibrozil, and danazol) and intolerance (with supporting documentation of trying a statin at least once within the last 5 years or diagnosis codes for myositis or toxic myopathy related to drugs)

G9508 Documentation that the patient is not on a statin medication

Ⓟ **G9509** Remission at twelve months as demonstrated by a twelve month (+/-30 days) phq-9 score of less than 5

Ⓟ **G9510** Remission at twelve months not demonstrated by a twelve month (+/-30 days) phq-9 score of less than five; either phq-9 score was not assessed or is greater than or equal to 5

Ⓟ **G9511** Index date phq-9 score greater than 9 documented during the twelve month denominator identification period

Ⓟ **G9512** Individual had a PDC of 0.8 or greater

Ⓟ **G9513** Individual did not have a PDC of 0.8 or greater

Ⓟ **G9514** Patient required a return to the operating room within 90 days of surgery

Ⓟ **G9515** Patient did not require a return to the operating room within 90 days of surgery

Ⓟ **G9516** Patient achieved an improvement in visual acuity, from their preoperative level, within 90 days of surgery

Ⓟ **G9517** Patient did not achieve an improvement in visual acuity, from their preoperative level, within 90 days of surgery, reason not given

G9518 Documentation of active injection drug use

▲Ⓟ **G9519** Patient achieves final refraction (spherical equivalent) +/- 0.5 diopters of their planned refraction within 90 days of surgery

▲Ⓟ **G9520** Patient does not achieve final refraction (spherical equivalent) +/- 0.5 diopters of their planned refraction within 90 days of surgery

Ⓟ **G9521** Total number of emergency department visits and inpatient hospitalizations less than two in the past 12 months

Ⓟ **G9522** Total number of emergency department visits and inpatient hospitalizations equal to or greater than two in the past 12 months or patient not screened, reason not given

Ⓟ **G9523** Patient discontinued from hemodialysis or peritoneal dialysis

Ⓟ **G9524** Patient was referred to hospice care

Ⓟ **G9525** Documentation of patient reason(s) for not referring to hospice care (e.g., patient declined, other patient reasons)

Ⓟ **G9526** Patient was not referred to hospice care, reason not given

Ⓟ **G9529** Patient with minor blunt head trauma had an appropriate indication(s) for a head ct

Ⓟ **G9530** Patient presented within 24 hours of a minor blunt head trauma with a GCS score of 15 and had a head ct ordered for trauma by an emergency care provider

▲Ⓟ **G9531** Patient has documentation of ventricular shunt, brain tumor, multisystem trauma, pregnancy, or is currently taking an antiplatelet medication including: asa/dipyridamole, clopidogrel, prasugrel, ticlopidine, ticagrelor or cilostazol)

▲Ⓟ **G9532** Patient's head injury occurred greater than 24 hours before presentation to the emergency department, or has a GCS score less than 15 or does not have a GCS score documented, or had a head ct for trauma ordered by someone other than an emergency care provider, or was ordered for a reason other than trauma

Ⓟ **G9533** Patient with minor blunt head trauma did not have an appropriate indication(s) for a head ct

Ⓟ **G9534** Advanced brain imaging (CTA, ct, MRA or MRI) was not ordered

Ⓟ **G9535** Patients with a normal neurological examination

Ⓟ **G9536** Documentation of medical reason(s) for ordering an advanced brain imaging study (i.e., patient has an abnormal neurological examination; patient has the coexistence of seizures, or both; recent onset of severe headache; change in the type of headache; signs of increased intracranial pressure (e.g., papilledema, absent venous pulsations on funduscopic examination, altered mental status, focal neurologic deficits, signs of meningeal irritation); hiv-positive patients with a new type of headache; immunocompromised patient with unexplained headache symptoms; patient on coagulopathy/anti-coagulation or anti-platelet therapy; very young patients with unexplained headache symptoms)

Ⓟ **G9537** Documentation of system reason(s) for ordering an advanced brain imaging study (i.e., needed as part of a clinical trial; other clinician ordered the study)

Ⓟ **G9538** Advanced brain imaging (CTA, ct, MRA or MRI) was ordered

Ⓟ **G9539** Intent for potential removal at time of placement

Ⓟ **G9540** Patient alive 3 months post procedure

Ⓟ **G9541** Filter removed within 3 months of placement

Ⓟ **G9542** Documented re-assessment for the appropriateness of filter removal within 3 months of placement

Ⓟ **G9543** Documentation of at least two attempts to reach the patient to arrange a clinical re-assessment for the appropriateness of filter removal within 3 months of placement

Ⓟ **G9544** Patients that do not have the filter removed, documented re-assessment for the appropriateness of filter removal, or documentation of at least two attempts to reach the patient to arrange a clinical re-assessment for the appropriateness of filter removal within 3 months of placement

▲Ⓟ **G9547** Incidental finding: liver lesion <= 0.5 cm, cystic kidney lesion < 1.0 cm or adrenal lesion <= 1.0 cm

Ⓟ **G9548** Final reports for abdominal imaging studies with follow-up imaging recommended

▲Ⓟ **G9549** Documentation of medical reason(s) that follow-up imaging is indicated (e.g., patient has a known malignancy that can metastasize, other medical reason(s) such as fever in an immunocompromised patient)

Ⓟ **G9550** Final reports for abdominal imaging studies with follow-up imaging not recommended

▲Ⓟ **G9551** Final reports for abdominal imaging studies without an incidentally found lesion noted: liver lesion <= 0.5 cm, cystic kidney lesion < 1.0 cm or adrenal lesion <= 1.0 cm noted or no lesion found

Ⓟ **G9552** Incidental thyroid nodule < 1.0 cm noted in report

G9553 Prior thyroid disease diagnosis

▲Ⓟ **G9554** Final reports for ct, CTA, MRI or MRA of the chest or neck or ultrasound of the neck with follow-up imaging recommended

▲Ⓟ **G9555** Documentation of medical reason(s) for recommending follow up imaging (e.g., patient has multiple endocrine neoplasia, patient has cervical lymphadenopathy, other medical reason(s))

▲Ⓟ **G9556** Final reports for ct, CTA, MRI or MRA of the chest or neck or ultrasound of the neck with follow-up imaging not recommended

▲Ⓟ **G9557** Final reports for ct, CTA, MRI or MRA studies of the chest or neck or ultrasound of the neck without an incidentally found thyroid nodule < 1.0 cm noted or no nodule found

Ⓟ **G9558** Patient treated with a beta-lactam antibiotic as definitive therapy

Ⓟ **G9559** Documentation of medical reason(s) for not prescribing a beta-lactam antibiotic (e.g., allergy, intolerance to beta -lactam antibiotics)

Ⓟ **G9560** Patient not treated with a beta-lactam antibiotic as definitive therapy, reason not given

Ⓟ **G9561** Patients prescribed opiates for longer than six weeks

Ⓟ **G9562** Patients who had a follow-up evaluation conducted at least every three months during opioid therapy

Ⓟ **G9563** Patients who did not have a follow-up evaluation conducted at least every three months during opioid therapy

(**G9572** Code deleted December 31, 2016).

Ⓟ **G9573** Remission at six months as demonstrated by a six month (+/-30 days) phq-9 score of less than five

Ⓟ **G9574** Remission at six months not demonstrated by a six month (+/-30 days) phq-9 score of less than five. either phq-9 score was not assessed or is greater than or equal to five

Ⓟ **G9577** Patients prescribed opiates for longer than six weeks

Ⓟ **G9578** Documentation of signed opioid treatment agreement at least once during opioid therapy

Ⓟ **G9579** No documentation of signed an opioid treatment agreement at least once during opioid therapy

Ⓟ **G9580** Door to puncture time of less than 2 hours

(**G9581** Code deleted December 31, 2016).

Ⓟ **G9582** Door to puncture time of greater than 2 hours, no reason given

Ⓟ **G9583** Patients prescribed opiates for longer than six weeks

▲Ⓟ **G9584** Patient evaluated for risk of misuse of opiates by using a brief validated instrument (e.g., opioid risk tool, soapp-r) or patient interviewed at least once during opioid therapy

Ⓟ **G9585** Patient not evaluated for risk of misuse of opiates by using a brief validated instrument (e.g., opioid risk tool, soaap-r) or patient not interviewed at least once during opioid therapy

Ⓟ **G9593** Pediatric patient with minor blunt head trauma classified as low risk according to the PECARN prediction rules

Ⓟ **G9594** Patient presented within 24 hours of a minor blunt head trauma with a GCS score of 15 and had a head ct ordered for trauma by an emergency care provider

▲Ⓟ **G9595** Patient has documentation of ventricular shunt, brain tumor, coagulopathy, including thrombocytopenia

▲Ⓟ **G9596** Pediatric patient's head injury occurred greater than 24 hours before presentation to the emergency department, or has a GCS score less than 15 or does not have a GCS score documented, or had a head ct for trauma ordered by someone other than an emergency care provider, or was ordered for a reason other than trauma

Ⓟ **G9597** Pediatric patient with minor blunt head trauma not classified as low risk according to the PECARN prediction rules

G9598 Aortic aneurysm 5.5 - 5.9 cm maximum diameter on centerline formatted ct or minor diameter on axial formatted ct

G9599 Aortic aneurysm 6.0 cm or greater maximum diameter on centerline formatted ct or minor diameter on axial formatted ct

Ⓟ **G9600** Symptomatic AAAS that required urgent/emergent (non-elective) repair

Ⓟ **G9601** Patient discharge to home no later than post-operative day #7

Ⓟ **G9602** Patient not discharged to home by post-operative day #7

Ⓟ **G9603** Patient survey score improved from baseline following treatment

Ⓟ **G9604** Patient survey results not available

Ⓟ **G9605** Patient survey score did not improve from baseline following treatment

Ⓟ **G9606** Intraoperative cystoscopy performed to evaluate for lower tract injury

▲ⓟ **G9607** Documented medical reasons for not performing intraoperative cystoscopy (e.g., urethral pathology precluding cystoscopy, any patient who has a congenital or acquired absence of the urethra)

ⓟ **G9608** Intraoperative cystoscopy not performed to evaluate for lower tract injury

▲ⓟ **G9609** Documentation of an order for anti-platelet agents

▲ⓟ **G9610** Documentation of medical reason(s) in the patient's record for not ordering anti-platelet agents

▲ⓟ **G9611** Order for anti-platelet agents was not documented in the patient's record, reason not given

ⓟ **G9612** Photodocumentation of one or more cecal landmarks to establish a complete examination

ⓟ **G9613** Documentation of post-surgical anatomy (e.g., right hemicolectomy, ileocecal resection, etc.)

ⓟ **G9614** No photodocumentation of cecal landmarks to establish a complete examination

ⓟ **G9615** Preoperative assessment documented

ⓟ **G9616** Documentation of reason(s) for not documenting a preoperative assessment (e.g., patient with a gynecologic or other pelvic malignancy noted at the time of surgery)

ⓟ **G9617** Preoperative assessment not documented, reason not given

ⓟ **G9618** Documentation of screening for uterine malignancy or those that had an ultrasound and/or endometrial sampling of any kind

(**G9619** Code deleted December 31, 2016).

ⓟ **G9620** Patient not screened for uterine malignancy, or those that have not had an ultrasound and/or endometrial sampling of any kind, reason not given

ⓟ **G9621** Patient identified as an unhealthy alcohol user when screened for unhealthy alcohol use using a systematic screening method and received brief counseling

ⓟ **G9622** Patient not identified as an unhealthy alcohol user when screened for unhealthy alcohol use using a systematic screening method

ⓟ **G9623** Documentation of medical reason(s) for not screening for unhealthy alcohol use (e.g., limited life expectancy, other medical reasons)

ⓟ **G9624** Patient not screened for unhealthy alcohol screening using a systematic screening method or patient did not receive brief counseling, reason not given

▲ⓟ **G9625** Patient sustained bladder injury at the time of surgery or discovered subsequently up to 1 month post-surgery

▲ⓟ **G9626** Documented medical reason for not reporting bladder injury (e.g., gynecologic or other pelvic malignancy documented, concurrent surgery involving bladder pathology, injury that occurs during urinary incontinence procedure, patient death from non-medical causes not related to surgery, patient died during procedure without evidence of bladder injury)

ⓟ **G9627** Patient did not sustained bladder injury at the time of surgery or subsequently up to 1 month post-surgery

▲Ⓟ **G9628** Patient sustained bowel injury at the time of surgery or discovered subsequently up to 1 month post-surgery

▲Ⓟ **G9629** Documented medical reasons for not reporting bowel injury (e.g., gynecologic or other pelvic malignancy documented, planned (e.g., not due to an unexpected bowel injury)

resection and/or re-anastomosis of bowel, or patient death from non-medical causes not related to surgery, patient died during procedure without evidence of bowel injury)

▲Ⓟ **G9630** Patient did not sustain a bowel injury at the time of surgery nor discovered subsequently up to 1 month post-surgery

Ⓟ **G9631** Patient sustained ureter injury at the time of surgery or discovered subsequently up to 1 month post-surgery

▲Ⓟ **G9632** Documented medical reasons for not reporting ureter injury (e.g., gynecologic or other pelvic malignancy documented, concurrent surgery involving bladder pathology, injury that occurs during a urinary incontinence procedure, patient death from non-medical causes not related to surgery, patient died during procedure without evidence of ureter injury)

▲Ⓟ **G9633** Patient did not sustain ureter injury at the time of surgery nor discovered subsequently up to 1 month post-surgery

Ⓟ **G9634** Health-related quality of life assessed with tool during at least two visits and quality of life score remained the same or improved

Ⓟ **G9635** Health-related quality of life not assessed with tool for documented reason(s) (e.g., patient has a cognitive or neuropsychiatric impairment that impairs his/her ability to complete the HRQOL survey, patient has the inability to read and/or write in order to complete the HRQOL questionnaire)

Ⓟ **G9636** Health-related quality of life not assessed with tool during at least two visits or quality of life score declined

Ⓟ **G9637** Final reports with documentation of one or more dose reduction techniques (e.g., automated exposure control, adjustment of the ma and/or kv according to patient size, use of iterative reconstruction technique)

Ⓟ **G9638** Final reports without documentation of one or more dose reduction techniques (e.g., automated exposure control, adjustment of the ma and/or kv according to patient size, use of iterative reconstruction technique)

Ⓟ **G9639** Major amputation or open surgical bypass not required within 48 hours of the index endovascular lower extremity revascularization procedure

Ⓟ **G9640** Documentation of planned hybrid or staged procedure

Ⓟ **G9641** Major amputation or open surgical bypass required within 48 hours of the index endovascular lower extremity revascularization procedure

▲Ⓟ **G9642** Current smokers (e.g., cigarette, cigar, pipe, e-cigarette or marijuana)

Ⓟ **G9643** Elective surgery

Ⓟ **G9644** Patients who abstained from smoking prior to anesthesia on the day of surgery or procedure

Ⓟ **G9645** Patients who did not abstain from smoking prior to anesthesia on the day of surgery or procedure

Ⓟ **G9646** Patients with 90 day MRS score of 0 to 2

Ⓟ **G9647** Patients in whom MRS score could not be obtained at 90 day follow-up

Ⓟ **G9648** Patients with 90 day MRS score greater than 2

Ⓟ **G9649** Psoriasis assessment tool documented meeting any one of the specified benchmarks (e.g., (pga; 6-point scale), body surface area (BSA), psoriasis area and severity index (PASI) and/or dermatology life quality index) (DLQI))

(**G9650** Code deleted December 31, 2016).

Ⓟ **G9651** Psoriasis assessment tool documented not meeting any one of the specified benchmarks (e.g., (pga; 6-point scale), body surface area (BSA), psoriasis area and severity index (PASI) and/or dermatology life quality index) (DLQI)) or psoriasis assessment tool not documented

(**G9652** Code deleted December 31, 2016).

(**G9653** Code deleted December 31, 2016).

Ⓟ **G9654** Monitored anesthesia care (mac)

Ⓟ **G9655** A transfer of care protocol or handoff tool/checklist that includes the required key handoff elements is used

Ⓟ **G9656** Patient transferred directly from anesthetizing location to PACU

(**G9657** Code deleted December 31, 2016).

Ⓟ **G9658** A transfer of care protocol or handoff tool/checklist that includes the required key handoff elements is not used

Ⓟ **G9659** Patients greater than 85 years of age who did not have a history of colorectal cancer or valid medical reason for the colonoscopy, including: iron deficiency anemia, lower gastrointestinal bleeding, Crohn's disease (i.e., regional enteritis), familial adenomatous polyposis, lynch syndrome (i.e., hereditary non-polyposis colorectal cancer), inflammatory bowel disease, ulcerative colitis, abnormal finding of gastrointestinal tract, or changes in bowel habits

Ⓟ **G9660** Documentation of medical reason(s) for a colonoscopy performed on a patient greater than 85 years of age (eg., last colonoscopy incomplete, last colonoscopy had inadequate prep, iron deficiency anemia, lower gastrointestinal bleeding, Crohn's disease (i.e., regional enteritis), familial history of adenomatous polyposis, lynch syndrome (i.e., hereditary non-polyposis colorectal cancer), inflammatory bowel disease, ulcerative colitis, abnormal finding of gastrointestinal tract, or changes in bowel habits)

Ⓟ **G9661** Patients greater than 85 years of age who received a routine colonoscopy for a reason other than the following: an assessment of signs/symptoms of GI tract illness, and/or the patient is considered high risk, and/or to follow-up on previously diagnoses advance lesions

Ⓟ **G9662** Previously diagnosed or have an active diagnosis of clinical ASCVD

Ⓟ **G9663** Any fasting or direct LDL-c laboratory test result = 190 mg/dl

Ⓟ **G9664** Patients who are currently statin therapy users or received an order (prescription) for statin therapy

Ⓟ **G9665** Patients who are not currently statin therapy users or did not receive an order (prescription) for statin therapy

Ⓟ **G9666** The highest fasting or direct LDL-c laboratory test result of 70?189 mg/dl in the measurement period or two years prior to the beginning of the measurement period

(**G9667** Code deleted December 31, 2016).

G9668 Documentation of medical reason (s) for not currently being a statin therapy user or receive an order (prescription) for statin therapy (e.g., patient with adverse effect, allergy or intolerance to statin medication therapy, patients who have an active diagnosis of pregnancy or who are breastfeeding, patients who are receiving palliative care, patients with active liver disease or hepatic disease or insufficiency, patients with end stage renal disease (ESRD), and patients with diabetes who have a fasting or direct LDL-c laboratory test result < 70 mg/dl and are not taking statin therapy)

G9669 I intend to report the multiple chronic conditions measures group

G9670 All quality actions for the applicable measures in the multiple chronic conditions measures group have been performed for this patient

(**G9671** Code deleted December 31, 2016).

(**G9672** Code deleted December 31, 2016).

(**G9673** Code deleted December 31, 2016).

G9674 Patients with clinical ASCVD diagnosis

G9675 Patients who have ever had a fasting or direct laboratory result of LDL-c = 190 mg/dl

G9676 Patients aged 40 to 75 years at the beginning of the measurement period with type 1 or type 2 diabetes and with an LDL-c result of 70?189 mg/dl recorded as the highest fasting or direct laboratory test result in the measurement year or during the two years prior to the beginning of the measurement period

(**G9677** Code deleted December 31, 2016).

• **G9678** Oncology Care Model (OCM) Monthly Enhanced Oncology Services (MEOS) payment for enhanced care management services for OCM beneficiaries. MEOS covers care management services for Medicare beneficiaries in a 6-month OCM Episode of Care triggered by the administration of chemotherapy. Enhanced care management services include services driven by the OCM practice requirements, including: 24/7 clinician access, use of an ONC-certified Electronic Health Record, utilization of data for quality improvement, patient navigation, documentation of care plans, and use of clinical guidelines. (G9678 may only be billed for OCM beneficiaries by OCM practitioners)

• **G9679** Onsite acute care treatment of a nursing facility resident with pneumonia. May only be billed once per day per beneficiary. (10/1/2016)

• **G9680** Onsite acute care treatment of a nursing facility resident with CHF. May only be billed once per day per beneficiary. (10/1/2016)

• **G9681** Onsite acute care treatment of a resident with COPD or asthma. May only be billed once per day per beneficiary. (10/1/2016)

- **G9682** Onsite acute care treatment a nursing facility resident with a skin infection. May only be billed once per day per beneficiary (10/1/2016)
- **G9683** Onsite acute care treatment of a nursing facility resident with fluid or electrolyte disorder or dehydration (similar pattern). May only be billed once per day per beneficiary. (10/1/2016)
- **G9684** Onsite acute care treatment of a nursing facility resident for a UTI. May only be billed once per day per beneficiary. (10/1/2016)
- **G9685** Evaluation and management of a beneficiary's acute change in condition in a nursing facility (10/1/2016)
- **G9686** Onsite nursing facility conference, that is separate and distinct from an evaluation and management visit, including qualified practitioner and at least one member of the nursing facility interdisciplinary care team
- **G9687** Hospice services provided to patient any time during the measurement period
- **G9688** Patients using hospice services any time during the measurement period
- **G9689** Patient admitted for performance of elective carotid intervention
- **G9690** Patient receiving hospice services any time during the measurement period
- **G9691** Patient had hospice services any time during the measurement period
- **G9692** Hospice services received by patient any time during the measurement period
- **G9693** Patient use of hospice services any time during the measurement period
- **G9694** Hospice services utilized by patient any time during the measurement period
- **G9695** Long-acting inhaled bronchodilator prescribed
- **G9696** Documentation of medical reason(s) for not prescribing a long-acting inhaled bronchodilator
- **G9697** Documentation of patient reason(s) for not prescribing a long-acting inhaled bronchodilator
- **G9698** Documentation of system reason(s) for not prescribing a long-acting inhaled bronchodilator
- **G9699** Long-acting inhaled bronchodilator not prescribed, reason not otherwise specified
- **G9700** Patients who use hospice services any time during the measurement period
- **G9701** Children who are taking antibiotics in the 30 days prior to the date of the encounter during which the diagnosis was established
- **G9702** Patients who use hospice services any time during the measurement period
- **G9703** Children who are taking antibiotics in the 30 days prior to the diagnosis of pharyngitis
- **G9704** AJCC breast cancer stage i: t1 mic or t1a documented
- **G9705** AJCC breast cancer stage i: t1b (tumor > 0.5 cm but <= 1 cm in greatest dimension) documented
- **G9706** Low (or very low) risk of recurrence, prostate cancer

- **G9707** Patient received hospice services any time during the measurement period
- **G9708** Women who had a bilateral mastectomy or who have a history of a bilateral mastectomy or for whom there is evidence of a right and a left unilateral mastectomy
- **G9709** Hospice services used by patient any time during the measurement period
- **G9710** Patient was provided hospice services any time during the measurement period
- **G9711** Patients with a diagnosis or past history of total colectomy or colorectal cancer
- **G9712** Documentation of medical reason(s) for prescribing or dispensing antibiotic (e.g., intestinal infection, pertussis, bacterial infection, lyme disease, otitis media, acute sinusitis, acute pharyngitis, acute tonsillitis, chronic sinusitis, infection of the pharynx/larynx/tonsils/adenoids, prostatitis, cellulitis/ mastoiditis/bone infections, acute lymphadenitis, impetigo, skin staph infections, pneumonia, gonococcal infections/ venereal disease (syphilis, chlamydia, inflammatory diseases [female reproductive organs]), infections of the kidney, cystitis/UTI, acne, HIV disease/asymptomatic hiv, cystic fibrosis, disorders of the immune system, malignancy neoplasms, chronic bronchitis, emphysema, bronchiectasis, extrinsic allergic alveolitis, chronic airway obstruction, chronic obstructive asthma, pneumoconiosis and other lung disease due to external agents, other diseases of the respiratory system, and tuberculosis
- **G9713** Patients who use hospice services any time during the measurement period
- **G9714** Patient is using hospice services any time during the measurement period
- **G9715** Patients who use hospice services any time during the measurement period
- **G9716** BMI is documented as being outside of normal limits, follow-up plan is not completed for documented reason
- **G9717** Documentation stating the patient has an active diagnosis of depression or has a diagnosed bipolar disorder, therefore screening or follow-up not required
- **G9718** Hospice services for patient provided any time during the measurement period
- **G9719** Patient is not ambulatory, bed ridden, immobile, confined to chair, wheelchair bound, dependent on helper pushing wheelchair, independent in wheelchair or minimal help in wheelchair
- **G9720** Hospice services for patient occurred any time during the measurement period
- **G9721** Patient not ambulatory, bed ridden, immobile, confined to chair, wheelchair bound, dependent on helper pushing wheelchair, independent in wheelchair or minimal help in wheelchair
- **G9722** Documented history of renal failure or baseline serum creatinine = 4.0 mg/dl; renal transplant recipients are not considered to have preoperative renal failure, unless, since transplantation the cr has been or is 4.0 or higher
- **G9723** Hospice services for patient received any time during the measurement period
- **G9724** Patients who had documentation of use of anticoagulant medications overlapping the measurement year
- **G9725** Patients who use hospice services any time during the measurement period
- **G9726** Patient refused to participate
- **G9727** Patient unable to complete the FOTO knee intake prom at admission and discharge due to

blindness, illiteracy, severe mental incapacity or language incompatibility and an adequate proxy is not available

- **G9728** Patient refused to participate
- **G9729** Patient unable to complete the FOTO hip intake prom at admission and discharge due to blindness, illiteracy, severe mental incapacity or language incompatibility and an adequate proxy is not available
- **G9730** Patient refused to participate
- **G9731** Patient unable to complete the FOTO foot or ankle intake prom at admission and discharge due to blindness, illiteracy, severe mental incapacity or language incompatibility and an adequate proxy is not available
- **G9732** Patient refused to participate
- **G9733** Patient unable to complete the FOTO lumbar intake prom at admission and discharge due to blindness, illiteracy, severe mental incapacity or language incompatibility and an adequate proxy is not available
- **G9734** Patient refused to participate
- **G9735** Patient unable to complete the FOTO shoulder intake prom at admission and discharge due to blindness, illiteracy, severe mental incapacity or language incompatibility and an adequate proxy is not available
- **G9736** Patient refused to participate
- **G9737** Patient unable to complete the FOTO elbow, wrist or hand intake prom at admission and discharge due to blindness, illiteracy, severe mental incapacity or language incompatibility and an adequate proxy is not available
- **G9738** Patient refused to participate
- **G9739** Patient unable to complete the FOTO general orthopedic intake prom at admission and discharge due to blindness, illiteracy, severe mental incapacity or language incompatibility and an adequate proxy is not available
- **G9740** Hospice services given to patient any time during the measurement period
- **G9741** Patients who use hospice services any time during the measurement period
- **G9742** Psychiatric symptoms assessed
- **G9743** Psychiatric symptoms not assessed, reason not otherwise specified
- **G9744** Patient not eligible due to active diagnosis of hypertension
- **G9745** Documented reason for not screening or recommending a follow-up for high blood pressure
- **G9746** Patient has mitral stenosis or prosthetic heart valves or patient has transient or reversible cause of af (e.g., pneumonia, hyperthyroidism, pregnancy, cardiac surgery)
- **G9747** Patient is undergoing palliative dialysis with a catheter
- **G9748** Patient approved by a qualified transplant program and scheduled to receive a living donor kidney transplant
- **G9749** Patient is undergoing palliative dialysis with a catheter

- **G9750** Patient approved by a qualified transplant program and scheduled to receive a living donor kidney transplant
- **G9751** Patient died at any time during the 24-month measurement period
- **G9752** Emergency surgery
- **G9753** Documentation of medical reason for not conducting a search for DICOM format images for prior patient ct imaging studies completed at non-affiliated external healthcare facilities or entities within the past 12 months that are available through a secure, authorized, media-free, shared archive (e.g., trauma, acute myocardial infarction, stroke, aortic aneurysm where time is of the essence)
- **G9754** A finding of an incidental pulmonary nodule
- **G9755** Documentation of medical reason(s) that follow-up imaging is indicated (e.g., patient has a known malignancy that can metastasize, other medical reason(s)
- **G9756** Surgical procedures that included the use of silicone oil
- **G9757** Surgical procedures that included the use of silicone oil
- **G9758** Patient in hospice and in terminal phase
- **G9759** History of preoperative posterior capsule rupture
- **G9760** Patients who use hospice services any time during the measurement period
- **G9761** Patients who use hospice services any time during the measurement period
- **G9762** Patient had at least three HPV vaccines on or between the patient's 9th and 13th birthdays
- **G9763** Patient did not have at least three HPV vaccines on or between the patient's 9th and 13th birthdays
- **G9764** Patient has been treated with an oral systemic or biologic medication for psoriasis
- **G9765** Documentation that the patient declined therapy change, has documented contraindications, or has not been treated with an oral systemic or biologic for at least six consecutive months (e.g., experienced adverse effects or lack of efficacy with all other therapy options) in order to achieve better disease control as measured by pga, bsa, pasi, or dlqi
- **G9766** Patients who are transferred from one institution to another with a known diagnosis of CVA for endovascular stroke treatment
- **G9767** Hospitalized patients with newly diagnosed CVA considered for endovascular stroke treatment
- **G9768** Patients who utilize hospice services any time during the measurement period
- **G9769** Patient had a bone mineral density test in the past two years or received osteoporosis medication or therapy in the past 12 months
- **G9770** Peripheral nerve block (PNB)
- **G9771** At least 1 body temperature measurement equal to or greater than 35.5 degrees celsius (or 95.9 degrees Fahrenheit) achieved within the 30 minutes immediately before or the 15 minutes immediately after anesthesia end time
- **G9772** Documentation of one of the following medical reason(s) for not achieving at least 1

body temperature measurement equal to or greater than 35.5 degrees celsius (or 95.9 degrees Fahrenheit) achieved within the 30 minutes immediately before or the 15 minutes immediately after anesthesia end time (e.g., emergency cases, intentional hypothermia, etc.)

• **G9773** At least 1 body temperature measurement equal to or greater than 35.5 degrees celsius (or 95.9 degrees Fahrenheit) not achieved within the 30 minutes immediately before or the 15 minutes immediately after anesthesia end time

• **G9774** Patients who have had a hysterectomy

• **G9775** Patient received at least 2 prophylactic pharmacologic anti-emetic agents of different classes preoperatively and/or intraoperatively

• **G9776** Documentation of medical reason for not receiving at least 2 prophylactic pharmacologic anti-emetic agents of different classes preoperatively and/or intraoperatively (e.g., intolerance or other medical reason)

• **G9777** Patient did not receive at least 2 prophylactic pharmacologic anti-emetic agents of different classes preoperatively and/or intraoperatively

• **G9778** Patients who have a diagnosis of pregnancy

• **G9779** Patients who are breastfeeding

• **G9780** Patients who have a diagnosis of rhabdomyolysis

• **G9781** Documentation of medical reason(s) for not currently being a statin therapy user or receive an order (prescription) for statin therapy (e.g., patient with adverse effect, allergy or intolerance to statin medication therapy, patients who are receiving palliative care, patients with active liver disease or hepatic disease or insufficiency, and patients with end stage renal disease (ESRD))

• **G9782** History of or active diagnosis of familial or pure hypercholesterolemia

• **G9783** Documentation of patients with diabetes who have a most recent fasting or direct LDL- c laboratory test result < 70 mg/dl and are not taking statin therapy

• **G9784** Pathologists/dermatopathologists providing a second opinion on a biopsy

• **G9785** Pathology report diagnosing cutaneous basal cell carcinoma or squamous cell carcinoma (to include in situ disease) sent from the pathologist/dermatopathologist to the biopsying clinician for review within 7 business days from the time when the tissue specimen was received by the pathologist

• **G9786** Pathology report diagnosing cutaneous basal cell carcinoma or squamous cell carcinoma (to include in situ disease) was not sent from the pathologist/dermatopathologist to the biopsying clinician for review within 7 business days from the time when the tissue specimen was received by the pathologist

• **G9787** Patient alive as of the last day of the measurement year

• **G9788** Most recent bp is less than or equal to 140/90 mm hg

• **G9789** Blood pressure recorded during inpatient stays, emergency room visits, urgent care visits, and patient self-reported bp's (home and health fair bp results)

• **G9790** Most recent bp is greater than 140/90 mm hg, or blood pressure not documented

• **G9791** Most recent tobacco status is tobacco free

- **G9792** Most recent tobacco status is not tobacco free
- **G9793** Patient is currently on a daily aspirin or other antiplatelet
- **G9794** Documentation of medical reason(s) for not on a daily aspirin or other antiplatelet (e.g. history of gastrointestinal bleed or intra-cranial bleed or documentation of active anticoagulant use during the measurement period
- **G9795** Patient is not currently on a daily aspirin or other antiplatelet
- **G9796** Patient is currently on a statin therapy
- **G9797** Patient is not on a statin therapy
- **G9798** Discharge(s) for AMI between July 1 of the year prior measurement year to June 30 of the measurement period
- **G9799** Patients with a medication dispensing event indicator of a history of asthma any time during the patient's history through the end of the measure period
- **G9800** Patients who are identified as having an intolerance or allergy to beta-blocker therapy
- **G9801** Hospitalizations in which the patient was transferred directly to a non-acute care facility for any diagnosis`
- **G9802** Patients who use hospice services any time during the measurement period
- **G9803** Patient prescribed a 180-day course of treatment with beta-blockers post discharge for AMI
- **G9804** Patient was not prescribed a 180-day course of treatment with beta-blockers post discharge for AMI
- **G9805** Patients who use hospice services any time during the measurement period
- **G9806** Patients who received cervical cytology or an HPV test
- **G9807** Patients who did not receive cervical cytology or an HPV test
- **G9808** Any patients who had no asthma controller medications dispensed during the measurement year
- **G9809** Patients who use hospice services any time during the measurement period
- **G9810** Patient achieved a PDC of at least 75% for their asthma controller medication
- **G9811** Patient did not achieve a PDC of at least 75% for their asthma controller medication
- **G9812** Patient died including all deaths occurring during the hospitalization in which the operation was performed, even if after 30 days, and those deaths occurring after discharge from the hospital, but within 30 days of the procedure
- **G9813** Patient did not die within 30 days of the procedure or during the index hospitalization
- **G9814** Death occurring during hospitalization
- **G9815** Death did not occur during hospitalization
- **G9816** Death occurring 30 days post procedure
- **G9817** Death did not occur 30 days post procedure
- **G9818** Documentation of sexual activity

- **G9819** Patients who use hospice services any time during the measurement period
- **G9820** Documentation of a chlamydia screening test with proper follow-up
- **G9821** No documentation of a chlamydia screening test with proper follow-up
- **G9822** Women who had an endometrial ablation procedure during the year prior to the index date (exclusive of the index date)
- **G9823** Endometrial sampling or hysteroscopy with biopsy and results documented
- **G9824** Endometrial sampling or hysteroscopy with biopsy and results not documented
- **G9825** Her-2/neu negative or undocumented/unknown
- **G9826** Patient transferred to practice after initiation of chemotherapy
- **G9827** Her2-targeted therapies not administered during the initial course of treatment
- **G9828** Her2-targeted therapies administered during the initial course of treatment
- **G9829** Breast adjuvant chemotherapy administered
- **G9830** Her-2/neu positive
- **G9831** AJCC stage at breast cancer diagnosis = ii or iii
- **G9832** AJCC stage at breast cancer diagnosis = i (ia or ib) and t-stage at breast cancer diagnosis does not equal = t1, t1a, t1b
- **G9833** Patient transfer to practice after initiation of chemotherapy
- **G9834** Patient has metastatic disease at diagnosis
- **G9835** Trastuzumab administered within 12 months of diagnosis
- **G9836** Reason for not administering trastuzumab documented (e.g. patient declined, patient died, patient transferred, contraindication or other clinical exclusion, neoadjuvant chemotherapy or radiation not complete)
- **G9837** Trastuzumab not administered within 12 months of diagnosis
- **G9838** Patient has metastatic disease at diagnosis
- **G9839** Anti-EGFR monoclonal antibody therapy
- **G9840** KRAS gene mutation testing performed before initiation of anti-EGFR MoAb
- **G9841** KRAS gene mutation testing not performed before initiation of anti-EGFR MoAb
- **G9842** Patient has metastatic disease at diagnosis
- **G9843** KRAS gene mutation
- **G9844** Patient did not receive anti-EGFR monoclonal antibody therapy
- **G9845** Patient received anti-EGFR monoclonal antibody therapy
- **G9846** Patients who died from cancer
- **G9847** Patient received chemotherapy in the last 14 days of life
- **G9848** Patient did not receive chemotherapy in the last 14 days of life

- **G9849** Patients who died from cancer
- **G9850** Patient had more than one emergency department visit in the last 30 days of life
- **G9851** Patient had one or less emergency department visits in the last 30 days of life
- **G9852** Patients who died from cancer
- **G9853** Patient admitted to the ICU in the last 30 days of life
- **G9854** Patient was not admitted to the ICU in the last 30 days of life
- **G9855** Patients who died from cancer
- **G9856** Patient was not admitted to hospice
- **G9857** Patient admitted to hospice
- **G9858** Patient enrolled in hospice
- **G9859** Patients who died from cancer
- **G9860** Patient spent less than three days in hospice care
- **G9861** Patient spent greater than or equal to three days in hospice care
- **G9862** Documentation of medical reason(s) for not recommending at least a 10 year follow-up interval (e.g., inadequate prep, familial or personal history of colonic polyps, patient had no adenoma and age is = 66 years old, or life expectancy < 10 years old, other medical reasons)

REHABILITATIVE SERVICES

Rehabilitative Services

H0001 Alcohol and/or drug assessment

H0002 Behavioral health screening to determine eligibility for admission to treatment program

H0003 Alcohol and/or drug screening; laboratory analysis of specimens for presence of alcohol and/or drugs

H0004 Behavioral health counseling and therapy, per 15 minutes

H0005 Alcohol and/or drug services; group counseling by a clinician

H0006 Alcohol and/or drug services; case management

H0007 Alcohol and/or drug services; crisis intervention (outpatient)

H0008 Alcohol and/or drug services; sub-acute detoxification (hospital inpatient)

H0009 Alcohol and/or drug services; acute detoxification (hospital inpatient)

H0010 Alcohol and/or drug services; sub-acute detoxification (residential addiction program inpatient)

H0011 Alcohol and/or drug services; acute detoxification (residential addiction program inpatient)

H0012 Alcohol and/or drug services; sub-acute detoxification (residential addiction program outpatient)

H0013 Alcohol and/or drug services; acute detoxification (residential addiction program outpatient)

H0014 Alcohol and/or drug services; ambulatory detoxification

H0015 Alcohol and/or drug services; intensive outpatient (treatment program that operates at least 3 hours/day and at least 3 days/week and is based on an individualized treatment plan), including assessment, counseling; crisis intervention, and activity therapies or education

H0016 Alcohol and/or drug services; medical/somatic (medical intervention in ambulatory setting)

H0017 Behavioral health; residential (hospital residential treatment program), without room and board, per diem

H0018 Behavioral health; short-term residential (non-hospital residential treatment program), without room and board, per diem

H0019 Behavioral health; long-term residential (non-medical, non-acute care in a residential treatment program where stay is typically longer than 30 days), without room and board, per diem

H0020 Alcohol and/or drug services; methadone administration and/or service (provision of the drug by a licensed program)

H0021 Alcohol and/or drug training service (for staff and personnel not employed by providers)

H0022 Alcohol and/or drug intervention service (planned facilitation)

H0023 Behavioral health outreach service (planned approach to reach a targeted population)

H0024 Behavioral health prevention information dissemination service (one-way direct or non-direct contact with service audiences to affect knowledge and attitude)

H0025 Behavioral health prevention education service (delivery of services with target population to affect knowledge, attitude and/or behavior)

H0026 Alcohol and/or drug prevention process service, community-based (delivery of services to develop skills of impactors)

H0027 Alcohol and/or drug prevention environmental service (broad range of external activities geared toward modifying systems in order to mainstream prevention through policy and law)

H0028 Alcohol and/or drug prevention problem identification and referral service (e.g., student assistance and employee assistance programs), does not include assessment

H0029 Alcohol and/or drug prevention alternatives service (services for populations that exclude alcohol and other drug use e.g., alcohol free social events)

H0030 Behavioral health hotline service

H0031 Mental health assessment, by non-physician

H0032 Mental health service plan development by non-physician

H0033 Oral medication administration, direct observation

H0034 Medication training and support, per 15 minutes

H0035 Mental health partial hospitalization, treatment, less than 24 hours

H0036 Community psychiatric supportive treatment, face-to-face, per 15 minutes

H0037 Community psychiatric supportive treatment program, per diem

H0038 Self-help/peer services, per 15 minutes

H0039 Assertive community treatment, face-to-face, per 15 minutes

H0040 Assertive community treatment program, per diem

H0041 Foster care, child, non-therapeutic, per diem

H0042 Foster care, child, non-therapeutic, per month

H0043 Supported housing, per diem

H0044 Supported housing, per month

H0045 Respite care services, not in the home, per diem

H0046 Mental health services, not otherwise specified

H0047 Alcohol and/or other drug abuse services, not otherwise specified

H0048 Alcohol and/or other drug testing: collection and handling only, specimens other than blood

H0049 Alcohol and/or drug screening

H0050 Alcohol and/or drug services, brief intervention, per 15 minutes

H1000 Prenatal care, at-risk assessment

H1001 Prenatal care, at-risk enhanced service; antepartum management

H1002 Prenatal care, at risk enhanced service; care coordination

H1003 Prenatal care, at-risk enhanced service; education

H1004 Prenatal care, at-risk enhanced service; follow-up home visit

H1005 Prenatal care, at-risk enhanced service package (includes h1001-h1004)

H1010 Non-medical family planning education, per session

H1011 Family assessment by licensed behavioral health professional for state defined purposes

H2000 Comprehensive multidisciplinary evaluation

H2001 Rehabilitation program, per 1/2 day

H2010 Comprehensive medication services, per 15 minutes

H2011 Crisis intervention service, per 15 minutes

H2012 Behavioral health day treatment, per hour

H2013 Psychiatric health facility service, per diem

H2014 Skills training and development, per 15 minutes

H2015 Comprehensive community support services, per 15 minutes

H2016 Comprehensive community support services, per diem

H2017 Psychosocial rehabilitation services, per 15 minutes

H2018 Psychosocial rehabilitation services, per diem

H2019 Therapeutic behavioral services, per 15 minutes

H2020 Therapeutic behavioral services, per diem

H2021 Community-based wrap-around services, per 15 minutes

H2022 Community-based wrap-around services, per diem

H2023 Supported employment, per 15 minutes

H2024 Supported employment, per diem

H2025 Ongoing support to maintain employment, per 15 minutes

H2026 Ongoing support to maintain employment, per diem

H2027 Psychoeducational service, per 15 minutes

H2028 Sexual offender treatment service, per 15 minutes

H2029 Sexual offender treatment service, per diem

H2030 Mental health clubhouse services, per 15 minutes

H2031 Mental health clubhouse services, per diem

H2032 Activity therapy, per 15 minutes

H2033 Multisystemic therapy for juveniles, per 15 minutes

H2034 Alcohol and/or drug abuse halfway house services, per diem

H2035 Alcohol and/or other drug treatment program, per hour

H2036 Alcohol and/or other drug treatment program, per diem

H2037 Developmental delay prevention activities, dependent child of client, per 15 minutes

DRUGS ADMINISTERED OTHER THAN ORAL METHOD

(EXCEPTION: ORAL IMMUNOSUPPRESSIVE DRUGS)

Guidelines

In addition to the information presented in the INTRODUCTION, several other items unique to this section are defined or identified here:

1. EXCEPTION: Oral immunosuppressive drugs are not included in this section.

2. ROUTE OF ADMINISTRATION: Unless otherwise specified, the drugs listed in this section may be injected either subcutaneously, intramuscularly or intravenously.

3. SUBSECTION INFORMATION: Some of the listed subheadings or subsections have special needs or instructions unique to that section. Where these are indicated, special "notes" will be presented preceding or following the listings. Those subsections within the DRUGS ADMINISTERED OTHER THAN ORAL METHOD section that have "notes" are as follows:

Subsection	Code Numbers
Drugs administered other than oral method	J0000-J8999
Immunosuppressive drugs	J7500-J7506
Chemotherapy drugs	J9000-J9999

4. UNLISTED SERVICE OR PROCEDURE: A service or procedure may be provided that is not listed in this edition of HCPCS. When reporting such a service, the appropriate "unlisted procedure" code may be used to indicate the service, identifying it by "special report" as defined below. HCPCS terminology is inconsistent in defining unlisted procedures. The procedure definition may include the term(s) "unlisted", "not otherwise classified", "unspecified", "unclassified", "other" and "miscellaneous". Prior to using these codes, try to determine if a Local Level III code or CPT code is available. The "unlisted procedures" and accompanying codes for DRUGS ADMINISTERED OTHER THAN ORAL METHOD are as follows:

   J3490 Unclassified drugs
   J9999 Not otherwise classified, antineoplastic drugs

5. SPECIAL REPORT: A service, material or supply that is rarely provided, unusual, variable or new may require a special report in determining medical appropriateness for reimbursement purposes. Pertinent information should include an adequate definition or description of the nature, extent, and need for the service, material or supply.

6. MODIFIERS: Listed services may be modified under certain circumstances. When appropriate, the modifying circumstance is identified by adding a modifier to the basic procedure code. CPT and HCPCS National Level II modifiers may be used with CPT and HCPCS National Level II procedure codes. Modifiers commonly used with DRUGS ADMINISTERED OTHER THAN ORAL METHOD are as follows:

   -AA Anesthesia services performed personally by anesthesiologist

-AD Medical supervision by a physician: more than four concurrent anesthesia procedures.

-CC Procedure code change (use "CC" when the procedure code submitted was changed either for administrative reasons or because an incorrect code was filed)

-G8 Monitored anesthesia care (MAC) for deep complex, complicated, or markedly invasive surgical procedure

-G9 Monitored anesthesia care (MAC) for patient who has history of severe cardio-pulmonary condition

-TC Technical component. Under certain circumstances, a charge may be made for the technical component alone. Under those circumstances, the technical component charge is identified by adding modifier -TC to the usual procedure code. Technical component charges are institutional charges and are not billed separately by physicians. However, portable x-ray suppliers bill only for the technical component and should use modifier -TC. The charge data from portable x-ray suppliers will then be used to build customary and prevailing profiles.

7. CPT CODE CROSS-REFERENCE: Unless otherwise specified, the equivalent CPT codes for all listings in this section fall within the range 90701-90799.

Drugs Administered Other Than Oral Method

The following list of drugs can be injected either subcutaneous, intramuscular, or intravenous. The brand name(s) of the drugs has been included as bold-type in brackets [ ] in some cases.

NOTE: Third party payers may wish to determine a threshold and pay up to a certain dollar limit before developing for the drug. Use procedure code J0110 for processing these cases.

J0120 Injection, tetracycline, up to 250 mg

MCM: 2049

J0129 Injection, abatacept, 10 mg (code may be used for Medicare when drug administered under the direct supervision of a physician, not for use when drug is self administered)

J0130 Injection abciximab, 10 mg

MCM: 2049

J0131 Injection, acetaminophen, 10 mg

J0132 Injection, acetylcysteine, 100 mg

J0133 Injection, acyclovir, 5 mg

J0135 Injection, adalimumab, 20 mg

J0153 Injection, adenosine, 1 mg (not to be used to report any adenosine phosphate compounds)

J0171 Injection, adrenalin, epinephrine, 0.1 mg

MCM: 2049

J0178 Injection, aflibercept, 1 mg

J0180 Injection, agalsidase beta, 1 mg

J0190 Injection, biperiden lactate, per 5 mg

MCM: 2049

J0200 Injection, alatrofloxacin mesylate, 100 mg

MCM: 2049.5

J0202 Injection, alemtuzumab, 1 mg

J0205 Injection, alglucerase, per 10 units

MCM: 2049

J0207 Injection, amifostine, 500 mg

MCM: 2049

J0210 Injection, methyldopate HCL, up to 250 mg

MCM: 2049

J0215 Injection, alefacept, 0.5 mg

J0220 Injection, alglucosidase alfa, 10 mg, not otherwise specified

J0221 Injection, alglucosidase alfa, (lumizyme), 10 mg

J0256 Injection, alpha 1 proteinase inhibitor (human), not otherwise specified, 10 mg

MCM: 2049

J0257 Injection, alpha 1 proteinase inhibitor (human), (glassia), 10 mg

MCM: 2049

J0270 Injection, alprostadil, 1.25 mcg (code may be used for Medicare when drug administered under the direct supervision of a physician, not for use when drug is self administered)

MCM: 2049

J0275 Alprostadil urethral suppository (code may be used for Medicare when drug administered under the direct supervision of a physician, not for use when drug is self administered)

MCM: 2049

J0278 Injection, amikacin sulfate, 100 mg

J0280 Injection, Aminophyllin, up to 250 mg

MCM: 2049

J0282 Injection, amiodarone hydrochloride, 30 mg

MCM: 2049

J0285 Injection, amphotericin b, 50 mg

MCM: 2049

J0287 Injection, amphotericin b lipid complex, 10 mg

MCM: 2049

J0288 Injection, amphotericin b cholesteryl sulfate complex, 10 mg
MCM: 2049

J0289 Injection, amphotericin b liposome, 10 mg
MCM: 2049

J0290 Injection, ampicillin sodium, 500 mg
MCM: 2049

J0295 Injection, ampicillin sodium/sulbactam sodium, per 1.5 gm
MCM: 2049

J0300 Injection, amobarbital, up to 125 mg
MCM: 2049

J0330 Injection, succinylcholine chloride, up to 20 mg
MCM: 2049

J0348 Injection, anidulafungin, 1 mg

J0350 Injection, anistreplase, per 30 units
MCM: 2049

J0360 Injection, hydralazine HCL, up to 20 mg
MCM: 2049

J0364 Injection, apomorphine hydrochloride, 1 mg

J0365 Injection, aprotinin, 10,000 kiu
MCM: 2049

J0380 Injection, metaraminol bitartrate, per 10 mg
MCM: 2049

J0390 Injection, chloroquine hydrochloride, up to 250 mg
MCM: 2049

J0395 Injection, arbutamine HCL, 1 mg
MCM: 2049

J0400 Injection, aripiprazole, intramuscular, 0.25 mg

J0401 Injection, aripiprazole, extended release, 1 mg

J0456 Injection, azithromycin, 500 mg
MCM: 2049.5

J0461 Injection, atropine sulfate, 0.01 mg
MCM: 2049

J0470 Injection, dimercaprol, per 100 mg
MCM: 2049

J0475 Injection, baclofen, 10 mg

MCM: 2049

J0476 Injection, baclofen, 50 mcg for intrathecal trial

MCM: 2049

J0480 Injection, basiliximab, 20 mg

MCM: 2049

J0485 Injection, Belatacept, 1 mg

J0490 Injection, belimumab, 10 mg

J0500 Injection, dicyclomine HCL, up to 20 mg

MCM: 2049

J0515 Injection, benztropine mesylate, per 1 mg

MCM: 2049

J0520 Injection, bethanechol chloride, Myotonachol or urecholine, up to 5 mg

MCM: 2049

J0558 Injection, penicillin g benzathine and penicillin g procaine, 100,000 units

J0561 Injection, penicillin g benzathine, 100,000 units

MCM: 2049

• **J0570** Buprenorphine implant, 74.2 mg

J0571 Buprenorphine/naloxone, oral, less than or equal to 3 mg buprenorphine

J0572 Buprenorphine/naloxone, oral, less than or equal to 3 mg buprenorphine

▲ **J0573** Buprenorphine/naloxone, oral, greater than 3 mg, but less than or equal to 6 mg buprenorphine

J0574 Buprenorphine/naloxone, oral, greater than 6 mg, but less than or equal to 10 mg buprenorphine

J0575 Buprenorphine/naloxone, oral, greater than 10 mg buprenorphine

J0583 Injection, bivalirudin, 1 mg

J0585 Injection, onabotulinumtoxinA, 1 unit

MCM: 2049

J0586 Injection, abobotulinumtoxinA, 5 units

J0587 Injection, rimabotulinumtoxinB, 100 units

MCM: 2049

J0588 Injection, incobotulinumtoxin a, 1 unit

J0592 Injection, buprenorphine hydrochloride, 0.1 mg

MCM: 2049

J0594 injection, busulfan, 1 mg

J0595 Injection, butorphanol tartrate, 1 mg

J0596 Injection, c1 esterase inhibitor (recombinant), ruconest, 10 units

J0597 Injection, c-1 esterase inhibitor (human), Berinert, 10 units

J0598 Injection, c-1 esterase inhibitor (human), Cinryze, 10 units

J0600 Injection, edetate calcium disodium, up to 1000 mg

MCM: 2049

J0610 Injection, calcium gluconate, per 10 ml

MCM: 2049

J0620 Injection, calcium glycerophosphate and calcium lactate, per 10 ml

MCM: 2049

J0630 Injection, calcitonin salmon, up to 400 units

MCM: 2049

J0636 Injection, calcitriol, 0.1 mcg

MCM: 2049

J0637 Injection, caspofungin acetate, 5 mg

J0638 Injection, canakinumab, 1 mg

J0640 Injection, leucovorin calcium, per 50 mg

MCM: 2049

J0641 Injection, levoleucovorin calcium, 0.5 mg

J0670 Injection, mepivacaine hydrochloride, per 10 ml

MCM: 2049

J0690 Injection, cefazolin sodium, 500 mg

MCM: 2049

J0692 Injection, cefepime hydrochloride, 500 mg

J0694 Injection, cefoxitin sodium, 1 gm

MCM: 2049,

J0695 Injection, Ceftolozane 50 mg and tazobactam 25 mg

J0696 Injection, ceftriaxone sodium, per 250 mg

MCM: 2049

J0697 Injection, sterile cefuroxime sodium, per 750 mg

MCM: 2049

J0698 Injection, cefotaxime sodium, per gm

MCM: 2049

J0702 Injection, betamethasone acetate 3 mg and betamethasone sodium phosphate 3 mg

MCM: 2049

J0706 Injection, caffeine citrate, 5 mg

J0710 Injection, cephapirin sodium, up to 1 gm

MCM: 2049

J0712 Injection, Ceftaroline fosamil, 10 mg

J0713 Injection, ceftazidime, per 500 mg

MCM: 2049

J0714 Injection, ceftazidime and Avibactam, 0.5 g/0.125 g

J0715 Injection, ceftizoxime sodium, per 500 mg

MCM: 2049

J0716 Injection, Centruroides immune f(ab)2, up to 120 milligrams

J0717 Injection, Certolizumab pegol, 1 mg (code may be used for Medicare when drug administered under the direct supervision of a physician, not for use when drug is self administered)

J0720 Injection, chloramphenicol sodium succinate, up to 1 gm

MCM: 2049

J0725 Injection, chorionic gonadotropin, per 1,000 USP units

MCM: 2049

J0735 Injection, clonidine hydrochloride, 1 mg

MCM: 2049

J0740 Injection, cidofovir, 375 mg

MCM: 2049

J0743 Injection, cilastatin sodium; imipenem, per 250 mg

MCM: 2049

J0744 Injection, ciprofloxacin for intravenous infusion, 200 mg

J0745 Injection, codeine phosphate, per 30 mg

MCM: 2049

(**J0760** Code deleted December 31, 2016).

J0770 Injection, colistimethate sodium, up to 150 mg

MCM: 2049

J0775 Injection, collagenase, clostridium histolyticum, 0.01 mg

J0780 Injection, prochlorperazine, up to 10 mg

MCM: 2049

J0795 Injection, corticorelin ovine triflutate, 1 microgram

MCM: 2049

J0800 Injection, corticotropin, up to 40 units

MCM: 2049

J0833 Injection, cosyntropin, not otherwise specified, 0.25 mg

J0834 Injection, cosyntropin (Cortrosyn), 0.25 mg

J0840 Injection, Crotalidae polyvalent immune fab (ovine), up to 1 gram

J0850 Injection, cytomegalovirus immune globulin intravenous (human), per vial

MCM: 2049

J0875 Injection, dalbavancin, 5mg

J0878 Injection, daptomycin, 1 mg

J0881 Injection, darbepoetin alfa, 1 microgram (non-ESRD use)

J0882 Injection, darbepoetin alfa, 1 microgram (for ESRD on dialysis)

MCM: 4273.1

• **J0883** Injection, argatroban, 1 mg (for non-ESRD use)

MCM: 2049, 4273.1

• **J0884** Injection, argatroban, 1 mg (for ESRD on dialysis)

MCM: 2049, 4273.1

J0885 Injection, epoetin alfa, (for non-ESRD use), 1000 units

MCM: 2049

(**J0886** Code deleted December 31, 2015.)

J0887 Injection, epoetin beta, 1 microgram, (for ESRD on dialysis)

J0888 Injection, epoetin beta, 1 microgram, (for non ESRD use)

J0890 Injection, Peginesatide, 0.1 mg (for ESRD on dialysis)

J0894 Injection, decitabine, 1 mg

J0895 Injection, deferoxamine mesylate, 500 mg

MCM: 2049,

J0897 Injection, denosumab, 1 mg

J0945 Injection, brompheniramine maleate, per 10 mg

MCM: 2049

J1000 Injection, depo-estradiol cypionate, up to 5 mg

MCM: 2049

J1020 Injection, methylprednisolone acetate, 20 mg

MCM: 2049

J1030 Injection, methylprednisolone acetate, 40 mg

MCM: 2049

J1040 Injection, methylprednisolone acetate, 80 mg

MCM: 2049

J1050 Injection, medroxyprogesterone acetate, 1 mg

J1071 Injection, testosterone cypionate, 1 mg

J1094 Injection, dexamethasone acetate, 1 mg

MCM: 2049

J1100 Injection, dexamethasone sodium phosphate, 1 mg

MCM: 2049

J1110 Injection, dihydroergotamine mesylate, per 1 mg

MCM: 2049

J1120 Injection, acetazolamide sodium, up to 500 mg

MCM: 2049

• **J1130** Injection, diclofenac sodium, 0.5 mg

J1160 Injection, digoxin, up to 0.5 mg

MCM: 2049

J1162 Injection, digoxin immune fab (ovine), per vial

MCM: 2049

J1165 Injection, phenytoin sodium, per 50 mg

MCM: 2049

J1170 Injection, hydromorphone, up to 4 mg

MCM: 2049

J1180 Injection, dyphylline, up to 500 mg

MCM: 2049

J1190 Injection, dexrazoxane hydrochloride, per 250 mg

MCM: 2049

J1200 Injection, diphenhydramine HCL, up to 50 mg

MCM: 2049

J1205 Injection, chlorothiazide sodium, per 500 mg

MCM: 2049

J1212 Injection, DMSO, dimethyl sulfoxide, 50%, 50 ml

CIM: 45-23

MCM: 2049

J1230 Injection, methadone HCL, up to 10 mg

MCM: 2049

J1240 Injection, dimenhydrinate, up to 50 mg
MCM: 2049

J1245 Injection, dipyridamole, per 10 mg
MCM: 15030, 2049

J1250 Injection, dobutamine hydrochloride, per 250 mg
MCM: 2049

J1260 Injection, dolasetron mesylate, 10 mg
MCM: 2049

J1265 Injection, dopamine HCL, 40 mg

J1267 Injection, doripenem, 10 mg

J1270 Injection, doxercalciferol, 1 mcg

J1290 Injection, ecallantide, 1 mg

J1300 Injection, eculizumab, 10 mg

J1320 Injection, amitriptyline HCL, up to 20 mg
MCM: 2049

J1322 Injection, elosulfase alfa, 1 mg

J1324 Injection, enfuvirtide, 1 mg

J1325 Injection, epoprostenol, 0.5 mg
MCM: 2049

J1327 Injection, eptifibatide, 5 mg
MCM: 2049

J1330 Injection, ergonovine maleate, up to 0.2 mg
MCM: 2049

J1335 Injection, ertapenem sodium, 500 mg

J1364 Injection, erythromycin lactobionate, per 500 mg
MCM: 2049

J1380 Injection, estradiol valerate, up to 10 mg
MCM: 2049

J1410 Injection, estrogen conjugated, per 25 mg
MCM: 2049

J1430 Injection, ethanolamine oleate, 100 mg
MCM: 2049

J1435 Injection, estrone, per 1 mg
MCM: 2049

J1436 Injection, etidronate disodium, per 300 mg

MCM: 2049

J1438 Injection, etanercept, 25 mg (code may be used for Medicare when drug administered under the direct supervision of a physician, not for use when drug is self administered)

MCM: 2049

J1439 Injection, ferric Carboxymaltose, 1 mg

J1442 Injection, filgrastim (g-csf), excludes biosimilars, 1 microgram

J1443 Injection, ferric pyrophosphate citrate solution, 0.1 mg of iron

(**J1446** Code deleted December 31, 2015.)

J1447 Injection, tbo-filgrastim, 1 microgram

MCM: 2049.5

J1450 Injection fluconazole, 200 mg

MCM: 2049.5

J1451 Injection, fomepizole, 15 mg

MCM: 2049

J1452 Injection, fomivirsen sodium, intraocular, 1.65 mg

MCM: 2049.3

J1453 Injection, fosaprepitant, 1 mg

J1455 Injection, foscarnet sodium, per 1000 mg

MCM: 2049

J1457 Injection, gallium nitrate, 1 mg

J1458 Injection, galsulfase, 1 mg

J1459 Injection, immune globulin (Privigen), intravenous, non-lyophilized (e.g., liquid), 500 mg

J1460 Injection, gamma globulin, intramuscular, 1 cc

MCM: 2049

J1556 Injection, immune globulin (Bivigam), 500 mg

J1557 Injection, immune globulin, (Gammaplex), intravenous, non-lyophilized (e.g., liquid), 500 mg

J1559 Injection, immune globulin (Hizentra), 100 mg

J1560 Injection, gamma globulin, intramuscular, over 10 cc

MCM: 2049

J1561 Injection, immune globulin, (Gamunex-c/gammaked), non-lyophilized (e.g., liquid), 500 mg

MCM: 2049

J1562 Injection, immune globulin (Vivaglobin), 100 mg

J1566 Injection, immune globulin, intravenous, lyophilized (e.g., powder), not otherwise specified, 500 mg

MCM: 2049

J1568 Injection, immune globulin, (Octagam), intravenous, non-lyophilized (e.g., liquid), 500 mg

J1569 Injection, immune globulin, (Gammagard liquid), non-lyophilized, (e.g., liquid), 500 mg

MCM: 2049

J1570 Injection, ganciclovir sodium, 500 mg

MCM: 2049

J1571 Injection, hepatitis b immune globulin (HepaGam b), intramuscular, 0.5 ml

MCM: 2049

J1572 Injection, immune globulin, (Flebogamma/Flebogamma dif), intravenous, non-lyophilized (e.g., liquid), 500 mg

MCM: 2049

J1573 Injection, hepatitis b immune globulin (HepaGam b), intravenous, 0.5 ml

J1575 Injection, immune globulin/hyaluronidase, (hyqvia), 100 mg immunoglobulin

J1580 Injection, Garamycin, gentamicin, up to 80 mg

MCM: 2049

(**J1590** Code deleted December 31, 2016).

J1595 Injection, glatiramer acetate, 20 mg

MCM: 2049

J1599 Injection, immune globulin, intravenous, non-lyophilized (e.g., liquid), not otherwise specified, 500 mg

J1600 Injection, gold sodium thiomalate, up to 50 mg

MCM: 2049

J1602 Injection, golimumab, 1 mg, for intravenous use

J1610 Injection, glucagon hydrochloride, per 1 mg

MCM: 2049

J1620 Injection, gonadorelin hydrochloride, per 100 mcg

MCM: 2049

J1626 Injection, granisetron hydrochloride, 100 mcg

MCM: 2049

J1630 Injection, haloperidol, up to 5 mg

MCM: 2049

J1631 Injection, haloperidol decanoate, per 50 mg

MCM: 2049

J1640 Injection, hemin, 1 mg

MCM: 2049

J1642 Injection, heparin sodium, (heparin lock flush), per 10 units

MCM: 2049

J1644 Injection, heparin sodium, per 1000 units

MCM: 2049

J1645 Injection, dalteparin sodium, per 2500 iu

MCM: 2049

J1650 Injection, enoxaparin sodium, 10 mg

J1652 Injection, fondaparinux sodium, 0.5 mg

MCM: 2049

J1655 Injection, tinzaparin sodium, 1000 iu

J1670 Injection, tetanus immune globulin, human, up to 250 units

MCM: 2049

J1675 Injection, histrelin acetate, 10 micrograms

MCM: 2049

J1700 Injection, hydrocortisone acetate, up to 25 mg

MCM: 2049

J1710 Injection, hydrocortisone sodium phosphate, up to 50 mg

MCM: 2049

J1720 Injection, hydrocortisone sodium succinate, up to 100 mg

MCM: 2049

J1725 Injection, hydroxyprogesterone caproate, 1 mg

J1730 Injection, diazoxide, up to 300 mg

MCM: 2049

J1740 Injection, ibandronate sodium, 1 mg

J1741 Injection, ibuprofen, 100 mg

J1742 Injection, ibutilide fumarate, 1 mg

MCM: 2049

J1743 Injection, idursulfase, 1 mg

J1744 Injection, icatibant, 1 mg

▲ **J1745** Injection, infliximab, excludes biosimilar, 10 mg

MCM: 2049

J1750 Injection, iron dextran, 50 mg

MCM: 2049.5

J1756 Injection, iron sucrose, 1 mg

J1786 Injection, imiglucerase, 10 units

MCM: 2049

J1790 Injection, droperidol, up to 5 mg

MCM: 2049

J1800 Injection, propranolol HCL, up to 1 mg

MCM: 2049

J1810 Injection, droperidol and fentanyl citrate, up to 2 ml ampule

MCM: 2049

J1815 Injection, insulin, per 5 units

CIM: 60-14

MCM: 2049

J1817 Insulin for administration through DME (i.e., insulin pump) per 50 units

J1826 Injection, interferon beta-1a, 30 mcg

J1830 Injection interferon beta-1b, 0.25 mg (code may be used for Medicare when drug administered under the direct supervision of a physician, not for use when drug is self administered)

MCM: 2049

J1833 Injection, Isavuconazonium, 1 mg

J1835 Injection, itraconazole, 50 mg

J1840 Injection, kanamycin sulfate, up to 500 mg

MCM: 2049

J1850 Injection, kanamycin sulfate, up to 75 mg

MCM: 2049

J1885 Injection, ketorolac tromethamine, per 15 mg

MCM: 2049

J1890 Injection, cephalothin sodium, up to 1 gram

MCM: 2049

J1930 Injection, lanreotide, 1 mg

J1931 Injection, laronidase, 0.1 mg

J1940 Injection, furosemide, up to 20 mg

MCM: 2049

• **J1942** Injection, aripiprazole lauroxil, 1 mg

J1945 Injection, lepirudin, 50 mg

MCM: 2049

J1950 Injection, leuprolide acetate (for depot suspension), per 3.75 mg

MCM: 2049

J1953 Injection, levetiracetam, 10 mg

J1955 Injection, levocarnitine, per 1 gm

MCM: 2049

J1956 Injection, levofloxacin, 250 mg

MCM: 2049

J1960 Injection, levorphanol tartrate, up to 2 mg

MCM: 2049

J1980 Injection, hyoscyamine sulfate, up to 0.25 mg

MCM: 2049

J1990 Injection, chlordiazepoxide HCL, up to 100 mg

MCM: 2049

J2001 Injection, lidocaine HCL for intravenous infusion, 10 mg

MCM: 2049

J2010 Injection, lincomycin HCL, up to 300 mg

MCM: 2049

J2020 Injection, linezolid, 200 mg

J2060 Injection, lorazepam, 2 mg

MCM: 2049

J2150 Injection, mannitol, 25% in 50 ml

MCM: 2049

J2170 Injection, mecasermin, 1 mg

J2175 Injection, meperidine hydrochloride, per 100 mg

MCM: 2049

J2180 Injection, meperidine and promethazine HCL, up to 50 mg

MCM: 2049

• **J2182** Injection, mepolizumab, 1 mg

J2185 Injection, meropenem, 100 mg

J2210 Injection, methylergonovine maleate, up to 0.2 mg

MCM: 2049

J2212 Injection, methylnaltrexone, 0.1 mg

J2248 Injection, micafungin sodium, 1 mg

J2250 Injection, midazolam hydrochloride, per 1 mg

MCM: 2049

J2260 Injection, milrinone lactate, 5 mg

MCM: 2049

J2265 Injection, minocycline hydrochloride, 1 mg

J2270 Injection, morphine sulfate, up to 10 mg

MCM: 2049

J2274 Injection, morphine sulfate, preservative-free for epidural or intrathecal use, 10 mg

CIM: 60-14

MCM: 2049

J2278 Injection, ziconotide, 1 microgram

J2280 Injection, moxifloxacin, 100 mg

J2300 Injection, nalbuphine hydrochloride, per 10 mg

MCM: 2049

J2310 Injection, naloxone hydrochloride, per 1 mg

MCM: 2049

J2315 Injection, naltrexone, depot form, 1 mg

J2320 Injection, nandrolone decanoate, up to 50 mg

MCM: 2049

J2323 Injection, natalizumab, 1 mg

J2325 Injection, nesiritide, 0.1 mg

MCM: 2049

J2353 Injection, octreotide, depot form for intramuscular injection, 1 mg

J2354 Injection, octreotide, non-depot form for subcutaneous or intravenous injection, 25 mcg

J2355 Injection, oprelvekin, 5 mg

MCM: 2049

J2357 Injection, omalizumab, 5 mg

J2358 Injection, olanzapine, long-acting, 1 mg

J2360 Injection, orphenadrine citrate, up to 60 mg

MCM: 2049

J2370 Injection, phenylephrine HCL, up to 1 ml

MCM: 2049

J2400 Injection, chloroprocaine hydrochloride, per 30 ml

MCM: 2049

J2405 Injection, ondansetron hydrochloride, per 1 mg

MCM: 2049

J2407 Injection, oritavancin, 10 mg

MCM: 2049

J2410 Injection, oxymorphone HCL, up to 1 mg

MCM: 2049

J2425 Injection, palifermin, 50 micrograms

J2426 Injection, paliperidone palmitate extended release, 1 mg

J2430 Injection, pamidronate disodium, per 30 mg

MCM: 2049

J2440 Injection, papaverine HCL, up to 60 mg

MCM: 2049

J2460 Injection, oxytetracycline HCL, up to 50 mg

MCM: 2049

J2469 Injection, palonosetron HCL, 25 mcg

J2501 Injection, paricalcitol, 1 mcg

MCM: 2049

J2502 Injection, Pasireotide long acting, 1 mg

J2503 Injection, pegaptanib sodium, 0.3 mg

J2504 Injection, pegademase bovine, 25 iu

MCM: 2049

J2505 Injection, pegfilgrastim, 6 mg

J2507 Injection, pegloticase, 1 mg

J2510 Injection, penicillin g procaine, aqueous, up to 600,000 units

MCM: 2049

J2513 Injection, pentastarch, 10% solution, 100 ml

MCM: 2049

J2515 Injection, pentobarbital sodium, per 50 mg

MCM: 2049

J2540 Injection, penicillin g potassium, up to 600,000 units

MCM: 2049

J2543 Injection, piperacillin sodium/tazobactam sodium, 1 gram/0.125 grams (1.125 grams)

MCM: 2049

J2545 Pentamidine isethionate, inhalation solution,-approved final product, non-compounded, administered through DME, unit dose form, per 300 mg

J2547 Injection, peramivir, 1 mg

J2550 Injection, promethazine HCL, up to 50 mg

MCM: 2049

J2560 Injection, phenobarbital sodium, up to 120 mg

MCM: 2049

J2562 Injection, plerixafor, 1 mg

J2590 Injection, oxytocin, up to 10 units

MCM: 2049

J2597 Injection, desmopressin acetate, per 1 mcg

MCM: 2049

J2650 Injection, prednisolone acetate, up to 1 ml

MCM: 2049

J2670 Injection, tolazoline HCL, up to 25 mg

MCM: 2049

J2675 Injection, progesterone, per 50 mg

MCM: 2049

J2680 Injection, fluphenazine decanoate, up to 25 mg

MCM: 2049

J2690 Injection, procainamide HCL, up to 1 gm

MCM: 2049

J2700 Injection, oxacillin sodium, up to 250 mg

MCM: 2049

J2704 Injection, propofol, 10 mg

J2710 Injection, neostigmine methylsulfate, up to 0.5 mg

MCM: 2049

J2720 Injection, protamine sulfate, per 10 mg

MCM: 2049

J2724 Injection, protein c concentrate, intravenous, human, 10 iu

J2725 Injection, protirelin, per 250 mcg

MCM: 2049

J2730 Injection, pralidoxime chloride, up to 1 gm

MCM: 2049

J2760 Injection, phentolamine mesylate, up to 5 mg

MCM: 2049

J2765 Injection, metoclopramide HCL, up to 10 mg

MCM: 2049

J2770 Injection, quinupristin/dalfopristin, 500 mg (150/350)

MCM: 2049

J2778 Injection, ranibizumab, 0.1 mg

J2780 Injection, ranitidine hydrochloride, 25 mg

MCM: 2049

J2783 Injection, rasburicase, 0.5 mg

J2785 Injection, regadenoson, 0.1 mg

• **J2786** Injection, reslizumab, 1 mg

J2788 Injection, rho d immune globulin, human, minidose, 50 micrograms (250 i.u.)

MCM: 2049

J2790 Injection, rho d immune globulin, human, full dose, 300 micrograms (1500 i.u.)

MCM: 2049

J2791 Injection, rho(d) immune globulin (human), (Rhophylac), intramuscular or intravenous, 100 iu

MCM: 2049

J2792 Injection, rho d immune globulin, intravenous, human, solvent detergent, 100 iu

MCM: 2049

J2793 Injection, rilonacept, 1 mg

MCM: 2049

J2794 Injection, risperidone, long acting, 0.5 mg

J2795 Injection, ropivacaine hydrochloride, 1 mg

J2796 Injection, romiplostim, 10 micrograms

J2800 Injection, methocarbamol, up to 10 ml

MCM: 2049

J2805 Injection, sincalide, 5 micrograms

J2810 Injection, theophylline, per 40 mg

MCM: 2049

J2820 Injection, sargramostim (gm-csf), 50 mcg

MCM: 2049

• **J2840** Injection, sebelipase alfa, 1 mg

J2850 Injection, secretin, synthetic, human, 1 microgram

MCM: 2049

J2860 Injection, Siltuximab, 10 mg

J2910 Injection, aurothioglucose, up to 50 mg

MCM: 2049

J2916 Injection, sodium ferric gluconate complex in sucrose injection, 12.5 mg

MCM: 2049.2, 2049.4

J2920 Injection, methylprednisolone sodium succinate, up to 40 mg

MCM: 2049

J2930 Injection, methylprednisolone sodium succinate, up to 125 mg

MCM: 2049

J2940 Injection, somatrem, 1 mg

MCM: 2049

Statute: 1861s2b

J2941 Injection, somatropin, 1 mg

MCM: 2049

Statute: 1861s2b

J2950 Injection, promazine HCL, up to 25 mg

MCM: 2049

J2993 Injection, reteplase, 18.1 mg

MCM: 2049

J2995 Injection, streptokinase, per 250,000 iu

MCM: 2049

J2997 Injection, alteplase recombinant, 1 mg

MCM: 2049

J3000 Injection, streptomycin, up to 1 gm

MCM: 2049

J3010 Injection, fentanyl citrate, 0.1 mg

MCM: 2049

J3030 Injection, sumatriptan succinate, 6 mg (code may be used for Medicare when drug administered under the direct supervision of a physician, not for use when drug is self administered)

MCM: 2049

J3060 Injection, taliglucerase alfa, 10 units

J3070 Injection, pentazocine, 30 mg

MCM: 2049

J3090 Injection, Tedizolid phosphate, 1 mg

J3095 Injection, telavancin, 10 mg

J3101 Injection, tenecteplase, 1 mg

J3105 Injection, terbutaline sulfate, up to 1 mg

MCM: 2049

J3110 Injection, teriparatide, 10 mcg

J3121 Injection, testosterone enanthate, 1 mg

J3145 Injection, testosterone undecanoate, 1 mg

J3230 Injection, chlorpromazine HCL, up to 50 mg

MCM: 2049

J3240 Injection, thyrotropin alpha, 0.9 mg, provided in 1.1 mg vial

MCM: 2049

J3243 Injection, tigecycline, 1 mg

J3246 Injection, tirofiban HCL, 0.25 mg

J3250 Injection, trimethobenzamide HCL, up to 200 mg

MCM: 2049

J3260 Injection, tobramycin sulfate, up to 80 mg

MCM: 2049

J3262 Injection, tocilizumab, 1 mg

J3265 Injection, torsemide, 10 mg/ml

MCM: 2049

J3280 Injection, thiethylperazine maleate, up to 10 mg

MCM: 2049

J3285 Injection, treprostinil, 1 mg

J3300 Injection, triamcinolone acetonide, preservative free, 1 mg

J3301 Injection, triamcinolone acetonide, not otherwise specified, 10 mg

MCM: 2049

J3302 Injection, triamcinolone diacetate, per 5mg

MCM: 2049

J3303 Injection, triamcinolone hexacetonide, per 5mg

MCM: 2049

J3305 Injection, trimetrexate glucuronate, per 25 mg

MCM: 2049

J3310 Injection, perphenazine, up to 5 mg

MCM: 2049

J3315 Injection, triptorelin pamoate, 3.75 mg
MCM: 2049

J3320 Injection, spectinomycin dihydrochloride, up to 2 gm
MCM: 2049

J3350 Injection, urea, up to 40 gm
MCM: 2049

J3355 Injection, urofollitropin, 75 iu
MCM: 2049

▲ **J3357** Ustekinumab, for subcutaneous injection, 1 mg

J3360 Injection, diazepam, up to 5 mg
MCM: 2049

J3364 Injection, urokinase, 5000 iu vial
MCM: 2049

J3365 Injection, iv, urokinase, 250,000 i.u. vial
MCM: 2049,

J3370 Injection, vancomycin HCL, 500 mg
CIM: 60-14
MCM: 2049

J3380 Injection, vedolizumab, 1 mg

J3385 Injection, velaglucerase alfa, 100 units

J3396 Injection, verteporfin, 0.1 mg
MCM: 35-100, 45-30

J3400 Injection, triflupromazine HCL, up to 20 mg
MCM: 2049

J3410 Injection, hydroxyzine HCL, up to 25 mg
MCM: 2049

J3411 Injection, thiamine HCL, 100 mg

J3415 Injection, pyridoxine HCL, 100 mg

J3420 Injection, vitamin b-12 cyanocobalamin, up to 1000 mcg
CIM: 45-4
MCM: 2049

J3430 Injection, phytonadione (vitamin k), per 1 mg
MCM: 2049

J3465 Injection, voriconazole, 10 mg

MCM: 2049

J3470 Injection, hyaluronidase, up to 150 units

MCM: 2049

J3471 Injection, hyaluronidase, ovine, preservative free, per 1 USP unit (up to 999 USP units)

J3472 Injection, hyaluronidase, ovine, preservative free, per 1000 USP units

J3473 Injection, hyaluronidase, recombinant, 1 USP unit

MCM: 2049

J3475 Injection, magnesium sulfate, per 500 mg

MCM: 2049

J3480 Injection, potassium chloride, per 2 mEq

MCM: 2049

J3485 Injection, zidovudine, 10 mg

MCM: 2049

J3486 Injection, ziprasidone mesylate, 10 mg

J3489 Injection, zoledronic acid, 1 mg

J3490 Unclassified drugs

MCM: 2049

J3520 Edetate disodium, per 150 mg

CIM: 35-64, 45-20

J3530 Nasal vaccine inhalation

MCM: 2049

J3535 Drug administered through a metered dose inhaler

MCM: 2050.5

J3570 Laetrile, amygdalin, vitamin b17

CIM: 45-10

J3590 Unclassified biologics

J7030 Infusion, normal saline solution , 1000 cc

MCM: 2049

J7040 Infusion, normal saline solution, sterile (500 ml=1 unit)

MCM: 2049

J7042 5% dextrose/normal saline (500 ml = 1 unit)

MCM: 2049

J7050 Infusion, normal saline solution , 250 cc

MCM: 2049

J7060 5% dextrose/water (500 ml = 1 unit)

MCM: 2049

J7070 Infusion, d5w, 1000 cc

MCM: 2049

J7100 Infusion, dextran 40, 500 ml

MCM: 2049

J7110 Infusion, dextran 75, 500 ml

MCM: 2049

J7120 Ringers lactate infusion, up to 1000 cc

MCM: 2049

J7121 5% dextrose in lactated ringers infusion, up to 1000 cc

MCM: 2049

J7131 Hypertonic saline solution, 1 ml

MCM: 2049

• **J7175** Injection, factor x, (human), 1 i.u.

J7178 Injection, human fibrinogen concentrate, 1 mg

• **J7179** Injection, von Willebrand factor (recombinant), (vonvendi), 1 i.u. vwf:rco

J7180 Injection, factor xiii (antihemophilic factor, human), 1 i.u.

J7181 Injection, factor xiii a-subunit, (recombinant), per iu

J7182 Injection, factor viii, (antihemophilic factor, recombinant), (novo eight), per iu

J7183 Injection, von Willebrand factor complex (human), wilate, 1 i.u. vwf:rco

MCM: 2049

J7185 Injection, factor viii (antihemophilic factor, recombinant) (Xyntha), per i.u.

J7186 Injection, antihemophilic factor viii/von Willebrand factor complex (human), per factor viii i.u.

MCM: 2049

J7187 Injection, von Willebrand factor complex (Humate-p), per iu vwf:rco

MCM: 2049

J7188 Injection, factor viii (antihemophilic factor, recombinant), (obizur), per i.u.

MCM: 2049

J7189 Factor VIIa (antihemophilic factor, recombinant), per 1 microgram

MCM: 2049

J7190 Factor viii (antihemophilic factor, human) per i.u.

MCM: 2049

J7191 Factor viii (antihemophilic factor (porcine)), per i.u.

MCM: 2049

J7192 Factor viii (antihemophilic factor, recombinant) per i.u., not otherwise specified

MCM: 2049

J7193 Factor ix (antihemophilic factor, purified, non-recombinant) per i.u.

MCM: 2049

J7194 Factor ix, complex, per i.u.

MCM: 2049

J7195 Injection, factor ix (antihemophilic factor, recombinant) per iu, not otherwise specified

MCM: 2049

J7196 Injection, antithrombin recombinant, 50 i.u.

J7197 Antithrombin iii (human), per i.u.

MCM: 2049

J7198 Anti-inhibitor, per i.u.

CIM: 45-24

MCM: 2049

J7199 Hemophilia clotting factor, not otherwise classified

CIM: 45-24

MCM: 2049

J7200 Injection, factor ix, (antihemophilic factor, recombinant), rixubis, per iu

MCM: 2049

▲ **J7201** Injection, factor ix, Fc fusion protein, (recombinant), alprolix, 1 i.u.

MCM: 2049

• **J7202** Injection, factor ix, albumin fusion protein, (recombinant), idelvion, 1 i.u.

J7205 Injection, factor viii Fc fusion (recombinant), per iu

• **J7207** Injection, factor viii, (antihemophilic factor, recombinant), pegylated, 1 i.u.

• **J7209** Injection, factor viii, (antihemophilic factor, recombinant), (nuwiq), 1 i.u.

▲ **J7297** Levonorgestrel-releasing intrauterine contraceptive system (liletta), 52 mg

Statute: 1862(a)(1)

▲ **J7298** Levonorgestrel-releasing intrauterine contraceptive system (Mirena), 52 mg

Statute: 1862(a)(1)

J7300 Intrauterine copper contraceptive

Statute: 1862A1

▲ **J7301** Levonorgestrel-releasing intrauterine contraceptive system (skyla), 13.5 mg

Statute: 1862(a)(1)

(**J7302** Code deleted December 31, 2015.)

J7303 Contraceptive supply, hormone containing vaginal ring, each

Statute: 1862.1

J7304 Contraceptive supply, hormone containing patch, each

Statute: 1862.1

J7306 Levonorgestrel (contraceptive) implant system, including implants and supplies

J7307 Etonogestrel (contraceptive) implant system, including implant and supplies

J7308 Aminolevulinic acid HCL for topical administration, 20%, single unit dosage form (354 mg)

J7309 Methyl aminolevulinate (mal) for topical administration, 16.8%, 1 gram

J7310 Ganciclovir, 4.5 mg, long-acting implant

MCM: 2049

J7311 Fluocinolone acetonide, intravitreal implant

J7312 Injection, dexamethasone, intravitreal implant, 0.1 mg

J7313 Injection, fluocinolone acetonide, intravitreal implant, 0.01 mg

J7315 Mitomycin, ophthalmic, 0.2 mg

J7316 Injection, Ocriplasmin, 0.125 mg

• **J7320** Hyaluronan or derivative, genvisc 850, for intra-articular injection, 1 mg

J7321 Hyaluronan or derivative, Hyalgan or Supartz, for intra-articular injection, per dose

• **J7322** Hyaluronan or derivative, hymovis, for intra-articular injection, 1 mg

J7323 Hyaluronan or derivative, Euflexxa, for intra-articular injection, per dose

J7324 Hyaluronan or derivative, Orthovisc, for intra-articular injection, per dose

J7325 Hyaluronan or derivative, Synvisc or Synvisc-one, for intra-articular injection, 1 mg

J7326 Hyaluronan or derivative, gel-one, for intra-articular injection, per dose

J7327 Hyaluronan or derivative, monovisc, for intra-articular injection, per dose

J7328 Hyaluronan or derivative, gel-syn, for intra-articular injection, 0.1 mg

J7330 Autologous cultured chondrocytes, implant

J7336 Capsaicin 8% patch, per square centimeter

▲ **J7340** Carbidopa 5 mg/levodopa 20 mg enteral suspension, 100 ml

• **J7342** Installation, ciprofloxacin otic suspension, 6 mg

Immunosuppressive Drugs (Includes Non-Injectibles)

J7500 Azathioprine, oral, 50 mg

MCM: 2049.5

J7501 Azathioprine, parenteral, 100 mg

MCM: 2049

J7502 Cyclosporine, oral, 100 mg

MCM: 2049.5

J7503 Tacrolimus, extended release, (envarsus XR), oral, 0.25 mg

MCM: 2049.5

J7504 Lymphocyte immune globulin, antithymocyte globulin, equine, parenteral, 250 mg

CIM: 45-22

MCM: 2049

J7505 Muromonab-cd3, parenteral, 5 mg

MCM: 2049

(**J7506** Code deleted December 31, 2015.)

J7507 Tacrolimus, immediate release, oral, 1 mg

MCM: 2049.5

J7508 Tacrolimus, extended release, (Astagraf xl), oral, 0.1 mg

MCM: 2049.5

J7509 Methylprednisolone oral, per 4 mg

MCM: 2049.5

J7510 Prednisolone oral, per 5 mg

MCM: 2049.5

J7511 Lymphocyte immune globulin, antithymocyte globulin, rabbit, parenteral, 25 mg

J7512 Prednisone, immediate release or delayed release, oral, 1 mg

MCM: 2049.5

J7513 Daclizumab, parenteral, 25 mg

MCM: 2049.5

J7515 Cyclosporine, oral, 25 mg

J7516 Cyclosporin, parenteral, 250 mg

J7517 Mycophenolate mofetil, oral, 250 mg

J7518 Mycophenolic acid, oral, 180 mg

MCM: 2050.5, 4471, 5249

J7520 Sirolimus, oral, 1 mg

MCM: 2049.5

J7525 Tacrolimus, parenteral, 5 mg

MCM: 2049.5

J7527 Everolimus, oral, 0.25 mg

MCM: 2049.5

J7599 Immunosuppressive drug, not otherwise classified

MCM: 2049.5

J7604 Acetylcysteine, inhalation solution, compounded product, administered through DME, unit dose form, per gram

J7605 Arformoterol, inhalation solution, approved final product, non-compounded, administered through DME, unit dose form, 15 micrograms

J7606 Formoterol fumarate, inhalation solution, approved final product, non-compounded, administered through DME, unit dose form, 20 micrograms

J7607 Levalbuterol, inhalation solution, compounded product, administered through DME, concentrated form, 0.5 mg

J7608 Acetylcysteine, inhalation solution,-approved final product, non-compounded, administered through DME, unit dose form, per gram

J7609 Albuterol, inhalation solution, compounded product, administered through DME, unit dose, 1 mg

J7610 Albuterol, inhalation solution, compounded product, administered through DME, concentrated form, 1 mg

J7611 Albuterol, inhalation solution,-approved final product, non-compounded, administered through DME, concentrated form, 1 mg

MCM: 2100.5

J7612 Levalbuterol, inhalation solution,-approved final product, non-compounded, administered through DME, concentrated form, 0.5 mg

MCM: 2100.5

J7613 Albuterol, inhalation solution,-approved final product, non-compounded, administered through DME, unit dose, 1 mg

MCM: 2100.5

J7614 Levalbuterol, inhalation solution,-approved final product, non-compounded, administered through DME, unit dose, 0.5 mg

MCM: 2100.5

J7615 Levalbuterol, inhalation solution, compounded product, administered through DME, unit dose, 0.5 mg

J7620 Albuterol, up to 2.5 mg and ipratropium bromide, up to 0.5 mg,-approved final product, non-compounded, administered through DME

J7622 Beclomethasone, inhalation solution, compounded product, administered through DME, unit dose form, per milligram

J7624 Betamethasone, inhalation solution, compounded product, administered through DME, unit dose form, per milligram

J7626 Budesonide, inhalation solution,-approved final product, non-compounded, administered through DME, unit dose form, up to 0.5 mg

J7627 Budesonide, inhalation solution, compounded product, administered through DME, unit dose form, up to 0.5 mg

J7628 Bitolterol mesylate, inhalation solution, compounded product, administered through DME, concentrated form, per milligram

J7629 Bitolterol mesylate, inhalation solution, compounded product, administered through DME, unit dose form, per milligram

J7631 Cromolyn sodium, inhalation solution,-approved final product, non-compounded, administered through DME, unit dose form, per 10 milligrams

J7632 Cromolyn sodium, inhalation solution, compounded product, administered through DME, unit dose form, per 10 milligrams

J7633 Budesonide, inhalation solution,-approved final product, non-compounded, administered through DME, concentrated form, per 0.25 milligram

J7634 Budesonide, inhalation solution, compounded product, administered through DME, concentrated form, per 0.25 milligram

J7635 Atropine, inhalation solution, compounded product, administered through DME, concentrated form, per milligram

J7636 Atropine, inhalation solution, compounded product, administered through DME, unit dose form, per milligram

J7637 Dexamethasone, inhalation solution, compounded product, administered through DME, concentrated form, per milligram

J7638 Dexamethasone, inhalation solution, compounded product, administered through DME, unit dose form, per milligram

J7639 Dornase alfa, inhalation solution,-approved final product, non-compounded, administered through DME, unit dose form, per milligram

J7640 Formoterol, inhalation solution, compounded product, administered through DME, unit dose form, 12 micrograms

J7641 Flunisolide, inhalation solution, compounded product, administered through DME, unit dose, per milligram

J7642 Glycopyrrolate, inhalation solution, compounded product, administered through DME, concentrated form, per milligram

J7643 Glycopyrrolate, inhalation solution, compounded product, administered through DME, unit dose form, per milligram

J7644 Ipratropium bromide, inhalation solution,-approved final product, non-compounded, administered through DME, unit dose form, per milligram

J7645 Ipratropium bromide, inhalation solution, compounded product, administered through DME, unit dose form, per milligram

J7647 Isoetharine HCL, inhalation solution, compounded product, administered through DME, concentrated form, per milligram

J7648 Isoetharine HCL, inhalation solution,-approved final product, non-compounded, administered through DME, concentrated form, per milligram

J7649 Isoetharine HCL, inhalation solution,-approved final product, non-compounded, administered through DME, unit dose form, per milligram

J7650 Isoetharine HCL, inhalation solution, compounded product, administered through DME, unit dose form, per milligram

J7657 Isoproterenol HCL, inhalation solution, compounded product, administered through DME, concentrated form, per milligram

J7658 Isoproterenol HCL, inhalation solution,-approved final product, non-compounded, administered through DME, concentrated form, per milligram

J7659 Isoproterenol HCL, inhalation solution,-approved final product, non-compounded, administered through DME, unit dose form, per milligram

J7660 Isoproterenol HCL, inhalation solution, compounded product, administered through DME, unit dose form, per milligram

J7665 Mannitol, administered through an inhaler, 5 mg

J7667 Metaproterenol sulfate, inhalation solution, compounded product, concentrated form, per 10 milligrams

J7668 Metaproterenol sulfate, inhalation solution,-approved final product, non-compounded, administered through DME, concentrated form, per 10 milligrams

J7669 Metaproterenol sulfate, inhalation solution,-approved final product, non-compounded, administered through DME, unit dose form, per 10 milligrams

J7670 Metaproterenol sulfate, inhalation solution, compounded product, administered through DME, unit dose form, per 10 milligrams

J7674 Methacholine chloride administered as inhalation solution through a nebulizer, per 1 mg

J7676 Pentamidine isethionate, inhalation solution, compounded product, administered through DME, unit dose form, per 300 mg

J7680 Terbutaline sulfate, inhalation solution, compounded product, administered through DME, concentrated form, per milligram

J7681 Terbutaline sulfate, inhalation solution, compounded product, administered through DME, unit dose form, per milligram

J7682 Tobramycin, inhalation solution,-approved final product, non-compounded, unit dose form, administered through DME, per 300 milligrams

J7683 Triamcinolone, inhalation solution, compounded product, administered through DME, concentrated form, per milligram

J7684 Triamcinolone, inhalation solution, compounded product, administered through DME, unit dose form, per milligram

J7685 Tobramycin, inhalation solution, compounded product, administered through DME, unit dose form, per 300 milligrams

J7686 Treprostinil, inhalation solution,-approved final product, non-compounded, administered through DME, unit dose form, 1.74 mg

J7699 Noc drugs, inhalation solution administered through DME

J7799 Noc drugs, other than inhalation drugs, administered through DME

MCM: 2100.5

J7999 Compounded drug, not otherwise classified

J8498 Antiemetic drug, rectal/suppository, not otherwise specified

Statute: 1861s2T

J8499 Prescription drug, oral, non chemotherapeutic, nos

MCM: 2049

J8501 Aprepitant, oral, 5 mg

J8510 Busulfan; oral, 2 mg

MCM: 2049.5

J8515 Cabergoline, oral, 0.25 mg

MCM: 2049.5

J8520 Capecitabine, oral, 150 mg

MCM: 2049.5

J8521 Capecitabine, oral, 500 mg

MCM: 2049.5

J8530 Cyclophosphamide; oral, 25 mg

MCM: 2049.5

J8540 Dexamethasone, oral, 0.25 mg

Statute: 1861(s)2T

J8560 Etoposide; oral, 50 mg

MCM: 2049.5

J8562 Fludarabine phosphate, oral, 10 mg

J8565 Gefitinib, oral, 250 mg

J8597 Antiemetic drug, oral, not otherwise specified

Statute: 1861s2T

J8600 Melphalan; oral, 2 mg

MCM: 2049.5

J8610 Methotrexate; oral, 2.5 mg

MCM: 2049.5

J8650 Nabilone, oral, 1 mg

J8655 Netupitant 300 mg and palonosetron 0.5 mg

• **J8670** Rolapitant, oral, 1 mg

J8700 Temozolomide, oral, 5 mg

MCM: 2049.5C

J8705 Topotecan, oral, 0.25 mg

J8999 Prescription drug, oral, chemotherapeutic, nos

MCM: 2049.5

CHEMOTHERAPY DRUGS

Guidelines

In addition to the information presented in the INTRODUCTION, several other items unique to this section are defined or identified here:

1. EXCEPTION: Oral immunosuppressive drugs are not included in this section.

2. ROUTE OF ADMINISTRATION: Unless otherwise specified, the drugs listed in this section may be injected either subcutaneously, intramuscularly or intravenously.

3. DRUG COST ONLY: The codes listed in this section include the cost of the chemotherapy drug only and do not include the administration of the drug.

4. SUBSECTION INFORMATION: Some of the listed subheadings or subsections have special needs or instructions unique to that section. Where these are indicated, special "notes" will be presented preceding or following the listings. Those subsections within the CHEMOTHERAPY DRUGS section that have "notes" are as follows:

Subsection	Code Numbers
Chemotherapy drugs	J9000-J9999

5. UNLISTED SERVICE OR PROCEDURE: A service or procedure may be provided that is not listed in this edition of HCPCS. When reporting such a service, the appropriate "unlisted procedure" code may be used to indicate the service, identifying it by "special report" as defined below. HCPCS terminology is inconsistent in defining unlisted procedures. The procedure definition may include the term(s) "unlisted", "not otherwise classified", "unspecified", "unclassified", "other" and "miscellaneous". Prior to using these codes, try to determine if a Local Level III code or CPT code is available. The "unlisted procedures" and accompanying codes for CHEMOTHERAPY DRUGS are as follows:

   J9999 Not otherwise classified, antineoplastic drugs

6. SPECIAL REPORT: A service, material or supply that is rarely provided, unusual, variable or new may require a special report in determining medical appropriateness for reimbursement purposes. Pertinent information should include an adequate definition or description of the nature, extent, and need for the service, material or supply.

7. MODIFIERS: Listed services may be modified under certain circumstances. When appropriate, the modifying circumstance is identified by adding a modifier to the basic procedure code. CPT and HCPCS National Level II modifiers may be used with CPT and HCPCS National Level II procedure codes. Modifiers commonly used with CHEMOTHERAPY DRUGS are as follows:

   -CC Procedure code change (used when the procedure code submitted was changed either for administrative reasons or because an incorrect code was filed)

   -TC Technical component. Under certain circumstances, a charge may be made for the technical component alone. Under these circumstances, the technical component charge is identified by adding the modifier -TC to the usual procedure code. Technical component charges are institutional charges and are not billed separately by physicians. Portable x-ray suppliers bill only for the technical component however, and should use modifier -TC.

8. CPT CODE CROSS-REFERENCE: Unless otherwise specified, the equivalent CPT code for all listings in this section is 96545.

Chemotherapy Drugs

J9000 Injection, doxorubicin hydrochloride, 10 mg

MCM: 2049

(**J9010** Code deleted December 31, 2015.) Use J0202

J9015 Injection, aldesleukin, per single use vial

MCM: 2049

J9017 Injection, arsenic trioxide, 1 mg

J9019 Injection, asparaginase (Erwinase), 1,000 iu

MCM: 2049

J9020 Injection, asparaginase, not otherwise specified, 10,000 units

MCM: 2049

J9025 Injection, azacitidine, 1 mg

J9027 Injection, clofarabine, 1 mg

J9031 BCG (intravesical) per instillation

MCM: 2049

J9032 Injection, Belinostat, 10 mg

▲ **J9033** Injection, bendamustine HCL (Treanda), 1 mg

• **J9034** Injection, bendamustine HCL (bendeka), 1 mg

J9035 Injection, bevacizumab, 10 mg

J9039 Injection, blinatumomab, 1 microgram

J9040 Injection, bleomycin sulfate, 15 units

MCM: 2049

J9041 Injection, bortezomib, 0.1 mg

J9042 Injection, Brentuximab Vedotin, 1 mg

J9043 Injection, cabazitaxel, 1 mg

J9045 Injection, carboplatin, 50 mg

MCM: 2049

J9047 Injection, carfilzomib, 1 mg

J9050 Injection, carmustine, 100 mg

MCM: 2049

J9055 Injection, cetuximab, 10 mg

J9060 Injection, cisplatin, powder or solution, 10 mg

MCM: 2049

J9065 Injection, cladribine, per 1 mg

MCM: 2049

J9070 Cyclophosphamide, 100 mg

MCM: 2049

J9098 Injection, cytarabine liposome, 10 mg

J9100 Injection, cytarabine, 100 mg

MCM: 2049

J9120 Injection, dactinomycin, 0.5 mg

MCM: 2049

J9130 Dacarbazine, 100 mg

MCM: 2049

• **J9145** Injection, daratumumab, 10 mg

MCM: 2049

J9150 Injection, daunorubicin, 10 mg

MCM: 2049

J9151 Injection, daunorubicin citrate, liposomal formulation, 10 mg

MCM: 2049

J9155 Injection, degarelix, 1 mg

J9160 Injection, denileukin diftitox, 300 micrograms

J9165 Injection, diethylstilbestrol diphosphate, 250 mg

MCM: 2049

J9171 Injection, docetaxel, 1 mg

MCM: 2049

J9175 Injection, Elliotts' b solution, 1 ml

MCM: 2049

• **J9176** Injection, elotuzumab, 1 mg

J9178 Injection, epirubicin HCL, 2 mg

J9179 Injection, Eribulin mesylate, 0.1 mg

J9181 Injection, etoposide, 10 mg

MCM: 2049

J9185 Injection, fludarabine phosphate, 50 mg

MCM: 2049

J9190 Injection, fluorouracil, 500 mg

MCM: 2049

J9200 Injection, floxuridine, 500 mg

MCM: 2049

J9201 Injection, gemcitabine hydrochloride, 200 mg

MCM: 2049

J9202 Goserelin acetate implant, per 3.6 mg

MCM: 2049

• **J9205** Injection, irinotecan liposome, 1 mg

MCM: 2049

J9206 Injection, irinotecan, 20 mg

MCM: 2049

J9207 Injection, ixabepilone, 1 mg

J9208 Injection, ifosfamide, 1 gram

MCM: 2049

J9209 Injection, mesna, 200 mg

MCM: 2049

J9211 Injection, idarubicin hydrochloride, 5 mg

MCM: 2049

J9212 Injection, interferon alfacon-1, recombinant, 1 microgram

MCM: 2049

J9213 Injection, interferon, alfa-2a, recombinant, 3 million units

MCM: 2049

J9214 Injection, interferon, alfa-2b, recombinant, 1 million units

MCM: 2049

J9215 Injection, interferon, alfa-n3, (human leukocyte derived), 250,000 iu

MCM: 2049

J9216 Injection, interferon, gamma 1-b, 3 million units

MCM: 2049

J9217 Leuprolide acetate (for depot suspension), 7.5 mg

MCM: 2049

J9218 Leuprolide acetate, per 1 mg

MCM: 2049

J9219 Leuprolide acetate implant, 65 mg

MCM: 2049

J9225 Histrelin implant (Vantas), 50 mg

MCM: 2049

J9226 Histrelin implant (Supprelin la), 50 mg

MCM: 2049

J9228 Injection, ipilimumab, 1 mg

J9230 Injection, mechlorethamine hydrochloride, (nitrogen mustard), 10 mg

MCM: 2049

J9245 Injection, melphalan hydrochloride, 50 mg

MCM: 2049

J9250 Methotrexate sodium, 5 mg

MCM: 2049

J9260 Methotrexate sodium, 50 mg

MCM: 2049

J9261 Injection, nelarabine, 50 mg

J9262 Injection, omacetaxine mepesuccinate, 0.01 mg

J9263 Injection, oxaliplatin, 0.5 mg

J9264 Injection, paclitaxel protein-bound particles, 1 mg

J9266 Injection, pegaspargase, per single dose vial

MCM: 2049

J9267 Injection, paclitaxel, 1 mg

J9268 Injection, pentostatin, 10 mg

MCM: 2049

J9270 Injection, plicamycin, 2.5 mg

MCM: 2049

J9271 Injection, Pembrolizumab, 1 mg

J9280 Injection, mitomycin, 5 mg

MCM: 2049

J9293 Injection, mitoxantrone hydrochloride, per 5 mg

MCM: 2049

• **J9295** Injection, necitumumab, 1 mg

J9299 Injection, nivolumab, 1 mg

J9300 Injection, gemtuzumab ozogamicin, 5 mg

J9301 Injection, obinutuzumab, 10 mg

J9302 Injection, ofatumumab, 10 mg

J9303 Injection, panitumumab, 10 mg

J9305 Injection, pemetrexed, 10 mg

J9306 Injection, pertuzumab, 1 mg

J9307 Injection, pralatrexate, 1 mg

J9308 Injection, ramucirumab, 5 mg

J9310 Injection, rituximab, 100 mg

MCM: 2049

J9315 Injection, romidepsin, 1 mg

J9320 Injection, streptozocin, 1 gram

MCM: 2049

• **J9325** Injection, talimogene laherparepvec, per 1 million plaque forming units

J9328 Injection, temozolomide, 1 mg

J9330 Injection, temsirolimus, 1 mg

J9340 Injection, thiotepa, 15 mg

MCM: 2049

J9351 Injection, topotecan, 0.1 mg

• **J9352** Injection, trabectedin, 0.1 mg

J9354 Injection, ado-trastuzumab Emtansine, 1 mg

J9355 Injection, trastuzumab, 10 mg

J9357 Injection, valrubicin, intravesical, 200 mg

MCM: 2049

J9360 Injection, vinblastine sulfate, 1 mg

MCM: 2049

J9370 Vincristine sulfate, 1 mg

MCM: 2049

J9371 Injection, vincristine sulfate liposome, 1 mg

J9390 Injection, vinorelbine tartrate, 10 mg

MCM: 2049

J9395 Injection, fulvestrant, 25 mg

J9400 Injection, Ziv-aflibercept, 1 mg

J9600 Injection, porfimer sodium, 75 mg

MCM: 2049

J9999 Not otherwise classified, antineoplastic drugs

CIM: 45-16

MCM: 2049

K CODES: FOR DME-MACs USE ONLY

Guidelines

In addition to the information presented in the INTRODUCTION, several other items unique to this section are defined or identified here:

1. EXCLUSIVE USE BY DME-MACs: The codes listed in this section are assigned by CMS on a temporary basis and are for the exclusive use of the Durable Medical Equipment Medicare Administrative Contractors (DME-MACs). These codes are not to be used by providers for reporting purposes unless specifically instructed to do so by the local carrier.

2. UNLISTED SERVICE OR PROCEDURE: A service or procedure may be provided that is not listed in this edition of HCPCS. When reporting such a service, the appropriate "unlisted procedure" code may be used to indicate the service, identifying it by "special report" as defined below. HCPCS terminology is inconsistent in defining unlisted procedures. The procedure definition may include the term(s) "unlisted", "not otherwise classified", "unspecified", "unclassified", "other" and "miscellaneous". Prior to using these codes, try to determine if a Local Level III code or CPT code is available.

3. SPECIAL REPORT: A service, material or supply that is rarely provided, unusual, variable or new may require a special report in determining medical appropriateness for reimbursement purposes. Pertinent information should include an adequate definition or description of the nature, extent, and need for the service, material or supply.

4. CPT CODE CROSS-REFERENCE: Unless otherwise specified, the equivalent CPT code for all listings in this section is 99070.

Temporary Codes for DMERCS

K0001 Standard wheelchair

K0002 Standard hemi (low seat) wheelchair

K0003 Lightweight wheelchair

K0004 High strength, lightweight wheelchair

K0005 Ultra lightweight wheelchair

K0006 Heavy duty wheelchair

K0007 Extra heavy duty wheelchair

K0008 Custom manual wheelchair/base

K0009 Other manual wheelchair/base

K0010 Standard - weight frame motorized/power wheelchair

K0011 Standard - weight frame motorized/power wheelchair with programmable control parameters for speed adjustment, tremor dampening, acceleration control and braking

	K0012	Lightweight portable motorized/power wheelchair
	K0013	Custom motorized/power wheelchair base
	K0014	Other motorized/power wheelchair base
	K0015	Detachable, non-adjustable height armrest, each
	K0017	Detachable, adjustable height armrest, base, replacement only, each
	K0018	Detachable, adjustable height armrest, upper portion, replacement only, each
▲	K0019	Arm pad, replacement only, each
	K0020	Fixed, adjustable height armrest, pair
▲	K0037	High mount flip-up footrest, replacement only, each
	K0038	Leg strap, each
	K0039	Leg strap, h style, each
	K0040	Adjustable angle footplate, each
	K0041	Large size footplate, each
▲	K0042	Standard size footplate, replacement only, each
▲	K0043	Footrest, lower extension tube, replacement only, each
▲	K0044	Footrest, upper hanger bracket, replacement only, each
▲	K0045	Footrest, complete assembly, replacement only, each
▲	K0046	Elevating leg rest, lower extension tube, replacement only, each
▲	K0047	Elevating leg rest, upper hanger bracket, replacement only, each
▲	K0050	Ratchet assembly, replacement only
▲	K0051	Cam release assembly, footrest or leg rest, replacement only, each
▲	K0052	Swing-Away, detachable footrests, replacement only, each
	K0053	Elevating footrests, articulating (telescoping), each
	K0056	Seat height less than 17" or equal to or greater than 21" for a high strength, lightweight, or ultra lightweight wheelchair
	K0065	Spoke protectors, each
▲	K0069	Rear wheel assembly, complete, with solid tire, spokes or molded, replacement only, each
	K0070	Rear wheel assembly, complete, with pneumatic tire, spokes or molded, each
▲	K0071	Front caster assembly, complete, with pneumatic tire, replacement only, each
▲	K0072	Front caster assembly, complete, with semi-pneumatic tire, replacement only, each
	K0073	Caster pin lock, each
▲	K0077	Front caster assembly, complete, with solid tire, replacement only, each
▲	K0098	Drive belt for power wheelchair, replacement only
	K0105	IV hanger, each

K0108 Wheelchair component or accessory, not otherwise specified

K0195 Elevating leg rests, pair (for use with capped rental wheelchair base)

CIM: 60-9

K0455 Infusion pump used for uninterrupted parenteral administration of medication, (e.g., epoprostenol or treprostinil)

CIM: 60-14

K0462 Temporary replacement for patient owned equipment being repaired, any type

MCM: 5102.3

▲ **K0552** Supplies for external non-insulin drug infusion pump, syringe type cartridge, sterile, each

CIM: 60-14

K0601 Replacement battery for external infusion pump owned by patient, silver oxide, 1.5 volt, each

K0602 Replacement battery for external infusion pump owned by patient, silver oxide, 3 volt, each

K0603 Replacement battery for external infusion pump owned by patient, alkaline, 1.5 volt, each

K0604 Replacement battery for external infusion pump owned by patient, lithium, 3.6 volt, each

K0605 Replacement battery for external infusion pump owned by patient, lithium, 4.5 volt, each

K0606 Automatic external defibrillator, with integrated electrocardiogram analysis, garment type

K0607 Replacement battery for automated external defibrillator, garment type only, each

K0608 Replacement garment for use with automated external defibrillator, each

K0609 Replacement electrodes for use with automated external defibrillator, garment type only, each

K0669 Wheelchair accessory, wheelchair seat or back cushion, does not meet specific code criteria or no written coding verification from DME PDAC

K0672 Addition to lower extremity orthosis, removable soft interface, all components, replacement only, each

K0730 Controlled dose inhalation drug delivery system

K0733 Power wheelchair accessory, 12 to 24 amp hour sealed lead acid battery, each (e.g., gel cell, absorbed glassmat)

K0738 Portable gaseous oxygen system, rental; home compressor used to fill portable oxygen cylinders; includes portable containers, regulator, flowmeter, humidifier, cannula or mask, and tubing

K0739 Repair or nonroutine service for durable medical equipment other than oxygen equipment requiring the skill of a technician, labor component, per 15 minutes

K0740 Repair or nonroutine service for oxygen equipment requiring the skill of a technician, labor component, per 15 minutes

K0743 Suction pump, home model, portable, for use on wounds

K0744 Absorptive wound dressing for use with suction pump, home model, portable, pad size 16 square inches or less

K0745 Absorptive wound dressing for use with suction pump, home model, portable, pad size more than 16 square inches but less than or equal to 48 square inches

K0746 Absorptive wound dressing for use with suction pump, home model, portable, pad size greater than 48 square inches

K0800 Power operated vehicle, group 1 standard, patient weight capacity up to and including 300 pounds

K0801 Power operated vehicle, group 1 heavy duty, patient weight capacity 301 to 450 pounds

K0802 Power operated vehicle, group 1 very heavy duty, patient weight capacity 451 to 600 pounds

K0806 Power operated vehicle, group 2 standard, patient weight capacity up to and including 300 pounds

K0807 Power operated vehicle, group 2 heavy duty, patient weight capacity 301 to 450 pounds

K0808 Power operated vehicle, group 2 very heavy duty, patient weight capacity 451 to 600 pounds

K0812 Power operated vehicle, not otherwise classified

K0813 Power wheelchair, group 1 standard, portable, sling/solid seat and back, patient weight capacity up to and including 300 pounds

K0814 Power wheelchair, group 1 standard, portable, captains chair, patient weight capacity up to and including 300 pounds

K0815 Power wheelchair, group 1 standard, sling/solid seat and back, patient weight capacity up to and including 300 pounds

K0816 Power wheelchair, group 1 standard, captains chair, patient weight capacity up to and including 300 pounds

K0820 Power wheelchair, group 2 standard, portable, sling/solid seat/back, patient weight capacity up to and including 300 pounds

K0821 Power wheelchair, group 2 standard, portable, captains chair, patient weight capacity up to and including 300 pounds

K0822 Power wheelchair, group 2 standard, sling/solid seat/back, patient weight capacity up to and including 300 pounds

K0823 Power wheelchair, group 2 standard, captains chair, patient weight capacity up to and including 300 pounds

K0824 Power wheelchair, group 2 heavy duty, sling/solid seat/back, patient weight capacity 301 to 450 pounds

K0825 Power wheelchair, group 2 heavy duty, captains chair, patient weight capacity 301 to 450 pounds

K0826 Power wheelchair, group 2 very heavy duty, sling/solid seat/back, patient weight capacity 451 to 600 pounds

K0827 Power wheelchair, group 2 very heavy duty, captains chair, patient weight capacity 451 to 600 pounds

K0828 Power wheelchair, group 2 extra heavy duty, sling/solid seat/back, patient weight capacity 601 pounds or more

K0829 Power wheelchair, group 2 extra heavy duty, captains chair, patient weight 601 pounds or more

K0830 Power wheelchair, group 2 standard, seat elevator, sling/solid seat/back, patient weight capacity up to and including 300 pounds

K0831 Power wheelchair, group 2 standard, seat elevator, captains chair, patient weight capacity up to and including 300 pounds

K0835 Power wheelchair, group 2 standard, single power option, sling/solid seat/back, patient weight capacity up to and including 300 pounds

K0836 Power wheelchair, group 2 standard, single power option, captains chair, patient weight capacity up to and including 300 pounds

K0837 Power wheelchair, group 2 heavy duty, single power option, sling/solid seat/back, patient weight capacity 301 to 450 pounds

K0838 Power wheelchair, group 2 heavy duty, single power option, captains chair, patient weight capacity 301 to 450 pounds

K0839 Power wheelchair, group 2 very heavy duty, single power option, sling/solid seat/back, patient weight capacity 451 to 600 pounds

K0840 Power wheelchair, group 2 extra heavy duty, single power option, sling/solid seat/back, patient weight capacity 601 pounds or more

K0841 Power wheelchair, group 2 standard, multiple power option, sling/solid seat/back, patient weight capacity up to and including 300 pounds

K0842 Power wheelchair, group 2 standard, multiple power option, captains chair, patient weight capacity up to and including 300 pounds

K0843 Power wheelchair, group 2 heavy duty, multiple power option, sling/solid seat/back, patient weight capacity 301 to 450 pounds

K0848 Power wheelchair, group 3 standard, sling/solid seat/back, patient weight capacity up to and including 300 pounds

K0849 Power wheelchair, group 3 standard, captains chair, patient weight capacity up to and including 300 pounds

K0850 Power wheelchair, group 3 heavy duty, sling/solid seat/back, patient weight capacity 301 to 450 pounds

K0851 Power wheelchair, group 3 heavy duty, captains chair, patient weight capacity 301 to 450 pounds

K0852 Power wheelchair, group 3 very heavy duty, sling/solid seat/back, patient weight capacity 451 to 600 pounds

K0853 Power wheelchair, group 3 very heavy duty, captains chair, patient weight capacity 451 to 600 pounds

K0854 Power wheelchair, group 3 extra heavy duty, sling/solid seat/back, patient weight capacity 601 pounds or more

K0855 Power wheelchair, group 3 extra heavy duty, captains chair, patient weight capacity 601 pounds or more

K0856 Power wheelchair, group 3 standard, single power option, sling/solid seat/back, patient weight capacity up to and including 300 pounds

K0857 Power wheelchair, group 3 standard, single power option, captains chair, patient weight capacity up to and including 300 pounds

K0858 Power wheelchair, group 3 heavy duty, single power option, sling/solid seat/back, patient weight 301 to 450 pounds

K0859 Power wheelchair, group 3 heavy duty, single power option, captains chair, patient weight capacity 301 to 450 pounds

K0860 Power wheelchair, group 3 very heavy duty, single power option, sling/solid seat/back, patient weight capacity 451 to 600 pounds

K0861 Power wheelchair, group 3 standard, multiple power option, sling/solid seat/back, patient weight capacity up to and including 300 pounds

K0862 Power wheelchair, group 3 heavy duty, multiple power option, sling/solid seat/back, patient weight capacity 301 to 450 pounds

K0863 Power wheelchair, group 3 very heavy duty, multiple power option, sling/solid seat/back, patient weight capacity 451 to 600 pounds

K0864 Power wheelchair, group 3 extra heavy duty, multiple power option, sling/solid seat/back, patient weight capacity 601 pounds or more

K0868 Power wheelchair, group 4 standard, sling/solid seat/back, patient weight capacity up to and including 300 pounds

K0869 Power wheelchair, group 4 standard, captains chair, patient weight capacity up to and including 300 pounds

K0870 Power wheelchair, group 4 heavy duty, sling/solid seat/back, patient weight capacity 301 to 450 pounds

K0871 Power wheelchair, group 4 very heavy duty, sling/solid seat/back, patient weight capacity 451 to 600 pounds

K0877 Power wheelchair, group 4 standard, single power option, sling/solid seat/back, patient weight capacity up to and including 300 pounds

K0878 Power wheelchair, group 4 standard, single power option, captains chair, patient weight capacity up to and including 300 pounds

K0879 Power wheelchair, group 4 heavy duty, single power option, sling/solid seat/back, patient weight capacity 301 to 450 pounds

K0880 Power wheelchair, group 4 very heavy duty, single power option, sling/solid seat/back, patient weight 451 to 600 pounds

K0884 Power wheelchair, group 4 standard, multiple power option, sling/solid seat/back, patient weight capacity up to and including 300 pounds

K0885 Power wheelchair, group 4 standard, multiple power option, captains chair, patient weight capacity up to and including 300 pounds

K0886 Power wheelchair, group 4 heavy duty, multiple power option, sling/solid seat/back, patient weight capacity 301 to 450 pounds

K0890 Power wheelchair, group 5 pediatric, single power option, sling/solid seat/back, patient weight capacity up to and including 125 pounds

K0891 Power wheelchair, group 5 pediatric, multiple power option, sling/solid seat/back, patient weight capacity up to and including 125 pounds

K0898 Power wheelchair, not otherwise classified

K0899 Power mobility device, not coded by DME PDAC or does not meet criteria

K0900 Customized durable medical equipment, other than wheelchair

(**K0901** Code deleted December 31, 2016). Use L1851.

(**K0902** Code deleted December 31, 2016). Use L1852

ORTHOTIC PROCEDURES

Guidelines

In addition to the information presented in the INTRODUCTION, several other items unique to this section are defined or identified here:

1. SUBSECTION INFORMATION: Some of the listed subheadings or subsections have special needs or instructions unique to that section. Where these are indicated, special "notes" will be presented preceding or following the listings. Those subsections within the ORTHOTIC PROCEDURES section that have "notes" are as follows:

Subsection	Code Numbers
Scoliosis procedures	L1000-L1499
Orthotic devices-lower limb	L1600-L2999
Lower limb-hip-knee-angle-foot (or any combination)	L2000-L2199
Orthotic devices-upper limb	L3650-L3999

2. UNLISTED SERVICE OR PROCEDURE: A service or procedure may be provided that is not listed in this edition of HCPCS. When reporting such a service, the appropriate "unlisted procedure" code may be used to indicate the service, identifying it by "special report" as defined below. HCPCS terminology is inconsistent in defining unlisted procedures. The procedure definition may include the term(s) "unlisted", "not otherwise classified", "unspecified", "unclassified", "other" and "miscellaneous". Prior to using these codes, try to determine if a Local Level III code or CPT code is available. The "unlisted procedures" and accompanying codes for ORTHOTIC PROCEDURES are as follows:

   L0999 Addition to spinal orthosis, not otherwise specified
   L1499 Spinal orthosis, not otherwise specified
   L2999 Lower extremity orthosis, not otherwise specified
   L3649 Orthopedic shoe, modification, addition or transfer, not otherwise specified
   L3999 Upper limb orthosis, not otherwise specified

3. SPECIAL REPORT: A service, material or supply that is rarely provided, unusual, variable or new may require a special report in determining medical appropriateness for reimbursement purposes. Pertinent information should include an adequate definition or description of the nature, extent, and need for the service, material or supply.

4. MODIFIERS: Listed services may be modified under certain circumstances. When appropriate, the modifying circumstance is identified by adding a modifier to the basic procedure code. CPT and HCPCS National Level II modifiers may be used with CPT and HCPCS National Level II procedure codes. Modifiers commonly used with ORTHOTIC PROCEDURES are as follows:

   -CC Procedure code change (use "CC" when the procedure code submitted was changed either for administrative reasons or because an incorrect code was filed)

   -LT Left side (used to identify procedures performed on the left side of the body)

   -RT Right side (used to identify procedures performed on the right side of the body)

-TC Technical component. Under certain circumstances, a charge may be made for the technical component alone. Under those circumstances, the technical component charge is identified by adding modifier -TC to the usual procedure number. Technical component charges are institutional charges and are not billed separately by physicians. However, portable x-ray suppliers bill only for the technical component and should use modifier -TC. The change data from portable x-ray suppliers will then be used to build customary and prevailing profiles.

5. CPT CODE CROSS-REFERENCE: Unless otherwise specified, the equivalent CPT code for all listings in this section is 99070.

6. DURABLE MEDICAL EQUIPMENT REGIONAL CARRIERS (DMERCS): Effective October 1, 1993, claims orthotics must be billed to one of four regional carriers depending upon the residence of the beneficiary. The transition dates for DMERC claims is from November 1, 1993 to March 1, 1994, depending upon the state you practice in. See the Introduction for a complete discussion of DMERCs.

Orthotic Devices Spinal – Cervical

L0112 Cranial cervical orthosis, congenital torticollis type, with or without soft interface material, adjustable range of motion joint, custom fabricated

L0113 Cranial cervical orthosis, torticollis type, with or without joint, with or without soft interface material, prefabricated, includes fitting and adjustment

L0120 Cervical, flexible, non-adjustable, prefabricated, off-the-shelf (foam collar)

L0130 Cervical, flexible, thermoplastic collar, molded to patient

L0140 Cervical, semi-rigid, adjustable (plastic collar)

L0150 Cervical, semi-rigid, adjustable molded chin cup (plastic collar with mandibular/occipital piece)

L0160 Cervical, semi-rigid, wire frame occipital/mandibular support, prefabricated, off-the-shelf

L0170 Cervical, collar, molded to patient model

L0172 Cervical, collar, semi-rigid thermoplastic foam, two-piece, prefabricated, off-the-shelf

L0174 Cervical, collar, semi-rigid, thermoplastic foam, two piece with thoracic extension, prefabricated, off-the-shelf

L0180 Cervical, multiple post collar, occipital/mandibular supports, adjustable

L0190 Cervical, multiple post collar, occipital/mandibular supports, adjustable cervical bars (SOMI, Guilford, Taylor types)

L0200 Cervical, multiple post collar, occipital/mandibular supports, adjustable cervical bars, and thoracic extension

Spinal - Thoracic-Lumbar-Sacral

L0220 Thoracic, rib belt, custom fabricated

L0450 TLSO, flexible, provides trunk support, upper thoracic region, produces intracavitary pressure to reduce load on the intervertebral disks with rigid stays or panel(s), includes shoulder straps and closures, prefabricated, off-the-shelf

L0452 TLSO, flexible, provides trunk support, upper thoracic region, produces intracavitary pressure to reduce load on the intervertebral disks with rigid stays or panel(s), includes shoulder straps and closures, custom fabricated

L0454 TLSO flexible, provides trunk support, extends from sacrococcygeal junction to above t-9 vertebra, restricts gross trunk motion in the sagittal plane, produces intracavitary pressure to reduce load on the intervertebral disks with rigid stays or panel(s), includes shoulder straps and closures, prefabricated item that has been trimmed, bent, molded, assembled, or otherwise customized to fit a specific patient by an individual with expertise

L0455 TLSO, flexible, provides trunk support, extends from sacrococcygeal junction to above t-9 vertebra, restricts gross trunk motion in the sagittal plane, produces intracavitary pressure to reduce load on the intervertebral disks with rigid stays or panel(s), includes shoulder straps and closures, prefabricated, off-the-shelf

L0456 TLSO, flexible, provides trunk support, thoracic region, rigid posterior panel and soft anterior apron, extends from the sacrococcygeal junction and terminates just inferior to the scapular spine, restricts gross trunk motion in the sagittal plane, produces intracavitary pressure to reduce load on the intervertebral disks, includes straps and closures, prefabricated item that has been trimmed, bent, molded, assembled, or otherwise customized to fit a specific patient by an individual with expertise

L0457 TLSO, flexible, provides trunk support, thoracic region, rigid posterior panel and soft anterior apron, extends from the sacrococcygeal junction and terminates just inferior to the scapular spine, restricts gross trunk motion in the sagittal plane, produces intracavitary pressure to reduce load on the intervertebral disks, includes straps and closures, prefabricated, off-the-shelf

L0458 TLSO, triplanar control, modular segmented spinal system, two rigid plastic shells, posterior extends from the sacrococcygeal junction and terminates just inferior to the scapular spine, anterior extends from the symphysis pubis to the xiphoid, soft liner, restricts gross trunk motion in the sagittal, coronal, and transverse planes, lateral strength is provided by overlapping plastic and stabilizing closures, includes straps and closures, prefabricated, includes fitting and adjustment

L0460 TLSO, triplanar control, modular segmented spinal system, two rigid plastic shells, posterior extends from the sacrococcygeal junction and terminates just inferior to the scapular spine, anterior extends from the symphysis pubis to the sternal notch, soft liner, restricts gross trunk motion in the sagittal, coronal, and transverse planes, lateral strength is provided by overlapping plastic and stabilizing closures, includes straps and closures, prefabricated item that has been trimmed, bent, molded, assembled, or otherwise customized to fit a specific patient by an individual with expertise

L0462 TLSO, triplanar control, modular segmented spinal system, three rigid plastic shells, posterior extends from the sacrococcygeal junction and terminates just inferior to the scapular spine, anterior extends from the symphysis pubis to the sternal notch, soft liner, restricts gross trunk motion in the sagittal, coronal, and transverse planes, lateral strength is provided by overlapping plastic and stabilizing closures, includes straps and closures, prefabricated, includes fitting and adjustment

L0464 TLSO, triplanar control, modular segmented spinal system, four rigid plastic shells, posterior extends from sacrococcygeal junction and terminates just inferior to scapular spine, anterior extends from symphysis pubis to the sternal notch, soft liner, restricts gross trunk motion in sagittal, coronal, and transverse planes, lateral strength is provided by overlapping plastic and stabilizing closures, includes straps and closures, prefabricated, includes fitting and adjustment

L0466 TLSO, sagittal control, rigid posterior frame and flexible soft anterior apron with straps, closures and padding, restricts gross trunk motion in sagittal plane, produces intracavitary pressure to reduce load on intervertebral disks, prefabricated item that has been trimmed, bent, molded, assembled, or otherwise customized to fit a specific patient by an individual with expertise

L0467 TLSO, sagittal control, rigid posterior frame and flexible soft anterior apron with straps, closures and padding, restricts gross trunk motion in sagittal plane, produces intracavitary pressure to reduce load on intervertebral disks, prefabricated, off-the-shelf

L0468 TLSO, sagittal-coronal control, rigid posterior frame and flexible soft anterior apron with straps, closures and padding, extends from sacrococcygeal junction over scapulae, lateral strength provided by pelvic, thoracic, and lateral frame pieces, restricts gross trunk motion in sagittal, and coronal planes, produces intracavitary pressure to reduce load on intervertebral disks, prefabricated item that has been trimmed, bent, molded, assembled, or otherwise customized to fit a specific patient by an individual with expertise

L0469 TLSO, sagittal-coronal control, rigid posterior frame and flexible soft anterior apron with straps, closures and padding, extends from sacrococcygeal junction over scapulae, lateral strength provided by pelvic, thoracic, and lateral frame pieces, restricts gross trunk motion in sagittal and coronal planes, produces intracavitary pressure to reduce load on intervertebral disks, prefabricated, off-the-shelf

L0470 TLSO, triplanar control, rigid posterior frame and flexible soft anterior apron with straps, closures and padding, extends from sacrococcygeal junction to scapula, lateral strength provided by pelvic, thoracic, and lateral frame pieces, rotational strength provided by subclavicular extensions, restricts gross trunk motion in sagittal, coronal, and transverse planes, provides intracavitary pressure to reduce load on the intervertebral disks, includes fitting and shaping the frame, prefabricated, includes fitting and adjustment

L0472 TLSO, triplanar control, hyperextension, rigid anterior and lateral frame extends from symphysis pubis to sternal notch with two anterior components (one pubic and one sternal), posterior and lateral pads with straps and closures, limits spinal flexion, restricts gross trunk motion in sagittal, coronal, and transverse planes, includes fitting and shaping the frame, prefabricated, includes fitting and adjustment

L0480 TLSO, triplanar control, one piece rigid plastic shell without interface liner, with multiple straps and closures, posterior extends from sacrococcygeal junction and terminates just inferior to scapular spine, anterior extends from symphysis pubis to sternal notch, anterior or posterior opening, restricts gross trunk motion in sagittal, coronal, and transverse planes, includes a carved plaster or cad-cam model, custom fabricated

L0482 TLSO, triplanar control, one piece rigid plastic shell with interface liner, multiple straps and closures, posterior extends from sacrococcygeal junction and terminates just inferior to scapular spine, anterior extends from symphysis pubis to sternal notch, anterior or posterior opening, restricts gross trunk motion in sagittal, coronal, and transverse planes, includes a carved plaster or cad-cam model, custom fabricated

L0484 TLSO, triplanar control, two piece rigid plastic shell without interface liner, with multiple straps and closures, posterior extends from sacrococcygeal junction and terminates just inferior to scapular spine, anterior extends from symphysis pubis to sternal notch, lateral strength is enhanced by overlapping plastic, restricts gross trunk motion in the sagittal, coronal, and transverse planes, includes a carved plaster or cad-cam model, custom fabricated

L0486 TLSO, triplanar control, two piece rigid plastic shell with interface liner, multiple straps and closures, posterior extends from sacrococcygeal junction and terminates just inferior to scapular spine, anterior extends from symphysis pubis to sternal notch, lateral strength is enhanced by overlapping plastic, restricts gross trunk motion in the sagittal, coronal, and transverse planes, includes a carved plaster or cad-cam model, custom fabricated

L0488 TLSO, triplanar control, one piece rigid plastic shell with interface liner, multiple straps and closures, posterior extends from sacrococcygeal junction and terminates just inferior to scapular spine, anterior extends from symphysis pubis to sternal notch, anterior or posterior opening, restricts gross trunk motion in sagittal, coronal, and transverse planes, prefabricated, includes fitting and adjustment

L0490 TLSO, sagittal-coronal control, one piece rigid plastic shell, with overlapping reinforced anterior, with multiple straps and closures, posterior extends from sacrococcygeal junction and terminates at or before the t-9 vertebra, anterior extends from symphysis pubis to xiphoid, anterior opening, restricts gross trunk motion in sagittal and coronal planes, prefabricated, includes fitting and adjustment

L0491 TLSO, sagittal-coronal control, modular segmented spinal system, two rigid plastic shells, posterior extends from the sacrococcygeal junction and terminates just inferior to the scapular spine, anterior extends from the symphysis pubis to the xiphoid, soft liner, restricts gross trunk motion in the sagittal and coronal planes, lateral strength is provided by overlapping plastic and stabilizing closures, includes straps and closures, prefabricated, includes fitting and adjustment

L0492 TLSO, sagittal-coronal control, modular segmented spinal system, three rigid plastic shells, posterior extends from the sacrococcygeal junction and terminates just inferior to the scapular spine, anterior extends from the symphysis pubis to the xiphoid, soft liner, restricts gross trunk motion in the sagittal and coronal planes, lateral strength is provided by overlapping plastic and stabilizing closures, includes straps and closures, prefabricated, includes fitting and adjustment

Spinal - Sacroiliac Semi-Rigid

L0621 Sacroiliac orthosis, flexible, provides pelvic-sacral support, reduces motion about the sacroiliac joint, includes straps, closures, may include pendulous abdomen design, prefabricated, off-the-shelf

L0622 Sacroiliac orthosis, flexible, provides pelvic-sacral support, reduces motion about the sacroiliac joint, includes straps, closures, may include pendulous abdomen design, custom fabricated

L0623 Sacroiliac orthosis, provides pelvic-sacral support, with rigid or semi-rigid panels over the sacrum and abdomen, reduces motion about the sacroiliac joint, includes straps, closures, may include pendulous abdomen design, prefabricated, off-the-shelf

L0624 Sacroiliac orthosis, provides pelvic-sacral support, with rigid or semi-rigid panels placed over the sacrum and abdomen, reduces motion about the sacroiliac joint, includes straps, closures, may include pendulous abdomen design, custom fabricated

L0625 Lumbar orthosis, flexible, provides lumbar support, posterior extends from l-1 to below l-5 vertebra, produces intracavitary pressure to reduce load on the intervertebral discs, includes straps, closures, may include pendulous abdomen design, shoulder straps, stays, prefabricated, off-the-shelf

L0626 Lumbar orthosis, sagittal control, with rigid posterior panel(s), posterior extends from l-1 to below l-5 vertebra, produces intracavitary pressure to reduce load on the intervertebral discs, includes straps, closures, may include padding, stays, shoulder straps, pendulous abdomen design, prefabricated item that has been trimmed, bent, molded, assembled, or otherwise customized to fit a specific patient by an individual with expertise

L0627 Lumbar orthosis, sagittal control, with rigid anterior and posterior panels, posterior extends from l-1 to below l-5 vertebra, produces intracavitary pressure to reduce load on the intervertebral discs, includes straps, closures, may include padding, shoulder straps, pendulous abdomen design, prefabricated item that has been trimmed, bent, molded, assembled, or otherwise customized to fit a specific patient by an individual with expertise

L0628 Lumbar-sacral orthosis, flexible, provides lumbo-sacral support, posterior extends from sacrococcygeal junction to t-9 vertebra, produces intracavitary pressure to reduce load on the intervertebral discs, includes straps, closures, may include stays, shoulder straps, pendulous abdomen design, prefabricated, off-the-shelf

L0629 Lumbar-sacral orthosis, flexible, provides lumbo-sacral support, posterior extends from sacrococcygeal junction to t-9 vertebra, produces intracavitary pressure to reduce load on the intervertebral discs, includes straps, closures, may include stays, shoulder straps, pendulous abdomen design, custom fabricated

L0630 Lumbar-sacral orthosis, sagittal control, with rigid posterior panel(s), posterior extends from sacrococcygeal junction to t-9 vertebra, produces intracavitary pressure to reduce load on the intervertebral discs, includes straps, closures, may include padding, stays, shoulder straps, pendulous abdomen design, prefabricated item that has been trimmed, bent, molded, assembled, or otherwise customized to fit a specific patient by an individual with expertise

L0631 Lumbar-sacral orthosis, sagittal control, with rigid anterior and posterior panels, posterior extends from sacrococcygeal junction to t-9 vertebra, produces intracavitary pressure to reduce load on the intervertebral discs, includes straps, closures, may include padding, shoulder straps, pendulous abdomen design, prefabricated item that has been trimmed, bent, molded, assembled, or otherwise customized to fit a specific patient by an individual with expertise

L0632 Lumbar-sacral orthosis, sagittal control, with rigid anterior and posterior panels, posterior extends from sacrococcygeal junction to t-9 vertebra, produces intracavitary pressure to reduce load on the intervertebral discs, includes straps, closures, may include padding, shoulder straps, pendulous abdomen design, custom fabricated

L0633 Lumbar-sacral orthosis, sagittal-coronal control, with rigid posterior frame/panel(s), posterior extends from sacrococcygeal junction to t-9 vertebra, lateral strength provided by rigid lateral frame/panels, produces intracavitary pressure to reduce load on intervertebral discs, includes straps, closures, may include padding, stays, shoulder straps, pendulous abdomen design, prefabricated item that has been trimmed, bent, molded, assembled, or otherwise customized to fit a specific patient by an individual with expertise

L0634 Lumbar-sacral orthosis, sagittal-coronal control, with rigid posterior frame/panel(s), posterior extends from sacrococcygeal junction to t-9 vertebra, lateral strength provided by rigid lateral frame/panel(s), produces intracavitary pressure to reduce load on intervertebral discs, includes straps, closures, may include padding, stays, shoulder straps, pendulous abdomen design, custom fabricated

L0635 Lumbar-sacral orthosis, sagittal-coronal control, lumbar flexion, rigid posterior frame/panel(s), lateral articulating design to flex the lumbar spine, posterior extends from sacrococcygeal junction to t-9 vertebra, lateral strength provided by rigid lateral frame/panel(s), produces intracavitary pressure to reduce load on intervertebral discs, includes straps, closures, may include padding, anterior panel, pendulous abdomen design, prefabricated, includes fitting and adjustment

L0636 Lumbar sacral orthosis, sagittal-coronal control, lumbar flexion, rigid posterior frame/panels, lateral articulating design to flex the lumbar spine, posterior extends from sacrococcygeal junction to t-9 vertebra, lateral strength provided by rigid lateral frame/panels, produces intracavitary pressure to reduce load on intervertebral discs, includes straps, closures, may include padding, anterior panel, pendulous abdomen design, custom fabricated

L0637 Lumbar-sacral orthosis, sagittal-coronal control, with rigid anterior and posterior frame/panels, posterior extends from sacrococcygeal junction to t-9 vertebra, lateral strength provided by rigid lateral frame/panels, produces intracavitary pressure to reduce load on intervertebral discs, includes straps, closures, may include padding, shoulder straps, pendulous abdomen design, prefabricated item that has been trimmed, bent, molded, assembled, or otherwise customized to fit a specific patient by an individual with expertise

L0638 Lumbar-sacral orthosis, sagittal-coronal control, with rigid anterior and posterior frame/panels, posterior extends from sacrococcygeal junction to t-9 vertebra, lateral strength provided by rigid lateral frame/panels, produces intracavitary pressure to reduce load on intervertebral discs, includes straps, closures, may include padding, shoulder straps, pendulous abdomen design, custom fabricated

L0639 Lumbar-sacral orthosis, sagittal-coronal control, rigid shell(s)/panel(s), posterior extends from sacrococcygeal junction to t-9 vertebra, anterior extends from symphysis pubis to xyphoid, produces intracavitary pressure to reduce load on the intervertebral discs, overall strength is provided by overlapping rigid material and stabilizing closures, includes straps, closures, may include soft interface, pendulous abdomen design, prefabricated item that has been trimmed, bent, molded, assembled, or otherwise customized to fit a specific patient by an individual with expertise

L0640 Lumbar-sacral orthosis, sagittal-coronal control, rigid shell(s)/panel(s), posterior extends from sacrococcygeal junction to t-9 vertebra, anterior extends from symphysis pubis to xyphoid, produces intracavitary pressure to reduce load on the intervertebral discs, overall strength is provided by overlapping rigid material and stabilizing closures, includes straps, closures, may include soft interface, pendulous abdomen design, custom fabricated

L0641 Lumbar orthosis, sagittal control, with rigid posterior panel(s), posterior extends from l-1 to below l-5 vertebra, produces intracavitary pressure to reduce load on the intervertebral discs, includes straps, closures, may include padding, stays, shoulder straps, pendulous abdomen design, prefabricated, off-the-shelf

L0642 Lumbar orthosis, sagittal control, with rigid anterior and posterior panels, posterior extends from l-1 to below l-5 vertebra, produces intracavitary pressure to reduce load on the intervertebral discs, includes straps, closures, may include padding, shoulder straps, pendulous abdomen design, prefabricated, off-the-shelf

L0643 Lumbar-sacral orthosis, sagittal control, with rigid posterior panel(s), posterior extends from sacrococcygeal junction to t-9 vertebra, produces intracavitary pressure to reduce load on the intervertebral discs, includes straps, closures, may include padding, stays, shoulder straps, pendulous abdomen design, prefabricated, off-the-shelf

L0648 Lumbar-sacral orthosis, sagittal control, with rigid anterior and posterior panels, posterior extends from sacrococcygeal junction to t-9 vertebra, produces intracavitary pressure to reduce load on the intervertebral discs, includes straps, closures, may include padding, shoulder straps, pendulous abdomen design, prefabricated, off-the-shelf

L0649 Lumbar-sacral orthosis, sagittal-coronal control, with rigid posterior frame/panel(s), posterior extends from sacrococcygeal junction to t-9 vertebra, lateral strength provided by rigid lateral frame/panels, produces intracavitary pressure to reduce load on intervertebral discs, includes straps, closures, may include padding, stays, shoulder straps, pendulous abdomen design, prefabricated, off-the-shelf

L0650 Lumbar-sacral orthosis, sagittal-coronal control, with rigid anterior and posterior frame/panel(s), posterior extends from sacrococcygeal junction to t-9 vertebra, lateral strength provided by rigid lateral frame/panel(s), produces intracavitary pressure to reduce load on intervertebral discs, includes straps, closures, may include padding, shoulder straps, pendulous abdomen design, prefabricated, off-the-shelf

L0651 Lumbar-sacral orthosis, sagittal-coronal control, rigid shell(s)/panel(s), posterior extends from sacrococcygeal junction to t-9 vertebra, anterior extends from symphysis pubis to xyphoid, produces intracavitary pressure to reduce load on the intervertebral discs, overall strength is provided by overlapping rigid material and stabilizing closures, includes straps, closures, may include soft interface, pendulous abdomen design, prefabricated, off-the-shelf

Spinal - Cervical-Thoracic-Lumbar-Sacral – Halo Procedure

L0700 Cervical-thoracic-lumbar-sacral-orthoses (CTLSO), anterior-posterior-lateral control, molded to patient model, (Minerva type)

L0710 CTLSO, anterior-posterior-lateral-control, molded to patient model, with interface material, (Minerva type)

L0810 Halo procedure, cervical halo incorporated into jacket vest

L0820 Halo procedure, cervical halo incorporated into plaster body jacket

L0830 Halo procedure, cervical halo incorporated into Milwaukee type orthosis

Additions to Spinal Orthoses

L0859 Addition to halo procedure, magnetic resonance image compatible systems, rings and pins, any material

L0861 Addition to halo procedure, replacement liner/interface material

L0970 TLSO, corset front

L0972 LSO, corset front

L0974 TLSO, full corset

L0976 LSO, full corset

L0978 Axillary crutch extension

L0980 Peroneal straps, prefabricated, off-the-shelf, pair

L0982 Stocking supporter grips, prefabricated, off-the-shelf, set of four (4)

L0984 Protective body sock, prefabricated, off-the-shelf, each

L0999 Addition to spinal orthosis, not otherwise specified

Orthotic Devices - Scoliosis Procedures

NOTE: The orthotic care of scoliosis differs from other orthotic care in that the treatment is more dynamic in nature and utilizes ongoing, continual modification of the orthosis to the patient's changing condition. This coding structure uses the proper names or eponyms of the procedures because they have historic and universal acceptance in the profession. It should be recognized that variations to the basic procedures described by the founders/developers are accepted in various medical and orthotic practices throughout the country. All procedures include model of patient when indicated.

L1000 Cervical-thoracic-lumbar-sacral orthosis (CTLSO) (Milwaukee), inclusive of furnishing initial orthosis, including model

L1001 Cervical thoracic lumbar sacral orthosis, immobilizer, infant size, prefabricated, includes fitting and adjustment

L1005 Tension based scoliosis orthosis and accessory pads, includes fitting and adjustment

L1010 Addition to cervical-thoracic-lumbar-sacral orthosis (CTLSO) or scoliosis orthosis, axilla sling

L1020 Addition to CTLSO or scoliosis orthosis, kyphosis pad

L1025 Addition to CTLSO or scoliosis orthosis, kyphosis pad, floating

L1030 Addition to CTLSO or scoliosis orthosis, lumbar bolster pad

L1040 Addition to CTLSO or scoliosis orthosis, lumbar or lumbar rib pad

L1050 Addition to CTLSO or scoliosis orthosis, sternal pad

L1060 Addition to CTLSO or scoliosis orthosis, thoracic pad

L1070 Addition to CTLSO or scoliosis orthosis, trapezius sling

L1080 Addition to CTLSO or scoliosis orthosis, outrigger

L1085 Addition to CTLSO or scoliosis orthosis, outrigger, bilateral with vertical extensions

L1090 Addition to CTLSO or scoliosis orthosis, lumbar sling

L1100 Addition to CTLSO or scoliosis orthosis, ring flange, plastic or leather

L1110 Addition to CTLSO or scoliosis orthosis, ring flange, plastic or leather, molded to patient model

L1120 Addition to CTLSO, scoliosis orthosis, cover for upright, each

L1200 Thoracic-lumbar-sacral-orthosis (TLSO), inclusive of furnishing initial orthosis only

L1210 Addition to TLSO, (low profile), lateral thoracic extension

L1220 Addition to TLSO, (low profile), anterior thoracic extension

L1230 Addition to TLSO, (low profile), Milwaukee type superstructure

L1240 Addition to TLSO, (low profile), lumbar derotation pad

L1250 Addition to TLSO, (low profile), anterior ASIS pad

L1260 Addition to TLSO, (low profile), anterior thoracic derotation pad

L1270 Addition to TLSO, (low profile), abdominal pad

L1280 Addition to TLSO, (low profile), rib gusset (elastic), each

L1290 Addition to TLSO, (low profile), lateral trochanteric pad

L1300 Other scoliosis procedure, body jacket molded to patient model

L1310 Other scoliosis procedure, post-operative body jacket

L1499 Spinal orthosis, not otherwise specified

Orthotic Devices - Lower Limb

NOTE: The procedures L1600-L2999 are considered as "base" or the "basic procedures" and may be modified by listing other procedures from the "additions" (L2200-L2999) section and adding them to the base procedure.

L1600 Hip orthosis, abduction control of hip joints, flexible, Frejka type with cover, prefabricated item that has been trimmed, bent, molded, assembled, or otherwise customized to fit a specific patient by an individual with expertise

L1610 Hip orthosis, abduction control of hip joints, flexible, (Frejka cover only), prefabricated item that has been trimmed, bent, molded, assembled, or otherwise customized to fit a specific patient by an individual with expertise

L1620 Hip orthosis, abduction control of hip joints, flexible, (Pavlik harness), prefabricated item that has been trimmed, bent, molded, assembled, or otherwise customized to fit a specific patient by an individual with expertise

L1630 Hip orthosis, abduction control of hip joints, semi-flexible (von Rosen type), custom fabricated

L1640 Hip orthosis, abduction control of hip joints, static, pelvic band or spreader bar, thigh cuffs, custom fabricated

L1650 Hip orthosis, abduction control of hip joints, static, adjustable, (Ilfeld type), prefabricated, includes fitting and adjustment

L1652 Hip orthosis, bilateral thigh cuffs with adjustable abductor spreader bar, adult size, prefabricated, includes fitting and adjustment, any type

L1660 Hip orthosis, abduction control of hip joints, static, plastic, prefabricated, includes fitting and adjustment

L1680 Hip orthosis, abduction control of hip joints, dynamic, pelvic control, adjustable hip motion control, thigh cuffs (rancho hip action type), custom fabricated

L1685 Hip orthosis, abduction control of hip joint, postoperative hip abduction type, custom fabricated

L1686 Hip orthosis, abduction control of hip joint, postoperative hip abduction type, prefabricated, includes fitting and adjustment

L1690 Combination, bilateral, lumbo-sacral, hip, femur orthosis providing adduction and internal rotation control, prefabricated, includes fitting and adjustment

L1700 Legg Perthes orthosis, (Toronto type), custom fabricated

L1710 Legg Perthes orthosis, (newington type), custom fabricated

L1720 Legg Perthes orthosis, trilateral, (Tachdjian type), custom fabricated

L1730 Legg Perthes orthosis, (Scottish rite type), custom fabricated

L1755 Legg Perthes orthosis, (patten bottom type), custom fabricated

L1810 Knee orthosis, elastic with joints, prefabricated item that has been trimmed, bent, molded, assembled, or otherwise customized to fit a specific patient by an individual with expertise

L1812 Knee orthosis, elastic with joints, prefabricated, off-the-shelf

L1820 Knee orthosis, elastic with condylar pads and joints, with or without patellar control, prefabricated, includes fitting and adjustment

L1830 Knee orthosis, immobilizer, canvas longitudinal, prefabricated, off-the-shelf

L1831 Knee orthosis, locking knee joint(s), positional orthosis, prefabricated, includes fitting and adjustment

L1832 Knee orthosis, adjustable knee joints (unicentric or polycentric), positional orthosis, rigid support, prefabricated item that has been trimmed, bent, molded, assembled, or otherwise customized to fit a specific patient by an individual with expertise

L1833 Knee orthosis, adjustable knee joints (unicentric or polycentric), positional orthosis, rigid support, prefabricated, off-the shelf

L1834 Knee orthosis, without knee joint, rigid, custom fabricated

L1836 Knee orthosis, rigid, without joint(s), includes soft interface material, prefabricated, off-the-shelf

L1840 Knee orthosis, derotation, medial-lateral, anterior cruciate ligament, custom fabricated

L1843 Knee orthosis, single upright, thigh and calf, with adjustable flexion and extension joint (unicentric or polycentric), medial-lateral and rotation control, with or without varus/valgus adjustment, prefabricated item that has been trimmed, bent, molded, assembled, or otherwise customized to fit a specific patient by an individual with expertise

L1844 Knee orthosis, single upright, thigh and calf, with adjustable flexion and extension joint (unicentric or polycentric), medial-lateral and rotation control, with or without varus/valgus adjustment, custom fabricated

L1845 Knee orthosis, double upright, thigh and calf, with adjustable flexion and extension joint (unicentric or polycentric), medial-lateral and rotation control, with or without varus/valgus adjustment, prefabricated item that has been trimmed, bent, molded, assembled, or otherwise customized to fit a specific patient by an individual with expertise

L1846 Knee orthosis, double upright, thigh and calf, with adjustable flexion and extension joint (unicentric or polycentric), medial-lateral and rotation control, with or without varus/valgus adjustment, custom fabricated

L1847 Knee orthosis, double upright with adjustable joint, with inflatable air support chamber(s), prefabricated item that has been trimmed, bent, molded, assembled, or otherwise customized to fit a specific patient by an individual with expertise

L1848 Knee orthosis, double upright with adjustable joint, with inflatable air support chamber(s), prefabricated, off-the-shelf

L1850 Knee orthosis, Swedish type, prefabricated, off-the-shelf

• **L1851** Knee orthosis (KO), single upright, thigh and calf, with adjustable flexion and extension joint (unicentric or polycentric), medial-lateral and rotation control, with or without varus/valgus adjustment, prefabricated, off-the-shelf

• **L1852** Knee orthosis (KO), double upright, thigh and calf, with adjustable flexion and extension joint (unicentric or polycentric), medial-lateral and rotation control, with or without varus/valgus adjustment, prefabricated, off-the-shelf

L1860 Knee orthosis, modification of supracondylar prosthetic socket, custom fabricated (sk)

L1900 Ankle foot orthosis, spring wire, dorsiflexion assist calf band, custom fabricated

L1902 Ankle orthosis, ankle gauntlet or similar, with or without joints, prefabricated, off-the-shelf

▲ **L1904** Ankle foot orthosis, multiligamentous ankle support, prefabricated, off-the-shelf

L1906 Ankle foot orthosis, multiligamentous ankle support, prefabricated, off-the-shelf

L1907 Ankle orthosis, supramalleolar with straps, with or without interface/pads, custom fabricated

L1910 Ankle foot orthosis, posterior, single bar, clasp attachment to shoe counter, prefabricated, includes fitting and adjustment

L1920 Ankle foot orthosis, single upright with static or adjustable stop (Phelps or Perlstein type), custom fabricated

L1930 Ankle foot orthosis, plastic or other material, prefabricated, includes fitting and adjustment

L1932 AFO, rigid anterior tibial section, total carbon fiber or equal material, prefabricated, includes fitting and adjustment

L1940 Ankle foot orthosis, plastic or other material, custom fabricated

L1945 Ankle foot orthosis, plastic, rigid anterior tibial section (floor reaction), custom fabricated

L1950 Ankle foot orthosis, spiral, (institute of rehabilitative medicine type), plastic, custom fabricated

L1951 Ankle foot orthosis, spiral, (institute of rehabilitative medicine type), plastic or other material, prefabricated, includes fitting and adjustment

L1960 Ankle foot orthosis, posterior solid ankle, plastic, custom fabricated

L1970 Ankle foot orthosis, plastic with ankle joint, custom fabricated

L1971 Ankle foot orthosis, plastic or other material with ankle joint, prefabricated, includes fitting and adjustment

L1980 Ankle foot orthosis, single upright free plantar dorsiflexion, solid stirrup, calf band/cuff (single bar 'BK' orthosis), custom fabricated

L1990 Ankle foot orthosis, double upright free plantar dorsiflexion, solid stirrup, calf band/cuff (double bar 'BK' orthosis), custom fabricated

L2000 Knee ankle foot orthosis, single upright, free knee, free ankle, solid stirrup, thigh and calf bands/cuffs (single bar 'AK' orthosis), custom fabricated

L2005 Knee ankle foot orthosis, any material, single or double upright, stance control, automatic lock and swing phase release, any type activation, includes ankle joint, any type, custom fabricated

L2010 Knee ankle foot orthosis, single upright, free ankle, solid stirrup, thigh and calf bands/cuffs (single bar 'AK' orthosis), without knee joint, custom fabricated

L2020 Knee ankle foot orthosis, double upright, free ankle, solid stirrup, thigh and calf bands/cuffs (double bar 'AK' orthosis), custom fabricated

L2030 Knee ankle foot orthosis, double upright, free ankle, solid stirrup, thigh and calf bands/cuffs, (double bar 'AK' orthosis), without knee joint, custom fabricated

L2034 Knee ankle foot orthosis, full plastic, single upright, with or without free motion knee, medial lateral rotation control, with or without free motion ankle, custom fabricated

L2035 Knee ankle foot orthosis, full plastic, static (pediatric size), without free motion ankle, prefabricated, includes fitting and adjustment

L2036 Knee ankle foot orthosis, full plastic, double upright, with or without free motion knee, with or without free motion ankle, custom fabricated

L2037 Knee ankle foot orthosis, full plastic, single upright, with or without free motion knee, with or without free motion ankle, custom fabricated

L2038 Knee ankle foot orthosis, full plastic, with or without free motion knee, multi-axis ankle, custom fabricated

Torsion Control

L2040 Hip knee ankle foot orthosis, torsion control, bilateral rotation straps, pelvic band/belt, custom fabricated

L2050 Hip knee ankle foot orthosis, torsion control, bilateral torsion cables, hip joint, pelvic band/belt, custom fabricated

L2060 Hip knee ankle foot orthosis, torsion control, bilateral torsion cables, ball bearing hip joint, pelvic band/ belt, custom fabricated

L2070 Hip knee ankle foot orthosis, torsion control, unilateral rotation straps, pelvic band/belt, custom fabricated

L2080 Hip knee ankle foot orthosis, torsion control, unilateral torsion cable, hip joint, pelvic band/belt, custom fabricated

L2090 Hip knee ankle foot orthosis, torsion control, unilateral torsion cable, ball bearing hip joint, pelvic band/ belt, custom fabricated

Fracture Orthoses and Additions

L2106 Ankle foot orthosis, fracture orthosis, tibial fracture cast orthosis, thermoplastic type casting material, custom fabricated

L2108 Ankle foot orthosis, fracture orthosis, tibial fracture cast orthosis, custom fabricated

L2112 Ankle foot orthosis, fracture orthosis, tibial fracture orthosis, soft, prefabricated, includes fitting and adjustment

L2114 Ankle foot orthosis, fracture orthosis, tibial fracture orthosis, semi-rigid, prefabricated, includes fitting and adjustment

L2116 Ankle foot orthosis, fracture orthosis, tibial fracture orthosis, rigid, prefabricated, includes fitting and adjustment

L2126 Knee ankle foot orthosis, fracture orthosis, femoral fracture cast orthosis, thermoplastic type casting material, custom fabricated

L2128 Knee ankle foot orthosis, fracture orthosis, femoral fracture cast orthosis, custom fabricated

L2132 KAFO, fracture orthosis, femoral fracture cast orthosis, soft, prefabricated, includes fitting and adjustment

L2134 KAFO, fracture orthosis, femoral fracture cast orthosis, semi-rigid, prefabricated, includes fitting and adjustment

L2136 KAFO, fracture orthosis, femoral fracture cast orthosis, rigid, prefabricated, includes fitting and adjustment

L2180 Addition to lower extremity fracture orthosis, plastic shoe insert with ankle joints

L2182 Addition to lower extremity fracture orthosis, drop lock knee joint

L2184 Addition to lower extremity fracture orthosis, limited motion knee joint

L2186 Addition to lower extremity fracture orthosis, adjustable motion knee joint, Lerman type

L2188 Addition to lower extremity fracture orthosis, quadrilateral brim

L2190 Addition to lower extremity fracture orthosis, waist belt

L2192 Addition to lower extremity fracture orthosis, hip joint, pelvic band, thigh flange, and pelvic belt

Additions To Lower Extremity Orthosis

L2200 Addition to lower extremity, limited ankle motion, each joint

L2210 Addition to lower extremity, dorsiflexion assist (plantar flexion resist), each joint

L2220 Addition to lower extremity, dorsiflexion and plantar flexion assist/resist, each joint

L2230 Addition to lower extremity, split flat caliper stirrups and plate attachment

L2232 Addition to lower extremity orthosis, rocker bottom for total contact ankle foot orthosis, for custom fabricated orthosis only

L2240 Addition to lower extremity, round caliper and plate attachment

L2250 Addition to lower extremity, foot plate, molded to patient model, stirrup attachment

L2260 Addition to lower extremity, reinforced solid stirrup (Scott-Craig type)

L2265 Addition to lower extremity, long tongue stirrup

L2270 Addition to lower extremity, varus/valgus correction ('t') strap, padded/lined or malleolus pad

L2275 Addition to lower extremity, varus/valgus correction, plastic modification, padded/lined

L2280 Addition to lower extremity, molded inner boot

L2300 Addition to lower extremity, abduction bar (bilateral hip involvement), jointed, adjustable

L2310 Addition to lower extremity, abduction bar-straight

L2320 Addition to lower extremity, non-molded lacer, for custom fabricated orthosis only

L2330 Addition to lower extremity, lacer molded to patient model, for custom fabricated orthosis only

L2335 Addition to lower extremity, anterior swing band

L2340 Addition to lower extremity, pre-tibial shell, molded to patient model

L2350 Addition to lower extremity, prosthetic type, (BK) socket, molded to patient model, (used for 'ptb' 'AFO' orthoses)

L2360 Addition to lower extremity, extended steel shank

L2370 Addition to lower extremity, patten bottom

L2375 Addition to lower extremity, torsion control, ankle joint and half solid stirrup

L2380 Addition to lower extremity, torsion control, straight knee joint, each joint

L2385 Addition to lower extremity, straight knee joint, heavy duty, each joint

L2387 Addition to lower extremity, polycentric knee joint, for custom fabricated knee ankle foot orthosis, each joint

L2390 Addition to lower extremity, offset knee joint, each joint

L2395 Addition to lower extremity, offset knee joint, heavy duty, each joint

L2397 Addition to lower extremity orthosis, suspension sleeve

Additions to Knee Joints

L2405 Addition to knee joint, drop lock, each

L2415 Addition to knee lock with integrated release mechanism (bail, cable, or equal), any material, each joint

L2425 Addition to knee joint, disc or dial lock for adjustable knee flexion, each joint

L2430 Addition to knee joint, ratchet lock for active and progressive knee extension, each joint

L2492 Addition to knee joint, lift loop for drop lock ring

Addition to Lower Extremity

L2500 Addition to lower extremity, thigh/weight bearing, gluteal/ ischial weight bearing, ring

L2510 Addition to lower extremity, thigh/weight bearing, quadri- lateral brim, molded to patient model

L2520 Addition to lower extremity, thigh/weight bearing, quadri- lateral brim, custom fitted

L2525 Addition to lower extremity, thigh/weight bearing, ischial containment/narrow m-l brim molded to patient model

L2526 Addition to lower extremity, thigh/weight bearing, ischial containment/narrow m-l brim, custom fitted

L2530 Addition to lower extremity, thigh-weight bearing, lacer, non-molded

L2540 Addition to lower extremity, thigh/weight bearing, lacer, molded to patient model

L2550 Addition to lower extremity, thigh/weight bearing, high roll cuff

L2570 Addition to lower extremity, pelvic control, hip joint, clevis type two position joint, each

L2580 Addition to lower extremity, pelvic control, pelvic sling

L2600 Addition to lower extremity, pelvic control, hip joint, clevis type, or thrust bearing, free, each

L2610 Addition to lower extremity, pelvic control, hip joint, clevis or thrust bearing, lock, each

L2620 Addition to lower extremity, pelvic control, hip joint, heavy duty, each

L2622 Addition to lower extremity, pelvic control, hip joint, adjustable flexion, each

L2624 Addition to lower extremity, pelvic control, hip joint, adjustable flexion, extension, abduction control, each

L2627 Addition to lower extremity, pelvic control, plastic, molded to patient model, reciprocating hip joint and cables

L2628 Addition to lower extremity, pelvic control, metal frame, reciprocating hip joint and cables

L2630 Addition to lower extremity, pelvic control, band and belt, unilateral

L2640 Addition to lower extremity, pelvic control, band and belt, bilateral

L2650 Addition to lower extremity, pelvic and thoracic control, gluteal pad, each

L2660 Addition to lower extremity, thoracic control, thoracic band

L2670 Addition to lower extremity, thoracic control, paraspinal uprights

L2680 Addition to lower extremity, thoracic control, lateral support uprights

L2750 Addition to lower extremity orthosis, plating chrome or nickel, per bar

L2755 Addition to lower extremity orthosis, high strength, lightweight material, all hybrid lamination/prepreg composite, per segment, for custom fabricated orthosis only

L2760 Addition to lower extremity orthosis, extension, per extension, per bar (for lineal adjustment for growth)

L2768 Orthotic side bar disconnect device, per bar

L2780 Addition to lower extremity orthosis, non-corrosive finish, per bar

L2785 Addition to lower extremity orthosis, drop lock retainer, each

L2795 Addition to lower extremity orthosis, knee control, full kneecap

L2800 Addition to lower extremity orthosis, knee control, knee cap, medial or lateral pull, for use with custom fabricated orthosis only

L2810 Addition to lower extremity orthosis, knee control, condylar pad

L2820 Addition to lower extremity orthosis, soft interface for molded plastic, below knee section

L2830 Addition to lower extremity orthosis, soft interface for molded plastic, above knee section

L2840 Addition to lower extremity orthosis, tibial length sock, fracture or equal, each

L2850 Addition to lower extremity orthosis, femoral length sock, fracture or equal, each

L2861 Addition to lower extremity joint, knee or ankle, concentric adjustable torsion style mechanism for custom fabricated orthotics only, each

L2999 Lower extremity orthoses, not otherwise specified

Foot- Insert and Arch Support

L3000 Foot, insert, removable, molded to patient model, 'UCB' type, Berkeley shell, each

MCM: 2323

L3001 Foot, insert, removable, molded to patient model, Spenco, each

MCM: 2323

L3002 Foot, insert, removable, molded to patient model, Plastazote or equal, each

MCM: 2323

L3003 Foot, insert, removable, molded to patient model, silicone gel, each

MCM: 2323

L3010 Foot, insert, removable, molded to patient model, longitudinal arch support, each

MCM: 2323

L3020 Foot, insert, removable, molded to patient model, longitudinal/ metatarsal support, each

MCM: 2323

L3030 Foot, insert, removable, formed to patient foot, each

MCM: 2323

L3031 Foot, insert/plate, removable, addition to lower extremity orthosis, high strength, lightweight material, all hybrid lamination/prepreg composite, each

L3040 Foot, arch support, removable, premolded, longitudinal, each

MCM: 2323

L3050 Foot, arch support, removable, premolded, metatarsal, each

MCM: 2323

L3060 Foot, arch support, removable, premolded, longitudinal/ metatarsal, each

MCM: 2323

L3070 Foot, arch support, non-removable attached to shoe, longitudinal, each

MCM: 2323

L3080 Foot, arch support, non-removable attached to shoe, metatarsal, each

MCM: 2323

L3090 Foot, arch support, non-removable attached to shoe, longitudinal/metatarsal, each

MCM: 2323

L3100 Hallus-valgus night dynamic splint, prefabricated, off-the-shelf

MCM: 2323

L3140 Foot, abduction rotation bar, including shoes

MCM: 2323

L3150 Foot, abduction rotatation bar, without shoes

MCM: 2323

L3160 Foot, adjustable shoe-styled positioning device

L3170 Foot, plastic, silicone or equal, heel stabilizer, prefabricated, off-the-shelf, each

MCM: 2323

Orthopedic Footwear

L3201 Orthopedic shoe, oxford with supinator or pronator, infant

MCM: 2323

L3202 Orthopedic shoe, oxford with supinator or pronator, child

MCM: 2323

L3203 Orthopedic shoe, oxford with supinator or pronator, junior
MCM: 2323

L3204 Orthopedic shoe, Hightop with supinator or pronator, infant
MCM: 2323

L3206 Orthopedic shoe, Hightop with supinator or pronator, child
MCM: 2323

L3207 Orthopedic shoe, Hightop with supinator or pronator, junior
MCM: 2323

L3208 Surgical boot, each, infant
MCM: 2079

L3209 Surgical boot, each, child
MCM: 2079

L3211 Surgical boot, each, junior
MCM: 2079

L3212 Benesch boot, pair, infant
MCM: 2079

L3213 Benesch boot, pair, child
MCM: 2079

L3214 Benesch boot, pair, junior
MCM: 2079

L3215 Orthopedic footwear, ladies shoe, oxford, each
Statute: 1862A8

L3216 Orthopedic footwear, ladies shoe, depth inlay, each
Statute: 1862A8

L3217 Orthopedic footwear, ladies shoe, Hightop, depth inlay, each
Statute: 1862A8

L3219 Orthopedic footwear, mens shoe, oxford, each
Statute: 1862A8

L3221 Orthopedic footwear, mens shoe, depth inlay, each
Statute: 1862A8

L3222 Orthopedic footwear, mens shoe, Hightop, depth inlay, each
Statute: 1862A8

L3224 Orthopedic footwear, woman's shoe, oxford, used as an integral part of a brace (orthosis)
MCM: 2323D

L3225 Orthopedic footwear, man's shoe, oxford, used as an integral part of a brace (orthosis)

MCM: 2323D

L3230 Orthopedic footwear, custom shoe, depth inlay, each

MCM: 2323

L3250 Orthopedic footwear, custom molded shoe, removable inner mold, prosthetic shoe, each

MCM: 2323

L3251 Foot, shoe molded to patient model, silicone shoe, each

MCM: 2323

L3252 Foot, shoe molded to patient model, Plastazote (or similar), custom fabricated, each

MCM: 2323

L3253 Foot, molded shoe Plastazote (or similar) custom fitted, each

MCM: 2323

L3254 Non-standard size or width

MCM: 2323

L3255 Non-standard size or length

MCM: 2323

L3257 Orthopedic footwear, additional charge for split size

MCM: 2323

L3260 Surgical boot/shoe, each

MCM: 2079

L3265 Plastazote sandal, each

Shoe Modification Lifts

L3300 Lift, elevation, heel, tapered to metatarsals, per inch

MCM: 2323

L3310 Lift, elevation, heel and sole, neoprene, per inch

MCM: 2323

L3320 Lift, elevation, heel and sole, cork, per inch

MCM: 2323

L3330 Lift, elevation, metal extension (skate)

MCM: 2323

L3332 Lift, elevation, inside shoe, tapered, up to one-half inch

MCM: 2323

L3334 Lift, elevation, heel, per inch

MCM: 2323

Wedges

L3340 Heel wedge, SACH

MCM: 2323

L3350 Heel wedge

MCM: 2323

L3360 Sole wedge, outside sole

MCM: 2323

L3370 Sole wedge, between sole

MCM: 2323

L3380 Clubfoot wedge

MCM: 2323

L3390 Outflare wedge

MCM: 2323

L3400 Metatarsal bar wedge, rocker

MCM: 2323

L3410 Metatarsal bar wedge, between sole

MCM: 2323

L3420 Full sole and heel wedge, between sole

MCM: 2323

Heels

L3430 Heel, counter, plastic reinforced

MCM: 2323

L3440 Heel, counter, leather reinforced

MCM: 2323

L3450 Heel, SACH cushion type

MCM: 2323

L3455 Heel, new leather, standard

MCM: 2323

L3460 Heel, new rubber, standard

MCM: 2323

L3465 Heel, Thomas with wedge

MCM: 2323

L3470 Heel, Thomas extended to ball

MCM: 2323

L3480 Heel, pad and depression for spur

MCM: 2323

L3485 Heel, pad, removable for spur

MCM: 2323

Orthopedic Shoe Additions

L3500 Orthopedic shoe addition, insole, leather

MCM: 2323

L3510 Orthopedic shoe addition, insole, rubber

MCM: 2323

L3520 Orthopedic shoe addition, insole, felt covered with leather

MCM: 2323

L3530 Orthopedic shoe addition, sole, half

MCM: 2323

L3540 Orthopedic shoe addition, sole, full

MCM: 2323

L3550 Orthopedic shoe addition, toe tap standard

MCM: 2323

L3560 Orthopedic shoe addition, toe tap, horseshoe

MCM: 2323

L3570 Orthopedic shoe addition, special extension to instep (leather with eyelets)

MCM: 2323

L3580 Orthopedic shoe addition, convert instep to Velcro closure

MCM: 2323

L3590 Orthopedic shoe addition, convert firm shoe counter to soft counter

MCM: 2323

L3595 Orthopedic shoe addition, march bar

MCM: 2323

Transfer or Replacement

L3600 Transfer of an orthosis from one shoe to another, caliper plate, existing

MCM: 2323

L3610 Transfer of an orthosis from one shoe to another, caliper plate, new

MCM: 2323

L3620 Transfer of an orthosis from one shoe to another, solid stirrup, existing

MCM: 2323

L3630 Transfer of an orthosis from one shoe to another, solid stirrup, new

MCM: 2323

L3640 Transfer of an orthosis from one shoe to another, Dennis Browne splint (Riveton), both shoes

MCM: 2323

L3649 Orthopedic shoe, modification, addition or transfer, not otherwise specified

MCM: 2323

Orthotic Devices – Upper Limb

L3650 Shoulder orthosis, figure of eight design abduction restrainer, prefabricated, off-the-shelf

L3660 Shoulder orthosis, figure of eight design abduction restrainer, canvas and webbing, prefabricated, off-the-shelf

L3670 Shoulder orthosis, acromio/clavicular (canvas and webbing type), prefabricated, off-the-shelf

L3671 Shoulder orthosis, shoulder joint design, without joints, may include soft interface, straps, custom fabricated, includes fitting and adjustment

L3674 Shoulder orthosis, abduction positioning (airplane design), thoracic component and support bar, with or without nontorsion joint/turnbuckle, may include soft interface, straps, custom fabricated, includes fitting and adjustment

L3675 Shoulder orthosis, vest type abduction restrainer, canvas webbing type or equal, prefabricated, off-the-shelf

L3677 Shoulder orthosis, shoulder joint design, without joints, may include soft interface, straps, prefabricated item that has been trimmed, bent, molded, assembled, or otherwise customized to fit a specific patient by an individual with expertise

MCM: 2130

L3678 Shoulder orthosis, shoulder joint design, without joints, may include soft interface, straps, prefabricated, off-the-shelf

L3702 Elbow orthosis, without joints, may include soft interface, straps, custom fabricated, includes fitting and adjustment

L3710 Elbow orthosis, elastic with metal joints, prefabricated, off-the-shelf

L3720 Elbow orthosis, double upright with forearm/arm cuffs, free motion, custom fabricated

L3730 Elbow orthosis, double upright with forearm/arm cuffs, extension/ flexion assist, custom fabricated

L3740 Elbow orthosis, double upright with forearm/arm cuffs, adjustable position lock with active control, custom fabricated

L3760 Elbow orthosis, with adjustable position locking joint(s), prefabricated, includes fitting and adjustments, any type

L3762 Elbow orthosis, rigid, without joints, includes soft interface material, prefabricated, off-the-shelf

L3763 Elbow wrist hand orthosis, rigid, without joints, may include soft interface, straps, custom fabricated, includes fitting and adjustment

L3764 Elbow wrist hand orthosis, includes one or more nontorsion joints, elastic bands, turnbuckles, may include soft interface, straps, custom fabricated, includes fitting and adjustment

L3765 Elbow wrist hand finger orthosis, rigid, without joints, may include soft interface, straps, custom fabricated, includes fitting and adjustment

L3766 Elbow wrist hand finger orthosis, includes one or more nontorsion joints, elastic bands, turnbuckles, may include soft interface, straps, custom fabricated, includes fitting and adjustment

L3806 Wrist hand finger orthosis, includes one or more nontorsion joint(s), turnbuckles, elastic bands/springs, may include soft interface material, straps, custom fabricated, includes fitting and adjustment

L3807 Wrist hand finger orthosis, without joint(s), prefabricated item that has been trimmed, bent, molded, assembled, or otherwise customized to fit a specific patient by an individual with expertise

L3808 Wrist hand finger orthosis, rigid without joints, may include soft interface material; straps, custom fabricated, includes fitting and adjustment

L3809 Wrist hand finger orthosis, without joint(s), prefabricated, off-the-shelf, any type

L3891 Addition to upper extremity joint, wrist or elbow, concentric adjustable torsion style mechanism for custom fabricated orthotics only, each

Wrist-Hand-Finger Orthoses

L3900 Wrist hand finger orthosis, dynamic flexor hinge, reciprocal wrist extension/ flexion, finger flexion/extension, wrist or finger driven, custom fabricated

L3901 Wrist hand finger orthosis, dynamic flexor hinge, reciprocal wrist extension/ flexion, finger flexion/extension, cable driven, custom fabricated

L3904 Wrist hand finger orthosis, external powered, electric, custom fabricated

L3905 Wrist hand orthosis, includes one or more nontorsion joints, elastic bands, turnbuckles, may include soft interface, straps, custom fabricated, includes fitting and adjustment

L3906 Wrist hand orthosis, without joints, may include soft interface, straps, custom fabricated, includes fitting and adjustment

L3908 Wrist hand orthosis, wrist extension control cock-up, non molded, prefabricated, off-the-shelf

L3912 Hand finger orthosis (HFO), flexion glove with elastic finger control, prefabricated, off-the-shelf

L3913 Hand finger orthosis, without joints, may include soft interface, straps, custom fabricated, includes fitting and adjustment

L3915 Wrist hand orthosis, includes one or more nontorsion joint(s), elastic bands, turnbuckles, may include soft interface, straps, prefabricated item that has been trimmed, bent, molded, assembled, or otherwise customized to fit a specific patient by an individual with expertise

L3916 Wrist hand orthosis, includes one or more nontorsion joint(s), elastic bands, turnbuckles, may include soft interface, straps, prefabricated, off-the-shelf

L3917 Hand orthosis, metacarpal fracture orthosis, prefabricated item that has been trimmed, bent, molded, assembled, or otherwise customized to fit a specific patient by an individual with expertise

L3918 Hand orthosis, metacarpal fracture orthosis, prefabricated, off-the-shelf

L3919 Hand orthosis, without joints, may include soft interface, straps, custom fabricated, includes fitting and adjustment

L3921 Hand finger orthosis, includes one or more nontorsion joints, elastic bands, turnbuckles, may include soft interface, straps, custom fabricated, includes fitting and adjustment

L3923 Hand finger orthosis, without joints, may include soft interface, straps, prefabricated item that has been trimmed, bent, molded, assembled, or otherwise customized to fit a specific patient by an individual with expertise

L3924 Hand finger orthosis, without joints, may include soft interface, straps, prefabricated, off-the-shelf

L3925 Finger orthosis, proximal interphalangeal (pip)/distal interphalangeal (dip), non torsion joint/spring, extension/flexion, may include soft interface material, prefabricated, off-the-shelf

L3927 Finger orthosis, proximal interphalangeal (pip)/distal interphalangeal (dip), without joint/spring, extension/flexion (e.g., static or ring type), may include soft interface material, prefabricated, off-the-shelf

L3929 Hand finger orthosis, includes one or more nontorsion joint(s), turnbuckles, elastic bands/springs, may include soft interface material, straps, prefabricated item that has been trimmed, bent, molded, assembled, or otherwise customized to fit a specific patient by an individual with expertise

L3930 Hand finger orthosis, includes one or more nontorsion joint(s), turnbuckles, elastic bands/springs, may include soft interface material, straps, prefabricated, off-the-shelf

L3931 Wrist hand finger orthosis, includes one or more nontorsion joint(s), turnbuckles, elastic bands/springs, may include soft interface material, straps, prefabricated, includes fitting and adjustment

L3933 Finger orthosis, without joints, may include soft interface, custom fabricated, includes fitting and adjustment

L3935 Finger orthosis, nontorsion joint, may include soft interface, custom fabricated, includes fitting and adjustment

L3956 Addition of joint to upper extremity orthosis, any material; per joint

Shoulder-Elbow-Wrist-Hand Orthoses (SEWHO)

L3960 Shoulder elbow wrist hand orthosis, abduction positioning, airplane design, prefabricated, includes fitting and adjustment

L3961 Shoulder elbow wrist hand orthosis, shoulder cap design, without joints, may include soft interface, straps, custom fabricated, includes fitting and adjustment

L3962 Shoulder elbow wrist hand orthosis, abduction positioning, Erb's palsy design, prefabricated, includes fitting and adjustment

L3967 Shoulder elbow wrist hand orthosis, abduction positioning (airplane design), thoracic component and support bar, without joints, may include soft interface, straps, custom fabricated, includes fitting and adjustment

L3971 Shoulder elbow wrist hand orthosis, shoulder cap design, includes one or more nontorsion joints, elastic bands, turnbuckles, may include soft interface, straps, custom fabricated, includes fitting and adjustment

L3973 Shoulder elbow wrist hand orthosis, abduction positioning (airplane design), thoracic component and support bar, includes one or more nontorsion joints, elastic bands, turnbuckles, may include soft interface, straps, custom fabricated, includes fitting and adjustment

L3975 Shoulder elbow wrist hand finger orthosis, shoulder cap design, without joints, may include soft interface, straps, custom fabricated, includes fitting and adjustment

L3976 Shoulder elbow wrist hand finger orthosis, abduction positioning (airplane design), thoracic component and support bar, without joints, may include soft interface, straps, custom fabricated, includes fitting and adjustment

L3977 Shoulder elbow wrist hand finger orthosis, shoulder cap design, includes one or more nontorsion joints, elastic bands, turnbuckles, may include soft interface, straps, custom fabricated, includes fitting and adjustment

L3978 Shoulder elbow wrist hand finger orthosis, abduction positioning (airplane design), thoracic component and support bar, includes one or more nontorsion joints, elastic bands, turnbuckles, may include soft interface, straps, custom fabricated, includes fitting and adjustment

Upper Limb – Fracture Orthoses

L3980 Upper extremity fracture orthosis, humeral, prefabricated, includes fitting and adjustment

L3981 Upper extremity fracture orthosis, humeral, prefabricated, includes shoulder cap design, with or without joints, forearm section, may include soft interface, straps, includes fitting and adjustments

L3982 Upper extremity fracture orthosis, radius/ulnar, prefabricated, includes fitting and adjustment

L3984 Upper extremity fracture orthosis, wrist, prefabricated, includes fitting and adjustment

L3995 Addition to upper extremity orthosis, sock, fracture or equal, each

L3999 Upper limb orthosis, not otherwise specified

Specific Repair

L4000 Replace girdle for spinal orthosis (CTLSO or so)

L4002 Replacement strap, any orthosis, includes all components, any length, any type

L4010 Replace trilateral socket brim

L4020 Replace quadrilateral socket brim, molded to patient model

L4030 Replace quadrilateral socket brim, custom fitted

L4040 Replace molded thigh lacer, for custom fabricated orthosis only

L4045 Replace non-molded thigh lacer, for custom fabricated orthosis only

L4050 Replace molded calf lacer, for custom fabricated orthosis only

L4055 Replace non-molded calf lacer, for custom fabricated orthosis only

L4060 Replace high roll cuff

L4070 Replace proximal and distal upright for KAFO

L4080 Replace metal bands KAFO, proximal thigh

L4090 Replace metal bands KAFO-AFO, calf or distal thigh

L4100 Replace leather cuff KAFO, proximal thigh

L4110 Replace leather cuff KAFO-AFO, calf or distal thigh

L4130 Replace pretibial shell

L4205 Repair of orthotic device, labor component, per 15 minutes

MCM: 2100.4

L4210 Repair of orthotic device, repair or replace minor parts

MCM: 2133, 2100.4, 2130D

Ancillary Orthotic Services

L4350 Ankle control orthosis, stirrup style, rigid, includes any type interface (e.g., pneumatic, gel), prefabricated, off-the-shelf

L4360 Walking boot, pneumatic and/or vacuum, with or without joints, with or without interface material, prefabricated item that has been trimmed, bent, molded, assembled, or otherwise customized to fit a specific patient by an individual with expertise

L4361 Walking boot, pneumatic and/or vacuum, with or without joints, with or without interface material, prefabricated, off-the-shelf

L4370 Pneumatic full leg splint, prefabricated, off-the-shelf

L4386 Walking boot, non-pneumatic, with or without joints, with or without interface material, prefabricated item that has been trimmed, bent, molded, assembled, or otherwise customized to fit a specific patient by an individual with expertise

L4387 Walking boot, non-pneumatic, with or without joints, with or without interface material, prefabricated, off-the-shelf

L4392 Replacement, soft interface material, static AFO

L4394 Replace soft interface material, foot drop splint

L4396 Static or dynamic ankle foot orthosis, including soft interface material, adjustable for fit, for positioning, may be used for minimal ambulation, prefabricated item that has been trimmed, bent, molded, assembled, or otherwise customized to fit a specific patient by an individual with expertise

L4397 Static or dynamic ankle foot orthosis, including soft interface material, adjustable for fit, for positioning, may be used for minimal ambulation, prefabricated, off-the-shelf

L4398 Foot drop splint, recumbent positioning device, prefabricated, off-the-shelf

L4631 Ankle foot orthosis, walking boot type, varus/valgus correction, rocker bottom, anterior tibial shell, soft interface, custom arch support, plastic or other material, includes straps and closures, custom fabricated

PROSTHETIC PROCEDURES

Guidelines

In addition to the information presented in the INTRODUCTION, several other items unique to this section are defined or identified here:

1. PROSTHETIC DEVICES: Prosthetic devices (other than dental) which replace all or part of an internal body organ (including contiguous tissue), or replace all or part of the function of a permanently inoperative or malfunctioning internal body organ, are covered when furnished upon a physician's order. This does not require a determination that there is no possibility that the patient's condition may improve in the future. If the medical record and the judgement of the attending physician indicate that the condition is of long and indefinite duration, the test of permanence is met. The device(s) may also be covered as a supply item when furnished incident to a physician's service.

2. SUBSECTION INFORMATION: Some of the listed subheadings or subsections have special needs or instructions unique to that section. Where these are indicated, special "notes" will be presented preceding or following the listings. Those subsections within the PROSTHETIC PROCEDURES section that have "notes" are as follows:

Subsection	Code Numbers
Prosthetic procedures-lower limb	L5000-L5999
Upper limb	L6000-L6590
Additions-upper limb	L6600-L6999

3. UNLISTED SERVICE OR PROCEDURE: A service or procedure may be provided that is not listed in this edition of HCPCS. When reporting such a service, the appropriate "unlisted procedure" code may be used to indicate the service, identifying it by "special report" as defined below. HCPCS terminology is inconsistent in defining unlisted procedures. The procedure definition may include the term(s) "unlisted", "not otherwise classified", "unspecified", "unclassified", "other" and "miscellaneous". Prior to using these codes, try to determine if a Local Level III code or CPT code is available. The "unlisted procedures" and accompanying codes for PROSTHETIC PROCEDURES are as follows:

   L5999 Lower extremity prosthesis, not otherwise specified
   L7499 Upper extremity prosthesis, not otherwise specified
   L8039 Breast prosthesis, not otherwise specified
   L8239 Gradient compression stocking, not otherwise specified
   L8499 Unlisted procedure for miscellaneous prosthetic services
   L8699 Prosthetic implant, not otherwise specified

4. SPECIAL REPORT: A service, material or supply that is rarely provided, unusual, variable or new may require a special report in determining medical appropriateness for reimbursement purposes. Pertinent information should include an adequate definition or description of the nature, extent, and need for the service, material or supply.

5. MODIFIERS: Listed services may be modified under certain circumstances. When appropriate, the modifying circumstance is identified by adding a modifier to the basic procedure code. CPT and HCPCS National Level II modifiers may be used with CPT and HCPCS National Level II procedure codes. Modifiers commonly used with PROSTHETIC PROCEDURES are as follows:

-CC Procedure code change (use "CC" when the procedure code submitted was changed either for administrative reasons or because an incorrect code was filed)

-LT Left side (used to identify procedures performed on the left side of the body)

-RT Right side (used to identify procedures performed on the right side of the body)

-TC Technical component. Under certain circumstances, a charge may be made for the technical component alone. Under those circumstances, the technical component charge is identified by adding modifier -TC to the usual procedure number. Technical component charges are institutional charges and are not billed separately by physicians. However, portable x-ray suppliers bill only for the technical component and should use modifier -TC. The charge data from portable x-ray suppliers will then be used to build customary and prevailing profiles.

6. CPT CODE CROSS-REFERENCE: Unless otherwise specified, the equivalent CPT code for all listings in this section is 99070.

7. DURABLE MEDICAL EQUIPMENT REGIONAL CARRIERS (DMERCS): Effective October 1, 1993 claims for prosthetics must be billed to one of four regional carriers depending upon the residence of the beneficiary. The transition dates for DMERC claims is from November 1, 1993 to March 1, 1994, depending upon the state you practice in. See the Introduction for a complete discussion of DMERCs.

Lower Limb

NOTE: The procedures in this section are considered as "base" or "basic" procedures, and they may be modified by listing items, procedures or special materials from the "additions" section, and adding them to the base procedure.

L5000 Partial foot, shoe insert with longitudinal arch, toe filler

MCM: 2323

L5010 Partial foot, molded socket, ankle height, with toe filler

MCM: 2323

L5020 Partial foot, molded socket, tibial tubercle height, with toe filler

MCM: 2323

L5050 Ankle, Symes, molded socket, SACH foot

L5060 Ankle, Symes, metal frame, molded leather socket, articulated ankle/foot

L5100 Below knee, molded socket, shin, SACH foot

L5105 Below knee, plastic socket, joints and thigh lacer, SACH foot

L5150 Knee disarticulation (or through knee), molded socket, external knee joints, shin, SACH foot

L5160 Knee disarticulation (or through knee), molded socket, bent knee configuration, external knee joints, shin, SACH foot

L5200 Above knee, molded socket, single axis constant friction knee, shin, SACH foot

L5210 Above knee, short prosthesis, no knee joint ('stubbies'), with foot blocks, no ankle joints, each

L5220 Above knee, short prosthesis, no knee joint ('stubbies'), with articulated ankle/foot, dynamically aligned, each

L5230 Above knee, for proximal femoral focal deficiency, constant friction knee, shin, SACH foot

L5250 Hip disarticulation, Canadian type; molded socket, hip joint, single axis constant friction knee, shin, SACH foot

L5270 Hip disarticulation, tilt table type; molded socket, locking hip joint, single axis constant friction knee, shin, SACH foot

L5280 Hemipelvectomy, Canadian type; molded socket, hip joint, single axis constant friction knee, shin, SACH foot

L5301 Below knee, molded socket, shin, SACH foot, endoskeletal system

L5312 Knee disarticulation (or through knee), molded socket, single axis knee, pylon, SACH foot, endoskeletal system

L5321 Above knee, molded socket, open end, SACH foot, endoskeletal system, single axis knee

L5331 Hip disarticulation, Canadian type, molded socket, endoskeletal system, hip joint, single axis knee, SACH foot

L5341 Hemipelvectomy, Canadian type, molded socket, endoskeletal system, hip joint, single axis knee, SACH foot

Immediate Post Surgical or Early Fitting Procedures

L5400 Immediate post surgical or early fitting, application of initial rigid dressing, including fitting, alignment, suspension, and one cast change, below knee

L5410 Immediate post surgical or early fitting, application of initial rigid dressing, including fitting, alignment and suspension, below knee, each additional cast change and realignment

L5420 Immediate post surgical or early fitting, application of initial rigid dressing, including fitting, alignment and suspension and one cast change 'AK' or knee disarticulation

L5430 Immediate post surgical or early fitting, application of initial rigid dressing, incl. fitting, alignment and suspension, 'AK' or knee disarticulation, each additional cast change and realignment

L5450 Immediate post surgical or early fitting, application of non-weight bearing rigid dressing, below knee

L5460 Immediate post surgical or early fitting, application of non-weight bearing rigid dressing, above knee

Initial Prosthesis

L5500 Initial, below knee 'ptb' type socket, non-alignable system, pylon, no cover, SACH foot, plaster socket, direct formed

L5505 Initial, above knee - knee disarticulation, ischial level socket, non-alignable system, pylon, no cover, SACH foot, plaster socket, direct formed

Preparatory Prosthesis

L5510 Preparatory, below knee 'ptb' type socket, non-alignable system, pylon, no cover, SACH foot, plaster socket, molded to model

L5520 Preparatory, below knee 'ptb' type socket, non-alignable system, pylon, no cover, SACH foot, thermoplastic or equal, direct formed

L5530 Preparatory, below knee 'ptb' type socket, non-alignable system, pylon, no cover, SACH foot, thermoplastic or equal, molded to model

L5535 Preparatory, below knee 'ptb' type socket, non-alignable system, no cover, SACH foot, prefabricated, adjustable open end socket

L5540 Preparatory, below knee 'ptb' type socket, non-alignable system, pylon, no cover, SACH foot, laminated socket, molded to model

L5560 Preparatory, above knee- knee disarticulation, ischial level socket, non-alignable system, pylon, no cover, SACH foot, plaster socket, molded to model

L5570 Preparatory, above knee - knee disarticulation, ischial level socket, non-alignable system, pylon, no cover, SACH foot, thermoplastic or equal, direct formed

L5580 Preparatory, above knee - knee disarticulation ischial level socket, non-alignable system, pylon, no cover, SACH foot, thermoplastic or equal, molded to model

L5585 Preparatory, above knee - knee disarticulation, ischial level socket, non-alignable system, pylon, no cover, SACH foot, prefabricated adjustable open end socket

L5590 Preparatory, above knee - knee disarticulation ischial level socket, non-alignable system, pylon no cover, SACH foot, laminated socket, molded to model

L5595 Preparatory, hip disarticulation-hemipelvectomy, pylon, no cover, SACH foot, thermoplastic or equal, molded to patient model

L5600 Preparatory, hip disarticulation-hemipelvectomy, pylon, no cover, SACH foot, laminated socket, molded to patient model

Additions To Lower Extremity

L5610 Addition to lower extremity, endoskeletal system, above knee, Hydra-Cadence system

L5611 Addition to lower extremity, endoskeletal system, above knee - knee disarticulation, 4 bar linkage, with friction swing phase control

L5613 Addition to lower extremity, endoskeletal system, above knee-knee disarticulation, 4 bar linkage, with hydraulic swing phase control

L5614 Addition to lower extremity, exoskeletal system, above knee-knee disarticulation, 4 bar linkage, with pneumatic swing phase control

L5616 Addition to lower extremity, endoskeletal system, above knee, universal multiplex system, friction swing phase control

L5617 Addition to lower extremity, quick change self-aligning unit, above knee or below knee, each

Additions - Test Sockets and Socket Variations

L5618 Addition to lower extremity, test socket, Symes

L5620 Addition to lower extremity, test socket, below knee

L5622 Addition to lower extremity, test socket, knee disarticulation

L5624 Addition to lower extremity, test socket, above knee

L5626 Addition to lower extremity, test socket, hip disarticulation

L5628 Addition to lower extremity, test socket, hemipelvectomy

L5629 Addition to lower extremity, below knee, acrylic socket

L5630 Addition to lower extremity, Symes type, expandable wall socket

L5631 Addition to lower extremity, above knee or knee disarticulation, acrylic socket

L5632 Addition to lower extremity, Symes type, 'ptb' brim design socket

L5634 Addition to lower extremity, Symes type, posterior opening (Canadian) socket

L5636 Addition to lower extremity, Symes type, medial opening socket

L5637 Addition to lower extremity, below knee, total contact

L5638 Addition to lower extremity, below knee, leather socket

L5639 Addition to lower extremity, below knee, wood socket

L5640 Addition to lower extremity, knee disarticulation, leather socket

L5642 Addition to lower extremity, above knee, leather socket

L5643 Addition to lower extremity, hip disarticulation, flexible inner socket, external frame

L5644 Addition to lower extremity, above knee, wood socket

L5645 Addition to lower extremity, below knee, flexible inner socket, external frame

L5646 Addition to lower extremity, below knee, air, fluid, gel or equal, cushion socket

L5647 Addition to lower extremity, below knee suction socket

L5648 Addition to lower extremity, above knee, air, fluid, gel or equal, cushion socket

L5649 Addition to lower extremity, ischial containment/narrow m-l socket

L5650 Additions to lower extremity, total contact, above knee or knee disarticulation socket

L5651 Addition to lower extremity, above knee, flexible inner socket, external frame

L5652 Addition to lower extremity, suction suspension, above knee or knee disarticulation socket

L5653 Addition to lower extremity, knee disarticulation, expandable wall socket

Additions - Socket Insert and Suspension

L5654 Addition to lower extremity, socket insert, Symes, (Kemblo, Pelite, Aliplast, Plastazote or equal)

L5655 Addition to lower extremity, socket insert, below knee (Kemblo, Pelite, Aliplast, Plastazote or equal)

L5656 Addition to lower extremity, socket insert, knee disarticulation (Kemblo, Pelite, Aliplast, Plastazote or equal)

L5658 Addition to lower extremity, socket insert, above knee (Kemblo, Pelite, Aliplast, Plastazote or equal)

L5661 Addition to lower extremity, socket insert, multi-durometer Symes

L5665 Addition to lower extremity, socket insert, multi-durometer, below knee

L5666 Addition to lower extremity, below knee, cuff suspension

L5668 Addition to lower extremity, below knee, molded distal cushion

L5670 Addition to lower extremity, below knee, molded supracondylar suspension ('pts' or similar)

L5671 Addition to lower extremity, below knee / above knee suspension locking mechanism (shuttle, lanyard or equal), excludes socket insert

L5672 Addition to lower extremity, below knee, removable medial brim suspension

L5673 Addition to lower extremity, below knee/above knee, custom fabricated from existing mold or prefabricated, socket insert, silicone gel, elastomeric or equal, for use with locking mechanism

L5676 Additions to lower extremity, below knee, knee joints, single axis, pair

L5677 Additions to lower extremity, below knee, knee joints, polycentric, pair

L5678 Additions to lower extremity, below knee, joint covers, pair

L5679 Addition to lower extremity, below knee/above knee, custom fabricated from existing mold or prefabricated, socket insert, silicone gel, elastomeric or equal, not for use with locking mechanism

L5680 Addition to lower extremity, below knee, thigh lacer, non-molded

L5681 Addition to lower extremity, below knee/above knee, custom fabricated socket insert for congenital or atypical traumatic amputee, silicone gel, elastomeric or equal, for use with or without locking mechanism, initial only (for other than initial, use code l5673 or l5679)

L5682 Addition to lower extremity, below knee, thigh lacer, gluteal/ischial, molded

L5683 Addition to lower extremity, below knee/above knee, custom fabricated socket insert for other than congenital or atypical traumatic amputee, silicone gel, elastomeric or equal, for use with or without locking mechanism, initial only (for other than initial, use code l5673 or l5679)

L5684 Addition to lower extremity, below knee, fork strap

L5685 Addition to lower extremity prosthesis, below knee, suspension/sealing sleeve, with or without valve, any material, each

L5686 Addition to lower extremity, below knee, back check (extension control)

L5688 Addition to lower extremity, below knee, waist belt, webbing

L5690 Addition to lower extremity, below knee, waist belt, padded and lined

L5692 Addition to lower extremity, above knee, pelvic control belt, light

L5694 Addition to lower extremity, above knee, pelvic control belt, padded and lined

L5695 Addition to lower extremity, above knee, pelvic control, sleeve suspension, neoprene or equal, each

L5696 Addition to lower extremity, above knee or knee disarticulation, pelvic joint

L5697 Addition to lower extremity, above knee or knee disarticulation, pelvic band

L5698 Addition to lower extremity, above knee or knee disarticulation, Silesian bandage

L5699 All lower extremity prostheses, shoulder harness

L5700 Replacement, socket, below knee, molded to patient model

L5701 Replacement, socket, above knee/knee disarticulation, including attachment plate, molded to patient model

L5702 Replacement, socket, hip disarticulation, including hip joint, molded to patient model

L5703 Ankle, Symes, molded to patient model, socket without solid ankle cushion heel (SACH) foot, replacement only

L5704 Custom shaped protective cover, below knee

L5705 Custom shaped protective cover, above knee

L5706 Custom shaped protective cover, knee disarticulation

L5707 Custom shaped protective cover, hip disarticulation

Additions - Knee-Shin System Exoskeletal

L5710 Addition, exoskeletal knee-shin system, single axis, manual lock

L5711 Additions exoskeletal knee-shin system, single axis, manual lock, ultra-light material

L5712 Addition, exoskeletal knee-shin system, single axis, friction swing and stance phase control (safety knee)

L5714 Addition, exoskeletal knee-shin system, single axis, variable friction swing phase control

L5716 Addition, exoskeletal knee-shin system, polycentric, mechanical stance phase lock

L5718 Addition, exoskeletal knee-shin system, polycentric, friction swing and stance phase control

L5722 Addition, exoskeletal knee-shin system, single axis, pneumatic swing, friction stance phase control

L5724 Addition, exoskeletal knee-shin system, single axis, fluid swing phase control

L5726 Addition, exoskeletal knee-shin system, single axis, external joints fluid swing phase control

L5728 Addition, exoskeletal knee-shin system, single axis, fluid swing and stance phase control

L5780 Addition, exoskeletal knee-shin system, single axis, pneumatic/hydra pneumatic swing phase control

L5781 Addition to lower limb prosthesis, vacuum pump, residual limb volume management and moisture evacuation system

L5782 Addition to lower limb prosthesis, vacuum pump, residual limb volume management and moisture evacuation system, heavy duty

L5785 Addition, exoskeletal system, below knee, ultra-light material (titanium, carbon fiber or equal)

L5790 Addition, exoskeletal system, above knee, ultra-light material (titanium, carbon fiber or equal)

L5795 Addition, exoskeletal system, hip disarticulation, ultra-light material (titanium, carbon fiber or equal)

Endoskeletal

L5810 Addition, endoskeletal knee-shin system, single axis, manual lock

L5811 Addition, endoskeletal knee-shin system, single axis, manual lock, ultra-light material

L5812 Addition, endoskeletal knee-shin system, single axis, friction swing and stance phase control (safety knee)

L5814 Addition, endoskeletal knee-shin system, polycentric, hydraulic swing phase control, mechanical stance phase lock

L5816 Addition, endoskeletal knee-shin system, polycentric, mechanical stance phase lock

L5818 Addition, endoskeletal knee-shin system, polycentric, friction swing, and stance phase control

L5822 Addition, endoskeletal knee-shin system, single axis, pneumatic swing, friction stance phase control

L5824 Addition, endoskeletal knee-shin system, single axis, fluid swing phase control

L5826 Addition, endoskeletal knee-shin system, single axis, hydraulic swing phase control, with miniature high activity frame

L5828 Addition, endoskeletal knee-shin system, single axis, fluid swing and stance phase control

L5830 Addition, endoskeletal knee-shin system, single axis, pneumatic/ swing phase control

L5840 Addition, endoskeletal knee/shin system, 4-bar linkage or multiaxial, pneumatic swing phase control

L5845 Addition, endoskeletal, knee-shin system, stance flexion feature, adjustable

L5848 Addition to endoskeletal knee-shin system, fluid stance extension, dampening feature, with or without adjustability

L5850 Addition, endoskeletal system, above knee or hip disarticulation, knee extension assist

L5855 Addition, endoskeletal system, hip disarticulation, mechanical hip extension assist

L5856 Addition to lower extremity prosthesis, endoskeletal knee-shin system, microprocessor control feature, swing and stance phase, includes electronic sensor(s), any type

L5857 Addition to lower extremity prosthesis, endoskeletal knee-shin system, microprocessor control feature, swing phase only, includes electronic sensor(s), any type

L5858 Addition to lower extremity prosthesis, endoskeletal knee shin system, microprocessor control feature, stance phase only, includes electronic sensor(s), any type

L5859 Addition to lower extremity prosthesis, endoskeletal knee-shin system, powered and programmable flexion/extension assist control, includes any type motor(s)

L5910 Addition, endoskeletal system, below knee, alignable system

L5920 Addition, endoskeletal system, above knee or hip disarticulation, alignable system

L5925 Addition, endoskeletal system, above knee, knee disarticulation or hip disarticulation, manual lock

L5930 Addition, endoskeletal system, high activity knee control frame

L5940 Addition, endoskeletal system, below knee, ultra-light material (titanium, carbon fiber or equal)

L5950 Addition, endoskeletal system, above knee, ultra-light material (titanium, carbon fiber or equal)

L5960 Addition, endoskeletal system, hip disarticulation, ultra-light material (titanium, carbon fiber or equal)

L5961 Addition, endoskeletal system, polycentric hip joint, pneumatic or hydraulic control, rotation control, with or without flexion and/or extension control

L5962 Addition, endoskeletal system, below knee, flexible protective outer surface covering system

L5964 Addition, endoskeletal system, above knee, flexible protective outer surface covering system

L5966 Addition, endoskeletal system, hip disarticulation, flexible protective outer surface covering system

L5968 Addition to lower limb prosthesis, multiaxial ankle with swing phase active dorsiflexion feature

L5969 Addition, endoskeletal ankle-foot or ankle system, power assist, includes any type motor(s)

L5970 All lower extremity prostheses, foot, external keel, SACH foot

L5971 All lower extremity prosthesis, solid ankle cushion heel (SACH) foot, replacement only

L5972 All lower extremity prostheses, foot, flexible keel

L5973 Endoskeletal ankle foot system, microprocessor controlled feature, dorsiflexion and/or plantar flexion control, includes power source

L5974 All lower extremity prostheses, foot, single axis ankle/foot

L5975 All lower extremity prosthesis, combination single axis ankle and flexible keel foot

L5976 All lower extremity prostheses, energy storing foot (Seattle carbon copy ii or equal)

L5978 All lower extremity prostheses, foot, multiaxial ankle/foot

L5979 All lower extremity prosthesis, multi-axial ankle, dynamic response foot, one piece system

L5980 All lower extremity prostheses, flex foot system

L5981 All lower extremity prostheses, flex-walk system or equal

L5982 All exoskeletal lower extremity prostheses, axial rotation unit

L5984 All endoskeletal lower extremity prosthesis, axial rotation unit, with or without adjustability

L5985 All endoskeletal lower extremity prostheses, dynamic prosthetic pylon

L5986 All lower extremity prostheses, multi-axial rotation unit ('MCP' or equal)

L5987 All lower extremity prosthesis, shank foot system with vertical loading pylon

L5988 Addition to lower limb prosthesis, vertical shock reducing pylon feature

L5990 Addition to lower extremity prosthesis, user adjustable heel height

L5999 Lower extremity prosthesis, not otherwise specified

Upper Limb

NOTE: The procedures in L6000-L6599 are considered as "base" or "basic" procedures and may be modified by listing procedures from the "additions" sections. The base procedures include only standard friction wrist and control cable system unless otherwise specified.

L6000 Partial hand, thumb remaining

L6010 Partial hand, little and/or ring finger remaining

L6020 Partial hand, no finger remaining

L6026 Transcarpal/metacarpal or partial hand disarticulation prosthesis, external power, self-suspended, inner socket with removable forearm section, electrodes and cables, two batteries, charger, myoelectric control of terminal device, excludes terminal device(s)

L6050 Wrist disarticulation, molded socket, flexible elbow hinges, triceps pad

L6055 Wrist disarticulation, molded socket with expandable interface, flexible elbow hinges, triceps pad

L6100 Below elbow, molded socket, flexible elbow hinge, triceps pad

L6110 Below elbow, molded socket, (muenster or northwestern suspension types)

L6120 Below elbow, molded double wall split socket, step-up hinges, half cuff

L6130 Below elbow, molded double wall split socket, stump activated locking hinge, half cuff

L6200 Elbow disarticulation, molded socket, outside locking hinge, forearm

L6205 Elbow disarticulation, molded socket with expandable interface, outside locking hinges, forearm

L6250 Above elbow, molded double wall socket, internal locking elbow, forearm

L6300 Shoulder disarticulation, molded socket, shoulder bulkhead, humeral section, internal locking elbow, forearm

L6310 Shoulder disarticulation, passive restoration (complete prosthesis)

L6320 Shoulder disarticulation, passive restoration (shoulder cap only)

L6350 Interscapular thoracic, molded socket, shoulder bulkhead, humeral section, internal locking elbow, forearm

L6360 Interscapular thoracic, passive restoration (complete prosthesis)

L6370 Interscapular thoracic, passive restoration (shoulder cap only)

L6380 Immediate post surgical or early fitting, application of initial rigid dressing, including fitting alignment and suspension of components, and one cast change, wrist disarticulation or below elbow

L6382 Immediate post surgical or early fitting, application of initial rigid dressing including fitting alignment and suspension of components, and one cast change, elbow disarticulation or above elbow

L6384 Immediate post surgical or early fitting, application of initial rigid dressing including fitting alignment and suspension of components, and one cast change, shoulder disarticulation or interscapular thoracic

L6386 Immediate post surgical or early fitting, each additional cast change and realignment

L6388 Immediate post surgical or early fitting, application of rigid dressing only

L6400 Below elbow, molded socket, endoskeletal system, including soft prosthetic tissue shaping

L6450 Elbow disarticulation, molded socket, endoskeletal system, including soft prosthetic tissue shaping

L6500 Above elbow, molded socket, endoskeletal system, including soft prosthetic tissue shaping

L6550 Shoulder disarticulation, molded socket, endoskeletal system, including soft prosthetic tissue shaping

L6570 Interscapular thoracic, molded socket, endoskeletal system, including soft prosthetic tissue shaping

L6580 Preparatory, wrist disarticulation or below elbow, single wall plastic socket, friction wrist, flexible elbow hinges, figure of eight harness, humeral cuff, Bowden cable control, USMC or equal pylon, no cover, molded to patient model

L6582 Preparatory, wrist disarticulation or below elbow, single wall socket, friction wrist, flexible elbow hinges, figure of eight harness, humeral cuff, Bowden cable control, USMC or equal pylon, no cover, direct formed

L6584 Preparatory, elbow disarticulation or above elbow, single wall plastic socket, friction wrist, locking elbow, figure of eight harness, fair lead cable control, USMC or equal pylon, no cover, molded to patient model

L6586 Preparatory, elbow disarticulation or above elbow, single wall socket, friction wrist, locking elbow, figure of eight harness, fair lead cable control, USMC or equal pylon, no cover, direct formed

L6588 Preparatory, shoulder disarticulation or interscapular thoracic, single wall plastic socket, shoulder joint, locking elbow, friction wrist, chest strap, fair lead cable control, USMC or equal pylon, no cover, molded to patient model

L6590 Preparatory, shoulder disarticulation or interscapular thoracic, single wall socket, shoulder joint, locking elbow, friction wrist, chest strap, fair lead cable control, USMC or equal pylon, no cover, direct formed

Additions - Upper Limb

NOTE: The following procedures, modifications and/or components may be added to other base procedures. The items in this section should reflect the additional complexity of each modification procedure, in addition to base procedure, at the time of the original order.

L6600 Upper extremity additions, polycentric hinge, pair

L6605 Upper extremity additions, single pivot hinge, pair

L6610 Upper extremity additions, flexible metal hinge, pair

L6611 Addition to upper extremity prosthesis, external powered, additional switch, any type

L6615 Upper extremity addition, disconnect locking wrist unit

L6616 Upper extremity addition, additional disconnect insert for locking wrist unit, each

L6620 Upper extremity addition, flexion/extension wrist unit, with or without friction

L6621 Upper extremity prosthesis addition, flexion/extension wrist with or without friction, for use with external powered terminal device

L6623 Upper extremity addition, spring assisted rotational wrist unit with latch release

L6624 Upper extremity addition, flexion/extension and rotation wrist unit

L6625 Upper extremity addition, rotation wrist unit with cable lock

L6628 Upper extremity addition, quick disconnect hook adapter, otto bock or equal

L6629 Upper extremity addition, quick disconnect lamination collar with coupling piece, otto bock or equal

L6630 Upper extremity addition, stainless steel, any wrist

L6632 Upper extremity addition, latex suspension sleeve, each

L6635 Upper extremity addition, lift assist for elbow

L6637 Upper extremity addition, nudge control elbow lock

L6638 Upper extremity addition to prosthesis, electric locking feature, only for use with manually powered elbow

L6640 Upper extremity additions, shoulder abduction joint, pair

L6641 Upper extremity addition, excursion amplifier, pulley type

L6642 Upper extremity addition, excursion amplifier, lever type

L6645 Upper extremity addition, shoulder flexion-abduction joint, each

L6646 Upper extremity addition, shoulder joint, multipositional locking, flexion, adjustable abduction friction control, for use with body powered or external powered system

L6647 Upper extremity addition, shoulder lock mechanism, body powered actuator

L6648 Upper extremity addition, shoulder lock mechanism, external powered actuator

L6650 Upper extremity addition, shoulder universal joint, each

L6655 Upper extremity addition, standard control cable, extra

L6660 Upper extremity addition, heavy duty control cable

L6665 Upper extremity addition, Teflon, or equal, cable lining

L6670 Upper extremity addition, hook to hand, cable adapter

L6672 Upper extremity addition, harness, chest or shoulder, saddle type

L6675 Upper extremity addition, harness, (e.g., figure of eight type), single cable design

L6676 Upper extremity addition, harness, (e.g., figure of eight type), dual cable design

L6677 Upper extremity addition, harness, triple control, simultaneous operation of terminal device and elbow

L6680 Upper extremity addition, test socket, wrist disarticulation or below elbow

L6682 Upper extremity addition, test socket, elbow disarticulation or above elbow

L6684 Upper extremity addition, test socket, shoulder disarticulation or interscapular thoracic

L6686 Upper extremity addition, suction socket

L6687 Upper extremity addition, frame type socket, below elbow or wrist disarticulation

L6688 Upper extremity addition, frame type socket, above elbow or elbow disarticulation

L6689 Upper extremity addition, frame type socket, shoulder disarticulation

L6690 Upper extremity addition, frame type socket, interscapular-thoracic

L6691 Upper extremity addition, removable insert, each

L6692 Upper extremity addition, silicone gel insert or equal, each

L6693 Upper extremity addition, locking elbow, forearm counterbalance

L6694 Addition to upper extremity prosthesis, below elbow/above elbow, custom fabricated from existing mold or prefabricated, socket insert, silicone gel, elastomeric or equal, for use with locking mechanism

L6695 Addition to upper extremity prosthesis, below elbow/above elbow, custom fabricated from existing mold or prefabricated, socket insert, silicone gel, elastomeric or equal, not for use with locking mechanism

L6696 Addition to upper extremity prosthesis, below elbow/above elbow, custom fabricated socket insert for congenital or atypical traumatic amputee, silicone gel, elastomeric or equal, for use with or without locking mechanism, initial only (for other than initial, use code l6694 or l6695)

L6697 Addition to upper extremity prosthesis, below elbow/above elbow, custom fabricated socket insert for other than congenital or atypical traumatic amputee, silicone gel, elastomeric or equal, for use with or without locking mechanism, initial only (for other than initial, use code l6694 or l6695)

L6698 Addition to upper extremity prosthesis, below elbow/above elbow, lock mechanism, excludes socket insert

Terminal Devices Hooks

L6703 Terminal device, passive hand/mitt, any material, any size

L6704 Terminal device, sport/recreational/work attachment, any material, any size

L6706 Terminal device, hook, mechanical, voluntary opening, any material, any size, lined or unlined

L6707 Terminal device, hook, mechanical, voluntary closing, any material, any size, lined or unlined

L6708 Terminal device, hand, mechanical, voluntary opening, any material, any size

L6709 Terminal device, hand, mechanical, voluntary closing, any material, any size

L6711 Terminal device, hook, mechanical, voluntary opening, any material, any size, lined or unlined, pediatric

L6712 Terminal device, hook, mechanical, voluntary closing, any material, any size, lined or unlined, pediatric

L6713 Terminal device, hand, mechanical, voluntary opening, any material, any size, pediatric

L6714 Terminal device, hand, mechanical, voluntary closing, any material, any size, pediatric

L6715 Terminal device, multiple articulating digit, includes motor(s), initial issue or replacement

L6721 Terminal device, hook or hand, heavy duty, mechanical, voluntary opening, any material, any size, lined or unlined

L6722 Terminal device, hook or hand, heavy duty, mechanical, voluntary closing, any material, any size, lined or unlined

L6805 Addition to terminal device, modifier wrist unit

MCM: 2133

L6810 Addition to terminal device, precision pinch device

MCM: 2133

Hands, Gloves and Restoration

L6880 Electric hand, switch or myoelectric controlled, independently articulating digits, any grasp pattern or combination of grasp patterns, includes motor(s)

L6881 Automatic grasp feature, addition to upper limb electric prosthetic terminal device

L6882 Microprocessor control feature, addition to upper limb prosthetic terminal device

MCM: 2133

L6883 Replacement socket, below elbow/wrist disarticulation, molded to patient model, for use with or without external power

L6884 Replacement socket, above elbow/elbow disarticulation, molded to patient model, for use with or without external power

L6885 Replacement socket, shoulder disarticulation/interscapular thoracic, molded to patient model, for use with or without external power

L6890 Addition to upper extremity prosthesis, glove for terminal device, any material, prefabricated, includes fitting and adjustment

L6895 Addition to upper extremity prosthesis, glove for terminal device, any material, custom fabricated

L6900 Hand restoration (casts, shading and measurements included), partial hand, with glove, thumb or one finger remaining

L6905 Hand restoration (casts, shading and measurements included), partial hand, with glove, multiple fingers remaining

L6910 Hand restoration (casts, shading and measurements included), partial hand, with glove, no fingers remaining

L6915 Hand restoration (shading, and measurements included), replacement glove for above

External Power Devices and Batteries

L6920 Wrist disarticulation, external power, self-suspended inner socket, removable forearm shell, otto bock or equal, switch, cables, two batteries and one charger, switch control of terminal device

L6925 Wrist disarticulation, external power, self-suspended inner socket, removable forearm shell, otto bock or equal electrodes, cables, two batteries and one charger, myoelectronic control of terminal device

L6930 Below elbow, external power, self-suspended inner socket, removable forearm shell, otto bock or equal switch, cables, two batteries and one charger, switch control of terminal device

L6935 Below elbow, external power, self-suspended inner socket, removable forearm shell, otto bock or equal electrodes, cables, two batteries and one charger, myoelectronic control of terminal device

L6940 Elbow disarticulation, external power, molded inner socket, removable humeral shell, outside locking hinges, forearm, otto bock or equal switch, cables, two batteries and one charger, switch control of terminal device

L6945 Elbow disarticulation, external power, molded inner socket, removable humeral shell, outside locking hinges, forearm, otto bock or equal electrodes, cables, two batteries and one charger, myoelectronic control of terminal device

L6950 Above elbow, external power, molded inner socket, removable humeral shell, internal locking elbow, forearm, otto bock or equal switch, cables, two batteries and one charger, switch control of terminal device

L6955 Above elbow, external power, molded inner socket, removable humeral shell, internal locking elbow, forearm, otto bock or equal electrodes, cables, two batteries and one charger, myoelectronic control of terminal device

L6960 Shoulder disarticulation, external power, molded inner socket, removable shoulder shell, shoulder bulkhead, humeral section, mechanical elbow, forearm, otto bock or equal switch, cables, two batteries and one charger, switch control of terminal device

L6965 Shoulder disarticulation, external power, molded inner socket, removable shoulder shell, shoulder bulkhead, humeral section, mechanical elbow, forearm, otto bock or equal electrodes, cables, two batteries and one charger, myoelectronic control of terminal device

L6970 Interscapular-thoracic, external power, molded inner socket, removable shoulder shell, shoulder bulkhead, humeral section, mechanical elbow, forearm, otto bock or equal switch, cables, two batteries and one charger, switch control of terminal device

L6975 Interscapular-thoracic, external power, molded inner socket, removable shoulder shell, shoulder bulkhead, humeral section, mechanical elbow, forearm, otto bock or equal electrodes, cables, two batteries and one charger, myoelectronic control of terminal device

L7007 Electric hand, switch or myoelectric controlled, adult

L7008 Electric hand, switch or myoelectric, controlled, pediatric

L7009 Electric hook, switch or myoelectric controlled, adult

L7040 Prehensile actuator, switch controlled

L7045 Electric hook, switch or myoelectric controlled, pediatric

L7170 Electronic elbow, Hosmer or equal, switch controlled

L7180 Electronic elbow, microprocessor sequential control of elbow and terminal device

L7181 Electronic elbow, microprocessor simultaneous control of elbow and terminal device

L7185 Electronic elbow, adolescent, variety village or equal, switch controlled

L7186 Electronic elbow, child, variety village or equal, switch controlled

L7190 Electronic elbow, adolescent, variety village or equal, myoelectronically controlled

L7191 Electronic elbow, child, variety village or equal, myoelectronically controlled

L7259 Electronic wrist rotator, any type

L7360 Six volt battery, each

L7362 Battery charger, six volt, each

L7364 Twelve volt battery, each

L7366 Battery charger, twelve volt, each

L7367 Lithium ion battery, rechargeable, replacement

L7368 Lithium ion battery charger, replacement only

L7400 Addition to upper extremity prosthesis, below elbow/wrist disarticulation, ultralight material (titanium, carbon fiber or equal)

L7401 Addition to upper extremity prosthesis, above elbow disarticulation, ultralight material (titanium, carbon fiber or equal)

L7402 Addition to upper extremity prosthesis, shoulder disarticulation/interscapular thoracic, ultralight material (titanium, carbon fiber or equal)

L7403 Addition to upper extremity prosthesis, below elbow/wrist disarticulation, acrylic material

L7404 Addition to upper extremity prosthesis, above elbow disarticulation, acrylic material

L7405 Addition to upper extremity prosthesis, shoulder disarticulation/interscapular thoracic, acrylic material

L7499 Upper extremity prosthesis, not otherwise specified

Repairs

L7510 Repair of prosthetic device, repair or replace minor parts

MCM: 2100.4, 2130D, 2133

L7520 Repair prosthetic device, labor component, per 15 minutes

L7600 Prosthetic donning sleeve, any material, each

Statute: 1862(1)(a)

L7900 Male vacuum erection system

Statute: 1834a

L7902 Tension ring, for vacuum erection device, any type, replacement only, each

Statute: 1834a

General - Breast Prostheses

L8000 Breast prosthesis, mastectomy bra, without integrated breast prosthesis form, any size, any type

MCM: 2130A

L8001 Breast prosthesis, mastectomy bra, with integrated breast prosthesis form, unilateral, any size, any type

MCM: 2130A

L8002 Breast prosthesis, mastectomy bra, with integrated breast prosthesis form, bilateral, any size, any type

MCM: 2130A

L8010 Breast prosthesis, mastectomy sleeve

MCM: 2130A

L8015 External breast prosthesis garment, with mastectomy form, post mastectomy

MCM: 2130

L8020 Breast prosthesis, mastectomy form

MCM: 2130A

L8030 Breast prosthesis, silicone or equal, without integral adhesive

MCM: 2130A

L8031 Breast prosthesis, silicone or equal, with integral adhesive

MCM: 2130A

L8032 Nipple prosthesis, reusable, any type, each

L8035 Custom breast prosthesis, post mastectomy, molded to patient model

MCM: 2130

L8039 Breast prosthesis, not otherwise specified

General – Facial Prosthesis

L8040 Nasal prosthesis, provided by a non-physician

L8041 Midfacial prosthesis, provided by a non-physician

L8042 Orbital prosthesis, provided by a non-physician

L8043 Upper facial prosthesis, provided by a non-physician

L8044 Hemi-facial prosthesis, provided by a non-physician

L8045 Auricular prosthesis, provided by a non-physician

L8046 Partial facial prosthesis, provided by a non-physician

L8047 Nasal septal prosthesis, provided by a non-physician

L8048 Unspecified maxillofacial prosthesis, by report, provided by a non-physician

L8049 Repair or modification of maxillofacial prosthesis, labor component, 15 minute increments, provided by a non-physician

General - Trusses

L8300 Truss, single with standard pad

CIM: 70-1, 70-2

MCM: 2133

L8310 Truss, double with standard pads

CIM: 70-170-1, 70-2

MCM: 2133

L8320 Truss, addition to standard pad, water pad

CIM: 70-170-1, 70-2

MCM: 2133

L8330 Truss, addition to standard pad, scrotal pad

CIM: 70-170-1, 70-2

MCM: 2133

Prosthetic Socks

L8400 Prosthetic sheath, below knee, each

MCM: 2133

L8410 Prosthetic sheath, above knee, each

MCM: 2133

L8415 Prosthetic sheath, upper limb, each

MCM: 2133

L8417 Prosthetic sheath/sock, including a gel cushion layer, below knee or above knee, each

L8420 Prosthetic sock, multiple ply, below knee, each

MCM: 2133

L8430 Prosthetic sock, multiple ply, above knee, each

MCM: 2133

L8435 Prosthetic sock, multiple ply, upper limb, each

MCM: 2133

L8440 Prosthetic shrinker, below knee, each

MCM: 2133

L8460 Prosthetic shrinker, above knee, each

MCM: 2133

L8465 Prosthetic shrinker, upper limb, each

MCM: 2133

L8470 Prosthetic sock, single ply, fitting, below knee, each

MCM: 2133

L8480 Prosthetic sock, single ply, fitting, above knee, each

MCM: 2133

L8485 Prosthetic sock, single ply, fitting, upper limb, each

MCM: 2133

L8499 Unlisted procedure for miscellaneous prosthetic services

Prosthetic Implants

L8500 Artificial larynx, any type

CIM: 65-5

MCM: 2130,

L8501 Tracheostomy speaking valve

CIM: 65-16

L8505 Artificial larynx replacement battery / accessory, any type

L8507 Tracheo-esophageal voice prosthesis, patient inserted, any type, each

L8509 Tracheo-esophageal voice prosthesis, inserted by a licensed health care provider, any type

L8510 Voice amplifier

CIM: 65-5

L8511 Insert for indwelling tracheoesophageal prosthesis, with or without valve, replacement only, each

L8512 Gelatin capsules or equivalent, for use with tracheoesophageal voice prosthesis, replacement only, per 10

L8513 Cleaning device used with tracheoesophageal voice prosthesis, pipet, brush, or equal, replacement only, each

L8514 Tracheoesophageal puncture dilator, replacement only, each

L8515 Gelatin capsule, application device for use with tracheoesophageal voice prosthesis, each

Integumentary System

L8600 Implantable breast prosthesis, silicone or equal

CIM: 35-47

MCM: 2130,

L8603 Injectable bulking agent, collagen implant, urinary tract, 2.5 ml syringe, includes shipping and necessary supplies

CIM: 65.9

L8604 Injectable bulking agent, dextranomer/hyaluronic acid copolymer implant, urinary tract, 1 ml, includes shipping and necessary supplies

L8605 Injectable bulking agent, dextranomer/hyaluronic acid copolymer implant, anal canal, 1 ml, includes shipping and necessary supplies

L8606 Injectable bulking agent, synthetic implant, urinary tract, 1 ml syringe, includes shipping and necessary supplies

CIM: 65.9

L8607 Injectable bulking agent for vocal cord medialization, 0.1 ml, includes shipping and necessary supplies

MCM: 65.9

Head (Skull, Facial Bones, and Temporomandibular Joint)

L8609 Artificial cornea

L8610 Ocular implant

MCM: 2130

L8612 Aqueous shunt

MCM: 2130

L8613 Ossicula implant

MCM: 2130

L8614 Cochlear device, includes all internal and external components

CIM: 65-14

MCM: 2130,

L8615 Headset/headpiece for use with cochlear implant device, replacement

CIM: 65-14

L8616 Microphone for use with cochlear implant device, replacement

CIM: 65-14

L8617 Transmitting coil for use with cochlear implant device, replacement

CIM: 65-14

L8618 Transmitter cable for use with cochlear implant device, replacement

CIM: 65-14

L8619 Cochlear implant, external speech processor and controller, integrated system, replacement

CIM: 65-14

L8621 Zinc air battery for use with cochlear implant device and auditory osseointegrated sound processors, replacement, each

L8622 Alkaline battery for use with cochlear implant device, any size, replacement, each

L8623 Lithium ion battery for use with cochlear implant device speech processor, other than ear level, replacement, each

L8624 Lithium ion battery for use with cochlear implant device speech processor, ear level, replacement, each

L8627 Cochlear implant, external speech processor, component, replacement

CIM: 65-14

L8628 Cochlear implant, external controller component, replacement

CIM: 65-14

L8629 Transmitting coil and cable, integrated, for use with cochlear implant device, replacement

CIM: 65-14

Upper Extremity

L8630 Metacarpophalangeal joint implant

MCM: 2130

L8631 Metacarpal phalangeal joint replacement, two or more pieces, metal (e.g., stainless steel or cobalt chrome), ceramic-like material (e.g., pyrocarbon), for surgical implantation (all sizes, includes entire system)

MCM: 2130

Lower Extremity (Joint: Knee, Ankle, Toe)

L8641 Metatarsal joint implant

MCM: 2130

L8642 Hallux implant

MCM: 2130

Miscellaneous Muscular - Skeletal

L8658 Interphalangeal joint spacer, silicone or equal, each

MCM: 2130

L8659 Interphalangeal finger joint replacement, 2 or more pieces, metal (e.g., stainless steel or cobalt chrome), ceramic-like material (e.g., pyrocarbon) for surgical implantation, any size

MCM: 2130

Cardiovascular System

L8670 Vascular graft material, synthetic, implant

MCM: 2130

L8679 Implantable neurostimulator, pulse generator, any type

CIM: 65-8

L8680 Implantable neurostimulator electrode, each

L8681 Patient programmer (external) for use with implantable programmable neurostimulator pulse generator, replacement only

CIM: 65-8

L8682 Implantable neurostimulator radiofrequency receiver

CIM: 65-8

L8683 Radiofrequency transmitter (external) for use with implantable neurostimulator radiofrequency receiver

CIM: 65-8

L8684 Radiofrequency transmitter (external) for use with implantable sacral root neurostimulator receiver for bowel and bladder management, replacement

CIM: 65-8

L8685 Implantable neurostimulator pulse generator, single array, rechargeable, includes extension

L8686 Implantable neurostimulator pulse generator, single array, non-rechargeable, includes extension

L8687 Implantable neurostimulator pulse generator, dual array, rechargeable, includes extension

L8688 Implantable neurostimulator pulse generator, dual array, non-rechargeable, includes extension

L8689 External recharging system for battery (internal) for use with implantable neurostimulator, replacement only

CIM: 65-8

L8690 Auditory osseointegrated device, includes all internal and external components

L8691 Auditory osseointegrated device, external sound processor, replacement

L8692 Auditory osseointegrated device, external sound processor, used without osseointegration, body worn, includes headband or other means of external attachment

Statute: 1862(a)(7)

L8693 Auditory osseointegrated device abutment, any length, replacement only

L8695 External recharging system for battery (external) for use with implantable neurostimulator, replacement only

CIM: 65-8

L8696 Antenna (external) for use with implantable diaphragmatic/phrenic nerve stimulation device, replacement, each

Other

L8699 Prosthetic implant, not otherwise specified

L9900 Orthotic and prosthetic supply, accessory, and/or service component of another HCPCS "l" code

Guidelines

In addition to the information presented in the INTRODUCTION, several other items unique to this section are defined or identified here:

1. SUBSECTION INFORMATION: Some of the listed subheadings or subsections have special needs or instructions unique to that section. Where these are indicated, special "notes" will be presented preceding or following the listings. Those subsections within the MEDICAL SERVICES section that have "notes" are as follows:

Subsection	Code Numbers
Office services	M0000-M0009
End-stage renal disease services	M0900-M0999

2. SPECIAL REPORT: A service, material or supply that is rarely provided, unusual, variable or new may require a special report in determining medical appropriateness for reimbursement purposes. Pertinent information should include an adequate definition or description of the nature, extent, and need for the service, material or supply.

3. MODIFIERS: Listed services may be modified under certain circumstances. When appropriate, the modifying circumstance is identified by adding a modifier to the basic procedure code. CPT and HCPCS National Level II modifiers may be used with CPT and HCPCS National Level II procedure codes. Modifiers commonly used with MEDICAL SERVICES are as follows:

   -AH Clinical psychologist

   -AJ Clinical social worker

   -CC Procedure code change (use "CC" when the procedure code submitted was changed either for administrative reasons or because an incorrect code was filed)

   -EJ Subsequent claims for a defined course of therapy (eg., EPO, sodium hyaluronate, infliximab)

   -EM Emergency reserve supply (for ESRD benefit only)

   -EP Service provided as part of Medicaid early periodic screening diagnosis and treatment (EPSDT) program

   -FP Service provided as part of Medicaid family planning program

   -Q5 Service furnished by a substitute physician under a reciprocal billing arrangement

   -Q6 Service furnished by a locum tenens physician

   -QC Single channel monitoring

   -QD Recording and storage in solid state memory by a digital recorder

   -QT Recording and storage on tape by an analog tape recorder

-SF Second opinion ordered by a professional review organization (PRO) per section 9401, P.L. 99-272 (100 percent reimbursement; no Medicare deductible or coinsurance)

-TC Technical component. Under certain circumstances, a charge may be made for the technical component alone. Under those circumstances, the technical component charge is identified by adding modifier -TC to the usual procedure number. Technical component charges are institutional charges and are not billed separately by physicians. However, portable x-ray suppliers bill only for the technical component and should use modifier -TC. The charge data from portable x-ray suppliers will then be used to build customary and prevailing profiles.

4. CPT CODE CROSS-REFERENCE: See sections for equivalent CPT code(s) for listings in this section.

Other Medical Services

M0075 Cellular therapy

CIM: 35-5

M0076 Prolotherapy

CIM: 35-13

M0100 Intragastric hypothermia using gastric freezing

CIM: 35-65

M0300 IV chelation therapy (chemical endarterectomy)

CIM: 35-64

M0301 Fabric wrapping of abdominal aneurysm

CIM: 35-34

PATHOLOGY AND LABORATORY

Guidelines

In addition to the information presented in the INTRODUCTION, several other items unique to this section are defined or identified here:

1. SPECIAL REPORT: A service, material or supply that is rarely provided, unusual, variable or new may require a special report in determining medical appropriateness for reimbursement purposes. Pertinent information should include an adequate definition or description of the nature, extent, and need for the service, material or supply.

2. MODIFIERS: Listed services may be modified under certain circumstances. When appropriate, the modifying circumstance is identified by adding a modifier to the basic procedure code. CPT and HCPCS National Level II modifiers may be used with CPT and HCPCS National Level II procedure codes. Modifiers commonly used with PATHOLOGY AND LABORATORY SERVICES are as follows:

   -CC Procedure code change (use "CC" when the procedure code submitted was changed either for administrative reasons or because an incorrect code was filed)

   -LR Laboratory round trip

   -TC Technical component. Under certain circumstances, a charge may be made for the technical component alone. Under these circumstances, the technical component charge is identified by adding the modifier -TC to the usual procedure code. Technical component charges are institutional charges and are not billed separately by physicians. Portable x-ray suppliers bill only for the technical component however, and should use modifier -TC. The charge data from portable x-ray suppliers will then be used to build customary and prevailing profiles.

3. CPT CODE CROSS-REFERENCE: See sections for equivalent CPT code(s) for all listings in this section.

Chemistry and Toxicology Tests

P2028 Cephalin flocculation, blood

CIM: 50-34

P2029 Congo red, blood

CIM: 50-34

P2031 Hair analysis (excluding arsenic)

CIM: 50-24

P2033 Thymol turbidity, blood

CIM: 50-34

P2038 Mucoprotein, blood (seromucoid) (medical necessity procedure)

CIM: 50-34

Pathology Screening Tests

P3000 Screening Papanicolaou smear, cervical or vaginal, up to three smears, by technician under physician supervision

CIM: 50-20

P3001 Screening Papanicolaou smear, cervical or vaginal, up to three smears, requiring interpretation by physician

CIM: 50-20

Miscellaneous Pathology and Laboratory Tests

P7001 Culture, bacterial, urine; quantitative, sensitivity study CPT

P9010 Blood (whole), for transfusion, per unit

MCM: 2455A

P9011 Blood, split unit

MCM: 2455A

P9012 Cryoprecipitate, each unit

MCM: 2455 B

P9016 Red blood cells, leukocytes reduced, each unit

MCM: 2455 B

P9017 Fresh frozen plasma (single donor), frozen within 8 hours of collection, each unit

MCM: 2455 B

P9019 Platelets, each unit

MCM: 2455 B

P9020 Platelet rich plasma, each unit

MCM: 2455 B

P9021 Red blood cells, each unit

MCM: 2455A

P9022 Red blood cells, washed, each unit

MCM: 2455A

P9023 Plasma, pooled multiple donor, solvent/detergent treated, frozen, each unit

MCM: 2455 B

P9031 Platelets, leukocytes reduced, each unit

MCM: 2455

P9032 Platelets, irradiated, each unit

MCM: 2455

P9033 Platelets, leukocytes reduced, irradiated, each unit

MCM: 2455

P9034 Platelets, pheresis, each unit

MCM: 2455

P9035 Platelets, pheresis, leukocytes reduced, each unit

MCM: 2455

P9036 Platelets, pheresis, irradiated, each unit

MCM: 2455

P9037 Platelets, pheresis, leukocytes reduced, irradiated, each unit

MCM: 2455

P9038 Red blood cells, irradiated, each unit

MCM: 2455

P9039 Red blood cells, deglycerolized, each unit

MCM: 2455

P9040 Red blood cells, leukocytes reduced, irradiated, each unit

MCM: 2455

P9041 Infusion, albumin (human), 5%, 50 ml

P9043 Infusion, plasma protein fraction (human), 5%, 50 ml

MCM: 2455B

P9044 Plasma, cryoprecipitate reduced, each unit

MCM: 2455.B

P9045 Infusion, albumin (human), 5%, 250 ml

P9046 Infusion, albumin (human), 25%, 20 ml

P9047 Infusion, albumin (human), 25%, 50 ml

P9048 Infusion, plasma protein fraction (human), 5%, 250 ml

P9050 Granulocytes, pheresis, each unit

P9051 Whole blood or red blood cells, leukocytes reduced, CMV-negative, each unit

Statute: 1833T

P9052 Platelets, HLA-matched leukocytes reduced, apheresis/pheresis, each unit

Statute: 1833T

P9053 Platelets, pheresis, leukocytes reduced, CMV-negative, irradiated, each unit

Statute: 1833T

P9054 Whole blood or red blood cells, leukocytes reduced, frozen, deglycerol, washed, each unit

Statute: 1833T

P9055 Platelets, leukocytes reduced, CMV-negative, apheresis/pheresis, each unit

Statute: 1833T

P9056 Whole blood, leukocytes reduced, irradiated, each unit

Statute: 1833T

P9057 Red blood cells, frozen/deglycerolized/washed, leukocytes reduced, irradiated, each unit

Statute: 1833T

P9058 Red blood cells, leukocytes reduced, CMV-negative, irradiated, each unit

Statute: 1833T

P9059 Fresh frozen plasma between 8-24 hours of collection, each unit

Statute: 1833T

P9060 Fresh frozen plasma, donor retested, each unit

Statute: 1833T

P9070 Plasma, pooled multiple donor, pathogen reduced, frozen, each unit

Statute: 1833T

P9071 Plasma (single donor), pathogen reduced, frozen, each unit

MCM: 2455B

Statute: 1833T

▲ **P9072** Platelets, pheresis, pathogen reduced or rapid bacterial tested, each unit

MCM: 2455B

Statute: 1833T

P9603 Travel allowance one way in connection with medically necessary laboratory specimen collection drawn from home bound or nursing home bound patient; prorated miles actually travelled

MCM: 51141K

P9604 Travel allowance one way in connection with medically necessary laboratory specimen collection drawn from home bound or nursing home bound patient; prorated trip charge.

MCM: 51141K

P9612 Catheterization for collection of specimen, single patient, all places of service

MCM: 5114.1D

P9615 Catheterization for collection of specimen(s) (multiple patients)

MCM: 51141D

Guidelines

In addition to the information presented in the INTRODUCTION, several other items unique to this section are defined or identified here:

1. SUBSECTION INFORMATION: Some of the listed subheadings or subsections have special needs or instructions unique to that section. Where these are indicated, special "notes" will be presented preceding or following the listings. Those subsections within the TEMPORARY CODES section that have "notes" are as follows:

Subsection	Code Numbers
Temporary codes	Q0000-Q9999

2. SPECIAL REPORT: A service, material or supply that is rarely provided, unusual, variable or new may require a special report in determining medical appropriateness for reimbursement purposes. Pertinent information should include an adequate definition or description of the nature, extent, and need for the service, material or supply.

3. MODIFIERS: Listed services may be modified under certain circumstances. When appropriate, the modifying circumstance is identified by adding a modifier to the basic procedure code. CPT and HCPCS National Level II modifiers may be used with CPT and HCPCS National Level II procedure codes. Modifiers commonly used with TEMPORARY CODES are as follows:

   -CC Procedure code change (use "CC" when the procedure code submitted was changed either for administrative reasons or because an incorrect code was filed)

   -LL Lease/rental (used when DME equipment rental is to be applied against the purchase price)

   -LR Laboratory round trip

   -QC Single channel monitoring

   -QD Recording and storage in solid state memory by a digital recorder

   -QE Prescribed amount of oxygen is less than 1 liter per minute (LPM)

   -QF Prescribed amount of oxygen exceeds 4 liters per minute (LPM) and portable oxygen is prescribed

   -QG Prescribed amount of oxygen is greater than 4 liters per minute (LPM)

   -QH Oxygen conserving device is being used with an oxygen delivery system

   -QT Recording and storage on tape by an analog tape recorder

   -RP Replacement and repair (may be used to indicate replacement of DME, orthotic and prosthetic devices that have been in use for some time. The claim shows the code for the part, followed by the "RP" modifier and the charge for the part.)

-RR Rental (used when DME is to be rented)

-TC Technical component. Under certain circumstances, a charge may be made for the technical component alone. Under these circumstances, the technical component charge is identified by adding the modifier -TC to the usual procedure code. Technical component charges are institutional charges and are not billed separately by physicians. Portable x-ray suppliers bill only for the technical component however, and should use modifier -TC. The charge data from portable x-ray suppliers will then be used to build customary and prevailing profiles.

-UE Used durable medical equipment

4. CPT CODE CROSS-REFERENCE: See sections for equivalent CPT code(s) for all listings in this section.

Temporary Codes

NOTE: Temporary codes are national codes given by CMS on a temporary basis. The list contains current codes, as well as those which have been superseded by permanent alphanumeric codes as indicated by the cross-reference.

Q0035 Cardiokymography

CIM: 50-50

Q0081 Infusion therapy, using other than chemotherapeutic drugs, per visit

CIM: 60-14

Q0083 Chemotherapy administration by other than infusion technique only (e.g., subcutaneous, intramuscular, push), per visit

Q0084 Chemotherapy administration by infusion technique only, per visit

CIM: 60-14

Q0085 Chemotherapy administration by both infusion technique and other technique(s) (e.g., subcutaneous, intramuscular, push), per visit

Q0091 Screening Papanicolaou smear; obtaining, preparing and conveyance of cervical or vaginal smear to laboratory

CIM: 50-20

Q0092 Set-up portable x-ray equipment

MCM: 2070.4

Q0111 Wet mounts, including preparations of vaginal, cervical or skin specimens

Q0112 All potassium hydroxide (KOH) preparations

Q0113 Pinworm examinations

Q0114 Fern test

Q0115 Post-coital direct, qualitative examinations of vaginal or cervical mucous

Q0138 Injection, ferumoxytol, for treatment of iron deficiency anemia, 1 mg (non-ESRD use)

Q0139 Injection, ferumoxytol, for treatment of iron deficiency anemia, 1 mg (for ESRD on dialysis)

Q0144 Azithromycin dihydrate, oral, capsules/powder, 1 gram

Q0161 Chlorpromazine hydrochloride, 5 mg, oral, approved prescription anti-emetic, for use as a complete therapeutic substitute for an iv anti-emetic at the time of chemotherapy treatment, not to exceed a 48 hour dosage regimen

Q0162 Ondansetron 1 mg, oral, approved prescription anti-emetic, for use as a complete therapeutic substitute for an iv anti-emetic at the time of chemotherapy treatment, not to exceed a 48 hour dosage regimen

Statute: 4557

Q0163 Diphenhydramine hydrochloride, 50 mg, oral, approved prescription anti-emetic, for use as a complete therapeutic substitute for an iv anti-emetic at time of chemotherapy treatment not to exceed a 48 hour dosage regimen

Statute: 4557

Q0164 Prochlorperazine maleate, 5 mg, oral, approved prescription anti-emetic, for use as a complete therapeutic substitute for an iv anti-emetic at the time of chemotherapy treatment, not to exceed a 48 hour dosage regimen

Statute: 4557

Q0166 Granisetron hydrochloride, 1 mg, oral, approved prescription anti-emetic, for use as a complete therapeutic substitute for an iv anti-emetic at the time of chemotherapy treatment, not to exceed a 24 hour dosage regimen

Statute: 4557

Q0167 Dronabinol, 2.5 mg, oral, approved prescription anti-emetic, for use as a complete therapeutic substitute for an iv anti-emetic at the time of chemotherapy treatment, not to exceed a 48 hour dosage regimen

Statute: 4557

Q0169 Promethazine hydrochloride, 12.5 mg, oral, approved prescription anti-emetic, for use as a complete therapeutic substitute for an iv anti-emetic at the time of chemotherapy treatment, not to exceed a 48 hour dosage regimen

Statute: 4557

Q0173 Trimethobenzamide hydrochloride, 250 mg, oral, approved prescription anti-emetic, for use as a complete therapeutic substitute for an iv anti-emetic at the time of chemotherapy treatment, not to exceed a 48 hour dosage regimen

Statute: 4557

Q0174 Thiethylperazine maleate, 10 mg, oral, approved prescription anti-emetic, for use as a complete therapeutic substitute for an iv anti-emetic at the time of chemotherapy treatment, not to exceed a 48 hour dosage regimen

Statute: 4557

Q0175 Perphenazine, 4 mg, oral, approved prescription anti-emetic, for use as a complete therapeutic substitute for an iv anti-emetic at the time of chemotherapy treatment, not to exceed a 48 hour dosage regimen

Statute: 4557

Q0177 Hydroxyzine pamoate, 25 mg, oral, approved prescription anti-emetic, for use as a complete therapeutic substitute for an iv anti-emetic at the time of chemotherapy treatment, not to exceed a 48 hour dosage regimen

Statute: 4557

Q0180 Dolasetron mesylate, 100 mg, oral, approved prescription anti-emetic, for use as a complete therapeutic substitute for an iv anti-emetic at the time of chemotherapy treatment, not to exceed a 24 hour dosage regimen

Statute: 4557

Q0181 Unspecified oral dosage form, approved prescription anti-emetic, for use as a complete therapeutic substitute for a iv anti-emetic at the time of chemotherapy treatment, not to exceed a 48 hour dosage regimen

Statute: 4557

Q0478 Power adapter for use with electric or electric/pneumatic ventricular assist device, vehicle type

Q0479 Power module for use with electric or electric/pneumatic ventricular assist device, replacement only

Q0480 Driver for use with pneumatic ventricular assist device, replacement only

Q0481 Microprocessor control unit for use with electric ventricular assist device, replacement only

Q0482 Microprocessor control unit for use with electric/pneumatic combination ventricular assist device, replacement only

Q0483 Monitor/display module for use with electric ventricular assist device, replacement only

Q0484 Monitor/display module for use with electric or electric/pneumatic ventricular assist device, replacement only

Q0485 Monitor control cable for use with electric ventricular assist device, replacement only

Q0486 Monitor control cable for use with electric/pneumatic ventricular assist device, replacement only

Q0487 Leads (pneumatic/electrical) for use with any type electric/pneumatic ventricular assist device, replacement only

Q0488 Power pack base for use with electric ventricular assist device, replacement only

Q0489 Power pack base for use with electric/pneumatic ventricular assist device, replacement only

Q0490 Emergency power source for use with electric ventricular assist device, replacement only

Q0491 Emergency power source for use with electric/pneumatic ventricular assist device, replacement only

Q0492 Emergency power supply cable for use with electric ventricular assist device, replacement only

Q0493 Emergency power supply cable for use with electric/pneumatic ventricular assist device, replacement only

Q0494 Emergency hand pump for use with electric or electric/pneumatic ventricular assist device, replacement only

Q0495 Battery/power pack charger for use with electric or electric/pneumatic ventricular assist device, replacement only

Q0496 Battery, other than lithium-ion, for use with electric or electric/pneumatic ventricular assist device, replacement only

Q0497 Battery clips for use with electric or electric/pneumatic ventricular assist device, replacement only

Q0498 Holster for use with electric or electric/pneumatic ventricular assist device, replacement only

Q0499 Belt/vest/bag for use to carry external peripheral components of any type ventricular assist device, replacement only

Q0500 Filters for use with electric or electric/pneumatic ventricular assist device, replacement only

Q0501 Shower cover for use with electric or electric/pneumatic ventricular assist device, replacement only

Q0502 Mobility cart for pneumatic ventricular assist device, replacement only

Q0503 Battery for pneumatic ventricular assist device, replacement only, each

Q0504 Power adapter for pneumatic ventricular assist device, replacement only, vehicle type

Q0506 Battery, lithium-ion, for use with electric or electric/pneumatic ventricular assist device, replacement only

Q0507 Miscellaneous supply or accessory for use with an external ventricular assist device

Q0508 Miscellaneous supply or accessory for use with an implanted ventricular assist device

Q0509 Miscellaneous supply or accessory for use with any implanted ventricular assist device for which payment was not made under Medicare part a

Q0510 Pharmacy supply fee for initial immunosuppressive drug(s), first month following transplant

Q0511 Pharmacy supply fee for oral anti-cancer, oral anti-emetic or immunosuppressive drug(s); for the first prescription in a 30-day period

Q0512 Pharmacy supply fee for oral anti-cancer, oral anti-emetic or immunosuppressive drug(s); for a subsequent prescription in a 30-day period

Q0513 Pharmacy dispensing fee for inhalation drug(s); per 30 days

Q0514 Pharmacy dispensing fee for inhalation drug(s); per 90 days

Q0515 Injection, sermorelin acetate, 1 microgram

MCM: 2049

Q1004 New technology intraocular lens category 4 as defined in federal register notice

Q1005 New technology intraocular lens category 5 as defined in federal register notice

Q2004 Irrigation solution for treatment of bladder calculi, for example Renacidin, per 500 ml

MCM: 2049

Statute: 1861S2B

Q2009 Injection, fosphenytoin, 50 mg phenytoin equivalent

MCM: 2049

Statute: 1861S2B

Q2017 Injection, teniposide, 50 mg

MCM: 2049

Statute: 1861S2B

Q2026 Injection, Radiesse, 0.1 ml

Q2028 Injection, Sculptra, 0.5 mg

Q2034 Influenza virus vaccine, split virus, for intramuscular use (Agriflu)

MCM: 2049.4

Q2035 Influenza virus vaccine, split virus, when administered to individuals 3 years of age and older, for intramuscular use (Afluria)

MCM: 2049.4

Q2036 Influenza virus vaccine, split virus, when administered to individuals 3 years of age and older, for intramuscular use (FluLaval)

MCM: 2049.4

Q2037 Influenza virus vaccine, split virus, when administered to individuals 3 years of age and older, for intramuscular use (Fluvirin)

MCM: 2049.4

Q2038 Influenza virus vaccine, split virus, when administered to individuals 3 years of age and older, for intramuscular use (Fluzone)

MCM: 2049.4

▲ **Q2039** Influenza virus vaccine, not otherwise specified

MCM: 2049.4

Q2043 Sipuleucel-t, minimum of 50 million autologous cd54+ cells activated with pap-gm-csf, including leukapheresis and all other preparatory procedures, per infusion

Q2049 Injection, doxorubicin hydrochloride, liposomal, imported Lipidox, 10 mg

Q2050 Injection, doxorubicin hydrochloride, liposomal, not otherwise specified, 10 mg

MCM: 2049.4

Q2052 Services, supplies and accessories used in the home under the Medicare intravenous immune globulin (IVIG) demonstration

Q3001 Radioelements for brachytherapy, any type, each

MCM: 15022

Q3014 Telehealth originating site facility fee

Q3027 Injection, interferon beta-1a, 1 mcg for intramuscular use

MCM: 2049

Q3028 Injection, interferon beta-1a, 1 mcg for subcutaneous use

Q3031 Collagen skin test

CIM: 65-9

Q4001 Casting supplies, body cast adult, with or without head, plaster

Q4002 Cast supplies, body cast adult, with or without head, fiberglass

Q4003 Cast supplies, shoulder cast, adult (11 years +), plaster

Q4004 Cast supplies, shoulder cast, adult (11 years +), fiberglass

Q4005 Cast supplies, long arm cast, adult (11 years +), plaster

Q4006 Cast supplies, long arm cast, adult (11 years +), fiberglass

Q4007 Cast supplies, long arm cast, pediatric (0-10 years), plaster

Q4008 Cast supplies, long arm cast, pediatric (0-10 years), fiberglass

Q4009 Cast supplies, short arm cast, adult (11 years +), plaster

Q4010 Cast supplies, short arm cast, adult (11 years +), fiberglass

Q4011 Cast supplies, short arm cast, pediatric (0-10 years), plaster

Q4012 Cast supplies, short arm cast, pediatric (0-10 years), fiberglass

Q4013 Cast supplies, gauntlet cast (includes lower forearm and hand), adult (11 years +), plaster

Q4014 Cast supplies, gauntlet cast (includes lower forearm and hand), adult (11 years +), fiberglass

Q4015 Cast supplies, gauntlet cast (includes lower forearm and hand), pediatric (0-10 years), plaster

Q4016 Cast supplies, gauntlet cast (includes lower forearm and hand), pediatric (0-10 years), fiberglass

Q4017 Cast supplies, long arm splint, adult (11 years +), plaster

Q4018 Cast supplies, long arm splint, adult (11 years +), fiberglass

Q4019 Cast supplies, long arm splint, pediatric (0-10 years), plaster

Q4020 Cast supplies, long arm splint, pediatric (0-10 years), fiberglass

Q4021 Cast supplies, short arm splint, adult (11 years +), plaster

Q4022 Cast supplies, short arm splint, adult (11 years +), fiberglass

Q4023 Cast supplies, short arm splint, pediatric (0-10 years), plaster

Q4024 Cast supplies, short arm splint, pediatric (0-10 years), fiberglass

Q4025 Cast supplies, hip spica (one or both legs), adult (11 years +), plaster

Q4026 Cast supplies, hip spica (one or both legs), adult (11 years +), fiberglass

Q4027 Cast supplies, hip spica (one or both legs), pediatric (0-10 years), plaster

Q4028 Cast supplies, hip spica (one or both legs), pediatric (0-10 years), fiberglass

Q4029 Cast supplies, long leg cast, adult (11 years +), plaster

Q4030 Cast supplies, long leg cast, adult (11 years +), fiberglass

Q4031 Cast supplies, long leg cast, pediatric (0-10 years), plaster

Q4032 Cast supplies, long leg cast, pediatric (0-10 years), fiberglass

Q4033 Cast supplies, long leg cylinder cast, adult (11 years +), plaster

Q4034 Cast supplies, long leg cylinder cast, adult (11 years +), fiberglass

Q4035 Cast supplies, long leg cylinder cast, pediatric (0-10 years), plaster

Q4036 Cast supplies, long leg cylinder cast, pediatric (0-10 years), fiberglass

Q4037 Cast supplies, short leg cast, adult (11 years +), plaster

Q4038 Cast supplies, short leg cast, adult (11 years +), fiberglass

Q4039 Cast supplies, short leg cast, pediatric (0-10 years), plaster

Q4040 Cast supplies, short leg cast, pediatric (0-10 years), fiberglass

Q4041 Cast supplies, long leg splint, adult (11 years +), plaster

Q4042 Cast supplies, long leg splint, adult (11 years +), fiberglass

Q4043 Cast supplies, long leg splint, pediatric (0-10 years), plaster

Q4044 Cast supplies, long leg splint, pediatric (0-10 years), fiberglass

Q4045 Cast supplies, short leg splint, adult (11 years +), plaster

Q4046 Cast supplies, short leg splint, adult (11 years +), fiberglass

Q4047 Cast supplies, short leg splint, pediatric (0-10 years), plaster

Q4048 Cast supplies, short leg splint, pediatric (0-10 years), fiberglass

Q4049 Finger splint, static

Q4050 Cast supplies, for unlisted types and materials of casts

Q4051 Splint supplies, miscellaneous (includes thermoplastics, strapping, fasteners, padding and other supplies)

Q4074 Iloprost, inhalation solution,-approved final product, non-compounded, administered through DME, unit dose form, up to 20 micrograms

Injection Codes for EPO

Q4081 Injection, epoetin alfa, 100 units (for ESRD on dialysis)

MCM: 4273.1

Q4082 Drug or biological, not otherwise classified, part b drug competitive acquisition program (cap)

Q4100 Skin substitute, not otherwise specified

Q4101 Apligraf, per square centimeter

Q4102 Oasis wound matrix, per square centimeter

Q4103 Oasis burn matrix, per square centimeter

Q4104 Integra bilayer matrix wound dressing (BMWD), per square centimeter

▲ **Q4105** Integra dermal regeneration template (DRT) or Integra omnigraft dermal regeneration matrix, per square centimeter

Q4106 Dermagraft, per square centimeter

Q4107 Graftjacket, per square centimeter

Q4108 Integra matrix, per square centimeter

Q4110 Primatrix, per square centimeter

Q4111 Gammagraft, per square centimeter

Q4112 Cymetra, injectable, 1 cc

Q4113 Graftjacket xpress, injectable, 1 cc

Q4114 Integra flowable wound matrix, injectable, 1 cc

Q4115 Alloskin, per square centimeter

Q4116 AlloDerm, per square centimeter

Q4117 Hyalomatrix, per square centimeter

Q4118 Matristem micromatrix, 1 mg

(**Q4119** Code deleted December 31, 2016).

(**Q4120** Code deleted December 31, 2016).

Q4121 Theraskin, per square centimeter

Q4122 Dermacell, per square centimeter

Q4123 Alloskin rt, per square centimeter

Q4124 Oasis ultra tri-layer wound matrix, per square centimeter

Q4125 Arthroflex, per square centimeter

Q4126 Memoderm, dermaspan, TranZgraft or integuply, per square centimeter

Q4127 Talymed, per square centimeter

Q4128 Flex hd, allopatch hd, or matrix hd, per square centimeter

(**Q4129** Code deleted December 31, 2016).

Q4130 Strattice tm, per square centimeter

▲ **Q4131** Epifix or epicord, per square centimeter

Q4132 Grafix core, per square centimeter

Q4133 Grafix prime, per square centimeter

Q4134 Hmatrix, per square centimeter

Q4135 Mediskin, per square centimeter

Q4136 Ez-derm, per square centimeter

Q4137 Amnioexcel or biodexcel, per square centimeter

Q4138 Biodefense dryflex, per square centimeter

Q4139 Amniomatrix or Biomatrix, injectable, 1 cc

Q4140 Biodefense, per square centimeter

Q4141 Alloskin ac, per square centimeter

Q4142 Xcm biologic tissue matrix, per square centimeter

Q4143 Repriza, per square centimeter

Q4145 Epifix, injectable, 1 mg

Q4146 Tensix, per square centimeter

Q4147 Architect, architect px, or architect fx, extracellular matrix, per square centimeter

Q4148 Neox 1k, per square centimeter

Q4149 Excellagen, 0.1 cc

Q4150 Allowrap DS or dry, per square centimeter

Q4151 Amnioband or guardian, per square centimeter

Q4152 Dermapure, per square centimeter

Q4153 Dermavest and Plurivest, per square centimeter

Q4154 Biovance, per square centimeter

Q4155 Neoxflo or Clarixflo, 1 mg

Q4156 Neox 100, per square centimeter

Q4157 Revitalon, per square centimeter

Q4158 Marigen, per square centimeter

Q4159 Affinity, per square centimeter

Q4160 Nushield, per square centimeter

Q4161 Bio-connekt wound matrix, per square centimeter

Q4162 Amniopro flow, BioSkin flow, Biorenew flow, Woundex flow, Aminogen-a, Aminogen-c, 0.5 cc

Q4163 Amniopro, BioSkin, Biorenew, Woundex, amniogen-45, amniogen-200, per square centimeter

Q4164 Helicoll, per square centimeter

Q4165 Keramatrix, per square centimeter

• **Q4166** Cytal, per square centimeter

• **Q4167** Truskin, per square centimeter

• **Q4168** Amnioband, 1 mg

• **Q4169** Artacent wound, per square centimeter

• **Q4170** Cygnus, per square centimeter

- **Q4171** Interfyl, 1 mg
- **Q4172** PuraPly or PuraPly am, per square centimeter
- **Q4173** Palingen or Palingen xplus, per square centimeter
- **Q4174** Palingen or Promatrx, 0.36 mg per 0.25 cc
- **Q4175** Miroderm, per square centimeter

Hospice or Home Health Care

Q5001 Hospice or home health care provided in patient's home/residence

Q5002 Hospice or home health care provided in assisted living facility

Q5003 Hospice care provided in nursing long term care facility (LTC) or non-skilled nursing facility (NF)

Q5004 Hospice care provided in skilled nursing facility (snf)

Q5005 Hospice care provided in inpatient hospital

Q5006 Hospice care provided in inpatient hospice facility

Q5007 Hospice care provided in long term care facility

Q5008 Hospice care provided in inpatient psychiatric facility

Q5009 Hospice or home health care provided in place not otherwise specified (nos)

Q5010 Hospice home care provided in a hospice facility

Miscellaneous and Osmolar Contrast Material

Q5101 Injection, filgrastim (g-csf), biosimilar, 1 microgram

- **Q5102** Injection, infliximab, biosimilar, 10 mg

  MCM: 2049

Q9950 Injection, sulfur hexafluoride lipid microspheres, per ml

Q9951 Low osmolar contrast material, 400 or greater mg/ml iodine concentration, per ml

MCM: 15022

Q9953 Injection, iron-based magnetic resonance contrast agent, per ml

MCM: 15022

Q9954 Oral magnetic resonance contrast agent, per 100 ml

MCM: 15022

Q9955 Injection, perflexane lipid microspheres, per ml

Q9956 Injection, octafluoropropane microspheres, per ml

Q9957 Injection, perflutren lipid microspheres, per ml

Q9958 High osmolar contrast material, up to 149 mg/ml iodine concentration, per ml

MCM: 15022

Q9959 High osmolar contrast material, 150-199 mg/ml iodine concentration, per ml
MCM: 15022

Q9960 High osmolar contrast material, 200-249 mg/ml iodine concentration, per ml
MCM: 15022

Q9961 High osmolar contrast material, 250-299 mg/ml iodine concentration, per ml
MCM: 15022

Q9962 High osmolar contrast material, 300-349 mg/ml iodine concentration, per ml
MCM: 15022

Q9963 High osmolar contrast material, 350-399 mg/ml iodine concentration, per ml
MCM: 15022

Q9964 High osmolar contrast material, 400 or greater mg/ml iodine concentration, per ml
MCM: 15022

Q9965 Low osmolar contrast material, 100-199 mg/ml iodine concentration, per ml
MCM: 15022

Q9966 Low osmolar contrast material, 200-299 mg/ml iodine concentration, per ml
MCM: 15022

Q9967 Low osmolar contrast material, 300-399 mg/ml iodine concentration, per ml
MCM: 15022

Q9968 Injection, non-radioactive, non-contrast, visualization adjunct (e.g., methylene blue, isosulfan blue), 1 mg

Q9969 Tc-99m from non-highly enriched uranium source, full cost recovery add-on, per study dose

(**Q9975** Code deleted December 31, 2015.) Use J7205

(**Q9976** Code deleted December 31, 2015.) Use J1443

(**Q9977** Code deleted December 31, 2015.)

(**Q9978** Code deleted December 31, 2015.) Use J8655

(**Q9979** Code deleted December 31, 2015.) Use J0202

(**Q9980** Code deleted December 31, 2016).

(**Q9981** Code deleted December 31, 2016). Use J8670.

• **Q9982** Flutemetamol f18, diagnostic, per study dose, up to 5 millicuries

• **Q9983** Florbetaben f18, diagnostic, per study dose, up to 8.1 millicuries

DIAGNOSTIC RADIOLOGY SERVICES

Guidelines

In addition to the information presented in the INTRODUCTION, several other items unique to this section are defined or identified here:

1. SPECIAL REPORT: A service, material or supply that is rarely provided, unusual, variable or new may require a special report in determining medical appropriateness for reimbursement purposes. Pertinent information should include an adequate definition or description of the nature, extent, and need for the service, material or supply.

2. MODIFIERS: Listed services may be modified under certain circumstances. When appropriate, the modifying circumstance is identified by adding a modifier to the basic procedure code. CPT and HCPCS National Level II modifiers may be used with CPT and HCPCS National Level II procedure codes. Modifiers commonly used with DIAGNOSTIC RADIOLOGY SERVICES are as follows:

   -CC Procedure code change (use "CC" when the procedure code submitted was changed either for administrative reasons or because an incorrect code was filed)

   -LT Left side (used to identify procedures performed on the left side of the body)

   -RT Right side (used to identify procedures performed on the right side of the body)

   -TC Technical component. Under certain circumstances, a charge may be made for the technical component alone. Under those circumstances, the technical component charge is identified by adding modifier -TC to the usual procedure number. Technical component charges are institutional charges and are not billed separately by physicians. However, portable x-ray suppliers bill only for the technical component and should use modifier -TC. The charge data from portable x-ray suppliers will then be used to build customary and prevailing profiles.

3. CPT CODE CROSS-REFERENCE: There are no equivalent CPT codes for procedures listed in this section.

Diagnostic Radiology Services

R0070 Transportation of portable x-ray equipment and personnel to home or nursing home, per trip to facility or location, one patient seen

MCM: 2070.4, 5244.B

R0075 Transportation of portable x-ray equipment and personnel to home or nursing home, per trip to facility or location, more than one patient seen

MCM: 2070.4, 5244.B

R0076 Transportation of portable ekg to facility or location, per patient

CIM: 50-15

MCM: 2070.1, 2070.4

PRIVATE PAYER CODES

Guidelines

HCPCS "S" codes are temporary national codes established by the private payers for private payer use. Prior to using "S" codes on insurance claims to private payers, you should consult with the payer to confirm that the "S" codes are acceptable. "S" codes are not valid for Medicare use.

In addition to the information presented in the INTRODUCTION, several other items unique to this section are defined or identified here.

1. SPECIAL REPORT: A service, material or supply that is rarely provided, unusual, variable or new may require a special report in determining medical appropriateness for reimbursement purposes. Pertinent information should include an adequate definition or description of the nature, extent, and need for the service, material or supply.

2. MODIFIERS: Listed services may be modified under certain circumstances. When appropriate, the modifying circumstance is identified by adding a modifier to the basic procedure code. CPT and HCPCS National Level II modifiers may be used with CPT and HCPCS National Level II procedure codes.

Private Payer Codes

S0012 Butorphanol tartrate, nasal spray, 25 mg

S0014 Tacrine hydrochloride, 10 mg

S0017 Injection, aminocaproic acid, 5 grams

S0020 Injection, Bupivicaine hydrochloride, 30 ml

S0021 Injection, cefoperazone sodium, 1 gram

S0023 Injection, cimetidine hydrochloride, 300 mg

S0028 Injection, famotidine, 20 mg

S0030 Injection, metronidazole, 500 mg

S0032 Injection, nafcillin sodium, 2 grams

S0034 Injection, ofloxacin, 400 mg

S0039 Injection, sulfamethoxazole and trimethoprim, 10 ml

S0040 Injection, ticarcillin disodium and clavulanate potassium, 3.1 grams

S0073 Injection, aztreonam, 500 mg

S0074 Injection, cefotetan disodium, 500 mg

S0077 Injection, clindamycin phosphate, 300 mg

S0078 Injection, fosphenytoin sodium, 750 mg

S0080 Injection, pentamidine isethionate, 300 mg

S0081 Injection, piperacillin sodium, 500 mg

S0088 Imatinib, 100 mg

S0090 Sildenafil citrate, 25 mg

S0091 Granisetron hydrochloride, 1 mg (for circumstances falling under the Medicare statute, use Q0166)

S0092 Injection, hydromorphone hydrochloride, 250 mg (loading dose for infusion pump)

S0093 Injection, morphine sulfate, 500 mg (loading dose for infusion pump)

S0104 Zidovudine, oral, 100 mg

S0106 Bupropion HCL sustained release tablet, 150 mg, per bottle of 60 tablets

S0108 Mercaptopurine, oral, 50 mg

S0109 Methadone, oral, 5 mg

S0117 Tretinoin, topical, 5 grams

S0119 Ondansetron, oral, 4 mg (for circumstances falling under the Medicare statute, use HCPCS q code)

S0122 Injection, menotropins, 75 iu

S0126 Injection, follitropin alfa, 75 iu

S0128 Injection, follitropin beta, 75 iu

S0132 Injection, ganirelix acetate, 250 mcg

S0136 Clozapine, 25 mg

S0137 Didanosine (ddi), 25 mg

S0138 Finasteride, 5 mg

S0139 Minoxidil, 10 mg

S0140 Saquinavir, 200 mg

S0142 Colistimethate sodium, inhalation solution administered through DME, concentrated form, per mg

S0145 Injection, pegylated interferon alfa-2a, 180 mcg per ml

S0148 Injection, pegylated interferon alfa-2b, 10 mcg

S0155 Sterile dilutant for epoprostenol, 50 ml

S0156 Exemestane, 25 mg

S0157 Becaplermin gel 0.01%, 0.5 gm

S0160 Dextroamphetamine sulfate, 5 mg

S0164 Injection, pantoprazole sodium, 40 mg

S0166 Injection, olanzapine, 2.5 mg

S0169 Calcitrol, 0.25 microgram

S0170 Anastrozole, oral, 1 mg

S0171 Injection, bumetanide, 0.5 mg

S0172 Chlorambucil, oral, 2 mg

S0174 Dolasetron mesylate, oral 50 mg (for circumstances falling under the Medicare statute, use Q0180)

S0175 Flutamide, oral, 125 mg

S0176 Hydroxyurea, oral, 500 mg

S0177 Levamisole hydrochloride, oral, 50 mg

S0178 Lomustine, oral, 10 mg

S0179 Megestrol acetate, oral, 20 mg

S0182 Procarbazine hydrochloride, oral, 50 mg

S0183 Prochlorperazine maleate, oral, 5 mg (for circumstances falling under the Medicare statute, use Q0164)

S0187 Tamoxifen citrate, oral, 10 mg

S0189 Testosterone pellet, 75 mg

S0190 Mifepristone, oral, 200 mg

S0191 Misoprostol, oral, 200 mcg

S0194 Dialysis/stress vitamin supplement, oral, 100 capsules

(**S0195** Code deleted December 31, 2015.)

S0197 Prenatal vitamins, 30-day supply

S0199 Medically induced abortion by oral ingestion of medication including all associated services and supplies (e.g., patient counseling, office visits, confirmation of pregnancy by hcg, ultrasound to confirm duration of pregnancy, ultrasound to confirm completion of abortion) except drugs

S0201 Partial hospitalization services, less than 24 hours, per diem

S0207 Paramedic intercept, non-hospital-based ALS service (non-voluntary), non-transport

S0208 Paramedic intercept, hospital-based ALS service (non-voluntary), non-transport

S0209 Wheelchair van, mileage, per mile

S0215 Non-emergency transportation; mileage, per mile

S0220 Medical conference by a physician with interdisciplinary team of health professionals or representatives of community agencies to coordinate activities of patient care (patient is present); approximately 30 minutes

S0221 Medical conference by a physician with interdisciplinary team of health professionals or representatives of community agencies to coordinate activities of patient care (patient is present); approximately 60 minutes

S0250 Comprehensive geriatric assessment and treatment planning performed by assessment team

S0255 Hospice referral visit (advising patient and family of care options) performed by nurse, social worker, or other designated staff

S0257 Counseling and discussion regarding advance directives or end of life care planning and decisions, with patient and/or surrogate (list separately in addition to code for appropriate evaluation and management service)

S0260 History and physical (outpatient or office) related to surgical procedure (list separately in addition to code for appropriate evaluation and management service)

S0265 Genetic counseling, under physician supervision, each 15 minutes

S0270 Physician management of patient home care, standard monthly case rate (per 30 days)

S0271 Physician management of patient home care, hospice monthly case rate (per 30 days)

S0272 Physician management of patient home care, episodic care monthly case rate (per 30 days)

S0273 Physician visit at member's home, outside of a capitation arrangement

S0274 Nurse practitioner visit at member's home, outside of a capitation arrangement

S0280 Medical home program, comprehensive care coordination and planning, initial plan

S0281 Medical home program, comprehensive care coordination and planning, maintenance of plan

S0302 Completed early periodic screening diagnosis and treatment (EPSDT) service (list in addition to code for appropriate evaluation and management service)

S0310 Hospitalist services (list separately in addition to code for appropriate evaluation and management service)

• **S0311** Comprehensive management and care coordination for advanced illness, per calendar month

S0315 Disease management program; initial assessment and initiation of the program

S0316 Disease management program, follow-up/reassessment

S0317 Disease management program; per diem

S0320 Telephone calls by a registered nurse to a disease management program member for monitoring purposes; per month

S0340 Lifestyle modification program for management of coronary artery disease, including all supportive services; first quarter / stage

S0341 Lifestyle modification program for management of coronary artery disease, including all supportive services; second or third quarter / stage

S0342 Lifestyle modification program for management of coronary artery disease, including all supportive services; fourth quarter / stage

S0353 Treatment planning and care coordination management for cancer, initial treatment

S0354 Treatment planning and care coordination management for cancer, established patient with a change of regimen

S0390 Routine foot care; removal and/or trimming of corns, calluses and/or nails and preventive maintenance in specific medical conditions (e.g., diabetes), per visit

S0395 Impression casting of a foot performed by a practitioner other than the manufacturer of the orthotic

Code	Description
S0400	Global fee for extracorporeal shock wave lithotripsy treatment of kidney stone(s)
S0500	Disposable contact lens, per lens
S0504	Single vision prescription lens (safety, athletic, or sunglass), per lens
S0506	Bifocal vision prescription lens (safety, athletic, or sunglass), per lens
S0508	Trifocal vision prescription lens (safety, athletic, or sunglass), per lens
S0510	Non-prescription lens (safety, athletic, or sunglass), per lens
S0512	Daily wear specialty contact lens, per lens
S0514	Color contact lens, per lens
S0515	Scleral lens, liquid bandage device, per lens
S0516	Safety eyeglass frames
S0518	Sunglasses frames
S0580	Polycarbonate lens (list this code in addition to the basic code for the lens)
S0581	Nonstandard lens (list this code in addition to the basic code for the lens)
S0590	Integral lens service, miscellaneous services reported separately
S0592	Comprehensive contact lens evaluation
S0595	Dispensing new spectacle lenses for patient supplied frame
S0596	Phakic intraocular lens for correction of refractive error
S0601	Screening proctoscopy
S0610	Annual gynecological examination, new patient
S0612	Annual gynecological examination, established patient
S0613	Annual gynecological examination; clinical breast examination without pelvic evaluation
S0618	Audiometry for hearing aid evaluation to determine the level and degree of hearing loss
S0620	Routine ophthalmological examination including refraction; new patient
S0621	Routine ophthalmological examination including refraction; established patient
S0622	Physical exam for college, new or established patient (list separately in addition to appropriate evaluation and management code)
S0630	Removal of sutures; by a physician other than the physician who originally closed the wound
S0800	Laser in situ keratomileusis (LASIK)
S0810	Photorefractive keratectomy (PRK)
S0812	Phototherapeutic keratectomy (ptk)
S1001	Deluxe item, patient aware (list in addition to code for basic item)
S1002	Customized item (list in addition to code for basic item)
S1015	IV tubing extension set

S1016 Non-pvc (polyvinyl chloride) intravenous administration set, for use with drugs that are not stable in pvc e.g., paclitaxel

S1030 Continuous noninvasive glucose monitoring device, purchase (for physician interpretation of data, use CPT code)

S1031 Continuous noninvasive glucose monitoring device, rental, including sensor, sensor replacement, and download to monitor (for physician interpretation of data, use CPT code)

S1034 Artificial pancreas device system (e.g., low glucose suspend (LGS) feature) including continuous glucose monitor, blood glucose device, insulin pump and computer algorithm that communicates with all of the devices

S1035 Sensor; invasive (e.g., subcutaneous), disposable, for use with artificial pancreas device system

S1036 Transmitter; external, for use with artificial pancreas device system

S1037 Receiver (monitor); external, for use with artificial pancreas device system

S1040 Cranial remolding orthosis, pediatric, rigid, with soft interface material, custom fabricated, includes fitting and adjustment(s)

S1090 Mometasone furoate sinus implant, 370 micrograms

S2053 Transplantation of small intestine and liver allografts

S2054 Transplantation of multivisceral organs

S2055 Harvesting of donor multivisceral organs, with preparation and maintenance of allografts; from cadaver donor

S2060 Lobar lung transplantation

S2061 Donor lobectomy (lung) for transplantation, living donor

S2065 Simultaneous pancreas kidney transplantation

S2066 Breast reconstruction with gluteal artery perforator (gap) flap, including harvesting of the flap, microvascular transfer, closure of donor site and shaping the flap into a breast, unilateral

S2067 Breast reconstruction of a single breast with "stacked" deep inferior epigastric perforator (diep) flap(s) and/or gluteal artery perforator (gap) flap(s), including harvesting of the flap(s), microvascular transfer, closure of donor site(s) and shaping the flap into a breast, unilateral

S2068 Breast reconstruction with deep inferior epigastric perforator (diep) flap or superficial inferior epigastric artery (siea) flap, including harvesting of the flap, microvascular transfer, closure of donor site and shaping the flap into a breast, unilateral

S2070 Cystourethroscopy, with ureteroscopy and/or pyeloscopy; with endoscopic laser treatment of ureteral calculi (includes ureteral catheterization)

S2079 Laparoscopic esophagomyotomy (Heller type)

S2080 Laser-assisted uvulopalatoplasty (LAUP)

S2083 Adjustment of gastric band diameter via subcutaneous port by injection or aspiration of saline

S2095 Transcatheter occlusion or embolization for tumor destruction, percutaneous, any method, using yttrium-90 microspheres

S2102 Islet cell tissue transplant from pancreas; allogeneic

S2103 Adrenal tissue transplant to brain

S2107 Adoptive immunotherapy i.e. development of specific anti-tumor reactivity (e.g., tumor-infiltrating lymphocyte therapy) per course of treatment

S2112 Arthroscopy, knee, surgical for harvesting of cartilage (chondrocyte cells)

S2115 Osteotomy, periacetabular, with internal fixation

S2117 Arthroereisis, subtalar

S2118 Metal-on-metal total hip resurfacing, including acetabular and femoral components

S2120 Low density lipoprotein (LDL) apheresis using heparin-induced extracorporeal LDL precipitation

S2140 Cord blood harvesting for transplantation, allogeneic

S2142 Cord blood-derived stem-cell transplantation, allogeneic

S2150 Bone marrow or blood-derived stem cells (peripheral or umbilical), allogeneic or autologous, harvesting, transplantation, and related complications; including: pheresis and cell preparation/storage; marrow ablative therapy; drugs, supplies, hospitalization with outpatient follow-up; medical/surgical, diagnostic, emergency, and rehabilitative services; and the number of days of pre-and post-transplant care in the global definition

S2152 Solid organ(s), complete or segmental, single organ or combination of organs; deceased or living donor(s), procurement, transplantation, and related complications; including: drugs; supplies; hospitalization with outpatient follow-up; medical/surgical, diagnostic, emergency, and rehabilitative services, and the number of days of pre- and post-transplant care in the global definition

S2202 Echosclerotherapy

S2205 Minimally invasive direct coronary artery bypass surgery involving mini-thoracotomy or mini-sternotomy surgery, performed under direct vision; using arterial graft(s), single coronary arterial graft

S2206 Minimally invasive direct coronary artery bypass surgery involving mini-thoracotomy or mini-sternotomy surgery, performed under direct vision; using arterial graft(s), two coronary arterial grafts

S2207 Minimally invasive direct coronary artery bypass surgery involving mini-thoracotomy or mini-sternotomy surgery, performed under direct vision; using venous graft only, single coronary venous graft

S2208 Minimally invasive direct coronary artery bypass surgery involving mini-thoracotomy or mini-sternotomy surgery, performed under direct vision; using single arterial and venous graft(s), single venous graft

S2209 Minimally invasive direct coronary artery bypass surgery involving mini-thoracotomy or mini-sternotomy surgery, performed under direct vision; using two arterial grafts and single venous graft

S2225 Myringotomy, laser-assisted

S2230 Implantation of magnetic component of semi-implantable hearing device on ossicles in middle ear

S2235 Implantation of auditory brain stem implant

S2260 Induced abortion, 17 to 24 weeks

S2265 Induced abortion, 25 to 28 weeks

S2266 Induced abortion, 29 to 31 weeks

S2267 Induced abortion, 32 weeks or greater

S2300 Arthroscopy, shoulder, surgical; with thermally-induced capsulorrhaphy

S2325 Hip core decompression

S2340 Chemodenervation of abductor muscle(s) of vocal cord

S2341 Chemodenervation of adductor muscle(s) of vocal cord

S2342 Nasal endoscopy for post-operative debridement following functional endoscopic sinus surgery, nasal and/or sinus cavity(s), unilateral or bilateral

S2348 Decompression procedure, percutaneous, of nucleus pulposus of intervertebral disc, using radiofrequency energy, single or multiple levels, lumbar

S2350 Diskectomy, anterior, with decompression of spinal cord and/or nerve root(s), including osteophytectomy; lumbar, single interspace

S2351 Diskectomy, anterior, with decompression of spinal cord and/or nerve root(s), including osteophytectomy; lumbar, each additional interspace (list separately in addition to code for primary procedure)

(**S2360** Code deleted December 31, 2015.)

(**S2361** Code deleted December 31, 2015.)

S2400 Repair, congenital diaphragmatic hernia in the fetus using temporary tracheal occlusion, procedure performed in utero

S2401 Repair, urinary tract obstruction in the fetus, procedure performed in utero

S2402 Repair, congenital cystic adenomatoid malformation in the fetus, procedure performed in utero

S2403 Repair, extralobar pulmonary sequestration in the fetus, procedure performed in utero

S2404 Repair, myelomeningocele in the fetus, procedure performed in utero

S2405 Repair of sacrococcygeal teratoma in the fetus, procedure performed in utero

S2409 Repair, congenital malformation of fetus, procedure performed in utero, not otherwise classified

S2411 Fetoscopic laser therapy for treatment of twin-to-twin transfusion syndrome

S2900 Surgical techniques requiring use of robotic surgical system (list separately in addition to code for primary procedure)

S3000 Diabetic indicator; retinal eye exam, dilated, bilateral

S3005 Performance measurement, evaluation of patient self assessment, depression

S3600 Stat laboratory request (situations other than s3601)

S3601 Emergency stat laboratory charge for patient who is homebound or residing in a nursing facility

S3620 Newborn metabolic screening panel, includes test kit, postage and the laboratory tests specified by the state for inclusion in this panel (e.g. galactose; hemoglobin, electrophoresis; hydroxyprogesterone, 17-d; phenylalanine (PKU); and thyroxine, total)

S3630 Eosinophil count, blood, direct

S3645 HIV-1 antibody testing of oral mucosal transudate

S3650 Saliva test, hormone level; during menopause

S3652 Saliva test, hormone level; to assess preterm labor risk

S3655 Antisperm antibodies test (immunobead)

S3708 Gastrointestinal fat absorption study

(**S3721** Code deleted December 31, 2015.)

S3722 Dose optimization by area under the curve (AUC) analysis, for infusional 5-fluorouracil

S3800 Genetic testing for amyotrophic lateral sclerosis (ALS)

S3840 DNA analysis for germline mutations of the ret proto-oncogene for susceptibility to multiple endocrine neoplasia type 2

S3841 Genetic testing for retinoblastoma

S3842 Genetic testing for von Hippel-Lindau disease

S3844 DNA analysis of the connexin 26 gene (gjb2) for susceptibility to congenital, profound deafness

S3845 Genetic testing for alpha-thalassemia

S3846 Genetic testing for hemoglobin e beta-thalassemia

S3849 Genetic testing for Niemann-pick disease

S3850 Genetic testing for sickle cell anemia

S3852 DNA analysis for apoe epsilon 4 allele for susceptibility to Alzheimer's disease

S3853 Genetic testing for myotonic muscular dystrophy

• **S3854** Gene expression profiling panel for use in the management of breast cancer treatment

S3861 Genetic testing, sodium channel, voltage-gated, type v, alpha subunit (scn5a) and variants for suspected Brugada syndrome

S3865 Comprehensive gene sequence analysis for hypertrophic cardiomyopathy

S3866 Genetic analysis for a specific gene mutation for hypertrophic cardiomyopathy (HCM) in an individual with a known HCM mutation in the family

S3870 Comparative genomic hybridization (CGH) microarray testing for developmental delay, autism spectrum disorder and/or intellectual disability

(**S3890** Code deleted December 31, 2015.)

S3900 Surface electromyography (EMG)

S3902 Ballistocardiogram

S3904 Masters two step

S4005 Interim labor facility global (labor occurring but not resulting in delivery)

S4011 In vitro fertilization; including but not limited to identification and incubation of mature oocytes, fertilization with sperm, incubation of embryo(s), and subsequent visualization for determination of development

S4013 Complete cycle, gamete intrafallopian transfer (gift), case rate

S4014 Complete cycle, zygote intrafallopian transfer (zift), case rate

S4015 Complete in vitro fertilization cycle, not otherwise specified, case rate

S4016 Frozen in vitro fertilization cycle, case rate

S4017 Incomplete cycle, treatment cancelled prior to stimulation, case rate

S4018 Frozen embryo transfer procedure cancelled before transfer, case rate

S4020 In vitro fertilization procedure cancelled before aspiration, case rate

S4021 In vitro fertilization procedure cancelled after aspiration, case rate

S4022 Assisted oocyte fertilization, case rate

S4023 Donor egg cycle, incomplete, case rate

S4025 Donor services for in vitro fertilization (sperm or embryo), case rate

S4026 Procurement of donor sperm from sperm bank

S4027 Storage of previously frozen embryos

S4028 Microsurgical epididymal sperm aspiration (mesa)

S4030 Sperm procurement and cryopreservation services; initial visit

S4031 Sperm procurement and cryopreservation services; subsequent visit

S4035 Stimulated intrauterine insemination (IUI), case rate

S4037 Cryopreserved embryo transfer, case rate

S4040 Monitoring and storage of cryopreserved embryos, per 30 days

S4042 Management of ovulation induction (interpretation of diagnostic tests and studies, non-face-to-face medical management of the patient), per cycle

S4981 Insertion of levonorgestrel-releasing intrauterine system

S4989 Contraceptive intrauterine device (e.g., Progestasert iud), including implants and supplies

S4990 Nicotine patches, legend

S4991 Nicotine patches, non-legend

S4993 Contraceptive pills for birth control

S4995 Smoking cessation gum

S5000 Prescription drug, generic

S5001 Prescription drug, brand name

S5010 5% dextrose and 0.45% normal saline, 1000 ml

(**S5011** Code deleted December 31, 2015.)

S5012 5% dextrose with potassium chloride, 1000 ml

S5013 5% dextrose/0.45% normal saline with potassium chloride and magnesium sulfate, 1000 ml

S5014 5% dextrose/0.45% normal saline with potassium chloride and magnesium sulfate, 1500 ml

S5035 Home infusion therapy, routine service of infusion device (e.g., pump maintenance)

S5036 Home infusion therapy, repair of infusion device (e.g., pump repair)

S5100 Day care services, adult; per 15 minutes

S5101 Day care services, adult; per half day

S5102 Day care services, adult; per diem

S5105 Day care services, center-based; services not included in program fee, per diem

S5108 Home care training to home care client, per 15 minutes

S5109 Home care training to home care client, per session

S5110 Home care training, family; per 15 minutes

S5111 Home care training, family; per session

S5115 Home care training, non-family; per 15 minutes

S5116 Home care training, non-family; per session

S5120 Chore services; per 15 minutes

S5121 Chore services; per diem

S5125 Attendant care services; per 15 minutes

S5126 Attendant care services; per diem

S5130 Homemaker service, nos; per 15 minutes

S5131 Homemaker service, nos; per diem

S5135 Companion care, adult (e.g., iadl/ADL); per 15 minutes

S5136 Companion care, adult (e.g., iadl/ADL); per diem

S5140 Foster care, adult; per diem

S5141 Foster care, adult; per month

S5145 Foster care, therapeutic, child; per diem

S5146 Foster care, therapeutic, child; per month

S5150 Unskilled respite care, not hospice; per 15 minutes

S5151 Unskilled respite care, not hospice; per diem

S5160 Emergency response system; installation and testing

S5161 Emergency response system; service fee, per month (excludes installation and testing)

S5162 Emergency response system; purchase only

S5165 Home modifications; per service

S5170 Home delivered meals, including preparation; per meal

S5175 Laundry service, external, professional; per order

S5180 Home health respiratory therapy, initial evaluation

S5181 Home health respiratory therapy, nos, per diem

S5185 Medication reminder service, non-face-to-face; per month

S5190 Wellness assessment, performed by non-physician

S5199 Personal care item, nos, each

S5497 Home infusion therapy, catheter care / maintenance, not otherwise classified; includes administrative services, professional pharmacy services, care coordination, and all necessary supplies and equipment (drugs and nursing visits coded separately), per diem

S5498 Home infusion therapy, catheter care / maintenance, simple (single lumen), includes administrative services, professional pharmacy services, care coordination and all necessary supplies and equipment, (drugs and nursing visits coded separately), per diem

S5501 Home infusion therapy, catheter care / maintenance, complex (more than one lumen), includes administrative services, professional pharmacy services, care coordination, and all necessary supplies and equipment (drugs and nursing visits coded separately), per diem

S5502 Home infusion therapy, catheter care / maintenance, implanted access device, includes administrative services, professional pharmacy services, care coordination and all necessary supplies and equipment, (drugs and nursing visits coded separately), per diem (use this code for interim maintenance of vascular access not currently in use)

S5517 Home infusion therapy, all supplies necessary for restoration of catheter patency or declotting

S5518 Home infusion therapy, all supplies necessary for catheter repair

S5520 Home infusion therapy, all supplies (including catheter) necessary for a peripherally inserted central venous catheter (PICC) line insertion

S5521 Home infusion therapy, all supplies (including catheter) necessary for a midline catheter insertion

S5522 Home infusion therapy, insertion of peripherally inserted central venous catheter (PICC), nursing services only (no supplies or catheter included)

S5523 Home infusion therapy, insertion of midline venous catheter, nursing services only (no supplies or catheter included)

S5550 Insulin, rapid onset, 5 units

S5551 Insulin, most rapid onset (lispro or aspart); 5 units

S5552 Insulin, intermediate acting (NPH or lente); 5 units

S5553 Insulin, long acting; 5 units

S5560 Insulin delivery device, reusable pen; 1.5 ml size

S5561 Insulin delivery device, reusable pen; 3 ml size

S5565 Insulin cartridge for use in insulin delivery device other than pump; 150 units

S5566 Insulin cartridge for use in insulin delivery device other than pump; 300 units

S5570 Insulin delivery device, disposable pen (including insulin); 1.5 ml size

S5571 Insulin delivery device, disposable pen (including insulin); 3 ml size

S8030 Scleral application of tantalum ring(s) for localization of lesions for proton beam therapy

(**S8032** Code deleted September 30, 2016). Use G0297

S8035 Magnetic source imaging

S8037 Magnetic resonance cholangiopancreatography (MRCP)

S8040 Topographic brain mapping

S8042 Magnetic resonance imaging (MRI), low-field

S8055 Ultrasound guidance for multifetal pregnancy reduction(s), technical component (only to be used when the physician doing the reduction procedure does not perform the ultrasound, guidance is included in the CPT code for multifetal pregnancy reduction - 59866)

S8080 Scintimammography (radioimmunoscintigraphy of the breast), unilateral, including supply of radiopharmaceutical

S8085 Fluorine-18 fluorodeoxyglucose (f-18 fdg) imaging using dual-head coincidence detection system (non-dedicated pet scan)

S8092 Electron beam computed tomography (also known as ultrafast ct, cine ct)

S8096 Portable peak flow meter

S8097 Asthma kit (including but not limited to portable peak expiratory flow meter, instructional video, brochure, and/or spacer)

S8100 Holding chamber or spacer for use with an inhaler or nebulizer; without mask

S8101 Holding chamber or spacer for use with an inhaler or nebulizer; with mask

S8110 Peak expiratory flow rate (physician services)

S8120 Oxygen contents, gaseous, 1 unit equals 1 cubic foot

S8121 Oxygen contents, liquid, 1 unit equals 1 pound

S8130 Interferential current stimulator, 2 channel

S8131 Interferential current stimulator, 4 channel

S8185 Flutter device

S8186 Swivel adapter

S8189 Tracheostomy supply, not otherwise classified

S8210 Mucus trap

(**S8262** Code deleted December 31, 2015.)

S8265 Haberman feeder for cleft lip/palate

S8270 Enuresis alarm, using auditory buzzer and/or vibration device

S8301 Infection control supplies, not otherwise specified

S8415 Supplies for home delivery of infant

S8420 Gradient pressure aid (sleeve and glove combination), custom made

S8421 Gradient pressure aid (sleeve and glove combination), ready made

S8422 Gradient pressure aid (sleeve), custom made, medium weight

S8423 Gradient pressure aid (sleeve), custom made, heavy weight

S8424 Gradient pressure aid (sleeve), ready made

S8425 Gradient pressure aid (glove), custom made, medium weight

S8426 Gradient pressure aid (glove), custom made, heavy weight

S8427 Gradient pressure aid (glove), ready made

S8428 Gradient pressure aid (gauntlet), ready made

S8429 Gradient pressure exterior wrap

S8430 Padding for compression bandage, roll

S8431 Compression bandage, roll

S8450 Splint, prefabricated, digit (specify digit by use of modifier)

S8451 Splint, prefabricated, wrist or ankle

S8452 Splint, prefabricated, elbow

S8460 Camisole, post-mastectomy

S8490 Insulin syringes (100 syringes, any size)

S8930 Electrical stimulation of auricular acupuncture points; each 15 minutes of personal one-on-one contact with the patient

S8940 Equestrian/hippotherapy, per session

S8948 Application of a modality (requiring constant provider attendance) to one or more areas; low-level laser; each 15 minutes

S8950 Complex lymphedema therapy, each 15 minutes

S8990 Physical or manipulative therapy performed for maintenance rather than restoration

S8999 Resuscitation bag (for use by patient on artificial respiration during power failure or other catastrophic event)

S9001 Home uterine monitor with or without associated nursing services

S9007 Ultrafiltration monitor

(**S9015** Code deleted December 31, 2015.)

S9024 Paranasal sinus ultrasound

S9025 Omnicardiogram/cardiointegram

S9034 Extracorporeal shockwave lithotripsy for gall stones (if performed with ERCP, use 43265)

S9055 Procuren or other growth factor preparation to promote wound healing

S9056 Coma stimulation per diem

S9061 Home administration of aerosolized drug therapy (e.g., pentamidine); administrative services, professional pharmacy services, care coordination, all necessary supplies and equipment (drugs and nursing visits coded separately), per diem

S9083 Global fee urgent care centers

S9088 Services provided in an urgent care center (list in addition to code for service)

S9090 Vertebral axial decompression, per session

S9097 Home visit for wound care

S9098 Home visit, phototherapy services (e.g., bili-lite), including equipment rental, nursing services, blood draw, supplies, and other services, per diem

S9110 Telemonitoring of patient in their home, including all necessary equipment; computer system, connections, and software; maintenance; patient education and support; per month

S9117 Back school, per visit

S9122 Home health aide or certified nurse assistant, providing care in the home; per hour

S9123 Nursing care, in the home; by registered nurse, per hour (use for general nursing care only, not to be used when CPT codes 99500-99602 can be used)

S9124 Nursing care, in the home; by licensed practical nurse, per hour

S9125 Respite care, in the home, per diem

S9126 Hospice care, in the home, per diem

S9127 Social work visit, in the home, per diem

S9128 Speech therapy, in the home, per diem

S9129 Occupational therapy, in the home, per diem

S9131 Physical therapy; in the home, per diem

S9140 Diabetic management program, follow-up visit to non-md provider

S9141 Diabetic management program, follow-up visit to md provider

S9145 Insulin pump initiation, instruction in initial use of pump (pump not included)

S9150 Evaluation by ocularist

S9152 Speech therapy, re-evaluation

S9208 Home management of preterm labor, including administrative services, professional pharmacy services, care coordination, and all necessary supplies or equipment (drugs and nursing visits coded separately), per diem (do not use this code with any home infusion per diem code)

S9209 Home management of preterm premature rupture of membranes (pprom), including administrative services, professional pharmacy services, care coordination, and all necessary supplies or equipment (drugs and nursing visits coded separately), per diem (do not use this code with any home infusion per diem code)

S9211 Home management of gestational hypertension, includes administrative services, professional pharmacy services, care coordination and all necessary supplies and equipment (drugs and nursing visits coded separately); per diem (do not use this code with any home infusion per diem code)

S9212 Home management of postpartum hypertension, includes administrative services, professional pharmacy services, care coordination, and all necessary supplies and equipment (drugs and nursing visits coded separately), per diem (do not use this code with any home infusion per diem code)

S9213 Home management of preeclampsia, includes administrative services, professional pharmacy services, care coordination, and all necessary supplies and equipment (drugs and nursing services coded separately); per diem (do not use this code with any home infusion per diem code)

S9214 Home management of gestational diabetes, includes administrative services, professional pharmacy services, care coordination, and all necessary supplies and equipment (drugs and nursing visits coded separately); per diem (do not use this code with any home infusion per diem code)

S9325 Home infusion therapy, pain management infusion; administrative services, professional pharmacy services, care coordination, and all necessary supplies and equipment, (drugs and nursing visits coded separately), per diem (do not use this code with s9326, s9327 or s9328)

S9326 Home infusion therapy, continuous (twenty-four hours or more) pain management infusion; administrative services, professional pharmacy services, care coordination and all necessary supplies and equipment (drugs and nursing visits coded separately), per diem

S9327 Home infusion therapy, intermittent (less than twenty-four hours) pain management infusion; administrative services, professional pharmacy services, care coordination, and all necessary supplies and equipment (drugs and nursing visits coded separately), per diem

S9328 Home infusion therapy, implanted pump pain management infusion; administrative services, professional pharmacy services, care coordination, and all necessary supplies and equipment (drugs and nursing visits coded separately), per diem

S9329 Home infusion therapy, chemotherapy infusion; administrative services, professional pharmacy services, care coordination, and all necessary supplies and equipment (drugs and nursing visits coded separately), per diem (do not use this code with s9330 or s9331)

S9330 Home infusion therapy, continuous (twenty-four hours or more) chemotherapy infusion; administrative services, professional pharmacy services, care coordination, and all necessary supplies and equipment (drugs and nursing visits coded separately), per diem

S9331 Home infusion therapy, intermittent (less than twenty-four hours) chemotherapy infusion; administrative services, professional pharmacy services, care coordination, and all necessary supplies and equipment (drugs and nursing visits coded separately), per diem

S9335 Home therapy, hemodialysis; administrative services, professional pharmacy services, care coordination, and all necessary supplies and equipment (drugs and nursing services coded separately), per diem

S9336 Home infusion therapy, continuous anticoagulant infusion therapy (e.g., heparin), administrative services, professional pharmacy services, care coordination and all necessary supplies and equipment (drugs and nursing visits coded separately), per diem

S9338 Home infusion therapy, immunotherapy, administrative services, professional pharmacy services, care coordination, and all necessary supplies and equipment (drugs and nursing visits coded separately), per diem

S9339 Home therapy; peritoneal dialysis, administrative services, professional pharmacy services, care coordination and all necessary supplies and equipment (drugs and nursing visits coded separately), per diem

S9340 Home therapy; enteral nutrition; administrative services, professional pharmacy services, care coordination, and all necessary supplies and equipment (enteral formula and nursing visits coded separately), per diem

S9341 Home therapy; enteral nutrition via gravity; administrative services, professional pharmacy services, care coordination, and all necessary supplies and equipment (enteral formula and nursing visits coded separately), per diem

S9342 Home therapy; enteral nutrition via pump; administrative services, professional pharmacy services, care coordination, and all necessary supplies and equipment (enteral formula and nursing visits coded separately), per diem

S9343 Home therapy; enteral nutrition via bolus; administrative services, professional pharmacy services, care coordination, and all necessary supplies and equipment (enteral formula and nursing visits coded separately), per diem

S9345 Home infusion therapy, anti-hemophilic agent infusion therapy (e.g., factor viii); administrative services, professional pharmacy services, care coordination, and all necessary supplies and equipment (drugs and nursing visits coded separately), per diem

S9346 Home infusion therapy, alpha-1-proteinase inhibitor (e.g., Prolastin); administrative services, professional pharmacy services, care coordination, and all necessary supplies and equipment (drugs and nursing visits coded separately), per diem

S9347 Home infusion therapy, uninterrupted, long-term, controlled rate intravenous or subcutaneous infusion therapy (e.g., epoprostenol); administrative services, professional pharmacy services, care coordination, and all necessary supplies and equipment (drugs and nursing visits coded separately), per diem

S9348 Home infusion therapy, sympathomimetic/inotropic agent infusion therapy (e.g., dobutamine); administrative services, professional pharmacy services, care coordination, all necessary supplies and equipment (drugs and nursing visits coded separately), per diem

S9349 Home infusion therapy, tocolytic infusion therapy; administrative services, professional pharmacy services, care coordination, and all necessary supplies and equipment (drugs and nursing visits coded separately), per diem

S9351 Home infusion therapy, continuous or intermittent anti-emetic infusion therapy; administrative services, professional pharmacy services, care coordination, and all necessary supplies and equipment (drugs and visits coded separately), per diem

S9353 Home infusion therapy, continuous insulin infusion therapy; administrative services, professional pharmacy services, care coordination, and all necessary supplies and equipment (drugs and nursing visits coded separately), per diem

S9355 Home infusion therapy, chelation therapy; administrative services, professional pharmacy services, care coordination, and all necessary

S9357 Home infusion therapy, enzyme replacement intravenous therapy; (e.g., imiglucerase); administrative services, professional pharmacy services, care coordination, and all necessary supplies and equipment (drugs and nursing visits coded separately), per diem

S9359 Home infusion therapy, anti-tumor necrosis factor intravenous therapy; (e.g., infliximab); administrative services, professional pharmacy services, care coordination, and all necessary supplies and equipment (drugs and nursing visits coded separately), per diem

S9361 Home infusion therapy, diuretic intravenous therapy; administrative services, professional pharmacy services, care coordination, and all necessary supplies and equipment (drugs and nursing visits coded separately), per diem

S9363 Home infusion therapy, anti-spasmotic therapy; administrative services, professional pharmacy services, care coordination, and all necessary supplies and equipment (drugs and nursing visits coded separately), per diem

S9364 Home infusion therapy, total parenteral nutrition (tpn); administrative services, professional pharmacy services, care coordination, and all necessary supplies and equipment including standard tpn formula (lipids, specialty amino acid formulas, drugs other than in standard formula and nursing visits coded separately), per diem (do not use with home infusion codes S9365-S9368 using daily volume scales)

S9365 Home infusion therapy, total parenteral nutrition (tpn); one liter per day, administrative services, professional pharmacy services, care coordination, and all necessary supplies and equipment including standard tpn formula (lipids, specialty amino acid formulas, drugs other than in standard formula and nursing visits coded separately), per diem

S9366 Home infusion therapy, total parenteral nutrition (tpn); more than one liter but no more than two liters per day, administrative services, professional pharmacy services, care coordination, and all necessary supplies and equipment including standard tpn formula (lipids, specialty amino acid formulas, drugs other than in standard formula and nursing visits coded separately), per diem

S9367 Home infusion therapy, total parenteral nutrition (tpn); more than two liters but no more than three liters per day, administrative services, professional pharmacy services, care coordination, and all necessary supplies and equipment including standard tpn formula (lipids, specialty amino acid formulas, drugs other than in standard formula and nursing visits coded separately), per diem

S9368 Home infusion therapy, total parenteral nutrition (tpn); more than three liters per day, administrative services, professional pharmacy services, care coordination, and all necessary supplies and equipment including standard tpn formula (lipids, specialty amino acid formulas, drugs other than in standard formula and nursing visits coded separately), per diem

S9370 Home therapy, intermittent anti-emetic injection therapy; administrative services, professional pharmacy services, care coordination, and all necessary supplies and equipment (drugs and nursing visits coded separately), per diem

S9372 Home therapy; intermittent anticoagulant injection therapy (e.g., heparin); administrative services, professional pharmacy services, care coordination, and all necessary supplies and equipment (drugs and nursing visits coded separately), per diem (do not use this code for flushing of infusion devices with heparin to maintain patency)

S9373 Home infusion therapy, hydration therapy; administrative services, professional pharmacy services, care coordination, and all necessary supplies and equipment (drugs and nursing visits coded separately), per diem (do not use with hydration therapy codes s9374-s9377 using daily volume scales)

S9374 Home infusion therapy, hydration therapy; one liter per day, administrative services, professional pharmacy services, care coordination, and all necessary supplies and equipment (drugs and nursing visits coded separately), per diem

S9375 Home infusion therapy, hydration therapy; more than one liter but no more than two liters per day, administrative services, professional pharmacy services, care coordination, and all necessary supplies and equipment (drugs and nursing visits coded separately), per diem

S9376 Home infusion therapy, hydration therapy; more than two liters but no more than three liters per day, administrative services, professional pharmacy services, care coordination, and all necessary supplies and equipment (drugs and nursing visits coded separately), per diem

S9377 Home infusion therapy, hydration therapy; more than three liters per day, administrative services, professional pharmacy services, care coordination, and all necessary supplies (drugs and nursing visits coded separately), per diem

S9379 Home infusion therapy, infusion therapy, not otherwise classified; administrative services, professional pharmacy services, care coordination, and all necessary supplies and equipment (drugs and nursing visits coded separately), per diem

S9381 Delivery or service to high risk areas requiring escort or extra protection, per visit

S9401 Anticoagulation clinic, inclusive of all services except laboratory tests, per session

S9430 Pharmacy compounding and dispensing services

S9433 Medical food nutritionally complete, administered orally, providing 100% of nutritional intake

S9434 Modified solid food supplements for inborn errors of metabolism

S9435 Medical foods for inborn errors of metabolism

S9436 Childbirth preparation/Lamaze classes, non-physician provider, per session

S9437 Childbirth refresher classes, non-physician provider, per session

S9438 Cesarean birth classes, non-physician provider, per session

S9439 VBAC (vaginal birth after cesarean) classes, non-physician provider, per session

S9441 Asthma education, non-physician provider, per session

S9442 Birthing classes, non-physician provider, per session

S9443 Lactation classes, non-physician provider, per session

S9444 Parenting classes, non-physician provider, per session

S9445 Patient education, not otherwise classified, non-physician provider, individual, per session

S9446 Patient education, not otherwise classified, non-physician provider, group, per session

S9447 Infant safety (including CPR) classes, non-physician provider, per session

S9449 Weight management classes, non-physician provider, per session

S9451 Exercise classes, non-physician provider, per session

S9452 Nutrition classes, non-physician provider, per session

S9453 Smoking cessation classes, non-physician provider, per session

S9454 Stress management classes, non-physician provider, per session

S9455 Diabetic management program, group session

S9460 Diabetic management program, nurse visit

S9465 Diabetic management program, dietitian visit

S9470 Nutritional counseling, dietitian visit

S9472 Cardiac rehabilitation program, non-physician provider, per diem

S9473 Pulmonary rehabilitation program, non-physician provider, per diem

S9474 Enterostomal therapy by a registered nurse certified in enterostomal therapy, per diem

S9475 Ambulatory setting substance abuse treatment or detoxification services, per diem

S9476 Vestibular rehabilitation program, non-physician provider, per diem

S9480 Intensive outpatient psychiatric services, per diem

S9482 Family stabilization services, per 15 minutes

S9484 Crisis intervention mental health services, per hour

S9485 Crisis intervention mental health services, per diem

S9490 Home infusion therapy, corticosteroid infusion; administrative services, professional pharmacy services, care coordination, and all necessary supplies and equipment (drugs and nursing visits coded separately), per diem

S9494 Home infusion therapy, antibiotic, antiviral, or antifungal therapy; administrative services, professional pharmacy services, care coordination, and all necessary supplies and equipment (drugs and nursing visits coded separately), per diem (do not use this code with home infusion codes for hourly dosing schedules s9497-s9504)

S9497 Home infusion therapy, antibiotic, antiviral, or antifungal therapy; once every 3 hours; administrative services, professional pharmacy services, care coordination, and all necessary supplies and equipment (drugs and nursing visits coded separately), per diem

S9500 Home infusion therapy, antibiotic, antiviral, or antifungal therapy; once every 24 hours; administrative services, professional pharmacy services, care coordination, and all necessary supplies and equipment (drugs and nursing visits coded separately), per diem

S9501 Home infusion therapy, antibiotic, antiviral, or antifungal therapy; once every 12 hours; administrative services, professional pharmacy services, care coordination, and all necessary supplies and equipment (drugs and nursing visits coded separately), per diem

S9502 Home infusion therapy, antibiotic, antiviral, or antifungal therapy; once every 8 hours, administrative services, professional pharmacy services, care coordination, and all necessary supplies and equipment (drugs and nursing visits coded separately), per diem

S9503 Home infusion therapy, antibiotic, antiviral, or antifungal; once every 6 hours; administrative services, professional pharmacy services, care coordination, and all necessary supplies and equipment (drugs and nursing visits coded separately), per diem

S9504 Home infusion therapy, antibiotic, antiviral, or antifungal; once every 4 hours; administrative services, professional pharmacy services, care coordination, and all necessary supplies and equipment (drugs and nursing visits coded separately), per diem

S9529 Routine venipuncture for collection of specimen(s), single home bound, nursing home, or skilled nursing facility patient

S9537 Home therapy; hematopoietic hormone injection therapy (e.g., erythropoietin, g-csf, gm-csf); administrative services, professional pharmacy services, care coordination, and all necessary supplies and equipment (drugs and nursing visits coded separately), per diem

S9538 Home transfusion of blood product(s); administrative services, professional pharmacy services, care coordination and all necessary supplies and equipment (blood products, drugs, and nursing visits coded separately), per diem

S9542 Home injectable therapy, not otherwise classified, including administrative services, professional pharmacy services, care coordination, and all necessary supplies and equipment (drugs and nursing visits coded separately), per diem

S9558 Home injectable therapy; growth hormone, including administrative services, professional pharmacy services, care coordination, and all necessary supplies and equipment (drugs and nursing visits coded separately), per diem

S9559 Home injectable therapy, interferon, including administrative services, professional pharmacy services, care coordination, and all necessary supplies and equipment (drugs and nursing visits coded separately), per diem

S9560 Home injectable therapy; hormonal therapy (e.g.; leuprolide, goserelin), including administrative services, professional pharmacy services, care coordination, and all necessary supplies and equipment (drugs and nursing visits coded separately), per diem

S9562 Home injectable therapy, palivizumab, including administrative services, professional pharmacy services, care coordination, and all necessary supplies and equipment (drugs and nursing visits coded separately), per diem

S9590 Home therapy, irrigation therapy (e.g., sterile irrigation of an organ or anatomical cavity); including administrative services, professional pharmacy services, care coordination, and all necessary supplies and equipment (drugs and nursing visits coded separately), per diem

S9810 Home therapy; professional pharmacy services for provision of infusion, specialty drug administration, and/or disease state management, not otherwise classified, per hour (do not use this code with any per diem code)

S9900 Services by a journal-listed Christian science practitioner for the purpose of healing, per diem

S9901 Services by a journal-listed Christian science nurse, per hour

S9960 Ambulance service, conventional air service, nonemergency transport, one way (fixed wing)

S9961 Ambulance service, conventional air service, nonemergency transport, one way (rotary wing)

S9970 Health club membership, annual

S9975 Transplant related lodging, meals and transportation, per diem

S9976 Lodging, per diem, not otherwise classified

S9977 Meals, per diem, not otherwise specified

S9981 Medical records copying fee, administrative

S9982 Medical records copying fee, per page

S9986 Not medically necessary service (patient is aware that service not medically necessary)

S9988 Services provided as part of a phase i clinical trial

S9989 Services provided outside of the united states of America (list in addition to code(s) for service(s))

S9990 Services provided as part of a phase ii clinical trial

S9991 Services provided as part of a phase iii clinical trial

S9992 Transportation costs to and from trial location and local transportation costs (e.g., fares for taxicab or bus) for clinical trial participant and one caregiver/companion

S9994 Lodging costs (e.g., hotel charges) for clinical trial participant and one caregiver/companion

S9996 Meals for clinical trial participant and one caregiver/companion

S9999 Sales tax

STATE MEDICAID AGENCY CODES

Guidelines

"T" codes were added to HCPCS in 2002. These codes are exclusively for the use of state Medicaid agencies. Prior to using "T" codes on health insurance claims to your state Medicaid processor, you should verify that these codes are acceptable. "T" codes are not valid for Medicare use.

In addition to the information presented in the INTRODUCTION, several other items unique to this section are defined or identified here.

1. SPECIAL REPORT: A service, material or supply that is rarely provided, unusual, variable or new may require a special report in determining medical appropriateness for reimbursement purposes. Pertinent information should include an adequate definition or description of the nature, extent, and need for the service, material or supply.

2. MODIFIERS: Listed services may be modified under certain circumstances. When appropriate, the modifying circumstance is identified by adding a modifier to the basic procedure code. CPT and HCPCS National Level II modifiers may be used with CPT and HCPCS National Level II procedure codes.

State Medicaid Agency Codes

T1000 Private duty / independent nursing service(s) - licensed, up to 15 minutes

T1001 Nursing assessment / evaluation

T1002 Rn services, up to 15 minutes

T1003 LPN/LVN services, up to 15 minutes

T1004 Services of a qualified nursing aide, up to 15 minutes

T1005 Respite care services, up to 15 minutes

T1006 Alcohol and/or substance abuse services, family/couple counseling

T1007 Alcohol and/or substance abuse services, treatment plan development and/or modification

T1009 Child sitting services for children of the individual receiving alcohol and/or substance abuse services

T1010 Meals for individuals receiving alcohol and/or substance abuse services (when meals not included in the program)

T1012 Alcohol and/or substance abuse services, skills development

T1013 Sign language or oral interpretive services, per 15 minutes

T1014 Telehealth transmission, per minute, professional services bill separately

T1015 Clinic visit/encounter, all-inclusive

T1016 Case management, each 15 minutes

T1017 Targeted case management, each 15 minutes

T1018 School-based individualized education program (iep) services, bundled

T1019 Personal care services, per 15 minutes, not for an inpatient or resident of a hospital, nursing facility, icf/mr or imd, part of the individualized plan of treatment (code may not be used to identify services provided by home health aide or certified nurse assistant)

T1020 Personal care services, per diem, not for an inpatient or resident of a hospital, nursing facility, icf/mr or imd, part of the individualized plan of treatment (code may not be used to identify services provided by home health aide or certified nurse assistant)

T1021 Home health aide or certified nurse assistant, per visit

T1022 Contracted home health agency services, all services provided under contract, per day

T1023 Screening to determine the appropriateness of consideration of an individual for participation in a specified program, project or treatment protocol, per encounter

T1024 Evaluation and treatment by an integrated, specialty team contracted to provide coordinated care to multiple or severely handicapped children, per encounter

T1025 Intensive, extended multidisciplinary services provided in a clinic setting to children with complex medical, physical, mental and psychosocial impairments, per diem

T1026 Intensive, extended multidisciplinary services provided in a clinic setting to children with complex medical, physical, medical and psychosocial impairments, per hour

T1027 Family training and counseling for child development, per 15 minutes

T1028 Assessment of home, physical and family environment, to determine suitability to meet patient's medical needs

T1029 Comprehensive environmental lead investigation, not including laboratory analysis, per dwelling

T1030 Nursing care, in the home, by registered nurse, per diem

T1031 Nursing care, in the home, by licensed practical nurse, per diem

• **T1040** Medicaid certified community behavioral health clinic services, per diem

• **T1041** Medicaid certified community behavioral health clinic services, per month

T1502 Administration of oral, intramuscular and/or subcutaneous medication by health care agency/professional, per visit

T1503 Administration of medication, other than oral and/or injectable, by a health care agency/professional, per visit

T1505 Electronic medication compliance management device, includes all components and accessories, not otherwise classified

T1999 Miscellaneous therapeutic items and supplies, retail purchases, not otherwise classified; identify product in "remarks"

T2001 Non-emergency transportation; patient attendant/escort

T2002 Non-emergency transportation; per diem

T2003 Non-emergency transportation; encounter/trip

T2004 Non-emergency transport; commercial carrier, multi-pass

T2005 Non-emergency transportation; stretcher van

T2007 Transportation waiting time, air ambulance and non-emergency vehicle, one-half (1/2) hour increments

T2010 Preadmission screening and resident review (pasrr) level i identification screening, per screen

T2011 Preadmission screening and resident review (pasrr) level ii evaluation, per evaluation

T2012 Habilitation, educational; waiver, per diem

T2013 Habilitation, educational, waiver; per hour

T2014 Habilitation, prevocational, waiver; per diem

T2015 Habilitation, prevocational, waiver; per hour

T2016 Habilitation, residential, waiver; per diem

T2017 Habilitation, residential, waiver; 15 minutes

T2018 Habilitation, supported employment, waiver; per diem

T2019 Habilitation, supported employment, waiver; per 15 minutes

T2020 Day habilitation, waiver; per diem

T2021 Day habilitation, waiver; per 15 minutes

T2022 Case management, per month

T2023 Targeted case management; per month

T2024 Service assessment/plan of care development, waiver

T2025 Waiver services; not otherwise specified (nos)

T2026 Specialized childcare, waiver; per diem

T2027 Specialized childcare, waiver; per 15 minutes

T2028 Specialized supply, not otherwise specified, waiver

T2029 Specialized medical equipment, not otherwise specified, waiver

T2030 Assisted living, waiver; per month

T2031 Assisted living; waiver, per diem

T2032 Residential care, not otherwise specified (nos), waiver; per month

T2033 Residential care, not otherwise specified (nos), waiver; per diem

T2034 Crisis intervention, waiver; per diem

T2035 Utility services to support medical equipment and assistive technology/devices, waiver

T2036 Therapeutic camping, overnight, waiver; each session

T2037 Therapeutic camping, day, waiver; each session

T2038 Community transition, waiver; per service

T2039 Vehicle modifications, waiver; per service

T2040 Financial management, self-directed, waiver; per 15 minutes

T2041 Supports brokerage, self-directed, waiver; per 15 minutes

T2042 Hospice routine home care; per diem

T2043 Hospice continuous home care; per hour

T2044 Hospice inpatient respite care; per diem

T2045 Hospice general inpatient care; per diem

T2046 Hospice long term care, room and board only; per diem

T2048 Behavioral health; long-term care residential (non-acute care in a residential treatment program where stay is typically longer than 30 days), with room and board, per diem

T2049 Non-emergency transportation; stretcher van, mileage; per mile

T2101 Human breast milk processing, storage and distribution only

T4521 Adult sized disposable incontinence product, brief/diaper, small, each

CIM: 60-9

T4522 Adult sized disposable incontinence product, brief/diaper, medium, each

CIM: 60-9

T4523 Adult sized disposable incontinence product, brief/diaper, large, each

CIM: 60-9

T4524 Adult sized disposable incontinence product, brief/diaper, extra large, each

CIM: 60-9

T4525 Adult sized disposable incontinence product, protective underwear/pull-on, small size, each

CIM: 60-9

T4526 Adult sized disposable incontinence product, protective underwear/pull-on, medium size, each

CIM: 60-9

T4527 Adult sized disposable incontinence product, protective underwear/pull-on, large size, each

CIM: 60-9

T4528 Adult sized disposable incontinence product, protective underwear/pull-on, extra large size, each

CIM: 60-9

T4529 Pediatric sized disposable incontinence product, brief/diaper, small/medium size, each

CIM: 60-9

T4530 Pediatric sized disposable incontinence product, brief/diaper, large size, each

CIM: 60-9

T4531 Pediatric sized disposable incontinence product, protective underwear/pull-on, small/medium size, each

CIM: 60-9

T4532 Pediatric sized disposable incontinence product, protective underwear/pull-on, large size, each

CIM: 60-9

T4533 Youth sized disposable incontinence product, brief/diaper, each

CIM: 60-9

T4534 Youth sized disposable incontinence product, protective underwear/pull-on, each

CIM: 60-9

T4535 Disposable liner/shield/guard/pad/undergarment, for incontinence, each

CIM: 60-9

T4536 Incontinence product, protective underwear/pull-on, reusable, any size, each

CIM: 60-9

T4537 Incontinence product, protective underpad, reusable, bed size, each

CIM: 60-9

T4538 Diaper service, reusable diaper, each diaper

CIM: 60-9

T4539 Incontinence product, diaper/brief, reusable, any size, each

CIM: 60-9

T4540 Incontinence product, protective underpad, reusable, chair size, each

CIM: 60-9

T4541 Incontinence product, disposable underpad, large, each

T4542 Incontinence product, disposable underpad, small size, each

T4543 Adult sized disposable incontinence product, protective brief/diaper, above extra large, each

CIM: 60-9

T4544 Adult sized disposable incontinence product, protective underwear/pull-on, above extra large, each

CIM: 60-9

T5001 Positioning seat for persons with special orthopedic needs

T5999 Supply, not otherwise specified

Guidelines

In addition to the information presented in the INTRODUCTION, several other items unique to this section are defined or identified here:

1. SUBSECTION INFORMATION: Some of the listed subheadings or subsections have special needs or instructions unique to that section. Where these are indicated, special "notes" will be presented preceding or following the listings. Those subsections within the VISION SERVICES section that have "notes" are as follows:

Subsection	Code Numbers
Spectacle lenses	V2100-V2499
Contact lenses	V2500-V2599
Low vision aids	V2600-V2615

2. UNLISTED SERVICE OR PROCEDURE: A service or procedure may be provided that is not listed in this edition of HCPCS. When reporting such a service, the appropriate "unlisted procedure" code may be used to indicate the service, identifying it by "special report" as defined below. HCPCS terminology is inconsistent in defining unlisted procedures. The procedure definition may include the term(s) "unlisted", "not otherwise classified", "unspecified", "unclassified", "other" and "miscellaneous". Prior to using these codes, try to determine if a Local Level III code or CPT code is available. The "unlisted procedures" and accompanying codes for VISION SERVICES are as follows:

   V2199 Not otherwise classified, single vision lens, bifocal, glass or plastic
   V2499 Variable sphericity lens, other type
   V2599 Not otherwise classified, contact lens
   V2629 Prosthetic eye, other type
   V2799 Vision service, miscellaneous

3. SPECIAL REPORT: A service, material or supply that is rarely provided, unusual, variable or new may require a special report in determining medical appropriateness for reimbursement purposes. Pertinent information should include an adequate definition or description of the nature, extent, and need for the service, material or supply.

4. MODIFIERS: Listed services may be modified under certain circumstances. When appropriate, the modifying circumstance is identified by adding a modifier to the basic procedure code. CPT and HCPCS National Level II modifiers may be used with CPT and HCPCS National Level II procedure codes. Modifiers commonly used with VISION SERVICES are as follows:

   -AP Determination of refractive state was not performed in the course of diagnostic ophthalmological examination

   -CC Procedure code change (use "CC" when the procedure code submitted was changed either for administrative reasons or because an incorrect code was filed)

   -LS FDA-monitored intraocular lens implant

-LT Left side (used to identify procedures performed on the left side of the body)

-PL Progressive addition lenses

-RT Right side (used to identify procedures performed on the right side of the body)

-SF Second opinion ordered by a professional review organization (PRO) per section 9401, P.L. 99-272. (100 percent reimbursement; no Medicare deductible or coinsurance)

-TC Technical component. Under certain circumstances, a charge may be made for the technical component alone. Under those circumstances, the technical component charge is identified by adding modifier -TC to the usual procedure number. Technical component charges are institutional charges and are not billed separately by physicians. However, portable x-ray suppliers bill only for the technical component and should use modifier -TC. The charge data from portable x-ray suppliers will then be used to build customary and prevailing profiles.

-VP Aphakic patient

5. CPT CODE CROSS-REFERENCE: See sections for equivalent CPT code(s) for all listings in this section.

Frames

V2020 Frames, purchases

MCM: 2130

V2025 Deluxe frame

MCM: 3045.4

Spectacle Lenses

NOTE: If CPT code 92390 or 92395 is reported, recode with the specific lens type listed below. For aphakic temporary spectacle correction, see CPT code 92358.

V2100 Sphere, single vision, plano to plus or minus 4.00, per lens

V2101 Sphere, single vision, plus or minus 4.12 to plus or minus 7.00d, per lens

V2102 Sphere, single vision, plus or minus 7.12 to plus or minus 20.00d, per lens

V2103 Spherocylinder, single vision, plano to plus or minus 4.00d sphere, .12 to 2.00d cylinder, per lens

V2104 Spherocylinder, single vision, plano to plus or minus 4.00d sphere, 2.12 to 4.00d cylinder, per lens

V2105 Spherocylinder, single vision, plano to plus or minus 4.00d sphere, 4.25 to 6.00d cylinder, per lens

V2106 Spherocylinder, single vision, plano to plus or minus 4.00d sphere, over 6.00d cylinder, per lens

V2107 Spherocylinder, single vision, plus or minus 4.25 to plus or minus 7.00 sphere, .12 to 2.00d cylinder, per lens

V2108 Spherocylinder, single vision, plus or minus 4.25d to plus or minus 7.00d sphere, 2.12 to 4.00d cylinder, per lens

V2109 Spherocylinder, single vision, plus or minus 4.25 to plus or minus 7.00d sphere, 4.25 to 6.00d cylinder, per lens

V2110 Spherocylinder, single vision, plus or minus 4.25 to 7.00d sphere, over 6.00d cylinder, per lens

V2111 Spherocylinder, single vision, plus or minus 7.25 to plus or minus 12.00d sphere, .25 to 2.25d cylinder, per lens

V2112 Spherocylinder, single vision, plus or minus 7.25 to plus or minus 12.00d sphere, 2.25d to 4.00d cylinder, per lens

V2113 Spherocylinder, single vision, plus or minus 7.25 to plus or minus 12.00d sphere, 4.25 to 6.00d cylinder, per lens

V2114 Spherocylinder, single vision, sphere over plus or minus 12.00d, per lens

V2115 Lenticular, (myodisc), per lens, single vision

V2118 Aniseikonic lens, single vision

V2121 Lenticular lens, per lens, single

MCM: 2130.B

V2199 Not otherwise classified, single vision lens

V2200 Sphere, bifocal, plano to plus or minus 4.00d, per lens

V2201 Sphere, bifocal, plus or minus 4.12 to plus or minus 7.00d, per lens

V2202 Sphere, bifocal, plus or minus 7.12 to plus or minus 20.00d, per lens

V2203 Spherocylinder, bifocal, plano to plus or minus 4.00d sphere, .12 to 2.00d cylinder, per lens

V2204 Spherocylinder, bifocal, plano to plus or minus 4.00d sphere, 2.12 to 4.00d cylinder, per lens

V2205 Spherocylinder, bifocal, plano to plus or minus 4.00d sphere, 4.25 to 6.00d cylinder, per lens

V2206 Spherocylinder, bifocal, plano to plus or minus 4.00d sphere, over 6.00d cylinder, per lens

V2207 Spherocylinder, bifocal, plus or minus 4.25 to plus or minus 7.00d sphere,.12 to 2.00d cylinder, per lens

V2208 Spherocylinder, bifocal, plus or minus 4.25 to plus or minus 7.00d sphere, 2.12 to 4.00d cylinder, per lens

V2209 Spherocylinder, bifocal, plus or minus 4.25 to plus or minus 7.00d sphere, 4.25 to 6.00d cylinder, per lens

V2210 Spherocylinder, bifocal, plus or minus 4.25 to plus or minus 7.00d sphere, over 6.00d cylinder, per lens

V2211 Spherocylinder, bifocal, plus or minus 7.25 to plus or minus 12.00d sphere, .25 to 2.25d cylinder, per lens

V2212 Spherocylinder, bifocal, plus or minus 7.25 to plus or minus 12.00d sphere, 2.25 to 4.00d cylinder, per lens

V2213 Spherocylinder, bifocal, plus or minus 7.25 to plus or minus 12.00d sphere, 4.25 to 6.00d cylinder, per lens

V2214 Spherocylinder, bifocal, sphere over plus or minus 12.00d, per lens

V2215 Lenticular (myodisc), per lens, bifocal

V2218 Aniseikonic, per lens, bifocal

V2219 Bifocal seg width over 28 mm

V2220 Bifocal add over 3.25d

V2221 Lenticular lens, per lens, bifocal

MCM: 2130.B

V2299 Specialty bifocal (by report)

V2300 Sphere, trifocal, plano to plus or minus 4.00d, per lens

V2301 Sphere, trifocal, plus or minus 4.12 to plus or minus 7.00d, per lens

V2302 Sphere, trifocal, plus or minus 7.12 to plus or minus 20.00, per lens

V2303 Spherocylinder, trifocal, plano to plus or minus 4.00d sphere, .12-2.00d cylinder, per lens

V2304 Spherocylinder, trifocal, plano to plus or minus 4.00d sphere, 2.25-4.00d cylinder, per lens

V2305 Spherocylinder, trifocal, plano to plus or minus 4.00d sphere, 4.25 to 6.00 cylinder, per lens

V2306 Spherocylinder, trifocal, plano to plus or minus 4.00d sphere, over 6.00d cylinder, per lens

V2307 Spherocylinder, trifocal, plus or minus 4.25 to plus or minus 7.00d sphere, .12 to 2.00d cylinder, per lens

V2308 Spherocylinder, trifocal, plus or minus 4.25 to plus or minus 7.00d sphere, 2.12 to 4.00d cylinder, per lens

V2309 Spherocylinder, trifocal, plus or minus 4.25 to plus or minus 7.00d sphere, 4.25 to 6.00d cylinder, per lens

V2310 Spherocylinder, trifocal, plus or minus 4.25 to plus or minus 7.00d sphere, over 6.00d cylinder, per lens

V2311 Spherocylinder, trifocal, plus or minus 7.25 to plus or minus 12.00d sphere, .25 to 2.25d cylinder, per lens

V2312 Spherocylinder, trifocal, plus or minus 7.25 to plus or minus 12.00d sphere, 2.25 to 4.00d cylinder, per lens

V2313 Spherocylinder, trifocal, plus or minus 7.25 to plus or minus 12.00d sphere, 4.25 to 6.00d cylinder, per lens

V2314 Spherocylinder, trifocal, sphere over plus or minus 12.00d, per lens

V2315 Lenticular, (myodisc), per lens, trifocal

V2318 Aniseikonic lens, trifocal

V2319 Trifocal seg width over 28 mm

V2320 Trifocal add over 3.25d

V2321 Lenticular lens, per lens, trifocal

MCM: 2130.B

V2399 Specialty trifocal (by report)

V2410 Variable asphericity lens, single vision, full field, glass or plastic, per lens

V2430 Variable asphericity lens, bifocal, full field, glass or plastic, per lens

V2499 Variable sphericity lens, other type

Contact Lenses (CPT 92391 or 92396)

NOTE: If CPT code 92391 or 92396 is reported, recode with specific lens type listed below, per lens.

V2500 Contact lens, PMMA, spherical, per lens

V2501 Contact lens, PMMA, toric or prism ballast, per lens

V2502 Contact lens, PMMA, bifocal, per lens

V2503 Contact lens, PMMA, color vision deficiency, per lens

V2510 Contact lens, gas permeable, spherical, per lens

V2511 Contact lens, gas permeable, toric, prism ballast, per lens

V2512 Contact lens, gas permeable, bifocal, per lens

V2513 Contact lens, gas permeable, extended wear, per lens

V2520 Contact lens, hydrophilic, spherical, per lens

CIM: 45-7, 65-1

V2521 Contact lens, hydrophilic, toric, or prism ballast, per lens

CIM: 45-7, 65-1

V2522 Contact lens, hydrophilic, bifocal, per lens

CIM: 45-7, 65-1

V2523 Contact lens, hydrophilic, extended wear, per lens

CIM: 45-7, 65-1

V2530 Contact lens, scleral, gas impermeable, per lens (for contact lens modification, see 92325)

V2531 Contact lens, scleral, gas permeable, per lens (for contact lens modification, see 92325)

CIM: 65-3

V2599 Contact lens, other type

Low Vision Aids (CPT 92392)

NOTE: If CPT code 92392 is reported, record with specific systems listed below.

V2600 Hand held low vision aids and other nonspectacle mounted aids

V2610 Single lens spectacle mounted low vision aids

V2615 Telescopic and other compound lens system, including distance vision telescopic, near vision telescopes and compound microscopic lens system

Prosthetic Eye (CPT 92330 or 92393)

V2623 Prosthetic eye, plastic, custom

MCM: 2133

V2624 Polishing/resurfacing of ocular prosthesis

V2625 Enlargement of ocular prosthesis

V2626 Reduction of ocular prosthesis

V2627 Scleral cover shell

CIM: 65-3

V2628 Fabrication and fitting of ocular conformer

V2629 Prosthetic eye, other type

Intraocular Lenses

V2630 Anterior chamber intraocular lens

MCM: 2130

V2631 Iris supported intraocular lens

MCM: 2130

V2632 Posterior chamber intraocular lens

MCM: 2130

Miscellaneous

V2700 Balance lens, per lens

V2702 Deluxe lens feature

MCM: 2130B

V2710 Slab off prism, glass or plastic, per lens

V2715 Prism, per lens

V2718 Press-on lens, Fresnell prism, per lens

V2730 Special base curve, glass or plastic, per lens

V2744 Tint, photochromatic, per lens

MCM: 2130B

V2745 Addition to lens; tint, any color, solid, gradient or equal, excludes photochromatic, any lens material, per lens

MCM: 2130.B

V2750 Anti-reflective coating, per lens

MCM: 2130B

V2755 U-V lens, per lens

MCM: 2130B

V2756 Eye glass case

V2760 Scratch resistant coating, per lens

V2761 Mirror coating, any type, solid, gradient or equal, any lens material, per lens

MCM: 2130.B

V2762 Polarization, any lens material, per lens

MCM: 2130.B

V2770 Occluder lens, per lens

V2780 Oversize lens, per lens

V2781 Progressive lens, per lens

V2782 Lens, index 1.54 to 1.65 plastic or 1.60 to 1.79 glass, excludes polycarbonate, per lens

MCM: 2130.B

V2783 Lens, index greater than or equal to 1.66 plastic or greater than or equal to 1.80 glass, excludes polycarbonate, per lens

MCM: 2130.B

V2784 Lens, polycarbonate or equal, any index, per lens

MCM: 2130.B

V2785 Processing, preserving and transporting corneal tissue

V2786 Specialty occupational multifocal lens, per lens

MCM: 2130.B

V2787 Astigmatism correcting function of intraocular lens

Statute: 1862(a)(7)

V2788 Presbyopia correcting function of intraocular lens

Statute: 1862(a)(7)

V2790 Amniotic membrane for surgical reconstruction, per procedure

V2797 Vision supply, accessory and/or service component of another HCPCS vision code

V2799 Vision item or service, miscellaneous

Guidelines

In addition to the information presented in the INTRODUCTION, several other items unique to this section are defined or identified here:

1. PROSTHETIC DEVICES: Prosthetic devices that replace all or part of an internal body organ or the function of a permanently inoperative or malfunctioning internal body organ are covered when furnished on a physician's order. If the medical record and attending physician indicate the condition will be indefinite, the test of permanence is met.

2. SPEECH PATHOLOGY: Services necessary for diagnosing and treating speech disorders that result in communication disabilities, and swallowing disorders, regardless of the presence of a disability, are covered Medicare services if reasonable and necessary. The services must be considered to be an effective treatment for the patient's condition, and the patient's condition must be at a level of severity that requires the service of a qualified speech pathologist.

3. UNLISTED SERVICE OR PROCEDURE: A service or procedure may be provided that is not listed in this edition of HCPCS. When reporting such a service, the appropriate "unlisted procedure" code may be used to indicate the service, identifying it by "special report" as defined below. HCPCS terminology is inconsistent in defining unlisted procedures. The procedure definition may include the term(s) "unlisted", "not otherwise classified", "unspecified", "unclassified", "other" and "miscellaneous". Prior to using these codes, try to determine if a Local Level III code or CPT code is available. The "unlisted procedures" and accompanying codes for HEARING SERVICES are as follows:

   V5299 Hearing service, miscellaneous

4. SPECIAL REPORT: A service, material or supply that is rarely provided, unusual, variable or new may require a special report in determining medical appropriateness for reimbursement purposes. Pertinent information should include an adequate definition or description of the nature, extent, and need for the service, material or supply.

5. MODIFIERS: Listed services may be modified under certain circumstances. When appropriate, the modifying circumstance is identified by adding a modifier to the basic procedure code. CPT and HCPCS National Level II modifiers may be used with CPT and HCPCS National Level II procedure codes. Modifiers commonly used with HEARING SERVICES are as follows:

   -CC Procedure code change (use "CC" when the procedure code submitted was changed either for administrative reasons or because an incorrect code was filed)

   -LT Left side (used to identify procedures performed on the left side of the body)

   -RT Right side (used to identify procedures performed on the right side of the body)

   -SF Second opinion ordered by a professional review organization (PRO) per section 9401, P.L. 99-272 (100 percent reimbursement; no Medicare deductible or coinsurance)

-TC Technical component. Under certain circumstances, a charge may be made for the technical component alone. Under those circumstances, the technical component charge is identified by adding modifier -TC to the usual procedure number. Technical component charges are institutional charges and are not billed separately by physicians. However, portable x-ray suppliers bill only for the technical component and should use modifier -TC. The charge data from portable x-ray suppliers will then be used to build customary and prevailing profiles.

6. CPT CODE CROSS-REFERENCE: See sections for equivalent CPT code(s) for all listings in this section.

Hearing Services

V5008 Hearing screening

MCM: 2320

V5010 Assessment for hearing aid

Statute: 1862A7

V5011 Fitting/orientation/checking of hearing aid

Statute: 1862A7

V5014 Repair/modification of a hearing aid

Statute: 1862A7

V5020 Conformity evaluation

Statute: 1862A7

V5030 Hearing aid, monaural, body worn, air conduction

Statute: 1862A7

V5040 Hearing aid, monaural, body worn, bone conduction

Statute: 1862A7

V5050 Hearing aid, monaural, in the ear

Statute: 1862A7

V5060 Hearing aid, monaural, behind the ear

Statute: 1862A7

V5070 Glasses, air conduction

Statute: 1862A7

V5080 Glasses, bone conduction

Statute: 1862A7

V5090 Dispensing fee, unspecified hearing aid

Statute: 1862A7

V5095 Semi-implantable middle ear hearing prosthesis

Statute: 1862A7

V5100 Hearing aid, bilateral, body worn

Statute: 1862A7

V5110 Dispensing fee, bilateral

Statute: 1862A7

V5120 Binaural, body

Statute: 1862A7

V5130 Binaural, in the ear

Statute: 1862A7

V5140 Binaural, behind the ear

Statute: 1862A7

V5150 Binaural, glasses

Statute: 1862A7

V5160 Dispensing fee, binaural

Statute: 1862A7

V5170 Hearing aid, cros, in the ear

Statute: 1862A7

V5180 Hearing aid, cros, behind the ear

Statute: 1862A7

V5190 Hearing aid, cros, glasses

Statute: 1862A7

V5200 Dispensing fee, cros

Statute: 1862A7

V5210 Hearing aid, bicros, in the ear

Statute: 1862A7

V5220 Hearing aid, bicros, behind the ear

Statute: 1862A7

V5230 Hearing aid, bicros, glasses

Statute: 1862A7

V5240 Dispensing fee, bicros

Statute: 1862A7

V5241 Dispensing fee, monaural hearing aid, any type

Statute: 1862A7

V5242 Hearing aid, analog, monaural, cic (completely in the ear canal)

Statute: 1862A7

V5243 Hearing aid, analog, monaural, itc (in the canal)

Statute: 1862A7

V5244 Hearing aid, digitally programmable analog, monaural, cic

Statute: 1862A7

V5245 Hearing aid, digitally programmable, analog, monaural, itc

Statute: 1862A7

V5246 Hearing aid, digitally programmable analog, monaural, ite (in the ear)

Statute: 1862A7

V5247 Hearing aid, digitally programmable analog, monaural, bte (behind the ear)

Statute: 1862A7

V5248 Hearing aid, analog, binaural, cic

Statute: 1862A7

V5249 Hearing aid, analog, binaural, itc

Statute: 1862A7

V5250 Hearing aid, digitally programmable analog, binaural, cic

Statute: 1862A7

V5251 Hearing aid, digitally programmable analog, binaural, itc

Statute: 1862A7

V5252 Hearing aid, digitally programmable, binaural, ite

Statute: 1862A7

V5253 Hearing aid, digitally programmable, binaural, bte

Statute: 1862A7

V5254 Hearing aid, digital, monaural, cic

Statute: 1862A7

V5255 Hearing aid, digital, monaural, itc

Statute: 1862A7

V5256 Hearing aid, digital, monaural, ite

Statute: 1862A7

V5257 Hearing aid, digital, monaural, bte

Statute: 1862A7

V5258 Hearing aid, digital, binaural, cic

Statute: 1862A7

V5259 Hearing aid, digital, binaural, itc

Statute: 1862A7

V5260 Hearing aid, digital, binaural, ite

Statute: 1862A7

V5261 Hearing aid, digital, binaural, bte

Statute: 1862A7

V5262 Hearing aid, disposable, any type, monaural

Statute: 1862A7

V5263 Hearing aid, disposable, any type, binaural

Statute: 1862A7

V5264 Ear mold/insert, not disposable, any type

Statute: 1862A7

V5265 Ear mold/insert, disposable, any type

Statute: 1862A7

V5266 Battery for use in hearing device

Statute: 1862A7

V5267 Hearing aid or assistive listening device/supplies/accessories, not otherwise specified

Statute: 1862A7

V5268 Assistive listening device, telephone amplifier, any type

Statute: 1862A7

V5269 Assistive listening device, alerting, any type

Statute: 1862A7

V5270 Assistive listening device, television amplifier, any type

Statute: 1862A7

V5271 Assistive listening device, television caption decoder

Statute: 1862A7

V5272 Assistive listening device, tdd

Statute: 1862A7

V5273 Assistive listening device, for use with cochlear implant

Statute: 1862A7

V5274 Assistive listening device, not otherwise specified

Statute: 1862A7

V5275 Ear impression, each

Statute: 1862A7

V5281 Assistive listening device, personal fm/dm system, monaural, (1 receiver, transmitter, microphone), any type

Statute: 1862a7

V5282 Assistive listening device, personal fm/dm system, binaural, (2 receivers, transmitter, microphone), any type

Statute: 1862a7

V5283 Assistive listening device, personal fm/dm neck, loop induction receiver

Statute: 1862a7

V5284 Assistive listening device, personal fm/dm, ear level receiver

Statute: 1862a7

V5285 Assistive listening device, personal fm/dm, direct audio input receiver

Statute: 1862a7

V5286 Assistive listening device, personal blue tooth fm/dm receiver

Statute: 1862a7

V5287 Assistive listening device, personal fm/dm receiver, not otherwise specified

Statute: 1862a7

V5288 Assistive listening device, personal fm/dm transmitter assistive listening device

Statute: 1862a7

V5289 Assistive listening device, personal fm/dm adapter/boot coupling device for receiver, any type

Statute: 1862a7

V5290 Assistive listening device, transmitter microphone, any type

Statute: 1862a7

V5298 Hearing aid, not otherwise classified

Statute: 1862A7

V5299 Hearing service, miscellaneous

MCM: 2320

V5336 Repair/modification of augmentative communicative system or device (excludes adaptive hearing aid)

Statute: 1862A7

V5362 Speech screening

Statute: 1862(a)(7)

V5363 Language screening

Statute: 1862(a)(7)

V5364 Dysphagia screening

Statute: 1862(a)(7)

ALPHABETIC INDEX

Questions regarding coding and billing guidance should be submitted to the insurer in whose jurisdiction a claim would be filed. For private sector health insurance systems, please contact the individual private insurance entity. For Medicaid systems, please contact the Medicaid Agency in the state in which the claim is being filed. For Medicare, contact the Medicare contractor.

A

B

C

D

E

F

G

H

I

J

K

L

M

N

O

P

Q

R

S

T

U

V

W

X

Y

Z

APPENDIX A: MODIFIERS

HCPCS National Level II Modifiers

The following list is the complete list of HCPCS National Level II modifiers and descriptions.

-A1 Dressing for one wound

-A2 Dressing for two wounds

-A3 Dressing for three wounds

-A4 Dressing for four wounds

-A5 Dressing for five wounds

-A6 Dressing for six wounds

-A7 Dressing for seven wounds

-A8 Dressing for eight wounds

-A9 Dressing for nine or more wounds

-AA Anesthesia services performed personally by anesthesiologist
MCM: 3350.5

-AD Medical supervision by a physician; more than four concurrent anesthesia procedures
MCM: 3350.5

-AE Registered dietician

-AF Specialty physician

-AG Primary physician

-AH Clinical psychologist
MCM: 2150, 5112

-AI Principal physician of record

-AJ Clinical social worker
MCM: 2152, 5113

-AK Non-participating physician

-AM Physician, team member service
MCM: 4105.7

-AO Alternate payment method declined by provider of service

-AP Determination of refractive state was not performed in the course of diagnostic ophthalmological examination

-AQ in an unlisted health professional shortage area (HPSA)

-AR Physician provider services in a physician scarcity area

-AS Physician assistant, nurse practitioner or clinical nurse specialist services for assistant at surgery

-AT Acute treatment (this modifier should be used when reporting service 98940, 98941, 98942)

-AU Item furnished in conjunction with a urological, ostomy, or tracheostomy supply

-AV Item furnished in conjunction with a prosthetic device, prosthetic or orthotic

-AW Item furnished in conjunction with a surgical dressing

-AX Item furnished in conjunction with dialysis services

-AY Item or service furnished to an ESRD patient that is not for the treatment of ESRD

-AZ Physician providing a service in a dental health professional shortage area for the purpose of an electronic health record incentive payment

-BA Item furnished in conjunction with parenteral enteral nutrition (PEN) services

-BL Special acquisition of blood and blood products

-BO Orally administered nutrition, not by feeding tube

-BP The beneficiary has been informed of the purchase and rental options and has elected to purchase the item

-BR The beneficiary has been informed of the purchase and rental options and has elected to rent the item

-BU The beneficiary has been informed of the purchase and rental options and after 30 days has not informed the supplier of his/her decision

-CA Procedure payable only in the inpatient setting when performed emergently on an outpatient who expires prior to admission

-CB Service ordered by a renal dialysis facility (RDF) physician as part of the ESRD beneficiary's dialysis benefit, is not part of the composite rate, and is separately reimbursable

-CC Procedure code change (use-CC when the procedure code submitted was changed either for administrative reasons or because an incorrect code was filed)

-CD AMCC test has been ordered by an ESRD facility or MCP physician that is part of the composite rate and is not separately billable

MCM: 4270.2

-CE AMCC test has been ordered by an ESRD facility or MCP physician that is a composite rate test but is beyond the normal frequency covered under the rate and is separately reimbursable based on medical necessity

MCM: 4270.2

-CF AMCC test has been ordered by an ESRD facility or MCP physician that is not part of the composite rate and is separately billable

MCM: 4270.2

-CG Policy criteria applied

-CH 0 percent impaired, limited or restricted

-CI At least 1 percent but less than 20 percent impaired, limited or restricted

-CJ At least 20 percent but less than 40 percent impaired, limited or restricted

-CK At least 40 percent but less than 60 percent impaired, limited or restricted

-CL At least 60 percent but less than 80 percent impaired, limited or restricted

-CM At least 80 percent but less than 100 percent impaired, limited or restricted

-CN 100 percent impaired, limited or restricted

-CP Adjunctive service related to a procedure assigned to a comprehensive ambulatory payment classification (c-apc) procedure, but reported on a different claim

-CR Catastrophe/disaster related

-CS Item or service related, in whole or in part, to an illness, injury, or condition that was caused by or exacerbated by the effects, direct or indirect, of the 2010 oil spill in the Gulf Of Mexico, including but not limited to subsequent clean-up activities

-CT Computed tomography services furnished using equipment that does not meet each of the attributes of the national electrical manufacturers association (nema) xr-29-2013 standard

-DA Oral health assessment by a licensed health professional other than a dentist

-E1 Upper left, eyelid

-E2 Lower left, eyelid

-E3 Upper right, eyelid

-E4 Lower right, eyelid

-EA Erythropoetic stimulating agent (ESA) administered to treat anemia due to anti-cancer chemotherapy

-EB Erythropoetic stimulating agent (ESA) administered to treat anemia due to anti-cancer radiotherapy

-EC Erythropoetic stimulating agent (ESA) administered to treat anemia not due to anti-cancer radiotherapy or anti-cancer chemotherapy

-ED Hematocrit level has exceeded 39% (or hemoglobin level has exceeded 13.0 g/dl) for 3 or more consecutive billing cycles immediately prior to and including the current cycle

-EE Hematocrit level has not exceeded 39% (or hemoglobin level has not exceeded 13.0 g/dl) for 3 or more consecutive billing cycles immediately prior to and including the current cycle

-EJ Subsequent claims for a defined course of therapy, e.g., EPO, sodium hyaluronate, infliximab

MCM: 4273.2

-EM Emergency reserve supply (for ESRD benefit only)

MCM: 3045.7

-EP Service provided as part of Medicaid early periodic screening, diagnosis, and treatment (EPSDT) program

-ET Emergency services

-EX Expatriate beneficiary

-EY No physician or other licensed health care provider order for this item or service

-F1 Left hand, second digit

-F2 Left hand, third digit

-F3 Left hand, fourth digit

-F4 Left hand, fifth digit

-F5 Right hand, thumb

-F6 Right hand, second digit

-F7 Right hand, third digit

-F8 Right hand, fourth digit

-F9 Right hand, fifth digit

-FA Left hand, thumb

-FB Item provided without cost to provider, supplier or practitioner, or full credit received for replaced device (examples, but not limited to: covered under warranty, replaced due to defect, free samples)

-FC Partial credit received for replaced device

-FP Service provided as part of family planning program

• **-FX** X-ray taken using film

-G1 Most recent URR reading of less than 60

-G2 Most recent URR reading of 60 to 64.9

-G3 Most recent URR reading of 65 to 69.9

-G4 Most recent URR reading of 70 to 74.9

-G5 Most recent URR reading of 75 or greater

-G6 ESRD patient for whom less than six dialysis sessions have been provided in a month

-G7 Pregnancy resulted from rape or incest or pregnancy certified by physician as life threatening

CIM: 35-99

MCM: 2005.1

-G8 Monitored anesthesia care (MAC) for deep complex, complicated, or markedly invasive surgical procedure

-G9 Monitored anesthesia care for patient who has history of severe cardio-pulmonary condition

-GA Waiver of liability statement issued as required by payer policy, individual case

-GB Claim being re-submitted for payment because it is no longer covered under a global payment demonstration

-GC This service has been performed in part by a resident under the direction of a teaching physician

MCM: 3350.5, 4116

-GD Units of service exceeds medically unlikely edit value and represents reasonable and necessary services

-GE This service has been performed by a resident without the presence of a teaching physician under the primary care exception

MCM: 4116

-GF Non-physician (eg., nurse practitioner (NP), certified registered nurse anesthetist (CRNA), certified registered nurse (CRN), clinical nurse specialist (CNS), physician assistant (PA)) services in a critical access hospital

-GG Performance and payment of a screening mammogram and diagnostic mammogram on the same patient, same day

-GH Diagnostic mammogram converted from screening mammogram on same day

-GJ "Opt Out" physician or practitioner emergency or urgent service

-GK Reasonable and necessary item/service associated with a-GA or-GZ modifier

-GL Medically unnecessary upgrade provided instead of non-upgraded item, no charge, no advance beneficiary notice (ABN)

-GM Multiple patients on one ambulance trip

-GN Services delivered under an outpatient speech language pathology plan of care

-GO Services delivered under an outpatient occupational therapy plan of care

-GP Services delivered under an outpatient physical therapy plan of care

-GQ Via asynchronous telecommunications system

-GR This service was performed in whole or in part by a resident in a department of veterans affairs medical center or clinic, supervised in accordance with VA policy

-GS Dosage of EPO or darbepoetin alfa has been reduced and maintained in response to hematocrit or hemoglobin level

MCM: 4273.1

-GT Via interactive audio and video telecommunication systems

-GU Waiver of liability statement issued as required by payer policy, routine notice

-GV Attending physician not employed or paid under arrangement by the patient's hospice provider

MCM: 4175-5

-GW Service not related to the hospice patient's terminal condition

MCM: 4175-5

-GX Notice of liability issued, voluntary under payer policy

-GY Item or service statutorily excluded, does not meet the definition of any Medicare benefit or, for non-Medicare insurers, is not a contract benefit

-GZ Item or service expected to be denied as not reasonable and necessary

MCM: 2000

-H9 Court-ordered

-HA Child/adolescent program

-HB Adult program, non geriatric

-HC Adult program, geriatric

-HD Pregnant/parenting women's program

-HE Mental health program

-HF Substance abuse program

-HG Opioid addiction treatment program

-HH Integrated mental health/substance abuse program

-HI Integrated mental health and intellectual disability/developmental disabilities program

-HJ Employee assistance program

-HK Specialized mental health programs for high-risk populations

-HL Intern

-HM Less than bachelor degree level

-HN Bachelors degree level

-HO Masters degree level

-HP Doctoral level

-HQ Group setting

-HR Family/couple with client present

-HS Family/couple without client present

-HT Multi-disciplinary team

-HU Funded by child welfare agency

-HV Funded state addictions agency

-HW Funded by state mental health agency

-HX Funded by county/local agency

-HY Funded by juvenile justice agency

-HZ Funded by criminal justice agency

-J1 Competitive acquisition program no-pay submission for a prescription number

-J2 Competitive acquisition program, restocking of emergency drugs after emergency administration

-J3 Competitive acquisition program (CAP), drug not available through CAP as written, reimbursed under average sales price methodology

-J4 DMEPOS item subject to DMEPOS competitive bidding program that is furnished by a hospital upon discharge

-JA Administered intravenously

-JB Administered subcutaneously

-JC Skin substitute used as a graft

-JD Skin substitute not used as a graft

-JE Administered via dialysate

(**-JF** Modifier deleted 06/30/2015.)

-JW Drug amount discarded/not administered to any patient

-K0 Lower extremity prosthesis functional level 0: Does not have the ability or potential to ambulate or transfer safely with or without assistance and a prosthesis does not enhance their quality of life or mobility

-K1 Lower extremity prosthesis functional level 1: Has the ability or potential to use a prosthesis for transfers or ambulation on level surfaces at fixed cadence. Typical of the limited and unlimited household ambulator.

-K2 Lower extremity prosthesis functional level 2: Has the ability or potential for ambulation with the ability to traverse low-level environmental barriers such as curbs, stairs or uneven surfaces. Typical of the limited community ambulator.

-K3 Lower extremity prosthesis functional level 3: Has the ability or potential for ambulation with variable cadence. Typical of the community ambulator who has the ability to traverse most environmental barriers and may have vocational, therapeutic or exercise activity that demands prosthetic utilization beyond simple locomotion.

-K4 Lower extremoty prosthesis functional level 4: Has the ability or potential for prosthetic ambulation that exceeds the basic ambulation skills, exhibiting high impact, stress or energy levels, typical of the prosthetic demands of the child, active adult, or athlete.

-KA Add on option/accessory for wheelchair

-KB Beneficiary requested upgrade for ABN, more than 4 modifiers identified on claim

-KC Replacement of special power wheelchair interface

-KD Drug or biological infused through DME

-KE Bid under round one of the DMEPOS competitive bidding program for use with non-competitive bid base equipment

-KF Item designated by FDA as class III device

-KG DMEPOS item subject to dmepos competitive bidding program number 1

-KH DMEPOS item, initial claim, purchase or first month rental

-KI DMEPOS item, second or third month rental

-KJ DMEPOS item, parenteral enteral nutrition (PEN) pump or capped rental, months four to fifteen

-KK DMEPOS item subject to dmepos competitive bidding program number 2

-KL DMEPOS item delivered via mail

-KM Replacement of facial prosthesis including new impression/ moulage

-KN Replacement of facial prosthesis using previous master model

-KO Single drug unit dose formulation

-KP First drug of a multiple drug unit dose formulation

-KQ Second or subsequent drug of a multiple drug unit dose formulation

-KR Rental item, billing for partial month

-KS Glucose monitor supply for diabetic beneficiary not treated with insulin

-KT Beneficiary resides in a competitive bidding area and travels outside that competitive bidding area and receives a competitive bid item

-KU DMEPOS item subject to dmepos competitive bidding program number 3

-KV DMEPOS item subject to dmepos competitive bidding program that is furnished as part of a professional service

-KW DMEPOS item subject to dmepos competitive bidding program number 4

-KX Requirements specified in the medical policy have been met

-KY DMEPOS item subject to dmepos competitive bidding program number 5

-KZ New coverage not implemented by managed care

(**-L1** Modifier deleted December 31, 2016.)

-LC Left circumflex coronary artery

-LD Left anterior descending coronary artery

-LL Lease/rental (use the-LL modifier when DME equipment rental is to be applied against the purchase price)

-LM Left main coronary artery

-LR Laboratory round trip

-LS FDA-monitored intraocular lens implant

CIM: 65-7

-LT Left side (used to identify procedures performed on the left side of the body)

-M2 Medicare secondary payer (MSP)

-MS Six-month maintenance and servicing fee for reasonable and necessary parts and labor which are not covered under any manufacturer or supplier warranty

-NB Nebulizer system, any type, FDA-cleared for use with specific drug

-NR New when rented (use the-NR modifier when DME which was new at the time of rental is subsequently purchased)

-NU New equipment

-P1 A normal healthy patient

-P2 A patient with mild systemic disease

-P3 A patient with severe systemic disease

-P4 A patient with severe systemic disease that is a constant threat to life

-P5 A moribund patient who is not expected to survive without the operation

-P6 A declared brain-dead patient whose organs are being removed for donor purposes

-PA Surgical or other invasive procedure on wrong body party

-PB Surgical or other invasive procedure on wrong patient

-PC Wrong surgery or other invasive procedure on patient

-PD Diagnostic or related non diagnostic item or service provided in a wholly owned or operated entity to a patient who is admitted as an inpatient within 3 days

-PI Positron emission tomography (PET) or PET/Computed Tomography (CT) to inform the initial treatment strategy of tumors that are biopsy proven or strongly suspected of being cancerous based on other diagnostic testing

-PL Progressive addition lenses

• **-PN** Non-excepted service provided at an off-campus, outpatient, provider-based department of a hospital

-PO Services, procedures and/or surgeries provided at off-campus provider-based outpatient departments

-PS Positron emission tomography (PET) or PET/Computed Tomography (CT) to inform the subsequent treatment strategy of cancerous tumors when the beneficiary's treating physician determines that the PET study is needed to inform subsequent anti-tumor strategy

-PT Colorectal cancer screening test; converted to diagnostic test or other procedure

-Q0 Investigational clinical service provided in a clinical research study that is in an approved clinical research study

-Q1 Routine clinical service provided in a clinical research study that is in an approved clinical research study

-Q2 HCFA/ORD demonstration project procedure/service

-Q3 Live kidney donor surgery and related services

-Q4 Service for ordering/referring physician qualifies as a service exemption

-Q5 Service furnished by a substitute physician under a reciprocal billing arrangement

MCM: 3060.6

-Q6 Service furnished by a locum tenens physician

MCM: 3060.7

-Q7 One class A finding

-Q8 Two class B findings

-Q9 One class B and two class C findings

-QC Single channel monitoring

-QD Recording and storage in solid state memory by a digital recorder

-QE Prescribed amount of oxygen is less than one liter per minute (LPM)

-QF Prescribed amount of oxygen exceeds 4 liters per minute (LPM) and portable oxygen is prescribed

-QG Prescribed amount of oxygen is greater than four liters per minute (LPM)

-QH Oxygen conserving device is being used with an oxygen delivery system

-QJ Services/items provided to a prisoner or patient in state or local custody, however the state or local government, as applicable, meets the requirements in 42 CFR 411.4 (B)

-QK Medical direction of two, three or four concurrent anesthesia procedures involving qualified individuals

MCM: 3350.5

-QL Patient pronounced dead after ambulance called

-QM Ambulance service provided under arrangement by a provider of services

-QN Ambulance service furnished directly by a provider of services

-QP Documentation is on file showing that the laboratory test(s) was ordered individually or ordered as a CPT-recognized panel other than automated profile codes 80002-80019, G0058, G0059, and G0060.

MCM: 7517.1

-QS Monitored anesthesia care service

CIM: 15018I

-QT Recording and storage on tape by an analog tape recorder

-QW CLIA waived test

-QX CRNA service: with medical direction by a physician

-QY Medical direction of one certified registered nurse anesthetist (CRNA) by an anesthesiologist

MCM: 3350.5

-QZ CRNA service: without medical direction by a physician

-RA Replacement of a DME, orthotic or prosthetic item

-RB Replacement of a part of a DME, orthotic or prosthetic item furnished as part of a repair

-RC Right coronary artery

-RD Drug provided to beneficiary, but not administered incident-to

-RE Furnished in full compliance with FDA-mandated risk evaluation and mitigation strategy (REMS)

-RI Ramus intermedius coronary artery

-RR Rental (use the-RR modifier when DME is to be rented)

-RT Right side (used to identify procedures performed on the right side of the body)

-SA Nurse practitioner rendering service in collaboration with a physician

-SB Nurse midwife

-SC Medically necessary service or supply

-SD Services provided by registered nurse with specialized, highly technical home infusion training

-SE State and/or federally funded programs/services

-SF Second opinion ordered by a professional review organization (PRO) per section 9401, P.L. 99-272 (100% reimbursement — no Medicare deductible or coinsurance)

-SG Ambulatory surgical center (ASC) facility service

-SH Second concurrently administered infusion therapy

-SJ Third or more concurrently administered infusion therapy

-SK Member of high-risk population (use only with codes for immunization)

-SL State supplied vaccine

-SM Second surgical opinion

-SN Third surgical opinion

-SQ Item ordered by home health

-SS Home infusion services provided in the infusion suite of the IV therapy provider

-ST Related to trauma or injury

-SU Procedure performed in physician's office (to denote use of facility and equipment)

-SV Pharmaceuticals delivered to patient's home but not utilized

-SW Services provided by a certified diabetic educator

-SY Persons who are in close contact with member of high-risk population (use only with codes for immunization)

-SZ Habilitative services

-T1 Left foot, second digit

-T2 Left foot, third digit

-T3 Left foot, fourth digit

-T4 Left foot, fifth digit

-T5 Right foot, great toe

-T6 Right foot, second digit

-T7 Right foot, third digit

-T8 Right foot, fourth digit

-T9 Right foot, fifth digit

-TA Left foot, great toe

-TC Technical component

Under certain circumstances, a charge may be made for the technical component alone. Under those circumstances the technical component charge is identified by adding modifier-TC to the usual procedure number. Technical component charges are institutional charges and not billed separately by physicians. However, portable x-ray suppliers only bill for technical component and should utilize modifier-TC. The charge data from portable x-ray suppliers will then be used to build customary and prevailing profiles.

-TD RN

-TE LPN/LVN

-TF Intermediate level of care

-TG Complex/high tech level of care

-TH Obstetrical treatment/services, prenatal or postpartum

-TJ Program group, child and/or adolescent

-TK Extra patient or passenger, non-ambulance

-TL Early intervention/individualized family services plan (IFSP)

-TM Individualized education program (IEP)

-TN Rural/outside providers customary service area

-TP Medical transport, unloaded vehicle

-TQ Basice life support (BLS) transport by a volunteer ambulance provider

-TR School-based individualized education program (IEP) services provided outside the public school district responsible for the student

-TS Follow-up service

-TT Individualized service provided to more than one patient in same setting

-TU Special payment rate, overtime

-TV Special payment rates, holidays/weekends

-TW Back-up equipment

-U1 Medicaid level of care 1, as defined by each state

-U2 Medicaid level of care 2, as defined by each state

-U3 Medicaid level of care 3, as defined by each state

-U4 Medicaid level of care 4, as defined by each state

-U5 Medicaid level of care 5, as defined by each state

-U6 Medicaid level of care 6, as defined by each state

-U7 Medicaid level of care 7, as defined by each state

-U8 Medicaid level of care 8, as defined by each state

-U9 Medicaid level of care 9, as defined by each state

-UA Medicaid level of care 10, as defined by each state

-UB Medicaid level of care 11, as defined by each state

-UC Medicaid level of care 12, as defined by each state

-UD Medicaid level of care 13, as defined by each state

-UE Used durable medical equipment

-UF Services provided in the morning

-UG Services provided in the afternoon

-UH Services provided in the evening

-UJ Services provided at night

-UK Services provided on behalf of the client to someone other than the client (collateral relationship)

-UN Two patients served

-UP Three patients served

-UQ Four patients served

-UR Five patients served

-US Six or more patients served

• **-V1** Demonstration modifier 1

• **-V2** Demonstration modifier 2

• **-V3** Demonstration modifier 3

-V5 Vascular catheter (alone or with any other vascular access)

-V6 Arteriovenous graft (or other vascular access not including a vascular catheter)

-V7 Arteriovenous fistula only (in use with two needles)

-VP Aphakic patient

-XE Separate encounter, a service that is distinct because it occurred during a separate encounter

-XP Separate practitioner, a service that is distinct because it was performed by a different practitioner

-XS Separate structure, a service that is distinct because it was performed on a separate organ/structure

-XU Unusual non-overlapping service, the use of a service that is distinct because it does not overlap usual components of the main service

• **-ZA** Novartis/sandoz

• **-ZB** Pfizer/Hospira (effective 7/1/2016)

AMBULANCE SERVICE MODIFIERS

For ambulance service, one-digit modifiers are combined to form a two-digit modifier that identifies the ambulance's place of origin with the first digit, and ambulance's destination with the second digit. They are used in items 12 and 13 on the CMS Form 1491.

One digit modifiers:

- **-D** Diagnostic or therapeutic site other than-P or-H when these are used as origin codes
- **-E** Residential, domiciliary, custodial facility (other than an 1819 facility)
- **-G** Hospital-based dialysis facility (hospital or hospital related)
- **-H** Hospital
- **-I** Site of transfer (for example, airport or helicopter pad) between types of ambulance
- **-J** Non-hospital-based dialysis facility
- **-N** Skilled nursing facility (SNF) (1819 facility)
- **-P** Physician's office (includes HMO non-hospital facility, clinic, etc.)
- **-R** Residence
- **-S** Scene of accident or acute event
- **-X** (Destination code only) Intermediate stop at physician's office on the way to the hospital (includes HMO non-hospital facility, clinic, etc.)

PET SCAN MODIFIERS

Use these single-digit alpha characters in combination as two-character modifiers to indicate the results of a current PET scan and a previous test.

- **-N** Negative
- **-E** Equivocal
- **-P** Positive, but not suggestive of extensive ischemia
- **-S** Positive and suggestive of extensive ischemia (>20 percent of the left ventricle)

APPENDIX B: SUMMARY OF CHANGES

Summary of Official HCPCS Additions, Changes, and Deletions for 2017

•	**-FX**	X-ray taken using film
(	**-L1**	Modifier deleted December 31, 2016.)
•	**-PN**	Non-excepted service provided at an off-campus, outpatient, provider-based department of a hospital
•	**-V1**	Demonstration modifier 1
•	**-V2**	Demonstration modifier 2
•	**-V3**	Demonstration modifier 3
•	**-ZA**	Novartis/Sandoz
•	**-ZB**	Pfizer/Hospira (effective July 1, 2016.)
▲	**A4221**	Supplies for maintenance of non-insulin drug infusion catheter, per week (list drugs separately)
•	**A4224**	Supplies for maintenance of insulin infusion catheter, per week
•	**A4225**	Supplies for external insulin infusion pump, syringe type cartridge, sterile, each
(	**A4466**	Code deleted December 31, 2016.)
•	**A4467**	Belt, strap, sleeve, garment, or covering, any type
•	**A4553**	Non-disposable underpads, all sizes
•	**A9285**	Inversion/eversion correction device
•	**A9286**	Hygienic item or device, disposable or non-disposable, any type, each
•	**A9515**	Choline c-11, diagnostic, per study dose up to 20 millicuries
(	**A9544**	Code deleted December 31, 2016.)
(	**A9545**	Code deleted December 31, 2016.)
•	**A9587**	Gallium ga-68, dotatate, diagnostic, 0.1 millicurie
•	**A9588**	Fluciclovine f-18, diagnostic, 1 millicurie
•	**A9597**	Positron emission tomography radiopharmaceutical, diagnostic, for tumor identification, not otherwise classified
•	**A9598**	Positron emission tomography radiopharmaceutical, diagnostic, for non-tumor identification, not otherwise classified
▲	**A9599**	Radiopharmaceutical, diagnostic, for beta-amyloid positron emission tomography (pet) imaging, per study dose, not otherwise specified
(	**B9000**	Code deleted December 31, 2016.)
▲	**B9002**	Enteral nutrition infusion pump, any type
•	**C1889**	Implantable/insertable device for device intensive procedure, not otherwise classified

(**C9121** Code deleted December 31, 2016.)

(**C9137** Code deleted December 31, 2016.)

(**C9138** Code deleted December 31, 2016.)

(**C9139** Code deleted December 31, 2016.)

• **C9140** Injection, factor viii (antihemophilic factor, recombinant) (afstyla), 1 i.u.

(**C9349** Code deleted December 31, 2016.)

(**C9458** Code deleted June 30, 2016.)

(**C9459** Code deleted June 30, 2016.)

(**C9461** Code deleted December 31, 2016.)

(**C9470** Code deleted December 31, 2016.)

(**C9471** Code deleted December 31, 2016.)

(**C9472** Code deleted December 31, 2016.)

(**C9473** Code deleted December 31, 2016.)

(**C9474** Code deleted December 31, 2016.)

(**C9475** Code deleted December 31, 2016.)

(**C9476** Code deleted December 31, 2016.)

(**C9477** Code deleted December 31, 2016.)

(**C9478** Code deleted December 31, 2016.)

(**C9479** Code deleted December 31, 2016.)

(**C9480** Code deleted December 31, 2016.)

(**C9481** Code deleted December 31, 2016.)

• **C9482** Injection, sotalol hydrochloride, 1 mg

• **C9483** Injection, atezolizumab, 10 mg

(**C9742** Code deleted December 31, 2016.)

(**C9743** Code deleted June 30, 2016.)

• **C9744** Ultrasound, abdominal, with contrast

(**C9800** Code deleted December 31, 2016.)

▲ **E0627** Seat lift mechanism, electric, any type

(**E0628** Code deleted December 31, 2016.)

▲ **E0629** Seat lift mechanism, non-electric, any type

▲ **E0740** Non-implanted pelvic floor electrical stimulator, complete system

▲ **E0967** Manual wheelchair accessory, hand rim with projections, any type, replacement only, each

▲ **E0995** Wheelchair accessory, calf rest/pad, replacement only, each

▲ **E2220** Manual wheelchair accessory, solid (rubber/plastic) propulsion tire, any size, replacement only, each

▲ **E2221** Manual wheelchair accessory, solid (rubber/plastic) caster tire (removable), any size, replacement only, each

▲ **E2222** Manual wheelchair accessory, solid (rubber/plastic) caster tire with integrated wheel, any size, replacement only, each

▲ **E2224** Manual wheelchair accessory, propulsion wheel excludes tire, any size, replacement only, each

(**G0154** Code deleted February 29, 2016.)

(**G0163** Code deleted December 31, 2016.)

(**G0164** Code deleted December 31, 2016.)

▲ **G0202** Screening mammography, bilateral (2-view study of each breast), including computer-aided detection (cad) when performed

▲ **G0204** Diagnostic mammography, including computer-aided detection (cad) when performed; bilateral

▲ **G0206** Diagnostic mammography, including computer-aided detection (cad) when performed; unilateral

(**G0389** Code deleted December 31, 2016.)

(**G0436** Code deleted September 30, 2016.)

(**G0437** Code deleted September 30, 2016.)

• **G0490** Face-to-face home health nursing visit by a rural health clinic (RHC) or federally qualified health center (fqhc) in an area with a shortage of home health agencies; (services limited to RN or LPN only)

• **G0491** Dialysis procedure at a medicare certified esrd facility for acute kidney injury without esrd

• **G0492** Dialysis procedure with single evaluation by a physician or other qualified health care professional for acute kidney injury without esrd

• **G0493** Skilled services of a registered nurse (RN) for the observation and assessment of the patient's condition, each 15 minutes (the change in the patient's condition requires skilled nursing personnel to identify and evaluate the patient's need for possible modification of treatment in the home health or hospice setting)

• **G0494** Skilled services of a licensed practical nurse (LPN) for the observation and assessment of the patient's condition, each 15 minutes (the change in the patient's condition requires skilled nursing personnel to identify and evaluate the patient's need for possible modification of treatment in the home health or hospice setting)

• **G0495** Skilled services of a registered nurse (RN), in the training and/or education of a patient or family member, in the home health or hospice setting, each 15 minutes

• **G0496** Skilled services of a licensed practical nurse (LPN), in the training and/or education of a patient or family member, in the home health or hospice setting, each 15 minutes

- • **G0499** Hepatitis b screening in non-pregnant, high risk individual includes hepatitis b surface antigen (HBsAg) followed by a neutralizing confirmatory test for initially reactive results, and antibodies to HBsAg (anti-HBs) and hepatitis b core antigen (anti-HBc)
- • **G0500** Moderate sedation services provided by the same physician or other qualified health care professional performing a gastrointestinal endoscopic service that sedation supports, requiring the presence of an independent trained observer to assist in the monitoring of the patient's level of consciousness and physiological status; initial 15 minutes of intra-service time; patient age 5 years or older (additional time may be reported with 99153, as appropriate)
- • **G0501** Resource-intensive services for patients for whom the use of specialized mobility-assistive technology (such as adjustable height chairs or tables, patient lift, and adjustable padded leg supports) is medically necessary and used during the provision of an office/outpatient, evaluation and management visit (list separately in addition to primary service)
- • **G0502** Initial psychiatric collaborative care management, first 70 minutes in the first calendar month of behavioral health care manager activities, in consultation with a psychiatric consultant, and directed by the treating physician or other qualified health care professional, with the following required elements: outreach to and engagement in treatment of a patient directed by the treating physician or other qualified health care professional; initial assessment of the patient, including administration of validated rating scales, with the development of an individualized treatment plan; review by the psychiatric consultant with modifications of the plan if recommended; entering patient in a registry and tracking patient follow-up and progress using the registry, with appropriate documentation, and participation in weekly caseload consultation with the psychiatric consultant; and provision of brief interventions using evidence-based techniques such as behavioral activation, motivational interviewing, and other focused treatment strategies
- • **G0503** Subsequent psychiatric collaborative care management, first 60 minutes in a subsequent month of behavioral health care manager activities, in consultation with a psychiatric consultant, and directed by the treating physician or other qualified health care professional, with the following required elements: tracking patient follow-up and progress using the registry, with appropriate documentation; participation in weekly caseload consultation with the psychiatric consultant; ongoing collaboration with and coordination of the patient's mental health care with the treating physician or other qualified health care professional and any other treating mental health providers; additional review of progress and recommendations for changes in treatment, as indicated, including medications, based on recommendations provided by the psychiatric consultant; provision of brief interventions using evidence-based techniques such as behavioral activation, motivational interviewing, and other focused treatment strategies; monitoring of patient outcomes using validated rating scales; and relapse prevention planning with patients as they achieve remission of symptoms and/or other treatment goals and are prepared for discharge from active treatment
- • **G0504** Initial or subsequent psychiatric collaborative care management, each additional 30 minutes in a calendar month of behavioral health care manager activities, in consultation with a psychiatric consultant, and directed by the treating physician or other qualified health care professional (list separately in addition to code for primary procedure); (use g0504 in conjunction with G0502, G0503)

- • **G0505** Cognition and functional assessment using standardized instruments with development of recorded care plan for the patient with cognitive impairment, history obtained from patient and/or caregiver, in office or other outpatient setting or home or domiciliary or rest home
- • **G0506** Comprehensive assessment of and care planning for patients requiring chronic care management services (list separately in addition to primary monthly care management service)
- • **G0507** Care management services for behavioral health conditions, at least 20 minutes of clinical staff time, directed by a physician or other qualified health care professional, per calendar month, with the following required elements: initial assessment or follow-up monitoring, including the use of applicable validated rating scales; behavioral health care planning in relation to behavioral/psychiatric health problems, including revision for patients who are not progressing or whose status changes; facilitating and coordinating treatment such as psychotherapy, pharmacotherapy, counseling and/or psychiatric consultation; and continuity of care with a designated member of the care team
- • **G0508** Telehealth consultation, critical care, initial , physicians typically spend 60 minutes communicating with the patient and providers via telehealth
- • **G0509** Telehealth consultation, critical care, subsequent, physicians typically spend 50 minutes communicating with the patient and providers via telehealth

(**G3001** Code deleted December 31, 2016.)

(**G8401** Code deleted December 31, 2016.)

▲ **G8427** Eligible clinician attests to documenting in the medical record they obtained, updated, or reviewed the patient's current medications

▲ **G8428** Current list of medications not documented as obtained, updated, or reviewed by the eligible clinician, reason not given

▲ **G8430** Eligible clinician attests to documenting in the medical record the patient is not eligible for a current list of medications being obtained, updated, or reviewed by the eligible clinician

▲ **G8431** Screening for depression is documented as being positive and a follow-up plan is documented

▲ **G8432** Depression screening not documented, reason not given

▲ **G8433** Screening for depression not completed, documented reason

(**G8458** Code deleted December 31, 2016.)

(**G8460** Code deleted December 31, 2016.)

(**G8461** Code deleted December 31, 2016.)

(**G8485** Code deleted December 31, 2016.)

(**G8486** Code deleted December 31, 2016.)

(**G8487** Code deleted December 31, 2016.)

(**G8489** Code deleted December 31, 2016.)

(**G8490** Code deleted December 31, 2016.)

(**G8491** Code deleted December 31, 2016.)

(**G8494** Code deleted December 31, 2016.)

(**G8495** Code deleted December 31, 2016.)

(**G8496** Code deleted December 31, 2016.)

(**G8497** Code deleted December 31, 2016.)

(**G8498** Code deleted December 31, 2016.)

(**G8499** Code deleted December 31, 2016.)

(**G8500** Code deleted December 31, 2016.)

▲ **G8510** Screening for depression is documented as negative, a follow-up plan is not required

▲ **G8511** Screening for depression documented as positive, follow-up plan not documented, reason not given

(**G8544** Code deleted December 31, 2016.)

(**G8545** Code deleted December 31, 2016.)

(**G8548** Code deleted December 31, 2016.)

(**G8549** Code deleted December 31, 2016.)

(**G8551** Code deleted December 31, 2016.)

▲ **G8598** Aspirin or another antiplatelet therapy used

▲ **G8599** Aspirin or another antiplatelet therapy not used, reason not given

(**G8634** Code deleted December 31, 2016.)

(**G8645** Code deleted December 31, 2016.)

(**G8646** Code deleted December 31, 2016.)

▲ **G8649** Risk-adjusted functional status change residual scores for the knee not measured because the patient did not complete foto's status survey near discharge, not appropriate

▲ **G8653** Risk-adjusted functional status change residual scores for the hip not measured because the patient did not complete follow up status survey near discharge, patient not appropriate

▲ **G8655** Risk-adjusted functional status change residual score for the foot or ankle successfully calculated and the score was equal to zero (0) or greater than zero (> 0)

▲ **G8656** Risk-adjusted functional status change residual score for the foot or ankle successfully calculated and the score was less than zero (< 0)

▲ **G8657** Risk-adjusted functional status change residual scores for the foot or ankle not measured because the patient did not complete foto's status survey near discharge, patient not appropriate

▲ **G8658** Risk-adjusted functional status change residual scores for the foot or ankle not measured because the patient did not complete foto's functional intake on admission and/or follow up status survey near discharge, reason not given

▲ **G8659** Risk-adjusted functional status change residual score for the lumbar impairment successfully calculated and the score was equal to zero (0) or greater than zero (> 0)

▲ **G8660** Risk-adjusted functional status change residual score for the lumbar impairment successfully calculated and the score was less than zero (< 0)

▲ **G8661** Risk-adjusted functional status change residual scores for the lumbar impairment not measured because the patient did not complete foto's status survey near discharge, patient not appropriate

▲ **G8662** Risk-adjusted functional status change residual scores for the lumbar impairment not measured because the patient did not complete foto's functional intake on admission and/or follow up status survey near discharge, reason not given

▲ **G8665** Risk-adjusted functional status change residual scores for the shoulder not measured because the patient did not complete foto's functional status survey near discharge, patient not appropriate

▲ **G8669** Risk-adjusted functional status change residual scores for the elbow, wrist or hand not measured because the patient did not complete foto's functional follow up status survey near discharge, patient not appropriate

▲ **G8671** Risk-adjusted functional status change residual score for the neck, cranium, mandible, thoracic spine, ribs, or other general orthopaedic impairment successfully calculated and the score was equal to zero (0) or greater than zero (> 0)

▲ **G8672** Risk-adjusted functional status change residual score for the neck, cranium, mandible, thoracic spine, ribs, or other general orthopaedic impairment successfully calculated and the score was less than zero (< 0)

▲ **G8673** Risk-adjusted functional status change residual scores for the neck, cranium, mandible, thoracic spine, ribs, or other general orthopaedic impairment not measured because the patient did not complete foto's functional follow up status survey near discharge, patient not appropriate

▲ **G8674** Risk-adjusted functional status change residual scores for the neck, cranium, mandible, thoracic spine, ribs, or other general orthopaedic impairment not measured because the patient did not complete foto's functional intake on admission and/or follow up status survey near discharge, reason not given

▲ **G8697** Antithrombotic therapy not prescribed for documented reasons (e.g., patient had stroke during hospital stay, patient expired during inpatient stay, other medical reason(s)); (e.g., patient left against medical advice, other patient reason(s))

(**G8725** Code deleted December 31, 2016.)

(**G8726** Code deleted December 31, 2016.)

(**G8728** Code deleted December 31, 2016.)

(**G8757** Code deleted December 31, 2016.)

(**G8758** Code deleted December 31, 2016.)

(**G8759** Code deleted December 31, 2016.)

(**G8761** Code deleted December 31, 2016.)

(**G8762** Code deleted December 31, 2016.)

(**G8765** Code deleted December 31, 2016.)

(**G8784** Code deleted December 31, 2016.)

▲ **G8815** Documented reason in the medical records for why the statin therapy was not prescribed (i.e., lower extremity bypass was for a patient with non-arthrosclerotic disease)

(**G8848** Code deleted December 31, 2016.)

(**G8853** Code deleted December 31, 2016.)

(**G8868** Code deleted December 31, 2016.)

(**G8898** Code deleted December 31, 2016.)

(**G8899** Code deleted December 31, 2016.)

(**G8900** Code deleted December 31, 2016.)

(**G8902** Code deleted December 31, 2016.)

(**G8903** Code deleted December 31, 2016.)

(**G8906** Code deleted December 31, 2016.)

▲ **G8924** Spirometry test results demonstrate fev1/fvc < 70%, fev < 60% predicted and patient has COPD symptoms (e.g., dyspnea, cough/sputum, wheezing)

▲ **G8925** Spirometry test results demonstrate fev1 >= 60% fev1/fvc >= 70%, predicted or patient does not have COPD symptoms

(**G8927** Code deleted December 31, 2016.)

(**G8928** Code deleted December 31, 2016.)

(**G8929** Code deleted December 31, 2016.)

(**G8940** Code deleted December 31, 2016.)

(**G8948** Code deleted December 31, 2016.)

(**G8953** Code deleted December 31, 2016.)

▲ **G8968** Documentation of medical reason(s) for not prescribing warfarin or another oral anticoagulant that is FDA approved for the prevention of thromboembolism (e.g., allergy, risk of bleeding, other medical reasons)

(**G8977** Code deleted December 31, 2016.)

(**G9203** Code deleted December 31, 2016.)

(**G9204** Code deleted December 31, 2016.)

(**G9205** Code deleted December 31, 2016.)

(**G9206** Code deleted December 31, 2016.)

(**G9207** Code deleted December 31, 2016.)

(**G9208** Code deleted December 31, 2016.)

(**G9209** Code deleted December 31, 2016.)

(**G9210** Code deleted December 31, 2016.)

(**G9211** Code deleted December 31, 2016.)

(**G9217** Code deleted December 31, 2016.)

(**G9219** Code deleted December 31, 2016.)

(**G9222** Code deleted December 31, 2016.)

▲ **G9229** Chlamydia, gonorrhea, and syphilis screening results not documented (patient refusal is the only allowed exception)

▲ **G9231** Documentation of end stage renal disease (esrd), dialysis, renal transplant before or during the measurement period or pregnancy during the measurement period

▲ **G9232** Clinician treating major depressive disorder did not communicate to clinician treating comorbid condition for specified patient reason (e.g., patient is unable to communicate the diagnosis of a comorbid condition; the patient is unwilling to communicate the diagnosis of a comorbid condition; or the patient is unaware of the comorbid condition, or any other specified patient reason)

(**G9233** Code deleted December 31, 2016.)

(**G9234** Code deleted December 31, 2016.)

(**G9235** Code deleted December 31, 2016.)

(**G9236** Code deleted December 31, 2016.)

(**G9237** Code deleted December 31, 2016.)

(**G9238** Code deleted December 31, 2016.)

▲ **G9239** Documentation of reasons for patient initiating maintenance hemodialysis with a catheter as the mode of vascular access (e.g., patient has a maturing AVF/avg, time-limited trial of hemodialysis, other medical reasons, patient declined AVF/avg, other patient reasons, patient followed by reporting nephrologist for fewer than 90 days, other system reasons)

(**G9244** Code deleted December 31, 2016.)

(**G9245** Code deleted December 31, 2016.)

▲ **G9264** Documentation of patient receiving maintenance hemodialysis for greater than or equal to 90 days with a catheter for documented reasons (e.g., other medical reasons, patient declined AVF/avg, other patient reasons)

▲ **G9307** No return to the operating room for a surgical procedure, for complications of the principal operative procedure, within 30 days of the principal operative procedure

▲ **G9308** Unplanned return to the operating room for a surgical procedure, for complications of the principal operative procedure, within 30 days of the principal operative procedure

(**G9324** Code deleted December 31, 2016.)

▲ **G9326** Ct studies performed not reported to a radiation dose index registry that is capable of collecting at a minimum all necessary data elements, reason not given

▲ **G9327** Ct studies performed reported to a radiation dose index registry that is capable of collecting at a minimum all necessary data elements

▲ **G9359** Documentation of negative or managed positive tb screen with further evidence that tb is not active within one year of patient visit

▲ **G9361** Medical indication for induction [documentation of reason(s) for elective delivery (c-section) or early induction (e.g., hemorrhage and placental complications, hypertension, preeclampsia and eclampsia, rupture of membranes-premature or prolonged, maternal conditions complicating pregnancy/delivery, fetal conditions complicating pregnancy/delivery, late pregnancy, prior uterine surgery, or participation in clinical trial)]

▲ **G9381** Documentation of medical reason(s) for not offering assistance with end of life issues (e.g., patient in hospice care, patient in terminal phase) during the measurement period

▲ **G9416** Patient had one tetanus, diphtheria toxoids and acellular pertussis vaccine (Tdap) on or between the patient's 10th and 13th birthdays

▲ **G9417** Patient did not have one tetanus, diphtheria toxoids and acellular pertussis vaccine (Tdap) on or between the patient's 10th and 13th birthdays

(**G9435** Code deleted December 31, 2016.)

(**G9436** Code deleted December 31, 2016.)

(**G9437** Code deleted December 31, 2016.)

(**G9438** Code deleted December 31, 2016.)

(**G9439** Code deleted December 31, 2016.)

(**G9440** Code deleted December 31, 2016.)

(**G9441** Code deleted December 31, 2016.)

(**G9442** Code deleted December 31, 2016.)

(**G9443** Code deleted December 31, 2016.)

(**G9463** Code deleted December 31, 2016.)

(**G9464** Code deleted December 31, 2016.)

(**G9465** Code deleted December 31, 2016.)

(**G9466** Code deleted December 31, 2016.)

(**G9467** Code deleted December 31, 2016.)

• **G9481** Remote in-home visit for the evaluation and management of a new patient for use only in the medicare-approved comprehensive care for joint replacement model, which requires these 3 key components:

- a problem focused history;
- a problem focused examination; and
- straightforward medical decision making, furnished in real time using interactive audio and video technology.

Counseling and coordination of care with other physicians, other qualified health care professionals or agencies are provided consistent with the nature of the problem(s) and the needs of the patient or the family or both. usually, the presenting problem(s) are self limited or minor. typically, 10 minutes are spent with the patient or family or both via real time, audio and video intercommunications technology

• **G9482** Remote in-home visit for the evaluation and management of a new patient for use only in the medicare-approved comprehensive care for joint replacement model, which requires these 3 key components:

- an expanded problem focused history;
- an expanded problem focused examination;

- straightforward medical decision making, furnished in real time using interactive audio and video technology.

Counseling and coordination of care with other physicians, other qualified health care professionals or agencies are provided consistent with the nature of the problem(s) and the needs of the patient or the family or both. usually, the presenting problem(s) are of low to moderate severity. typically, 20 minutes are spent with the patient or family or both via real time, audio and video intercommunications technology

• **G9483** Remote in-home visit for the evaluation and management of a new patient for use only in the medicare-approved comprehensive care for joint replacement model, which requires these 3 key components:

- a detailed history;
- a detailed examination;
- medical decision making of low complexity, furnished in real time using interactive audio and video technology.

Counseling and coordination of care with other physicians, other qualified health care professionals or agencies are provided consistent with the nature of the problem(s) and the needs of the patient or the family or both. usually, the presenting problem(s) are of moderate severity. typically, 30 minutes are spent with the patient or family or both via real time, audio and video intercommunications technology

• **G9484** Remote in-home visit for the evaluation and management of a new patient for use only in the medicare-approved comprehensive care for joint replacement model, which requires these 3 key components:

- a comprehensive history;
- a comprehensive examination;
- medical decision making of moderate complexity, furnished in real time using interactive audio and video technology.

Counseling and coordination of care with other physicians, other qualified health care professionals or agencies are provided consistent with the nature of the problem(s) and the needs of the patient or the family or both. usually, the presenting problem(s) are of moderate to high severity. typically, 45 minutes are spent with the patient or family or both via real time, audio and video intercommunications technology

• **G9485** Remote in-home visit for the evaluation and management of a new patient for use only in the medicare-approved comprehensive care for joint replacement model, which requires these 3 key components:

- a comprehensive history;
- a comprehensive examination;
- medical decision making of high complexity, furnished in real time using interactive audio and video technology.

Counseling and coordination of care with other physicians, other qualified health care professionals or agencies are provided consistent with the nature of the problem(s) and the needs of the patient or the family or both. usually, the presenting problem(s) are of moderate to high severity. typically, 60 minutes are spent with the patient or family or both via real time, audio and video intercommunications technology

• **G9486** Remote in-home visit for the evaluation and management of an established patient for use only in the medicare-approved comprehensive care for joint replacement model, which requires at least 2 of the following 3 key components:

- a problem focused history;
- a problem focused examination;
- straightforward medical decision making, furnished in real time using interactive audio and video technology.

Counseling and coordination of care with other physicians, other qualified health care professionals or agencies are provided consistent with the nature of the problem(s) and the needs of the patient or the family or both. usually, the presenting problem(s) are self limited or minor. typically, 10 minutes are spent with the patient or family or both via real time, audio and video intercommunications technology

• **G9487** Remote in-home visit for the evaluation and management of an established patient for use only in the medicare-approved comprehensive care for joint replacement model, which requires at least 2 of the following 3 key components:

- an expanded problem focused history;
- an expanded problem focused examination;
- medical decision making of low complexity, furnished in real time using interactive audio and video technology.

Counseling and coordination of care with other physicians, other qualified health care professionals or agencies are provided consistent with the nature of the problem(s) and the needs of the patient or the family or both. usually, the presenting problem(s) are of low to moderate severity. typically, 15 minutes are spent with the patient or family or both via real time, audio and video intercommunications technology

• **G9488** Remote in-home visit for the evaluation and management of an established patient for use only in the medicare-approved comprehensive care for joint replacement model, which requires at least 2 of the following 3 key components:

- a detailed history;
- a detailed examination;
- medical decision making of moderate complexity, furnished in real time using interactive audio and video technology.

Counseling and coordination of care with other physicians, other qualified health care professionals or agencies are provided consistent with the nature of the problem(s) and the needs of the patient or the family or both. usually, the presenting problem(s) are of moderate to high severity. typically, 25 minutes are spent with the patient or family or both via real time, audio and video intercommunications technology

• **G9489** Remote in-home visit for the evaluation and management of an established patient for use only in the medicare-approved comprehensive care for joint replacement model, which requires at least 2 of the following 3 key components:

- a comprehensive history;
- a comprehensive examination;
- medical decision making of high complexity, furnished in real time using interactive audio and video technology.

Counseling and coordination of care with other physicians, other qualified health care professionals or agencies are provided consistent with the nature of the problem(s) and the needs of the patient or the family or both. usually, the presenting problem(s) are of moderate to high severity. typically, 40 minutes are spent with the patient or family or both via real time, audio and video intercommunications technology

● **G9490** Comprehensive care for joint replacement model, home visit for patient assessment performed by clinical staff for an individual not considered homebound, including, but not necessarily limited to patient assessment of clinical status, safety/fall prevention, functional status/ambulation, medication reconciliation/management, compliance with orders/plan of care, performance of activities of daily living, and ensuring beneficiary connections to community and other services. (for use only in the medicare-approved cjr model); may not be billed for a 30 day period covered by a transitional care management code

▲ **G9497** Received instruction from the anesthesiologist or proxy prior to the day of surgery to abstain from smoking on the day of surgery

(**G9499** Code deleted December 31, 2016.)

▲ **G9500** Radiation exposure indices, or exposure time and number of fluorographic images in final report for procedures using fluoroscopy, documented

▲ **G9501** Radiation exposure indices, or exposure time and number of fluorographic images not documented in final report for procedure using fluoroscopy, reason not given

▲ **G9519** Patient achieves final refraction (spherical equivalent) 0.5 diopters of their planned refraction within 90 days of surgery

▲ **G9520** Patient does not achieve final refraction (spherical equivalent) 0.5 diopters of their planned refraction within 90 days of surgery

▲ **G9531** Patient has documentation of ventricular shunt, brain tumor, multisystem trauma, pregnancy, or is currently taking an antiplatelet medication including: asa/dipyridamole, clopidogrel, prasugrel, ticlopidine, ticagrelor or cilostazol)

▲ **G9532** Patient's head injury occurred greater than 24 hours before presentation to the emergency department, or has a GCS score less than 15 or does not have a GCS score documented, or had a head ct for trauma ordered by someone other than an emergency care provider, or was ordered for a reason other than trauma

▲ **G9547** Incidental finding: liver lesion <= 0.5 cm, cystic kidney lesion < 1.0 cm or adrenal lesion <= 1.0 cm

▲ **G9549** Documentation of medical reason(s) that follow-up imaging is indicated (e.g., patient has a known malignancy that can metastasize, other medical reason(s) such as fever in an immunocompromised patient)

▲ **G9551** Final reports for abdominal imaging studies without an incidentally found lesion noted: liver lesion <= 0.5 cm, cystic kidney lesion < 1.0 cm or adrenal lesion <= 1.0 cm noted or no lesion found

▲ **G9554** Final reports for ct, CTA, MRI or MRA of the chest or neck or ultrasound of the neck with follow-up imaging recommended

▲ **G9555** Documentation of medical reason(s) for recommending follow up imaging (e.g., patient has multiple endocrine neoplasia, patient has cervical lymphadenopathy, other medical reason(s))

▲ **G9556** Final reports for ct, CTA, MRI or MRA of the chest or neck or ultrasound of the neck with follow-up imaging not recommended

▲ **G9557** Final reports for ct, CTA, MRI or MRA studies of the chest or neck or ultrasound of the neck without an incidentally found thyroid nodule < 1.0 cm noted or no nodule found

(**G9572** Code deleted December 31, 2016.)

(**G9581** Code deleted December 31, 2016.)

▲ **G9584** Patient evaluated for risk of misuse of opiates by using a brief validated instrument (e.g., opioid risk tool, soapp-r) or patient interviewed at least once during opioid therapy

▲ **G9585** Patient not evaluated for risk of misuse of opiates by using a brief validated instrument (e.g., opioid risk tool, soapp-r) or patient not interviewed at least once during opioid therapy

▲ **G9595** Patient has documentation of ventricular shunt, brain tumor, coagulopathy, including thrombocytopenia

▲ **G9596** Pediatric patient's head injury occurred greater than 24 hours before presentation to the emergency department, or has a GCS score less than 15 or does not have a GCS score documented, or had a head ct for trauma ordered by someone other than an emergency care provider, or was ordered for a reason other than trauma

▲ **G9607** Documented medical reasons for not performing intraoperative cystoscopy (e.g., urethral pathology precluding cystoscopy, any patient who has a congenital or acquired absence of the urethra)

▲ **G9609** Documentation of an order for anti-platelet agents

▲ **G9610** Documentation of medical reason(s) in the patient's record for not ordering anti-platelet agents

▲ **G9611** Order for anti-platelet agents was not documented in the patient's record, reason not given

(**G9619** Code deleted December 31, 2016.)

▲ **G9625** Patient sustained bladder injury at the time of surgery or discovered subsequently up to 1 month post-surgery

▲ **G9626** Documented medical reason for not reporting bladder injury (e.g., gynecologic or other pelvic malignancy documented, concurrent surgery involving bladder pathology, injury that occurs during urinary incontinence procedure, patient death from non-medical causes not related to surgery, patient died during procedure without evidence of bladder injury)

▲ **G9627** Patient did not sustain bladder injury at the time of surgery nor discovered subsequently up to 1 month post-surgery

▲ **G9628** Patient sustained bowel injury at the time of surgery or discovered subsequently up to 1 month post-surgery

▲ **G9629** Documented medical reasons for not reporting bowel injury (e.g., gynecologic or other pelvic malignancy documented, planned (e.g., not due to an unexpected bowel injury) resection and/or re-anastomosis of bowel, or patient death from non-medical causes not related to surgery, patient died during procedure without evidence of bowel injury)

▲ **G9630** Patient did not sustain a bowel injury at the time of surgery nor discovered subsequently up to 1 month post-surgery

▲ **G9632** Documented medical reasons for not reporting ureter injury (e.g., gynecologic or other pelvic malignancy documented, concurrent surgery involving bladder pathology, injury that occurs during a urinary incontinence procedure, patient death from non-medical causes not related to surgery, patient died during procedure without evidence of ureter injury)

▲ **G9633** Patient did not sustain ureter injury at the time of surgery nor discovered subsequently up to 1 month post-surgery

▲ **G9642** Current smokers (e.g., cigarette, cigar, pipe, e-cigarette or marijuana)

(**G9650** Code deleted December 31, 2016.)

(**G9652** Code deleted December 31, 2016.)

(**G9653** Code deleted December 31, 2016.)

(**G9657** Code deleted December 31, 2016.)

(**G9667** Code deleted December 31, 2016.)

(**G9669** Code deleted December 31, 2016.)

(**G9670** Code deleted December 31, 2016.)

(**G9671** Code deleted December 31, 2016.)

(**G9672** Code deleted December 31, 2016.)

(**G9673** Code deleted December 31, 2016.)

(**G9677** Code deleted December 31, 2016.)

• **G9678** Oncology care model (OCM) monthly enhanced oncology services (MEOS) payment for OCM enhanced services. g9678 payments may only be made to OCM practitioners for OCM beneficiaries for the furnishing of enhanced services as defined in the OCM participation agreement

• **G9679** This code is for onsite acute care treatment of a nursing facility resident with pneumonia; may only be billed once per day per beneficiary

• **G9680** This code is for onsite acute care treatment of a nursing facility resident with CHF; may only be billed once per day per beneficiary

• **G9681** This code is for onsite acute care treatment of a resident with COPD or asthma; may only be billed once per day per beneficiary

• **G9682** This code is for the onsite acute care treatment a nursing facility resident with a skin infection; may only be billed once per day per beneficiary

• **G9683** This code is for the onsite acute care treatment of a nursing facility resident with fluid or electrolyte disorder or dehydration (similar pattern); may only be billed once per day per beneficiary

- **G9684** This code is for the onsite acute care treatment of a nursing facility resident for a UTI; may only be billed once per day per beneficiary
- **G9685** This code is for the evaluation and management of a beneficiary's acute change in condition in a nursing facility
- **G9686** Onsite nursing facility conference, that is separate and distinct from an evaluation and management visit, including qualified practitioner and at least one member of the nursing facility interdisciplinary care team
- **G9687** Hospice services provided to patient any time during the measurement period
- **G9688** Patients using hospice services any time during the measurement period
- **G9689** Patient admitted for performance of elective carotid intervention
- **G9690** Patient receiving hospice services any time during the measurement period
- **G9691** Patient had hospice services any time during the measurement period
- **G9692** Hospice services received by patient any time during the measurement period
- **G9693** Patient use of hospice services any time during the measurement period
- **G9694** Hospice services utilized by patient any time during the measurement period
- **G9695** Long-acting inhaled bronchodilator prescribed
- **G9696** Documentation of medical reason(s) for not prescribing a long-acting inhaled bronchodilator
- **G9697** Documentation of patient reason(s) for not prescribing a long-acting inhaled bronchodilator
- **G9698** Documentation of system reason(s) for not prescribing a long-acting inhaled bronchodilator
- **G9699** Long-acting inhaled bronchodilator not prescribed, reason not otherwise specified
- **G9700** Patients who use hospice services any time during the measurement period
- **G9701** Children who are taking antibiotics in the 30 days prior to the date of the encounter during which the diagnosis was established
- **G9702** Patients who use hospice services any time during the measurement period
- **G9703** Children who are taking antibiotics in the 30 days prior to the diagnosis of pharyngitis
- **G9704** AJCC breast cancer stage i: t1 mic or t1a documented
- **G9705** AJCC breast cancer stage i: t1b (tumor > 0.5 cm but <= 1 cm in greatest dimension) documented
- **G9706** Low (or very low) risk of recurrence, prostate cancer
- **G9707** Patient received hospice services any time during the measurement period
- **G9708** Women who had a bilateral mastectomy or who have a history of a bilateral mastectomy or for whom there is evidence of a right and a left unilateral mastectomy
- **G9709** Hospice services used by patient any time during the measurement period
- **G9710** Patient was provided hospice services any time during the measurement period
- **G9711** Patients with a diagnosis or past history of total colectomy or colorectal cancer

- **G9712** Documentation of medical reason(s) for prescribing or dispensing antibiotic (e.g., intestinal infection, pertussis, bacterial infection, lyme disease, otitis media, acute sinusitis, acute pharyngitis, acute tonsillitis, chronic sinusitis, infection of the pharynx/larynx/tonsils/ adenoids, prostatitis, cellulitis/ mastoiditis/bone infections, acute lymphadenitis, impetigo, skin staph infections, pneumonia, gonococcal infections/venereal disease (syphilis, chlamydia, inflammatory diseases [female reproductive organs]), infections of the kidney, cystitis/UTI, acne, hiv disease/asymptomatic hiv, cystic fibrosis, disorders of the immune system, malignancy neoplasms, chronic bronchitis, emphysema, bronchiectasis, extrinsic allergic alveolitis, chronic airway obstruction, chronic obstructive asthma, pneumoconiosis and other lung disease due to external agents, other diseases of the respiratory system, and tuberculosis
- **G9713** Patients who use hospice services any time during the measurement period
- **G9714** Patient is using hospice services any time during the measurement period
- **G9715** Patients who use hospice services any time during the measurement period
- **G9716** Bmi is documented as being outside of normal limits, follow-up plan is not completed for documented reason
- **G9717** Documentation stating the patient has an active diagnosis of depression or has a diagnosed bipolar disorder, therefore screening or follow-up not required
- **G9718** Hospice services for patient provided any time during the measurement period
- **G9719** Patient is not ambulatory, bed ridden, immobile, confined to chair, wheelchair bound, dependent on helper pushing wheelchair, independent in wheelchair or minimal help in wheelchair
- **G9720** Hospice services for patient occurred any time during the measurement period
- **G9721** Patient not ambulatory, bed ridden, immobile, confined to chair, wheelchair bound, dependent on helper pushing wheelchair, independent in wheelchair or minimal help in wheelchair
- **G9722** Documented history of renal failure or baseline serum creatinine = 4.0 mg/dl; renal transplant recipients are not considered to have preoperative renal failure, unless, since transplantation the cr has been or is 4.0 or higher
- **G9723** Hospice services for patient received any time during the measurement period
- **G9724** Patients who had documentation of use of anticoagulant medications overlapping the measurement year
- **G9725** Patients who use hospice services any time during the measurement period
- **G9726** Patient refused to participate
- **G9727** Patient unable to complete the FOTO knee intake prom at admission and discharge due to blindness, illiteracy, severe mental incapacity or language incompatibility and an adequate proxy is not available
- **G9728** Patient refused to participate
- **G9729** Patient unable to complete the FOTO hip intake prom at admission and discharge due to blindness, illiteracy, severe mental incapacity or language incompatibility and an adequate proxy is not available

- • **G9730** Patient refused to participate
- • **G9731** Patient unable to complete the FOTO foot or ankle intake prom at admission and discharge due to blindness, illiteracy, severe mental incapacity or language incompatibility and an adequate proxy is not available
- • **G9732** Patient refused to participate
- • **G9733** Patient unable to complete the FOTO lumbar intake prom at admission and discharge due to blindness, illiteracy, severe mental incapacity or language incompatibility and an adequate proxy is not available
- • **G9734** Patient refused to participate
- • **G9735** Patient unable to complete the FOTO shoulder intake prom at admission and discharge due to blindness, illiteracy, severe mental incapacity or language incompatibility and an adequate proxy is not available
- • **G9736** Patient refused to participate
- • **G9737** Patient unable to complete the FOTO elbow, wrist or hand intake prom at admission and discharge due to blindness, illiteracy, severe mental incapacity or language incompatibility and an adequate proxy is not available
- • **G9738** Patient refused to participate
- • **G9739** Patient unable to complete the FOTO general orthopedic intake prom at admission and discharge due to blindness, illiteracy, severe mental incapacity or language incompatibility and an adequate proxy is not available
- • **G9740** Hospice services given to patient any time during the measurement period
- • **G9741** Patients who use hospice services any time during the measurement period
- • **G9742** Psychiatric symptoms assessed
- • **G9743** Psychiatric symptoms not assessed, reason not otherwise specified
- • **G9744** Patient not eligible due to active diagnosis of hypertension
- • **G9745** Documented reason for not screening or recommending a follow-up for high blood pressure
- • **G9746** Patient has mitral stenosis or prosthetic heart valves or patient has transient or reversible cause of af (e.g., pneumonia, hyperthyroidism, pregnancy, cardiac surgery)
- • **G9747** Patient is undergoing palliative dialysis with a catheter
- • **G9748** Patient approved by a qualified transplant program and scheduled to receive a living donor kidney transplant
- • **G9749** Patient is undergoing palliative dialysis with a catheter
- • **G9750** Patient approved by a qualified transplant program and scheduled to receive a living donor kidney transplant
- • **G9751** Patient died at any time during the 24-month measurement period
- • **G9752** Emergency surgery

- **G9753** Documentation of medical reason for not conducting a search for DICOM format images for prior patient ct imaging studies completed at non-affiliated external healthcare facilities or entities within the past 12 months that are available through a secure, authorized, media-free, shared archive (e.g., trauma, acute myocardial infarction, stroke, aortic aneurysm where time is of the essence)
- **G9754** A finding of an incidental pulmonary nodule
- **G9755** Documentation of medical reason(s) that follow-up imaging is indicated (e.g., patient has a known malignancy that can metastasize, other medical reason(s)
- **G9756** Surgical procedures that included the use of silicone oil
- **G9757** Surgical procedures that included the use of silicone oil
- **G9758** Patient in hospice and in terminal phase
- **G9759** History of preoperative posterior capsule rupture
- **G9760** Patients who use hospice services any time during the measurement period
- **G9761** Patients who use hospice services any time during the measurement period
- **G9762** Patient had at least three HPV vaccines on or between the patient's 9th and 13th birthdays
- **G9763** Patient did not have at least three HPV vaccines on or between the patient's 9th and 13th birthdays
- **G9764** Patient has been treated with an oral systemic or biologic medication for psoriasis
- **G9765** Documentation that the patient declined therapy change, has documented contraindications, or has not been treated with an oral systemic or biologic for at least six consecutive months (e.g., experienced adverse effects or lack of efficacy with all other therapy options) in order to achieve better disease control as measured by PGA, BSA, PASI, or DLQI
- **G9766** Patients who are transferred from one institution to another with a known diagnosis of CVA for endovascular stroke treatment
- **G9767** Hospitalized patients with newly diagnosed CVA considered for endovascular stroke treatment
- **G9768** Patients who utilize hospice services any time during the measurement period
- **G9769** Patient had a bone mineral density test in the past two years or received osteoporosis medication or therapy in the past 12 months
- **G9770** Peripheral nerve block (PNB)
- **G9771** At least 1 body temperature measurement equal to or greater than 35.5 degrees celsius (or 95.9 degrees Fahrenheit) achieved within the 30 minutes immediately before or the 15 minutes immediately after anesthesia end time
- **G9772** Documentation of one of the following medical reason(s) for not achieving at least 1 body temperature measurement equal to or greater than 35.5 degrees celsius (or 95.9 degrees Fahrenheit) achieved within the 30 minutes immediately before or the 15 minutes immediately after anesthesia end time (e.g., emergency cases, intentional hypothermia, etc.)

- • **G9773** At least 1 body temperature measurement equal to or greater than 35.5 degrees celsius (or 95.9 degrees Fahrenheit) not achieved within the 30 minutes immediately before or the 15 minutes immediately after anesthesia end time
- • **G9774** Patients who have had a hysterectomy
- • **G9775** Patient received at least 2 prophylactic pharmacologic anti-emetic agents of different classes preoperatively and/or intraoperatively
- • **G9776** Documentation of medical reason for not receiving at least 2 prophylactic pharmacologic anti-emetic agents of different classes preoperatively and/or intraoperatively (e.g., intolerance or other medical reason)
- • **G9777** Patient did not receive at least 2 prophylactic pharmacologic anti-emetic agents of different classes preoperatively and/or intraoperatively
- • **G9778** Patients who have a diagnosis of pregnancy
- • **G9779** Patients who are breastfeeding
- • **G9780** Patients who have a diagnosis of rhabdomyolysis
- • **G9781** Documentation of medical reason(s) for not currently being a statin therapy user or receive an order (prescription) for statin therapy (e.g., patient with adverse effect, allergy or intolerance to statin medication therapy, patients who are receiving palliative care, patients with active liver disease or hepatic disease or insufficiency, and patients with end stage renal disease (esrd))
- • **G9782** History of or active diagnosis of familial or pure hypercholesterolemia
- • **G9783** Documentation of patients with diabetes who have a most recent fasting or direct LDL- c laboratory test result < 70 mg/dl and are not taking statin therapy
- • **G9784** Pathologists/dermatopathologists providing a second opinion on a biopsy
- • **G9785** Pathology report diagnosing cutaneous basal cell carcinoma or squamous cell carcinoma (to include in situ disease) sent from the pathologist/dermatopathologist to the biopsying clinician for review within 7 business days from the time when the tissue specimen was received by the pathologist
- • **G9786** Pathology report diagnosing cutaneous basal cell carcinoma or squamous cell carcinoma (to include in situ disease) was not sent from the pathologist/dermatopathologist to the biopsying clinician for review within 7 business days from the time when the tissue specimen was received by the pathologist
- • **G9787** Patient alive as of the last day of the measurement year
- • **G9788** Most recent bp is less than or equal to 140/90 mm hg
- • **G9789** Blood pressure recorded during inpatient stays, emergency room visits, urgent care visits, and patient self-reported bp's (home and health fair bp results)
- • **G9790** Most recent bp is greater than 140/90 mm hg, or blood pressure not documented
- • **G9791** Most recent tobacco status is tobacco free
- • **G9792** Most recent tobacco status is not tobacco free
- • **G9793** Patient is currently on a daily aspirin or other antiplatelet

- **G9794** Documentation of medical reason(s) for not on a daily aspirin or other antiplatelet (e.g. history of gastrointestinal bleed or intra-cranial bleed or documentation of active anticoagulant use during the measurement period
- **G9795** Patient is not currently on a daily aspirin or other antiplatelet
- **G9796** Patient is currently on a statin therapy
- **G9797** Patient is not on a statin therapy
- **G9798** Discharge(s) for AMI between July 1 of the year prior measurement year to June 30 of the measurement period
- **G9799** Patients with a medication dispensing event indicator of a history of asthma any time during the patient's history through the end of the measure period
- **G9800** Patients who are identified as having an intolerance or allergy to beta-blocker therapy
- **G9801** Hospitalizations in which the patient was transferred directly to a non-acute care facility for any diagnosis`
- **G9802** Patients who use hospice services any time during the measurement period
- **G9803** Patient prescribed a 180-day course of treatment with beta-blockers post discharge for AMI
- **G9804** Patient was not prescribed a 180-day course of treatment with beta-blockers post discharge for AMI
- **G9805** Patients who use hospice services any time during the measurement period
- **G9806** Patients who received cervical cytology or an HPV test
- **G9807** Patients who did not receive cervical cytology or an HPV test
- **G9808** Any patients who had no asthma controller medications dispensed during the measurement year
- **G9809** Patients who use hospice services any time during the measurement period
- **G9810** Patient achieved a PDC of at least 75% for their asthma controller medication
- **G9811** Patient did not achieve a PDC of at least 75% for their asthma controller medication
- **G9812** Patient died including all deaths occurring during the hospitalization in which the operation was performed, even if after 30 days, and those deaths occurring after discharge from the hospital, but within 30 days of the procedure
- **G9813** Patient did not die within 30 days of the procedure or during the index hospitalization
- **G9814** Death occurring during hospitalization
- **G9815** Death did not occur during hospitalization
- **G9816** Death occurring 30 days post procedure
- **G9817** Death did not occur 30 days post procedure
- **G9818** Documentation of sexual activity
- **G9819** Patients who use hospice services any time during the measurement period
- **G9820** Documentation of a chlamydia screening test with proper follow-up
- **G9821** No documentation of a chlamydia screening test with proper follow-up

- **G9822** Women who had an endometrial ablation procedure during the year prior to the index date (exclusive of the index date)
- **G9823** Endometrial sampling or hysteroscopy with biopsy and results documented
- **G9824** Endometrial sampling or hysteroscopy with biopsy and results not documented
- **G9825** Her-2/neu negative or undocumented/unknown
- **G9826** Patient transferred to practice after initiation of chemotherapy
- **G9827** Her2-targeted therapies not administered during the initial course of treatment
- **G9828** Her2-targeted therapies administered during the initial course of treatment
- **G9829** Breast adjuvant chemotherapy administered
- **G9830** Her-2/neu positive
- **G9831** AJCC stage at breast cancer diagnosis = ii or iii
- **G9832** AJCC stage at breast cancer diagnosis = i (ia or ib) and t-stage at breast cancer diagnosis does not equal = t1, t1a, t1b
- **G9833** Patient transfer to practice after initiation of chemotherapy
- **G9834** Patient has metastatic disease at diagnosis
- **G9835** Trastuzumab administered within 12 months of diagnosis
- **G9836** Reason for not administering trastuzumab documented (e.g. patient declined, patient died, patient transferred, contraindication or other clinical exclusion, neoadjuvant chemotherapy or radiation not complete)
- **G9837** Trastuzumab not administered within 12 months of diagnosis
- **G9838** Patient has metastatic disease at diagnosis
- **G9839** Anti-EGFR monoclonal antibody therapy
- **G9840** KRAS gene mutation testing performed before initiation of anti-EGFR MoAb
- **G9841** KRAS gene mutation testing not performed before initiation of anti-EGFR MoAb
- **G9842** Patient has metastatic disease at diagnosis
- **G9843** KRAS gene mutation
- **G9844** Patient did not receive anti-EGFR monoclonal antibody therapy
- **G9845** Patient received anti-EGFR monoclonal antibody therapy
- **G9846** Patients who died from cancer
- **G9847** Patient received chemotherapy in the last 14 days of life
- **G9848** Patient did not receive chemotherapy in the last 14 days of life
- **G9849** Patients who died from cancer
- **G9850** Patient had more than one emergency department visit in the last 30 days of life
- **G9851** Patient had one or less emergency department visits in the last 30 days of life
- **G9852** Patients who died from cancer

- • **G9853** Patient admitted to the ICU in the last 30 days of life
- • **G9854** Patient was not admitted to the ICU in the last 30 days of life
- • **G9855** Patients who died from cancer
- • **G9856** Patient was not admitted to hospice
- • **G9857** Patient admitted to hospice
- • **G9858** Patient enrolled in hospice
- • **G9859** Patients who died from cancer
- • **G9860** Patient spent less than three days in hospice care
- • **G9861** Patient spent greater than or equal to three days in hospice care
- • **G9862** Documentation of medical reason(s) for not recommending at least a 10 year follow-up interval (e.g., inadequate prep, familial or personal history of colonic polyps, patient had no adenoma and age is = 66 years old, or life expectancy < 10 years old, other medical reasons)
- • **J0570** Buprenorphine implant, 74.2 mg
- ▲ **J0573** Buprenorphine/naloxone, oral, greater than 3 mg, but less than or equal to 6 mg buprenorphine
- (**J0760** Code deleted December 31, 2016.)
- • **J0883** Injection, argatroban, 1 mg (for non-esrd use)
- • **J0884** Injection, argatroban, 1 mg (for esrd on dialysis)
- • **J1130** Injection, diclofenac sodium, 0.5 mg
- (**J1590** Code deleted December 31, 2016.)
- ▲ **J1745** Injection, infliximab, excludes biosimilar, 10 mg
- • **J1942** Injection, aripiprazole lauroxil, 1 mg
- • **J2182** Injection, mepolizumab, 1 mg
- • **J2786** Injection, reslizumab, 1 mg
- • **J2840** Injection, sebelipase alfa, 1 mg
- ▲ **J3357** Ustekinumab, for subcutaneous injection, 1 mg
- • **J7175** Injection, factor x, (human), 1 i.u.
- • **J7179** Injection, von Willebrand factor (recombinant), (Vonvendi), 1 i.u. vwf:rco
- ▲ **J7201** Injection, factor ix, Fc fusion protein, (recombinant), alprolix, 1 i.u.
- • **J7202** Injection, factor ix, albumin fusion protein, (recombinant), idelvion, 1 i.u.
- • **J7207** Injection, factor viii, (antihemophilic factor, recombinant), pegylated, 1 i.u.
- • **J7209** Injection, factor viii, (antihemophilic factor, recombinant), (Nuwiq), 1 i.u.
- ▲ **J7297** Levonorgestrel-releasing intrauterine contraceptive system (liletta), 52 mg
- ▲ **J7298** Levonorgestrel-releasing intrauterine contraceptive system (Mirena), 52 mg

▲ **J7301** Levonorgestrel-releasing intrauterine contraceptive system (skyla), 13.5 mg

• **J7320** Hyaluronan or derivative, genvisc 850, for intra-articular injection, 1 mg

• **J7322** Hyaluronan or derivative, hymovis, for intra-articular injection, 1 mg

▲ **J7340** Carbidopa 5 mg/levodopa 20 mg enteral suspension, 100 ml

• **J7342** Installation, ciprofloxacin otic suspension, 6 mg

• **J8670** Rolapitant, oral, 1 mg

▲ **J9033** Injection, bendamustine HCL (Treanda), 1 mg

• **J9034** Injection, bendamustine HCL (bendeka), 1 mg

• **J9145** Injection, daratumumab, 10 mg

• **J9176** Injection, elotuzumab, 1 mg

• **J9205** Injection, irinotecan liposome, 1 mg

• **J9295** Injection, necitumumab, 1 mg

• **J9325** Injection, talimogene laherparepvec, per 1 million plaque forming units

• **J9352** Injection, trabectedin, 0.1 mg

▲ **K0019** Arm pad, replacement only, each

▲ **K0037** High mount flip-up footrest, replacement only, each

▲ **K0042** Standard size footplate, replacement only, each

▲ **K0043** Footrest, lower extension tube, replacement only, each

▲ **K0044** Footrest, upper hanger bracket, replacement only, each

▲ **K0045** Footrest, complete assembly, replacement only, each

▲ **K0046** Elevating leg rest, lower extension tube, replacement only, each

▲ **K0047** Elevating leg rest, upper hanger bracket, replacement only, each

▲ **K0050** Ratchet assembly, replacement only

▲ **K0051** Cam release assembly, footrest or leg rest, replacement only, each

▲ **K0052** Swing-Away, detachable footrests, replacement only, each

▲ **K0069** Rear wheel assembly, complete, with solid tire, spokes or molded, replacement only, each

▲ **K0071** Front caster assembly, complete, with pneumatic tire, replacement only, each

▲ **K0072** Front caster assembly, complete, with semi-pneumatic tire, replacement only, each

▲ **K0077** Front caster assembly, complete, with solid tire, replacement only, each

▲ **K0098** Drive belt for power wheelchair, replacement only

▲ **K0552** Supplies for external non-insulin drug infusion pump, syringe type cartridge, sterile, each

(**K0901** Code deleted December 31, 2016.)

(**K0902** Code deleted December 31, 2016.)

- • **L1851** Knee orthosis (KO), single upright, thigh and calf, with adjustable flexion and extension joint (unicentric or polycentric), medial-lateral and rotation control, with or without varus/valgus adjustment, prefabricated, off-the-shelf
- • **L1852** Knee orthosis (KO), double upright, thigh and calf, with adjustable flexion and extension joint (unicentric or polycentric), medial-lateral and rotation control, with or without varus/valgus adjustment, prefabricated, off-the-shelf
- ▲ **L1906** Ankle foot orthosis, multiligamentous ankle support, prefabricated, off-the-shelf
- ▲ **P9072** Platelets, pheresis, pathogen reduced or rapid bacterial tested, each unit
- ▲ **Q2039** Influenza virus vaccine, not otherwise specified
- ▲ **Q4105** Integra dermal regeneration template (DRT) or Integra omnigraft dermal regeneration matrix, per square centimeter
- (**Q4119** Code deleted December 31, 2016.)
- (**Q4120** Code deleted December 31, 2016.)
- (**Q4129** Code deleted December 31, 2016.)
- ▲ **Q4131** Epifix or epicord, per square centimeter
- • **Q4166** Cytal, per square centimeter
- • **Q4167** Truskin, per square centimeter
- • **Q4168** Amnioband, 1 mg
- • **Q4169** Artacent wound, per square centimeter
- • **Q4170** Cygnus, per square centimeter
- • **Q4171** Interfyl, 1 mg
- • **Q4172** PuraPly or PuraPly am, per square centimeter
- • **Q4173** Palingen or Palingen xplus, per square centimeter
- • **Q4174** Palingen or promatrx, 0.36 mg per 0.25 cc
- • **Q4175** Miroderm, per square centimeter
- • **Q5102** Injection, infliximab, biosimilar, 10 mg
- (**Q9980** Code deleted December 31, 2016.)
- (**Q9981** Code deleted December 31, 2016.)
- • **Q9982** Flutemetamol f18, diagnostic, per study dose, up to 5 millicuries
- • **Q9983** Florbetaben f18, diagnostic, per study dose, up to 8.1 millicuries
- • **S0285** Colonoscopy consultation performed prior to a screening colonoscopy procedure
- • **S0311** Comprehensive management and care coordination for advanced illness, per calendar month
- (**S8032** Code deleted September 30, 2016.)
- • **T1040** Medicaid certified community behavioral health clinic services, per diem
- • **T1041** Medicaid certified community behavioral health clinic services, per month

APPENDIX C: TABLE OF DRUGS

HCPCS Table of Drugs

Directions for the Use of the Table:

1. All drugs are listed in strict alphabetical order by generic drug name.

2. HCPCS code numbers for drugs are listed only under the generic drug name. Users should first look for entries under generic names of drugs. When a drug is known only by brand name, look for the brand name and you will be directed to the generic name of the drug (see "generic name".

3. Information which is indented and appears beneath the first line for a drug is to be considered a continuation of the line preceding it. All drug entries should be checked for indented lines beneath it as a continuation of that entry.

4. When one drug has more than one entry as a result of different routes of administration or different amounts, the drug name is not repeated. All entries for the same drug are listed beneath that drug.

5. The following abbreviations are used in the "routes of administration" column:

   amp = ampule

   DME = durable medical equipment

   EPI = epidural

   G = gram

   IA = intra-arterial administration

   IM = intramuscular administration

   INF = infusion

   INH = administration by inhaled solution

   INJ = injection

   IO = intraocular

   IT = intrathecal

   IU = international unit

   IV = intravenous administration

   mcg = microgram

   mg = milligram

   ml = milliliter

   ORAL = administered orally

   OTH = other routes of administration

   PAR = parenteral

SC = subcutaneous administration

TABS = tablets

U = units

VAR = various routes of administration

DRUG	DOSE	ROUTE	HCPCS
A			
Abatacept	**10 mg**	**IV**	**J0129**
Abbokinase, *see* Urokinase			
Abbokinase, Open Cath, *see* Urokinase			
Abciximab	10 mg	IV	J0130
Abelcet, *see* Amphotericin B Lipid Complex			
ABLC, *see* Amphotericin B			
AbobotulinumtoxintypeA	5 units	IM	J0586
Acetaminophen	10 mg	IV	J0131
Acetazolamide sodium	up to 500 mg	IM, IV	J1120
Acetylcysteine, IVection	100 mg	IV	J0132
Acetylcysteine, unit dose form	per gram	INH	J7604, J7608
Achromycin, *see* Tetracycline			
Actemra, *see* Tocilizumab			
ACTH, *see* Corticotropin			
Acthar, *see* Corticotropin			
Actimmune, *see* Interferon gamma 1-B			
Activase, *see* Alteplase recombinant			
Acyclovir	5 mg		J0133
Adalimumab	20 mg	SC	J0135
Adcetis, *see* Brentuximab Vedotin			
Adenocard, *see* Adenosine			
Adenoscan, *see* Adenosine			
Adenosine	1 mg	IV	J0153
Ado-trastuzumab Emtansine	1 mg	IV	J9354
Adrenalin Chloride, *see* Adrenalin, epinephrine			
Adrenalin, epinephrine	0.1 mg	SC, IM	J0171
Adriamycin PFS, *see* Doxorubicin HCl			

DRUG	DOSE	ROUTE	HCPCS
Adriamycin RDF, *see* Doxorubicin HCl			
Adrucil, *see* Fluorouracil			
Aflibercept	1 mg	OTH	J0178
Agalsidase beta	1 mg	IV	J0180
Aggrastat, *see* Tirofiban hydrochloride			
A-hydroCort, *see* Hydrocortisone sodium phosphate			
Akineton, *see* Biperiden			
Alatrofloxacin mesylate, Ivection	100 mg	IV	J0200
Albuterol	0.5 mg	INH	J7620
Albuterol, concentrated form	1 mg	INH	J7610, J7611
Albuterol, unit dose form	1 mg	INH	J7609, J7613
Aldesleukin	per single use vial	IM, IV	J9015
Aldomet, *see* Methyldopate HCl			
Alefacept	0.5 mg	IM, IV	J0215
Alferon N, *see* Interferon alfa-n3			
Alglucerase	per 10 units	IV	J0205
Alglucosidase alfa	10 mg	IV	J0220, J0221
Alkaban-AQ, *see* Vinblastine sulfate			
Alkeran, *see* Melphalan, oral			
Alpha 1-proteinase inhibitor, human	10 mg	IV	J0256, J0257
Alphanate			J7186
Alprostadil, Ivection	1.25 mcg	OTH	J0270
Alprostadil, urethral suppository		OTH	J0275
Alteplase recombinant	1 mg	IV	J2997
Alupent, *see* Metaproterenol sulfate or Metaproterenol, compounded			
Amcort, *see* Triamcinolone diacetate			
A-methaPred, *see* Methylprednisolone sodium succinate			
Amgen, *see* Interferon alphacon-1			
Amifostine	500 mg	IV	J0207
Amikacin sulfate	100 mg		J0278
Aminolevulinic acid HCl unit dose	(354 mg)	OTH	J7308

DRUG	DOSE	ROUTE	HCPCS
Aminolevulinate	1 gm	OTH	J7309
Aminophylline/Aminophyllin	up to 250 mg	IV	J0280
Amiodarone HCl	30 mg	IV	J0282
Amitriptyline HCl	up to 20 mg	IM	J1320
Amobarbital	up to 125 mg	IM, IV	J0300
Amphocin, *see* Amphotericin B			
Amphotericin B 50 mg	IV	J0285	
Amphotericin B, lipid complex	10 mg	IV	J0287-J0289
Ampicillin sodium	up to 500 mg	IM, IV	J0290
Ampicillin sodium/sulbactam sodium	per 1.5 gm	IM, IV	J0295
Amygdalin, *see* Laetrile, Amygdalin, vitamin B-17			
Amytal, *see* Amobarbital			
Anabolin LA 100, *see* Nandrolone decanoate			
Anidulafungin	1 mg	IV	J0348
Anascorp, *see* Centruroides Immune F(ab)			
Ancef, *see* Cefazolin sodium			
Andrest 90-4, *see* Testosterone enanthate and estradiol valerate			
Andro-Cyp, *see* Testosterone cypionate			
Andro-Cyp 200, *see* Testosterone cypionate			
Andro L.A. 200, *see* Testosterone enanthate			
Andro-Estro 90-4, *see* Testosterone enanthate and estradiol valerate			
Andro/Fem, *see* Testosterone cypionate and estradiol cypionate			
Androgyn L.A., *see* Testosterone enanthate and estradiol valerate			
Androlone-50, *see* Nandrolone phenpropionate			
Androlone-D 100, *see* Nandrolone decanoate			
Andronaq-50, *see* Testosterone suspension			
Andronaq-LA, *see* Testosterone cypionate			
Andronate-200, *see* Testosterone cypionate			
Andronate-100, *see* Testosterone cypionate			
Andropository 100, *see* Testosterone enanthate			

DRUG	DOSE	ROUTE	HCPCS
Andryl 200, *see* Testosterone enanthate			
Anectine, *see* Succinylcholine chloride			
Anergan 25, *see* Promethazine HCl			
Anergan 50, *see* Promethazine HCl			
Anistreplase	30 units	IV	J0350
Anti-Inhibitor	per IU	IV	J7198
Antispas, *see* Dicyclomine HCl			
Antithrombin III (human)	per IU	IV	J7197
Antithrombin recombinant	50 IU	IV	J7196
Anzemet, *see* Dolasetron mesylate IVection			
A.P.L., *see* Chorionic gonadotropin			
Apomorphine Hydrochloride	1 mg	SC	J0364
Apresoline, *see* Hydralazine HCl			
Aprotinin	10,000 k	IU	J0365
AquaMEPHYTON, *see* Vitamin K			
Aralen, *see* Chloroquine HCl			
Aramine, *see* Metaraminol			
Aranesp, *see* Darbepoetin Alfa			
Arbutamine	1 mg	IV	J0395
Arcalyst, *see* Rilonacept			
Aredia, *see* Pamidronate disodium			
Arfonad, *see* Trimethaphan camsylate			
Arformoterol tartrate	15 mcg	INH	J7605
Argatroban (for non-ESRD use)	1 mg	IV	J0883
(for ESRD use)	1 mg	IV	J0884
Aridol, *see* Mannitol			
Aripiprazole 0.25 mg	IM	J0400	
Aripiprazole, extended release 1 mg	IV	J0401	
Aripiprazole lauroxil 1 mg	IV	J1942	
Aristocort Forte, *see* Triamcinolone diacetate			
Aristocort Intralesional, *see* Triamcinolone diacetate			
Aristospan Intra-Articular, *see* Triamcinolone hexacetonide			

DRUG	DOSE	ROUTE	HCPCS
Aristospan Intralesional, *see* Triamcinolone hexacetonide			
Arrestin, *see* Trimethobenzamide HCl			
Arsenic trioxide	1 mg	IV	J9017
Arzerra, *see* Ofatumumab			
Asparaginase	1,000 units	IV, IM	J9019
	10,000 units	IV, IM	J9020
Astramorph PF, *see* Morphine sulfate			
Atgam, *see* Lymphocyte immune globulin			
Ativan, *see* Lorazepam			
Atropine, concentrated form	per mg	INH	J7635
Atropine, unit dose form	per mg	INH	J7636
Atropine sulfate	0.01 mg	IV, IM, SC	J0461
Atrovent, *see* Ipratropium bromide			
Atryn, *see* Antithrombin recombinant			
Aurothioglucose	up to 50 mg	IM	J2910
Autologous cultured chondrocytes implant		OTH	J7330
Autoplex T, *see* Hemophilia clotting factors			
Avonex, *see* Interferon beta-1a			
Azacitidine	1 mg	SC	J9025
Azathioprine	50 mg	ORAL	J7500
Azathioprine, parenteral	100 mg	IV	J7501
Azithromycin, dihydrate	1 gm	ORAL	Q0144
Azithromycin, IVection	500 mg	IV	J0456
B			
Baclofen	10 mg	IT	J0475
Baclofen for intrathecal trial	50 mcg	OTH	J0476
Bactocill, *see* Oxacillin sodium			
BAL in oil, *see* Dimercaprol			
Banflex, *see* Orphenadrine citrate			
Basiliximab	20 mg		J0480
BCG (Bacillus Calmette and Guérin), live	per vial	IV	J9031
instillation			
Beclomethasone inhalation solution, unit dose form	per mg	INH	J7622

DRUG	DOSE	ROUTE	HCPCS
Belatacept	1 mg	IV	J0485
Belimumab	10 mg	IV	J0490
Belinostat	10 mg	IV	J9032
Bena-D 10, *see* Diphenhydramine HCl			
Bena-D 50, *see* Diphenhydramine HCl			
Benadryl, *see* Diphenhydramine HCl			
Benahist 10, *see* Diphenhydramine HCl			
Benahist 50, *see* Diphenhydramine HCl			
Ben-Allergin-50, *see* Diphenhydramine HCl			
Bendamustine HCl	1 mg	IV	J9033
BeneFIX, *see* Factor IX, recombinant			
Benlysta, *see* Belimumab			
Benoject-10, *see* Diphenhydramine HCl			
Benoject-50, *see* Diphenhydramine HCl			
Bentyl, *see* Dicyclomine			
Benztropine mesylate	per 1 mg	IM, IV	J0515
Berinert, *see* C-1 esterase inhibitor			
Berubigen, *see* Vitamin B-12 cyanocobalamin			
Beta amyloid	per study dose	OTH	A9599
Betalin 12, *see* Vitamin B-12 cyanocobalamin			
Betameth, *see* Betamethasone sodium phosphate			
Betamethasone acetate & betamethasone sodium phosphate	per 3 mg	IM	J0702
Betamethasone inhalation solution, unit doseform	per mg	INH	J7624
Betaseron, *see* Interferon beta-1b			
Bethanechol chloride	up to 5 mg	SC	J0520
Bevacizumab	10 mg	IV	J9035
Bicillin L-A, *see* Penicillin G benzathine			
Bicillin C-R 900/300, *see* Penicillin G procaine and penicillin G benzathine			
Bicillin C-R, *see* Penicillin G benzathine and penicillin G procaine			
BiCNU, *see* Carmustine			

DRUG	DOSE	ROUTE	HCPCS
Biperiden lactate	per 5 mg	IM, IV	J0190
Bitolterol mesylate, concentrated form	per mg	INH	J7628
Bitolterol mesylate, unit dose form	per mg	INH	J7629
Bivalirudin	1 mg	IV	J0583
Blenoxane, *see* Bleomycin sulfate			
Bleomycin sulfate	15 units	IM, IV, SC	J9040
Blinatumomab	1 microgram	IV	J9039
Bortezomib	0.1 mg	IV	J9041
Botox, *see* OnabotulinumtoxinA			
Brentuximab Vedotin	1 mg	IV	J9042
Brethine, *see* Terbutaline sulfate or Terbutaline, compounded			
Bricanyl Subcutaneous, *see* Terbutaline sulfate			
Brompheniramine maleate	per 10 mg	IM, SC, IV	J0945
Bronkephrine, *see* Ethylnorepinephrine HCl			
Bronkosol, *see* Isoetharine HCl			
Budesonide inhalation solution, concentrated form	0.25 mg	INH	J7633, J7634
Budesonide inhalation solution, unit dose form	0.5 mg	INH	J7626, J7627
Buprenorphine Hydrochloride	0.1 mg	IM	J0592
Buprenorphine/Naloxone	1 mg	ORAL	J0571
	< = 3 mg	ORAL	J0572
	> 3 mg but < = 6 mg	ORAL	J0573
	> 6 mg but < = 10 mg	ORAL	J0574
	> 10 mg	ORAL	J0575
Busulfan	1 mg	IV	J0594
Busulfan	2 mg	ORAL	J8510
Butorphanol tartrate	1 mg		J0595
C			
C1 Esterase Inhibitor	10 units	IV	J0596-J0598
Cabazitaxel	1 mg	IV	J9043
Cabergoline	.25 mg	ORAL	J8515
Cafcit, *see* Caffeine citrate			

DRUG	DOSE	ROUTE	HCPCS
Caffeine citrate	5 mg	IV	J0706
Caine-1, *see* Lidocaine HCl			
Caine-2, *see* Lidocaine HCl			
Calcijex, *see* Calcitriol			
Calcimar, *see* Calcitonin-salmon			
Calcitonin-salmon	up to 400 units	SC, IM	J0630
Calcitriol	0.1 mcg	IM	J0636
Calcium Disodium Versenate, *see* Edetate calcium disodium			
Calcium gluconate	per 10 ml	IV	J0610
Calcium glycerophosphate & calcium lactate	per 10 ml	IM, SC	J0620
Caldolor, *see* Ibuprofen			
Calphosan, *see* Calcium glycerophosphate and calcium lactate			
Camptosar, *see* Irinotecan			
Canakinumab	1 mg	SC	J0638
Capecitabine	150 mg	ORAL	J8520
	500 mg	ORAL	J8521
Capsaicin patch	per sq cm	OTH	J7336
Carbidopa 5 mg/levodopa 20 mg	enteral suspension	IV	J7340
Carbocaine with Neo-Cobefrin, *see* Mepivacaine			
Carbocaine, *see* Mepivacaine			
Carboplatin	50 mg	IV	J9045
Carfilzomib	1 mg	IV	J9047
Carmustine	100 mg	IV	J9050
Carnitor, *see* Levocarnitine			
Carticel, *see* Autologous cultured chondrocytes			
Caspofungin acetate	5 mg	IV	J0637
Cayston, *see* Aztreonam			
Cefadyl, *see* Cephapirin Sodium			
Cefazolin sodium	500 mg	IV, IM	J0690
Cefepime hydrochloride	500 mg	IV	J0692

DRUG	DOSE	ROUTE	HCPCS
Cefizox, *see* Ceftizoxime sodium			
Cefotaxime sodium	per 1 g	IV, IM	J0698
Cefoxitin sodium	1 g	IV, IM	J0694
Ceftaroline fosamil	1 mg		J0712
Ceftazidime	per 500 mg	IM, IV	J0713
Ceftazidime and Avibactam	0.5 g/0.125 g	IV	J0714
Ceftizoxime sodium	per 500 mg	IV, IM	J0715
Ceftriaxone sodium	per 250 mg	IV, IM	J0696
Ceftolozane 50 mg and tazobactam	25 mg	IV	J0695
Cefuroxime sodium, sterile	per 750 mg	IM, IV	J0697
Celestone Soluspan, *see* Betamethasone acetate and betamethasone sodium phosphate			
CellCept, *see* Mycophenolate mofetil			
Cel-U-Jec, *see* Betamethasone sodium phosphate			
Cenacort Forte, *see* Triamcinolone diacetate			
Cenacort A-40, *see* Triamcinolone acetonide			
Centruroides Immune F(ab)	up to 120 mg	IV	J0716
Cephalothin sodium	up to 1 g	IM, IV	J1890
Cephapirin sodium	up to 1 g	IV, IM	J0710
Ceredase, *see* Alglucerase			
Certolizumab pegol	1 mg	SC	J0717
Cerubidine, *see* Daunorubicin HCl			
Cetuximab	10 mg	IV	J9055
Chealamide, *see* Endrate ethylenediamine-tetra-acetic acid			
Chloramphenicol sodium succinate	up to 1 g	IV	J0720
Chlordiazepoxide HCl	up to 100 mg	IM, IV	J1990
Chloromycetin Sodium Succinate, *see* Chloramphenicol sodium succinate			
Chloroprocaine HCl	per 30 ml	VAR	J2400
Chlorpromazine	5 mg	ORAL	Q0161
Chloroquine HCl	up to 250 mg	IM	J0390
Chlorothiazide sodium	per 500 mg	IV	J1205
Chlorpromazine HCl	up to 50 mg	IM, IV	J3230

DRUG	DOSE	ROUTE	HCPCS
Chorex-5, *see* Chorionic gonadotropin			
Chorex-10, *see* Chorionic gonadotropin			
Chorignon, *see* Chorionic gonadotropin			
Chorionic gonadotropin	per 1,000 USP units	IM	J0725
Choron 10, *see* Chorionic gonadotropin			
Cidofovir	375 mg	IV	J0740
Cilastatin sodium, imipenem	per 250 mg	IV, IM	J0743
Cimzia, *see* Certolizumab pegol			
Cinryze, *see* C1 Esterase Inhibitor			
Cipro IV, *see* Ciprofloxacin			
Ciprofloxacin	200 mg	IV	J0706
octic suspension	6 mg	OTH	J7342
Cisplatin, powder or solution	per 10 mg	IV	J9060
Cladribine	per mg	IV	J9065
Claforan, *see* Cefotaxime sodium			
Clofarabine	1 mg	IV	J9027
Clonidine Hydrochloride	1 mg	epidural	J0735
Cobex, *see* Vitamin B-12 cyanocobalamin			
Codeine phosphate	per 30 mg	IM, IV, SC	J0745
Codimal-A, *see* Brompheniramine maleate			
Cogentin, *see* Benztropine mesylate			
Collagenase, Clostridium Histolyticum	0.01 mg	OTH	J0775
Colistimethate sodium	up to 150 mg	IM, IV	J0770
Coly-Mycin M, *see* Colistimethate sodium			
Compa-Z, *see* Prochlorperazine			
Compazine, *see* Prochlorperazine			
Compounded drug, not otherwise classified			J7999
Cophene-B, *see* Brompheniramine maleate			
Cop per contraceptive, intrauterine		OTH	J7300
Cordarone, *see* Amiodarone HCl			
Corgonject-5, *see* Chorionic gonadotropin			
Corticorelin ovine triflutate	1 mcg		J0795

DRUG	DOSE	ROUTE	HCPCS
Corticotropin	up to 40 units	IV, IM, SC	J0800
Cortrosyn, *see* Cosyntropin			
Cosmegen, *see* Dactinomycin			
Cosyntropin	per 0.25 mg	IM, IV	J0833, J0834
Cotranzine, *see* Prochlorperazine			
CroFab, *see* Crotalidae Polyvalent Immune Fab			
Cromolyn sodium, unit dose form	per 10 mg	INH	J7631, J7632
Crotalidae Polyvalent Immune Fab	up to 1 gram	IV	J0840
Crysticillin 300 A.S., *see* Penicillin G procaine			
Crysticillin 600 A.S., *see* Penicillin G procaine			
Cyclophosphamide	100 mg	IV	J9070
Cyclophosphamide, oral	25 mg	ORAL	J8530
Cyclosporine, oral	25 mg	ORAL	J7515
	100 mg	ORAL	J7502
Cyclosporine, parenteral	250 mg	IV	J7516
Cytarabine	100 mg	SC, IV	J9100
Cytarabine liposome	10 mg	IT	J9098
Cytomegalovirus immune globulin intravenous(human)	per vial	IV	J0850
Cytosar-U, *see* Cytarabine			
Cytovene, *see* Ganciclovir sodium			
Cytoxan, *see* Cyclophosphamide; cyclophosphamide, lyophilized; and cyclophosphamide, oral			
D			
D-5-W, infusion	1000 cc	IV	J7070
Dacarbazine	100 mg	IV	J9130
Daclizumab	25 mg	IV	J7513
Dactinomycin	0.5 mg	IV	J9120
Dalalone, *see* Dexamethasone sodium phosphate			
Dalalone L.A., *see* Dexamethasone acetate			
Dalbavancin	5 mg	IV	J0875
Dalteparin sodium	per 2500 IU	SC	J1645
Daptomycin	1 mg	IV	J0878
Daratumumab	10 mg	IV	J9145

DRUG	DOSE	ROUTE	HCPCS
Darbepoetin Alfa	1 mcg	IV, SC	J0881, J0882
Daunorubicin citrate, liposomal	10 mg	IV	J9151
formulation			
Daunorubicin HCl	10 mg	IV	J9150
DaunoXome, *see* Daunorubicin citrate			
DDAVP, *see* Desmopressin acetate			
Decadron Phosphate, *see* Dexamethasone sodium phosphate			
Decadron, *see* Dexamethasone sodium phosphate			
Decadron-LA, *see* Dexamethasone acetate			
Deca-Durabolin, *see* Nandrolone decanoate			
Decaject, *see* Dexamethasone sodium phosphate			
Decaject-L.A., *see* Dexamethasone acetate			
Decitabine	1 mg	IV	J0894
Decolone-50, *see* Nandrolone decanoate			
Decolone-100, *see* Nandrolone decanoate			
De-Comberol, *see* Testosterone cypionate and estradiol cypionate			
Deferoxamine mesylate	500 mg	IM, SC, IV	J0895
Degarelix	1 mg	SC	J9155
Dehist, *see* Brompheniramine maleate			
Deladumone OB, *see* Testosterone enanthate and estradiol valerate			
Deladumone, *see* Testosterone enanthate and estradiol valerate			
Delatest, *see* Testosterone enanthate			
Delatestadiol, *see* Testosterone enanthate and estradiol valerate			
Delatestryl, *see* Testosterone enanthate			
Delta-Cortef, *see* Prednisolone, oral			
Delestrogen, *see* Estradiol valerate			
Demadex, *see* Torsemide			
Demerol HCl, *see* Meperidine HCl			
Denileukin diftitox	300 mcg	IV	J9160
Denosumab	1 mg	SC	J0897

DRUG	DOSE	ROUTE	HCPCS
DepAndro 100, *see* Testosterone cypionate			
DepAndro 200, *see* Testosterone cypionate			
DepAndrogyn, *see* Testosterone cypionate and estradiol cypionate			
DepGynogen, *see* Depo-estradiol cypionate			
DepMedalone 40, *see* Methylprednisolone acetate			
DepMedalone 80, *see* Methylprednisolone acetate			
Depo-estradiol cypionate	up to 5 mg	IM	J1000
Depogen, *see* Depo-estradiol cypionate			
Depoject, *see* Methylprednisolone acetate			
Depo-Medrol, *see* Methylprednisolone acetate			
Depopred-40, *see* Methylprednisolone acetate			
Depopred-80, *see* Methylprednisolone acetate			
Depo-Provera, *see* Medroxyprogesterone acetate			
Depotest, *see* Testosterone cypionate			
Depo-Testadiol, *see* Testosterone cypionate and estradiol cypionate			
Depotestogen, *see* Testosterone cypionate and estradiol cypionate			
Depo-Testosterone, *see* Testosterone cypionate			
Desferal Mesylate, *see* Deferoxamine mesylate			
Desmopressin acetate	1 mcg	IV, SC	J2597
Dexacen LA-8, *see* Dexamethasone acetate			
Dexacen-4, *see* Dexamethasone sodium phosphate			
Dexamethasone, concentrated form	per mg	INH	J7637
Dexamethasone, unit form	per mg	INH	J7638
Dexamethasone, intravitreal implant	0.1 mg	OTH	J7312
Dexamethasone, oral	0.25 mg	ORAL	J8540
Dexamethasone acetate	1 mg	IM	J1094
Dexamethasone sodium phosphate	1 mg	IM, IV, OTH	J1100
Dexasone, *see* Dexamethasone sodium phosphate			
Dexasone L.A., *see* Dexamethasone acetate			
Dexferrum, *see* Iron Dextran			
Dexone, *see* Dexamethasone sodium phosphate			

DRUG	DOSE	ROUTE	HCPCS
Dexone LA, *see* Dexamethasone acetate			
Dexrazoxane hydrochloride	250 mg	IV	J1190
Dextran 40	500 ml	IV	J7100
Dextran 75	500 ml	IV	J7110
Dextrose 5%/normal saline solution,	500 ml = 1 unit	IV	J7042
Dextrose/water (5%)	500 ml = 1 unit	IV	J7060
D.H.E. 45, *see* Dihydroergotamine			
Diamox, *see* Acetazolamide sodium			
Diazepam	up to 5 mg	IM, IV	J3360
Diazoxide	up to 300 mg	IV	J1730
Dibent, *see* Dicyclomine HCl			
Diclofenac sodium	37.5 I	V	J1130
Dicyclomine HCl	up to 20 mg	IM	J0500
Didronel, *see* Etidronate disodium			
Diethylstilbestrol diphosphate	250 mg	IV	J9165
Diflucan, *see* Fluconazole			
Digoxin	up to 0.5 mg	IM, IV	J1160
Digoxin immune Fab (ovine)	per vial		J1162
Dihydrex, *see* Diphenhydramine HCl			
Dihydroergotamine mesylate	per 1 mg	IM, IV	J1110
Dilantin, *see* Phenytoin sodium			
Dilaudid, *see* Hydromorphone HCl			
Dilocaine, *see* Lidocaine HCl			
Dilomine, *see* Dicyclomine HCl			
Dilor, *see* Dyphylline			
Dimenhydrinate	up to 50 mg	IM, IV	J1240
Dimercaprol	per 100 mg	IM	J0470
Dimethyl sulfoxide, *see* DMSO, Dimethylsulfoxide			
Dinate, *see* Dimenhydrinate			
Dioval, *see* Estradiol valerate			
Dioval 40, *see* Estradiol valerate			
Dioval XX, *see* Estradiol valerate			

DRUG	DOSE	ROUTE	HCPCS
Diphenacen-50, *see* Diphenhydramine HCl			
Diphenhydramine HCl, IVection	up to 50 mg	IV, IM	J1200
Diphenhydramine HCl, oral	50 mg	ORAL	Q0163
Dipyridamole	per 10 mg	IV	J1245
Disotate, *see* Endrate ethylenediamine-tetra-acetic acid			
Di-Spaz, *see* Dicyclomine HCl			
Ditate-DS, *see* Testosterone enanthate and estradiol valerate			
Diuril Sodium, *see* Chlorothiazide sodium			
D-Med 80, *see* Methylprednisolone acetate			
DMSO, Dimethyl sulfoxide	50%, 50 ml	OTH	J1212
Dobutamine HCl	per 250 mg	IV	J1250
Dobutrex, *see* Dobutamine HCl			
Docetaxel	20 mg	IV	J9170
Dolasetron mesylate, IVection	10 mg	IV	J1260
Dolasetron mesylate, tablets	100 mg	ORAL	Q0180
Dolophine HCl, *see* Methadone HCl			
Dommanate, *see* Dimenhydrinate			
Donbax, *see* Doripenem			
Dopamine HCl	40 mg		J1265
Doribax, *see* Doripenem			
Doripenem	10 mg	IV	J1267
Dornase alpha, unit dose form	per mg	INH	J7639
Doxercalciferol	1 mcg	IV	J1270
Doxil, *see* Doxorubicin HCL, lipid			
Doxorubicin HCL	10 mg	IV	J9000
Dramamine, *see* Dimenhydrinate			
Dramanate, *see* Dimenhydrinate			
Dramilin, *see* Dimenhydrinate			
Dramocen, *see* Dimenhydrinate			
Dramoject, *see* Dimenhydrinate			
Dronabinol, oral	2.5 mg	ORAL	Q0167
Droperidol	up to 5 mg	IM, IV	J1790

DRUG	DOSE	ROUTE	HCPCS
Drug administered through a metered dose	inhaler	INH	J3535
Droperidol and fentanyl citrate	up to 2 ml ampule	IM, IV	J1810
DTIC-Dome, *see* Dacarbazine			
Dua-Gen L.A., *see* Testosterone enanthate and estradiol valerate cypionate			
Duoval P.A., *see* Testosterone enanthate and estradiol valerate			
Durabolin, *see* Nandrolone phenpropionate			
Duraclon, *see* Clonidine Hydrochloride			
Dura-Estrin, *see* Depo-estradiol cypionate			
Duracillin A.S., *see* Penicillin G procaine			
Duragen-10, *see* Estradiol valerate			
Duragen-20, *see* Estradiol valerate			
Duragen-40, *see* Estradiol valerate			
Duralone-40, *see* Methylprednisolone acetate			
Duralone-80, *see* Methylprednisolone acetate			
Duralutin, *see* Hydroxyprogesterone Caproate			
Duramorph, *see* Morphine sulfate			
Duratest-100, *see* Testosterone cypionate			
Duratest-200, *see* Testosterone cypionate			
Duratestrin, *see* Testosterone cypionate and estradiol cypionate			
Durathate-200, *see* Testosterone enanthate			
Dymenate, *see* Dimenhydrinate			
Dyphylline	up to 500 mg	IM	J1180
Dysport, *see* AbobotulinumtoxintypeA			
E			
Ecallantide	1 mg	SC	J1290
Eculizumab	10 mg	IV	J1300
Edetate calcium disodium	up to 1000 mg	IV, SC, IM	J0600
Edetate disodium	per 150 mg	IV	J3520
Elavil, *see* Amitriptyline HCl			
Ellence, *see* Epirubicin HCl			

DRUG	DOSE	ROUTE	HCPCS
Elliotts b solution	1 ml	OTH	J9175
Elosulfase alfa	1 mg	IV	J1322
Elotuzumab	1 mg	IV	J9176
Elspar, *see* Asparaginase			
Emend, *see* Fosaprepitant			
Emete-Con, *see* Benzquinamide			
Eminase, *see* Anistreplase			
Enbrel, *see* Etanercept			
Endrate ethylenediamine-tetra-acetic acid, *see* Edetate disodium			
Enfuvirtide	1 mg	SC	J1324
Enovil, *see* Amitriptyline HCl			
Enoxaparin sodium	10 mg	SC	J1650
Eovist, *see* Gadoxetate disodium			
Epinephrine, adrenalin	0.1 mg	SC, IM	J0171
Epirubicin hydrochloride	2 mg		J9178
Epoetin alfa	100 units	IV, SC	Q4081
Epoetin alfa, non-ESRD use	1000 units	IV	J0885
Epoetin beta, esrd use	1 mcg	IV	J0887
Epoetin beta, non-esrd use	1 mcg	IV	J0888
Epoprostenol	0.5 mg	IV	J1325
Eptifibatide, IVection	5 mg	IM, IV	J1327
Ergonovine maleate	up to 0.2 mg	IM, IV	J1330
Eribulin mesylate	0.1 mg	IV	J9179
Ertapenem sodium	500 mg	IM, IV	J1335
Erwinase, *see* Asparaginase			
Erythromycin lactobionate	500 mg	IV	J1364
Estra-D, *see* Depo-estradiol cypionate			
Estra-L 20, *see* Estradiol valerate			
Estra-L 40, *see* Estradiol valerate			
Estra-Testrin, *see* Testosterone enanthate and estradiol valerate			
Estradiol Cypionate, *see* Depo-estradiol cypionate			
Estradiol L.A., *see* Estradiol valerate			

DRUG	DOSE	ROUTE	HCPCS
Estradiol L.A. 20, *see* Estradiol valerate			
Estradiol L.A. 40, *see* Estradiol valerate			
Estradiol valerate	up to 10 mg	IM	J1380
Estro-Cyp, *see* Depo-estradiol cypionate			
Estrogen, conjugated	per 25 mg	IV, IM	J1410
Estroject-LA, *see* Depo-estradiol cypionate			
Estrone	per 1 mg	IM	J1435
Estrone 5, *see* Estrone			
Estrone Aqueous, *see* Estrone			
Estronol, *see* Estrone			
Estronol-L.A., *see* Depo-estradiol cypionate			
Etanercept, IVection	25 mg	IM, IV	J1438
Ethanolamine	100 mg		J1430
Ethyol, *see* Amifostine			
Etidronate disodium	per 300 mg	IV	J1436
Etonogestrel implant			J7307
Etopophos, *see* Etoposide			
Etoposide	10 mg	IV	J9181
Etoposide, oral	50 mg	ORAL	J8560
Euflexxa	per dose	OTH	J7323
Everolimus, oral	0.25 mg	ORAL	J7527
Everone, *see* Testosterone Enanthate			
Eylea, *see* Aflibercept			
F			
Factor VIIa (coagulation factor, recombinant)	1 mcg	IV	J7189
Factor VIII (anti-hemophilic factor, human)	per IU	IV	J7190
Factor VIII (anti-hemophilic factor, porcine)	per IU	IV	J7191
Factor VIII (anti-hemophilic factor, recombinant)	per IU	IV	J7182, J7185, J7192, J7188
Factor VIII fc fusion (recombinant)	per IU	IV	J7205, J7207, J7209
Factor IX (anti-hemophilic factor, purified, non-recombinant)	per IU	IV	J7193

DRUG	DOSE	ROUTE	HCPCS
Factor IX (anti-hemophilic factor, recombinant)	per IU	IV	J7195, J7200-J7202
Factor IX, complex	per IU	IV	J7194
Factor X (human)	per IU	IV	J7175
Factor XIII A-subunit (recombinant)	per IU	IV	J7181
Factors, other hemophilia clotting	per IU	IV	J7196
Factrel, *see* Gonadorelin HCl			
Feiba VH Immuno, *see* Factors, other hemophilia clotting			
Fentanyl citrate	0.1 mg	IM, IV	J3010
Feraheme, *see* Ferumoxytol			
Ferric Carboxymaltose	1 mg	IV	J1439
Ferric pyrophosphate citrate solution	0.1 mg of iron	IV	J1443
Ferrlecit, *see* Sodium ferric gluconate complex in sucrose IVection			
Ferumoxytol	1 mg		Q0138, Q0139
Filgrastim (G-CSF)	1 mcg	SC, IV	J1442, Q5101
Filgrastim (TBO)	1 mcg	IV	J1447
Firazyr, *see* Icatibant			
Firmagon, *see* Degarelix			
Flebogamma	500 mg	IV	J1572
Flexoject, *see* Orphenadrine citrate			
Flexon, *see* Orphenadrine citrate Flolan, *see* Epoprostenol			
Florbetaben f18, diagnostic	per study dose	IV	Q9983
Floxuridine	500 mg	IV	J9200
Fluconazole	200 mg	IV	J1450
Fludara, *see* Fludarabine phosphate			
Fludarabine phosphate	1 mg	ORAL	J8562
	50 mg	IV	J9185
Flunisolide inhalation solution, unit dose form	per mg	INH	J7641
Fluocinolone		OTH	J7311, J7313

DRUG	DOSE	ROUTE	HCPCS
Fluorouracil	500 mg	IV	J9190
Flutemetamol f18, diagnostic	per study dose	IV	Q9982
Folex, *see* Methotrexate sodium			
Folex PFS, *see* Methotrexate sodium			
Follutein, *see* Chorionic gonadotropin			
Folotyn, *see* Pralatrexate			
Fomepizole	15 mg		J1451
Fomivirsen sodium	1.65 mg	Intraocular	J1452
Fondaparinux sodium	0.5 mg	SC	J1652
Formoterol	12 mcg	INH	J7640
Formoterol fumarate	20 mcg	INH	J7606
Fortaz, *see* Ceftazidime			
Fosaprepitant	1 mg	IV	J1453
Foscarnet sodium	per 1,000 mg	IV	J1455
Foscavir, *see* Foscarnet sodium			
Fosphenytoin	50 mg	IV	Q2009
FUDR, *see* Floxuridine			
Fulvestrant	25 mg	IM	J9395
Fungizone Intravenous, *see* Amphotericin B			
Furomide M.D., *see* Furosemide			
Furosemide	up to 20 mg	IM, IV	J1940
G			
Gadoxetate disodium	1 ml	IV	A9581
Gallium nitrate	1 mg	IV	J1457
Galsulfase	1 mg	IV	J1458
GamaSTAN, *see* Gamma globulin and Immune globulin			
Gammagard Liquid	500 mg	IV	J1569
Gamma globulin	1 cc	IM	J1460
	over 10 cc	IM	J1560
Gammaplex	500 mg	IV	J1557
Gammar, *see* Gamma globulin and Immune globulin			

DRUG	DOSE	ROUTE	HCPCS
Gammar-IV, *see* Immune globulin intravenous (human)			
Gamulin RH, *see* Rho(D) immune globulin			
Gamunex	500 mg	IV	J1561
Ganciclovir, implant	4.5 mg	OTH	J7310
Ganciclovir sodium	500 mg	IV	J1570
Garamycin, gentamicin	up to 80 mg	IM, IV	J1580
Gatifloxacin	10 mg	IV	J1590
Gefitinib	250 mg	ORAL	J8565
Gel-One	per dose	OTH	J7326
Gemcitabine HCl	200 mg	IV	J9201
Gemsar, *see* Gemcitabine HCl			
Gemtuzumab ozogamicin	5 mg	IV	J9300
Gentamicin Sulfate, *see* Garamycin, gentamicin			
Gentran, *see* Dextran 40			
Gentran 75, *see* Dextran 75			
Gesterol 50, *see* Progesterone			
Glassia	10 mg	IV	J0257
Glatiramer Acetate	20 mg	SC	J1595
Glucagon HCl	per 1 mg	SC, IM, IV	J1610
Glukor, *see* Chorionic gonadotropin			
Glycopyrrolate, concentrated form	per 1 mg	INH	J7642
Glycopyrrolate, unit dose form	per 1 mg	INH	J7643
Gold sodium thiomalate	up to 50 mg	IM	J1600
Golimumab	1 mg	IV	J1602
Gonadorelin HCl	per 100 mcg	SC, IV	J1620
Gonic, *see* Chorionic gonadotropin			
Goserelin acetate implant	per 3.6 mg	SC	J9202
Granisetron HCl, IVection	100 mcg	IV	J1626
Granisetron HCl, oral	1 mg	ORAL	Q0166
Gynogen L.A. A10, @ *see* Estradiol valerate			
Gynogen L.A. A20, @ *see* Estradiol valerate			
Gynogen L.A. A40, @ *see* Estradiol valerate			
H			

DRUG	DOSE	ROUTE	HCPCS
Halaven, *see* Eribulin mesylate			
Haldol, *see* Haloperidol			
Haloperidol	up to 5 mg	IM, IV	J1630
Haloperidol decanoate	per 50 mg	IM	J1631
Hectorol, *see* Doxercalciferol			
Hemin	1 mg		J1640
Hemofil M, *see* Factor VIII			
Hemophilia clotting factors(e.g., anti-inhibitors)	per IU	IV	J7198
Hemophilia clotting factors, NOC	per IU	IV	J7199
HepaGam B	0.5 ml	IM	J1571
	0.5 ml	IV	J1573
Hep-Lock, *see* Heparin sodium (heparin lock flush)			
Hep-Lock U/P, *see* Heparin sodium (heparin lock flush)			
Heparin sodium	1,000 units	IV, SC	J1644
Heparin sodium (heparin lock flush)	10 units	IV	J1642
Herceptin, *see* Trastuzumab			
Hexadrol Phosphate, *see* Dexamethasone sodium phosphate			
Histaject, *see* Brompheniramine maleate			
Histerone 50, *see* Testosterone suspension			
Histerone 100, *see* Testosterone suspension			
Histrelin acetate	10 mcg		J1675
Histrelin implant	50 mg	OTH	J9225
Hizentra, *see* Immune globulin			
Human fibrinogen concentrate	100 mg	IV	J7178
Hyalgan		OTH	J7321
Hyaluronan or derivative	per dose	IV	J7327
Gel-Syn	0.1 mg	IA	J7328
Gen Visc 850	1 mg	IA	J7320
Hymovis	1 mg	IA	J7322
Hyaluronidase	up to 150 units	SC, IV	J3470

DRUG	DOSE	ROUTE	HCPCS
Hyaluronidase, ovine	up to 999 units	VAR	J3471
Hyaluronidase, ovine	per 1000 units	VAR	J3472
Hyaluronidase recombinant	1 usp	SC	J3473
Hyate:C, *see* Factor VIII (anti-hemophilic factor (porcine))			
Hybolin Improved, *see* Nandrolone phenpropionate			
Hybolin Decanoate, *see* Nandrolone decanoate Hycamtin, *see* Topotecan			
Hydralazine HCl	up to 20 mg	IV, IM	J0360
Hydrate, *see* Dimenhydrinate			
Hydrocortisone acetate	up to 25 mg	IV, IM, SC	J1700
Hydrocortisone sodium phosphate	up to 50 mg	IV, IM, SC	J1710
Hydrocortisone succinate sodium	up to 100 mg	IV, IM, SC	J1720
Hydrocortone Acetate, *see* Hydrocortisone acetate			
Hydrocortone Phosphate, *see* Hydrocortisone sodium phosphate			
Hydromorphone HCl	up to 4 mg	SC, IM, IV	J1170
Hydroxyprogesterone Caproate	1 mg	IM	J1725
Hydroxyzine HCl	up to 25 mg	IM	J3410
Hydroxyzine Pamoate	25 mg	ORAL	Q0177
Hylan G-F 20		OTH	J7322
Hyoscyamine sulfate	up to 0.25 mg	SC, IM, IV	J1980
Hyperstat IV, *see* Diazoxide			
Hyper-Tet, *see* Tetanus immune globulin, human			
HypRho-D, *see* Rho(D) immune globulin			
Hyrexin-50, *see* Diphenhydramine HCl			
Hyzine-50, *see* Hydroxyzine HCl			
I			
Ibandronate sodium	1 mg	IV	J1740
Ibuprofen	100 mg	IV	J1741
Ibutilide fumarate	1 mg	IV	J1742
Icatibant	1 mg	SC	J1744
Idamycin, *see* Idarubicin HCl			

DRUG	DOSE	ROUTE	HCPCS
Idarubicin HCl	5 mg	IV	J9211
Idursulfase	1 mg	IV	J1743
Ifex, *see* Ifosfamide			
Ifosfamide	1 g	IV	J9208
Ilaris, *see* Canakinumab			
Iloprost	20 mcg	INH	Q4074
Ilotycin, *see* Erythromycin gluceptate			
Imferon, *see* Iron dextran			
Imiglucerase	10 units	IV	J1786
Imitrex, *see* Sumatriptan succinate			
Immune globulin			
Bivigam	500 mg	IV	J1556
Flebogamma	500 mg	IV	J1572
Gammagard Liquid	500 mg	IV	J1569
Gammaplex	500 mg	IV	J1557
Gamunex	500 mg	IV	J1561
HepaGam B	0.5 ml	IM	J1571
HepaGam B	0.5 ml	IV	J1573
Hizentra	100 mg	SC	J1559
Hyaluronidase, (hyqvia)	100 mg	IV	J1575
NOS	500 mg	IV	J1566, J1599
Octagam	500 mg	IV	J1568
Privigen	500 mg	IV	J1459
Rhophylac	100 IU	IM	J2791
Subcutaneous	100 mg	SC	J1562
Immunosuppressive drug, not otherwise classified			J7599
Imuran, *see* Azathioprine			
Inapsine, *see* Droperidol			
Incobotulinumtoxin type A	1 unit	IM	J0588
Inderal, *see* Propranolol HCl			
INFeD, *see* Iron Dextran			
Infergen, *see* Interferon alfa-1			
Infliximab, IVection	10 mg	IM, IV	J1745, Q5102

DRUG	DOSE	ROUTE	HCPCS
Innohep, *see* Tinzaparin			
Innovar, *see* Droperidol with fentanyl citrate			
Insulin	5 units	SC	J1815
Insulin lispro	50 units	SC	J1817
Intal, *see* Cromolyn sodium or Cromolyn sodium, compounded			
Integrilin, IVection, *see* Eptifibatide			
Interferon alphacon-1, recombinant	1 mcg	SC	J9212
Interferon alfa-2a, recombinant	3 million units	SC, IM	J9213
Interferon alfa-2b, recombinant	1 million units	SC, IM	J9214
Interferon alfa-n3 (human leukocyte derived)	250,000 IU	IM	J9215
Interferon beta-1a	30 mcg	IM	J1826
Interferon beta-1a	1 mcg	IM	Q3027
Interferon beta-1a	1 mcg	SC	Q3028
Interferon beta-1b	0.25 mg	SC	J1830
Interferon gamma-1b	3 million units	SC	J9216
Intrauterine cop per contraceptive, *see* Cop per contraceptive, intrauterine			
Invega Sustenna, *see* Paliperidone Palmitate			
Ipilimumab	1 mg	IV	J9228
Ipratropium bromide, unit dose form	per mg	INH	J7644, J7645
Irinotecan	20 mg	IV	J9206, J9205
Iron dextran	50 mg	IV	J1750
Iron sucrose	1 mg	IV	J1756
Irrigation solution for Tx of bladder calculi	per 50 ml	OTH	Q2004
Isavuconazonium	1 mg	IV	J1833
Isocaine HCl, *see* Mepivacaine			
Isoetharine HCl, concentrated form	per mg	INH	J7647, J7648
Isoetharine HCl, unit dose form	per mg	INH	J7649, J7650
Isoproterenol HCl, concentrated form	per mg	INH	J7657, J7658
Isoproterenol HCl, unit dose form	per mg	INH	J7659, J7660
Istodax, *see* Romidepsin			

DRUG	DOSE	ROUTE	HCPCS
Isuprel, *see* Isoproterenol HCl			
Itraconazole	50 mg	IV	J1835
Ixabepilone	1 mg	IV	J9207
Ixempra, *see* Ixabepilone			
J			
Jenamicin, *see* Garamycin, gentamicin Jevtana, *see* Cabazitaxel			
K			
Kabikinase, *see* Streptokinase			
Kalbitor, *see* Ecallantide			
Kaleinate, *see* Calcium gluconate			
Kanamycin sulfate	up to 75 mg	IM, IV	J1850
Kanamycin sulfate	up to 500 mg	IM, IV	J1840
Kantrex, *see* Kanamycin sulfate			
Keflin, *see* Cephalothin sodium			
Kefurox, *see* Cefuroxime sodium			
Kefzol, *see* Cefazolin sodium			
Kenaject-40, *see* Triamcinolone acetonide			
Kenalog-10, *see* Triamcinolone acetonide			
Kenalog-40, *see* Triamcinolone acetonide			
Keppra, *see* Levetiracetam			
Kestrone 5, *see* Estrone			
Ketorolac tromethamine	per 15 mg	IM, IV	J1885
Key-Pred 25, *see* Prednisolone acetate			
Key-Pred 50, *see* Prednisolone acetate			
Key-Pred-SP, *see* Prednisolone sodium phosphate			
K-Flex, *see* Orphenadrine citrate			
Klebcil, *see* Kanamycin sulfate			
Koate-HP, *see* Factor VIII			
Kogenate, *see* Factor VIII			
Konakion, *see* Vitamin K, phytonadione, etc.			
Konyne-80, *see* Factor IX, complex			
Krystexxa, *see* Pegloticase			

DRUG	DOSE	ROUTE	HCPCS
Kytril, *see* Granisetron HCl			
L			
L.A.E. 20, *see* Estradiol valerate			
Laetrile, Amygdalin, vitamin B-17			J3570
Lanoxin, *see* Digoxin			
Lanreotide	1 mg	SC	J1930
Largon, *see* Propiomazine HCl			
Laronidase	0.1 mg	IV	J1931
Lasix, *see* Furosemide			
L-Caine, *see* Lidocaine HCl			
Lepirudin	50 mg		J1945
Leucovorin calcium	per 50 mg	IM, IV	J0640
Leukine, *see* Sargramostim (GM-CSF)			
Leuprolide acetate (for depot suspension)	per 3.75 mg	IM	J1950
	7.5 mg	IM	J9217
Leuprolide acetate	per 1 mg	IM	J9218
Leuprolide acetate implant	65 mg	OTH	J9219
Leustatin, *see* Cladribine			
Levalbuterol HCl, concentrated form	0.5 mg	INH	J7607, J7612
Levalbuterol HCl, unit dose	form 0.5 mg	INH	J7614, J7615
Levaquin I.U., *see* Levofloxacin			
Levetiracetam	10 mg	IV	J1953
Levocarnitine	per 1 gm	IV	J1955
Levo-Dromoran, *see* Levorphanol tartrate			
Levofloxacin	250 mg	IV	J1956
Levoleucovorin calcium	0.5 mg	IV	J0641
Levonorgestrel implant		OTH	J7306
Levonorgestrel releasing intrauterine contraceptive	52 mg	OTH	J7297, J7298
Levorphanol tartrate	up to 2 mg	SC, IV	J1960
Levsin, *see* Hyoscyamine sulfate			
Levulan Kerastick, *see* Aminolevulinic acid HCl			
Lexiscan, *see* Regadenoson			
Librium, *see* Chlordiazepoxide HCl			

DRUG	DOSE	ROUTE	HCPCS
Lidocaine HCl	10 mg	IV	J2001
Lidoject-1, *see* Lidocaine HCl			
Lidoject-2, *see* Lidocaine HCl			
Lincocin, *see* Lincomycin HCl			
Lincomycin HCl	up to 300 mg	IV	J2010
Linezolid	200 mg	IV	J2020
Liquaemin Sodium, *see* Heparin sodium			
Lioresal, *see* Baclofen			
LMD (10%), *see* Dextran 40			
Lovenox, *see* Enoxaparin sodium			
Lorazepam	2 mg	IM, IV	J2060
Lufyllin, *see* Dyphylline			
Luminal Sodium, *see* Phenobarbital sodium			
Lumizyme, *see* Alglucosidase alfa			
Lunelle, *see* Medroxyprogesterone acetate/estradiol cypionate			
Lupron, *see* Leuprolide acetate			
Lyophilized, *see* Cyclophosphamide, lyophilized			
M			
Magnesium sulfate	500 mg		J3475
Makena, *see* Hydroxyprogesterone Caproate			
Mannitol	25% in 50 ml	IV	J2150
	5mg	INH	J7665
Marmine, *see* Dimenhydrinate			
Maxipime, *see* Cefepime hydrochloride			
Mecasermin	1 mg	SC	J2170
Mechlorethamine HCl (nitrogen mustard), HN2	10 mg	IV	J9230
Medralone 40, *see* Methylprednisolone acetate			
Medralone 80, *see* Methylprednisolone acetate			
Medrol, *see* Methylprednisolone			
Medroxyprogesterone acetate	1 mg	IM	J1050
Mefoxin, *see* Cefoxitin sodium			
Melphalan HCl	50 mg	IV	J9245

DRUG	DOSE	ROUTE	HCPCS
Melphalan, oral	2 mg	ORAL	J8600
Menoject LA, *see* Testosterone cypionate and estradiol cypionate			
Mepergan IVection, *see* Meperidine and promethazine HCl			
Meperidine HCl	per 100 mg	IM, IV, SC	J2175
Meperidine and promethazine HCl	up to 50 mg	IM, IV	J2180
Mepivacaine HCL	per 10 ml	VAR	J0670
Mepolizumab	1 mg	IV	J2182
Meropenem	100 mg	IV	J2185
Mesna	200 mg	IV	J9209
Mesnex, *see* Mesna			
Metaprel, *see* Metaproterenol sulfate			
Metaproterenol sulfate, concentrated form	per 10 mg	INH	J7667, J7668
Metaproterenol sulfate, unit dose form	per 10 mg	INH	J7669, J7670
Metaraminol bitartrate	per 10 mg	IV, IM, SC	J0380
Metastron, *see* Strontium-89 chloride			
Methacholine chloride	1 mg	INH	J7674
Methadone HCl	up to 10 mg	IM, SC	J1230
Methergine, *see* Methylergonovine maleate			
Methocarbamol	up to 10 ml	IV, IM	J2800
Methotrexate, oral	2.5 mg	ORAL	J8610
Methotrexate sodium	5 mg	IV, IM, IT, IA	J9250
	50 mg	IV, IM, IT, IA	J9260
Methotrexate LPF, *see* Methotrexate sodium			
Methyldopate HCl	up to 250 mg	IV	J0210
Methylnaltrexone	0.1 mg	SC	J2212
Methylprednisolone, oral	per 4 mg	ORAL	J7509
Methylprednisolone acetate	20 mg	IM	J1020
	40 mg	IM	J1030
	80 mg	IM	J1040
Methylprednisolone sodium succinate	up to 40 mg	IM, IV	J2920

DRUG	DOSE	ROUTE	HCPCS
	up to 125 mg	IM, IV	J2930
Metoclopramide HCl	up to 10 mg	IV	J2765
Metvixia, *see* Aminolevulinate			
Miacalcin, *see* Calcitonin-salmon			
Micafungin sodium	1 mg		J2248
Midazolam HCl	per 1 mg	IM, IV	J2250
Milrinone lactate	5 mg	IV	J2260
Minocine, *see* Minocycline Hydrochloride			
Minocycline Hydrochloride	1 mg	IV	J2265
Mirena, *see* Levonorgestrel releasing intrauterine contraceptive			
Mithracin, *see* Plicamycin			
Mitomycin	0.2 mg	Ophthalmic	J7315
	5 mg	IV	J9280
Mitosol, *see* Mitomycin			
Mitoxantrone HCl	per 5 mg	IV	J9293
Monocid, *see* Cefonicid sodium			
Monoclate-P, *see* Factor VIII			
Monoclonal antibodies, parenteral	5 mg	IV	J7505
Mononine, *see* Factor IX, purified, non-recombinant			
Morphine sulfate	up to 10 mg	IM, IV, SC	J2270
Morphine sulfate, preservative-free	10 mg	SC, IM, IV	J2274
Moxifloxacin	100 mg	IV	J2280
Mozobil, *see* Plerixafor			
M-Prednisol-40, *see* Methylprednisolone acetate			
M-Prednisol-80, *see* Methylprednisolone acetate			
Mucomyst, *see* Acetylcysteine or Acetylcysteine, compounded			
Mucosol, *see* Acetylcysteine			
Muromonab-CD3	5 mg	IV	J7505
Muse, *see* Alprostadil			
Mustargen, *see* Mechlorethamine HCl			
Mutamycin, *see* Mitomycin			
Mycophenolic acid	180 mg	ORAL	J7518

DRUG	DOSE	ROUTE	HCPCS
Mycophenolate Mofetil	250 mg	ORAL	J7517
Myleran, *see* Busulfan			
Mylotarg, *see* Gemtuzumab ozogamicin			
Myobloc, *see* RimabotulinumtoxinB			
Myochrysine, *see* Gold sodium thiomalate			
Myolin, *see* Orphenadrine citrate			
N			
Nabilone	1 mg	ORAL	J8650
Nalbuphine HCl	per 10 mg	IM, IV, SC	J2300
Naloxone HCl	per 1 mg	IM, IV, SC	J2310
Naltrexone, depot form	1 mg	IM	J2315
Nandrobolic L.A., *see* Nandrolone decanoate			
Nandrolone decanoate	up to 50 mg	IM	J2320
Narcan, *see* Naloxone HCl			
Naropin, *see* Ropivacaine HCl			
Nasahist B, *see* Brompheniramine maleate			
Nasal vaccine inhalation		INH	J3530
Natalizumab	1 mg	IV	J2323
Navane, *see* Thiothixene			
Navelbine, *see* Vinorelbine tartrate			
ND Stat, *see* Brompheniramine maleate			
Nebcin, *see* Tobramycin sulfate			
NebuPent, *see* Pentamidine isethionate			
Necitumumab	1 mg	IV	J9295
Nelarabine	50 mg	IV	J9261
Nembutal Sodium Solution, *see* Pentobarbital sodium			
Neocyten, *see* Orphenadrine citrate			
Neo-Durabolic, *see* Nandrolone decanoate			
Neoquess, *see* Dicyclomine HCl			
Neosar, *see* Cyclophosphamide			
Neostigmine methylsulfate	up to 0.5 mg	IM, IV, SC	J2710
Neo-Synephrine, *see* Phenylephrine HCl			
Nervocaine 1%, *see* Lidocaine HCl			

DRUG	DOSE	ROUTE	HCPCS
Nervocaine 2%, *see* Lidocaine HCl			
Nesacaine, *see* Chloroprocaine HCL			
Nesacaine-MPF, *see* Chloroprocaine HCl			
Nesiritide	0.1 mg	IV	J2325
Neumega, *see* Oprelvekin			
Neupogen, *see* Filgrastim (G-CSF)			
Neutrexin, *see* Trimetrexate glucuronate			
Nipent, *see* Pentostatin			
Nivolumab	1 mg	IV	J9299
Nordryl, *see* Diphenhydramine HCl			
Norflex, *see* Orphenadrine citrate			
Norzine, *see* Thiethylperazine maleate			
Not otherwise classified drugs			J3490
Not otherwise classified drugs		other than INH administered thru DME	J7799
Not otherwise classified drugs		INH administered thru DME	J7699
Not otherwise classified drugs, anti-neoplastic			J9999
Not otherwise classified drugs, chemotherapeutic		ORAL	J8999
Not otherwise classified drugs, immunosuppressive			J7599
Not otherwise classified drugs, non-chemotherapeutic		ORAL	J8499
Novantrone, *see* Mitoxantrone HCl			
Novo Seven, *see* Factor VIIa			
NPH, *see* Insulin			
Nplate, *see* Romiplostim			
Nubain, *see* Nalbuphine HCl			
Nulicaine, *see* Lidocaine HCl			
Nulojix, *see* Belatacept			
Numorphan, *see* Oxymorphone HCl			
Numorphan H.P., *see* Oxymorphone HCl			
O			

DRUG	DOSE	ROUTE	HCPCS
Ocriplasmin	0.125 mg	IV	J7316
Octagam	500 mg	IV	J1568
Octreotide Acetate, IVection	1 mg	IM	J2353
	25 mcg	IV, SQ	J2354
Oculinum, *see* Botulinum toxin type A			
Ofatumumab	10 mg	IV	J9302
Ofirmev, *see* Acetaminophen			
O-Flex, *see* Orphenadrine citrate			
Oforta, *see* Fludarabine phosphate			
Olanzapine	1 mg	IM	J2358
Omacetaxine Mepesuccinate	0.01 mg	IV	J9262
Omalizumab	5 mg	SC	J2357
Omnipen-N, *see* Ampicillin			
Omontys, *see* Peginesatide			
OnabotulinumtoxinA	1 unit	IM	J0585
Oncaspar, *see* Pegaspargase			
Oncovin, *see* Vincristine sulfate			
Ondansetron HCI	1 mg	IV	J2405
Ondansetron HCl, oral	1 mg	ORAL	Q0162
Oprelvekin	5 mg	SC	J2355
Oraminic II, *see* Brompheniramine maleate			
Oritavancin	10 mg	IV	J2407
Ormazine, *see* Chlorpromazine HCl			
Orphenadrine citrate	up to 60 mg	IV, IM	J2360
Orphenate, *see* Orphenadrine citrate			
Orthovisc		OTH	J7324
Or-Tyl, *see* Dicyclomine			
Oxacillin sodium	up to 250 mg	IM, IV	J2700
Oxaliplatin	0.5 mg	IV	J9263
Oxymorphone HCl	up to 1 mg	IV, SC, IM	J2410
Oxytetracycline HCl	up to 50 mg	IM	J2460
Oxytocin	up to 10 units	IV, IM	J2590
Ozurdex, *see* Dexamethasone, intravitreal implant			

DRUG	DOSE	ROUTE	HCPCS
P			
Paclitaxel	1 mg	IV	J9267
Paclitaxel protein-bound particles	1 mg	IV	J9264
Palifermin	50 mcg	IV	J2425
Paliperidone Palmitate	1 mg	IM	J2426
Palonosetron HCl	25 mcg	IV	J2469
Netupitant 300 mg and palonosetron 0.5 mg		ORAL	J8655
Pamidronate disodium	per 30 mg	IV	J2430
Panitumumab	10 mg	IV	J9303
Papaverine HCl	up to 60 mg	IV, IM	J2440
ParaGard T 380 A, *see* Cop per contraceptive, intrauterine			
Paraplatin, *see* Carboplatin			
Paricalcitol, IVection	1 mcg	IV, IM	J2501
Pasireotide, long acting	1 mg	IV	J2502
Pegademase bovine	25 iu		J2504
Pegaptanib	0.3 mg	OTH	J2503
Pegaspargase	per single dose vial	IM, IV	J9266
Pegfilgrastim	6 mg	SC	J2505
Peginesatide	0.1 mg	IV, SC	J0890
Pegloticase	1 mg	IV	J2507
Pemetrexed	10 mg	IV	J9305
Pembrolizumab	1 mg	IV	J9271
Penicillin G benzathine	100,000 units	IM	J0561
Penicillin G benzathine and penicillin G procaine	100,000 units	IM	J0558
Penicillin G potassium	up to 600,000 units	IM, IV	J2540
Penicillin G procaine, aqueous	up to 600,000 units	IM, IV	J2510
Pentamidine isethionate	per 300 mg	INH	J2545,J7676
Pentastarch, 10%	100 ml		J2513
Pentazocine HCl	30 mg	IM, SC, IV	J3070
Pentobarbital sodium	per 50 mg	IM, IV, OTH	J2515

DRUG	DOSE	ROUTE	HCPCS
Pentostatin	per 10 mg	IV	J9268
Perforomist, *see* Formoterol fumarate			
Peramivir	1 mg	IV	J2547
Permapen, *see* Penicillin G benzathine			
Perphenazine, IVection	up to 5 mg	IM, IV	J3310
Perphenazine, tablets	4 mg	ORAL	Q0175
Persantine IV, *see* Dipyridamole			
Pertuzumab	1 mg	IV	J9306
Pet Imaging			
Gallium Ga-68, dotatate, diagnostic	0.1 millicurie	IV	A9587
Fluciclovine F-18, diagnostic	1 millicurie	IV	A9588
Positron emission tomography radiopharmaceutical, diagnostic			
for tumor identification, NOC		IV	A9597
for non-tumor identification, NOC		IV	A9598
Pfizerpen, *see* Penicillin G potassium			
Pfizerpen A.S., *see* Penicillin G procaine			
Phenazine 25, *see* Promethazine HCl			
Phenazine 50, *see* Promethazine HCl			
Phenergan, *see* Promethazine HCl			
Phenobarbital sodium	up to 120 mg	IM, IV	J2560
Phentolamine mesylate	up to 5 mg	IM, IV	J2760
Phenylephrine HCl	up to 1 ml	SC, IM, IV	J2370
Phenytoin sodium	per 50 mg	IM, IV	J1165
Photofrin, *see* Porfimer sodium			
Phytonadione (Vitamin K)	per 1 mg	IM, SC, IV	J3430
Piperacillin/Tazobactam Sodium, IVection	1.125 g	IV	J2543
Pitocin, *see* Oxytocin			
Platinol AQ, *see* Cisplatin			
Plas+SD, *see* Plasma, pooled multiple donor			
Plasma, cryoprecipitate reduced	each unit	IV	P9044
Plasma, pooled multiple donor, frozen,	each unit	IV	P9023, P9070
Plasma (single donor), pathogen reduced, frozen	each unit	IV	P9071

DRUG	DOSE	ROUTE	HCPCS
Platelets, pheresis, pathogen reduced	each unit	IV	P9072
Platinol, *see* Cisplatin			
Plerixafor	1 mg	SC	J2562
Plicamycin	2,500 mcg	IV	J9270
Polocaine, *see* Mepivacaine			
Polycillin-N, *see* Ampicillin			
Porfimer Sodium	75 mg	IV	J9600
Potassium chloride	per 2 mEq	IV	J3480
Pralatrexate	1 mg	IV	J9307
Pralidoxime chloride	up to 1 g	IV, IM, SC	J2730
Predalone-50, *see* Prednisolone acetate			
Predcor-25, *see* Prednisolone acetate			
Predcor-50, *see* Prednisolone acetate			
Predicort-50, *see* Prednisolone acetate			
Prednisone, immediate release or delayed release	1 mg	ORAL	J7512
Prednisolone, oral	5 mg	ORAL	J7510
Prednisolone acetate	up to 1 ml	IM	J2650
Predoject-50, *see* Prednisolone acetate			
Pregnyl, *see* Chorionic gonadotropin			
Premarin Intravenous, *see* Estrogen, conjugated			
Prescription, chemotherapeutic, not otherwise specified		ORAL	J8999
Prescription, nonchemotherapeutic, not otherwise specified		ORAL	J8499
Primacor, *see* Milrinone lactate			
Primaxin I.M., *see* Cilastatin sodium, imipenem			
Primaxin I.V., *see* Cilastatin sodium, imipenem			
Priscoline HCl, *see* Tolazoline HCl			
Privigen	500 mg	IV	J1459
Pro-Depo, *see* Hydroxyprogesterone Caproate			
Procainamide HCl	up to 1 g	IM, IV	J2690
Prochlorperazine	up to 10 mg	IM, IV	J0780
Prochlorperazine maleate, oral	5 mg	ORAL	Q0164
Profasi HP, *see* Chorionic gonadotropin			

DRUG	DOSE	ROUTE	HCPCS
Profilnine Heat-Treated, *see* Factor IX			
Progestaject, *see* Progesterone			
Progesterone	per 50 mg	IM	J2675
Prograf, *see* Tacrolimus, oral or parenteral			
Prokine, *see* Sargramostim (GM-CSF)			
Prolastin, *see* Alpha 1-proteinase inhibitor, human			
Proleukin, *see* Aldesleukin			
Prolixin Decanoate, *see* Fluphenazine decanoate			
Promazine HCl	up to 25 mg	IM	J2950
Promethazine HCl, IVection	up to 50 mg	IM, IV	J2550
Promethazine HCl, oral	12.5 mg	ORAL	Q0169
Pronestyl, *see* Procainamide HCl			
Proplex T, *see* Factor IX			
Proplex SX-T, *see* Factor IX			
Propofol	10 mg	IV	J2704
Propranolol HCl	up to 1 mg	IV	J1800
Prorex-25, *see* Promethazine HCl			
Prorex-50, *see* Promethazine HCl			
Prostaphlin, *see* Procainamide HCl			
Prostigmin, *see* Neostigmine methylsulfate			
Protamine sulfate	per 10 mg	IV	J2720
Protein C Concentrate	10 IU	IV	J2724
Protirelin	per 250 mcg	IV	J2725
Prothazine, *see* Promethazine HCl			
Protopam Chloride, *see* Pralidoxime chloride			
Proventil, *see* Albuterol sulfate, compounded			
Prozine-50, *see* Promazine HCl			
Pulmicort Respules, *see* Budesonide			
Pyridoxine HCl	100 mg		J3415
Q			
Quelicin, *see* Succinylcholine chloride			
Quinupristin/dalfopristin	500 mg (150/350)	IV	J2770
Qutenza, *see* Capsaicin patch			

DRUG	DOSE	ROUTE	HCPCS
R			
Ramucirumab	5 mg	IV	J9308
Ranibizumab	0.1 mg	OTH	J2778
Ranitidine HCL, IVection	25 mg	IV, IM	J2780
Rapamune, *see* Sirolimus			
Rasburicase	0.5 mg	IV	J2783
Recombinate, *see* Factor VIII			
Redisol, *see* Vitamin B-12 cyanocobalamin			
Regadenoson	0.1 mg	IV	J2785
Regitine, *see* Phentolamine mesylate			
Reglan, *see* Metoclopramide HCl			
Regular, *see* Insulin			
Relefact TRH, *see* Protirelin			
Relistor, *see* methylnaltrexone			
Remicade, *see* Infliximab, IVection			
Reo Pro, *see* Abciximab			
Rep-Pred 40, *see* Methylprednisolone acetate			
Rep-Pred 80, *see* Methylprednisolone acetate			
Reslizumab	1 mg	IV	J2786
RespiGam, *see* Respiratory Syncytial Virus			
Retavase, *see* Reteplase			
Reteplase	18.8 mg	IV	J2993
Retrovir, *see* Zidovudine			
Rheomacrodex, *see* Dextran 40			
Rhesonativ, *see* Rho(D) immune globulin, human			
Rheumatrex Dose Pack, *see* Methotrexate, oral			
Rho(D) immune globulin IM, IV			J2791
Rho(D) immune globulin, human	1 dose package, 300 mcg	IM	J2790
	50 mg	IM	J2788
Rho(D)immune globulin, human, solvent detergent	100 IU	IV	J2792
RhoGAM, *see* Rho(D) immune globulin, human			
Rhophylac	100 IU	IM, IV	J2791

DRUG	DOSE	ROUTE	HCPCS
RiaSTAP, *see* Human Fibrinogen concentrate			
Rilonacept	1 mg	SC	J2793
RimabotulinumtoxinB	100 units	IM	J0587
Ringers lactate infusion	up to 1,000 cc	IV	J7120, J7121
Risperidone	0.5 mg	IM	J2794
Rituxan, *see* Rituximab			
Rituximab	100 mg	IV	J9310
Robaxin, *see* Methocarbamol			
Rocephin, *see* Ceftriaxone sodium			
Roferon-A, *see* Interferon alfa-2A, recombinant			
Rolapitant, oral, 1 mg	1 mg	Oral	J8670
Romidepsin	1 mg	IV	J9315
Romiplostim	10 mcg	SC	J2796
Ropivacaine Hydrochloride	1 mg	OTH	J2795
Rubex, *see* Doxorubicin HCl			
Rubramin PC, *see* Vitamin B-12 cyanocobalamin			
S			
Saline solution	5% dextrose, 500 ml	IV	J7042
	infusion, 250 cc	IV	J7050
	infusion, 1,000 cc	IV	J7030
Saline solution, sterile	500 ml = 1 unit	IV, OTH	J7040
Sandimmune, *see* Cyclosporine			
Sandoglobulin, *see* Immune globulin intravenous (human)			
Sandostatin LAR Depot, *see* Octreotide			
Sargramostim (GM-CSF)	50 mcg	IV	J2820
Sculptra	0.5 mg	IV	Q2028
Sebelelipase alfa	1 mg	IV	J2840
Selestoject, *see* Betamethasone sodium phosphate			
Sermorelin acetate	1 mcg	SC	Q0515

DRUG	DOSE	ROUTE	HCPCS
Siltuximab	10 mg	IV	J2860
Sincalide	5 mcg	IV	J2805
Sinusol-B, *see* Brompheniramine maleate			
Sirolimus	1 mg	Oral	J7520
Skyla	13.5 mg	OTH	J7301
Sodium ferric gluconate in sucrose	12.5 mg		J2916
Sodium Hyaluronate			
Euflexxa			J7323
Hyalgan			J7321
Orthovisc			J7324
Supartz			J7321
Solganal, *see* Aurothioglucose			
Solu-Cortef, *see* Hydrocortisone sodium phosphate (J1710)			
Solu-Medrol, *see* Methylprednisolone sodium succinate			
Solurex, *see* Dexamethasone sodium phosphate			
Solurex LA, *see* Dexamethasone acetate			
Somatrem	1 mg	SC	J2940
Somatropin	1 mg	SC	J2941
Somatuline Depot, *see* Lanreotide			
Sparine, *see* Promazine HCl			
Spasmoject, *see* Dicyclomine HCl			
Spectinomycin HCl	up to 2 g	IM	J3320
Sporanox, *see* Itraconazole			
Staphcillin, *see* Methicillin sodium			
Stelara, *see* Ustekinumab			
Stilphostrol, *see* Diethylstilbestrol diphosphate			
Streptase, *see* Streptokinase			
Streptokinase	per 250,000 IU	IV	J2995
Streptomycin Sulfate, *see* Streptomycin			
Streptomycin	up to 1 g	IM	J3000
Streptozocin	1 gm	IV	J9320

DRUG	DOSE	ROUTE	HCPCS
Strontium-89 chloride	per millicurie		A9600
Sublimaze, *see* Fentanyl citrate			
Succinylcholine chloride	up to 20 mg	IV, IM	J0330
IVection, sulfur hexafluoride lipid microspheres	per ml	IV	Q9950
Sumatriptan succinate	6 mg	SC	J3030
Supartz		OTH	J7321
Surostrin, *see* Succinylcholine chloride			
Sus-Phrine, *see* Adrenalin, epinephrine			
Synercid, *see* Quinupristin/dalfopristin			
Synkavite, *see* Vitamin K, phytonadione, etc.			
Syntocionon, *see* Oxytocin			
Synvisc and Synvisc-One	1 mg	OTH	J7325
Sytobex, *see* Vitamin B-12 cyanocobalamin			
T			
Tacrolimus, oral, extended release	0.1 mg	ORAL	J7508
(Envarsus XR)	0.25 mg	ORAL	J7503
Tacrolimus, oral, immediate release	per 1 mg	ORAL	J7507
Tacrolimus, parenteral	5 mg	IV	J7525
Taliglucerase Alfa	10 units	IV	J3060
Talimogene laherparepvec	per 1 million plaque forming units	IV	J9325
Talwin, *see* Pentazocine HCl			
Taractan, *see* Chlorprothixene			
Taxol, *see* Paclitaxel			
Taxotere, *see* Docetaxel			
Tazidime, *see* Ceftazidime			
Technetium TC Sestamibi	per dose		A9500
Tedizolid phosphate	1 mg	IV	J3090
TEEV, *see* Testosterone enanthate and estradiol valerate			
Teflaro, *see* Ceftaroline fosamil			
Telavancin	10 mg	IV	J3095
Temozolomide	1 mg	IV	J9328

DRUG	DOSE	ROUTE	HCPCS
	5 mg	ORAL	J8700
Temsirolimus	1 mg	IV	J9330
Tenecteplase	1 mg	IV	J3101
Teniposide	50 mg		Q2017
Tequin, *see* Gatifloxacin			
Terbutaline sulfate	up to 1 mg	SC, IV	J3105
Terbutaline sulfate, concentrated form	per 1 mg	INH	J7680
Terbutaline sulfate, unit dose form	per 1 mg	INH	J7681
Teriparatide	10 mcg	SC	J3110
Terramycin IM, *see* Oxytetracycline HCl			
Testa-C, *see* Testosterone cypionate			
Testadiate, *see* Testosterone enanthate and estradiol valerate			
Testadiate-Depo, *see* Testosterone cypionate			
Testoject-LA, *see* Testosterone cypionate			
Testaqua, *see* Testosterone suspension			
Test-Estro Cypionates, *see* Testosterone cypionate and estradiol cypionate			
Test-Estro-C, *see* Testosterone cypionate and estradiol cypionate			
Testex, *see* Testosterone propionate			
Testoject-50, *see* Testosterone suspension			
Testoject-LA, *see* Testosterone cypionate			
Testone LA 200, *see* Testosterone enanthate			
Testone LA 100, *see* Testosterone enanthate			
Testosterone Aqueous, *see* Testosterone suspension			
Testosterone enanthate	1 mg	IM	J3121
Testosterone cypionate	1 mg	IM	J1071
Testosterone undecanoate	1 mg	IM	J3145
Testradiol 90/4, *see* Testosterone enanthate and estradiol valerate			
Testrin PA, *see* Testosterone enanthate			
Tetanus immune globulin, human	up to 250 units	IM	J1670
Tetracycline	up to 250 mg	IM, IV	J0120

DRUG	DOSE	ROUTE	HCPCS
Thallous Chloride TL 201	per MCI		A9505
Theelin Aqueous, *see* Estrone			
Theophylline	per 40 mg	IV	J2810
TheraCys, *see* BCG live			
Thiamine HCl	100 mg		J3411
Thiethylperazine maleate, IVection	up to 10 mg	IM	J3280
Thiethylperazine maleate, oral	10 mg	ORAL	Q0174
Thiotepa	15 mg	IV	J9340
Thorazine, *see* Chlorpromazine HCl			
Thymoglobulin, also *see* Immune globulin			
anti-thymocyte globulin, equine	250 mg	IV	J7504
anti-thymocyte globulin, rabbit	25 mg	IV	J7511
Thypinone, *see* Protirelin Thyrogen, *see* Thyrotropin Alfa			
Thyrotropin Alfa, IVection	0.9 mg	IM, SC	J3240
Tice BCG, *see* BCG live			
Ticon, *see* Trimethobenzamide HCl			
Tigan, *see* Trimethobenzamide HCl			
Tigecycline	1 mg	IV	J3243
Tiject-20, *see* Trimethobenzamide HCl			
Tinzaparin	1000 IU	SC	J1655
Tirofiban Hydrochloride, IVection	0.25 mg	IM, IV	J3246
TNKase, *see* Tenecteplase			
TOBI, *see* Tobramycin, inhalation solution			
Tobramycin, inhalation solution	300 mg	INH	J7682, J7685
Tobramycin sulfate	up to 80 mg	IM, IV	J3260
Tocilizumab	1 mg	IV	J3262
Tofranil, *see* Imipramine HCl			
Tolazoline HCl	up to 25 mg	IV	J2670
Topotecan	0.25 mg	Oral	J8705
	0.1 mg	IV	J9351
Toradol, *see* Ketorolac tromethamine			
Torecan, *see* Thiethylperazine maleate Torisel, *see* Temsirolimus			

DRUG	DOSE	ROUTE	HCPCS
Tornalate, *see* Bitolterol mesylate			
Torsemide	10 mg/ml	IV	J3265
Totacillin-N, *see* Ampicillin			
Trabectedin	0.1 mg	IV	J9352
Trastuzumab	10 mg	IV	J9355
Treanda, *see* Bendamustine HCl			
Treprostinil	1 mg		J3285
Tri-Kort, *see* Triamcinolone acetonide			
Triam-A, *see* Triamcinolone acetonide			
Triamcinolone, concentrated form	per 1 mg	INH	J7683
Triamcinolone, unit dose	per 1 mg	INH	J7684
Triamcinolone acetonide	1 mg		J3300
	per 10 mg	IM	J3301
Triamcinolone diacetate	per 5 mg	IM	J3302
Triamcinolone hexacetonide	per 5 mg	VAR	J3303
Triesence, *see* Triamcinolone acetonide			
Triflupromazine HCl	up to 20 mg	IM, IV	J3400
Trilafon, *see* Perphenazine			
Trilog, *see* Triamcinolone acetonide			
Trilone, *see* Triamcinolone diacetate			
Trimethobenzamide HCl, IVection	up to 200 mg	IM	J3250
Trimethobenzamide HCl, oral	250 mg	ORAL	Q0173
Trimetrexate glucuronate	per 25 mg	IV	J3305
Triptorelin Pamoate	3.75 mg	SC	J3315
Trisenox, *see* Arsenic trioxide			
Trobicin, *see* Spectinomycin HCl			
Trovan, *see* Alatrofloxacin mesylate			
Tysabri, *see* Natalizumab			
U			
Ultrazine-10, *see* Prochlorperazine			
Unasyn, *see* Ampicillin sodium/sulbactam sodium			
Unclassified drugs (see also Not elsewhere classified)			J3490
Unspecified oral antiemetic			Q0181

DRUG	DOSE	ROUTE	HCPCS
Urea	up to 40 g IV	J3350	
Ureaphil, *see* Urea			
Urecholine, *see* Bethanechol chloride			
Urofollitropin	75 IU		J3355
Urokinase	5,000 IU vial	IV	J3364
	250,000 IU vial	IV	J3365
Ustekinumab	1 mg	SC	J3357
V			
V-Gan 25, *see* Promethazine HCl			
V-Gan 50, *see* Promethazine HCl			
Valergen 10, *see* Estradiol valerate			
Valergen 20, *see* Estradiol valerate			
Valergen 40, *see* Estradiol valerate			
Valertest No. 1, *see* Testosterone enanthate and estradiol valerate			
Valertest No. 2, *see* Testosterone enanthate and estradiol valerate			
Valium, *see* Diazepam			
Valrubicin, intravesical	200 mg	OTH	J9357
Valstar, *see* Valrubicin			
Vancocin, *see* Vancomycin HCl			
Vancoled, *see* Vancomycin HCl			
Vancomycin HCl	500 mg	IV, IM	J3370
Vasoxyl, *see* Methoxamine HCl			
Vedolizumab	1 mg	IV	J3380
Velaglucerase alfa	100 units	IV	J3385
Velban, *see* Vinblastine sulfate			
Velsar, *see* Vinblastine sulfate			
Venofer, *see* Iron sucrose			
Ventolin, *see* Albuterol sulfate			
VePesid, *see* Etoposide and Etoposide, oral			
Versed, *see* Midazolam HCl			
Verteporfin	0.1 mg	IV	J3396

DRUG	DOSE	ROUTE	HCPCS
Vesprin, *see* Triflupromazine HCl			
Viadur, *see* Leuprolide acetate implant			
Vibativ, *see* Telavancin			
Vinblastine sulfate	1 mg	IV	J9360
Vincasar PFS, *see* Vincristine sulfate			
Vincristine sulfate	1 mg	IV	J9370
Vincristine sulfate Liposome	1 mg	IV	J9371
Vinorelbine tartrate	per 10 mg	IV	J9390
Vistaject-25, *see* Hydroxyzine HCl			
Vistaril, *see* Hydroxyzine HCl			
Vistide, *see* cidofovir			
Visudyne, *see* Verteporfin			
Vitamin K, phytonadione, menadione,			
menadiol sodium diphosphate	per 1 mg	IM, SC, IV	J3430
Vitamin B-12 cyanocobalamin	up to 1,000 mcg	IM, SC	J3420
Von Willebrand Factor Complex, human	per IU VWF:RCo	IV	J7187
	per IU VWF:RCo	IV	J7183
Vonvendi	per IU VWF:RCp	IV	J7179
Voriconazole	10 mg	IV	J3465
Vpriv, *see* Velaglucerase alfa			
W			
Wehamine, *see* Dimenhydrinate			
Wehydryl, *see* Diphenhydramine HCl			
Wellcovorin, *see* Leucovorin calcium			
Wilate, *see* Von Willebrand Factor complex (human)			
Win Rho SD, *see* Rho(D) immuglobulin, human, solvent detergent			
Wyamine Sulfate, *see* Mephentermine sulfate			
Wycillin, *see* Penicillin G procaine			
Wydase, *see* Hyaluronidase			

DRUG	DOSE	ROUTE	HCPCS
X			
Xeloda, *see* Capecitabine			
Xeomin, *see* Incobotulinumtoxin type A			
Xgeva, *see* Denosumab			
Xiaflex, *see* Collagenase			
Xopenex, *see* Albuterol			
Xylocaine HCl, *see* Lidocaine HCl			
Xyntha, *see* Factor VIII (anti-hemophilic factor, recombinant)			
Y			
Yervoy, *see* Ipilimumab			
Z			
Zanosar, *see* Streptozocin			
Zantac, *see* Ranitidine HCL			
Zemplar, *see* Paricalcitol			
Zenapax, *see* Daclizumab			
Zetran, *see* Diazepam			
Ziconotide	1 mcg	OTH	J2278
Zidovudine	10 mg	IV	J3485
Zinacef, *see* Cefuroxime sodium			
Ziprasidone Mesylate	10 mg	IM	J3486
Zithromax, *see* Azithromycin dihydrate			
Zithromax I.V., *see* Azithromycin, IVection			
Ziv-Aflibercept	1 mg	IV	J9400
Zofran, *see* Ondansetron HCl			
Zoladex, *see* Goserelin acetate implant			
Zoledronic Acid	1 mg	IV	J3489
Zolicef, *see* Cefazolin sodium			
Zortress, *see* Everolimus			
Zosyn, *see* Piperacillin			
Zyprexa Relprevv, *see* Olanzapine			
Zyvox, *see* Linezolid			

APPENDIX D: MEDICARE REFERENCES

COVERAGE INSTRUCTION MANUAL (CIM) REFERENCES

The following Medicare references refer to policy issues identified in the main body of the HCPCS code section. Coverage Instruction Manual references are identified with the term CIM: followed by the reference number(s).

35-10 HYPERBARIC OXYGEN THERAPY

For purposes of coverage under Medicare, hyperbaric oxygen (HBO) therapy is a modality in which the entire body is exposed to oxygen under increased atmospheric pressure.

A. Covered Conditions.—Program reimbursement for HBO therapy will be limited to that which is administered in a chamber (including the one man unit) and is limited to the following conditions:

1. Acute carbon monoxide intoxication, (ICD-9 -CM diagnosis 986).
2. Decompression illness, (ICD-9-CM diagnosis 993.2, 993.3).
3. Gas embolism, (ICD-9-CM diagnosis 958.0, 999.1).
4. Gas gangrene, (ICD-9-CM diagnosis 0400).
5. Acute traumatic peripheral ischemia. HBO therapy is an adjunctive treatment to be used in combination with accepted standard therapeutic measures when loss of function, limb, or life is threatened. (ICD-9-CM diagnosis 902.53, 903.01, 903.1, 904.0, 904.41.)
6. Crush injuries and suturing of severed limbs. As in the previous conditions, HBO therapy would be an adjunctive treatment when loss of function, limb, or life is threatened. (ICD-9-CM diagnosis 927.00-927.03, 927.09-927.11, 927.20-927.21, 927.8-927.9, 928.00-928.01, 928.10-928.11, 928.20-928.21, 928.3, 928.8-928.9, 929.0, 929.9, 996.90-996.99.)
7. Progressive necrotizing infections (necrotizing fasciitis), (ICD-9-CM diagnosis 728.86).
8. Acute peripheral arterial insufficiency, (ICD-9-CM diagnosis 444.21, 444.22, 444.81).
9. Preparation and preservation of compromised skin grafts (not for primary management of wounds), (ICD-9CM diagnosis 996.52; excludes artificial skin graft).
10. Chronic refractory osteomyelitis, unresponsive to conventional medical and surgical management, (ICD-9-CM diagnosis 730.10-730.19).
11. Osteoradionecrosis as an adjunct to conventional treatment, (ICD-9-CM diagnosis 526.89).
12. Soft tissue radionecrosis as an adjunct to conventional treatment, (ICD-9-CM diagnosis 990).
13. Cyanide poisoning, (ICD-9-CM diagnosis 987.7, 989.0).
14. Actinomycosis, only as an adjunct to conventional therapy when the disease process is refractory to antibiotics and surgical treatment, (ICD-9-CM diagnosis 039.0-039.4, 039.8, 039.9).
15. Diabetic wounds of the lower extremities in patients who meet the following three criteria:

    a) Patient has type I or type II diabetes and has a lower extremity wound that is due to diabetes;
    b) Patient has a wound classified as Wagner grade III or higher; and
    c) Patient has failed an adequate course of standard wound therapy.

    The use of HBO therapy is covered as adjunctive therapy only after there are no measurable signs of healing for at least 30-days of treatment with standard wound therapy and must be used in addition to standard wound care. Standard wound care in patients with diabetic wounds includes: assessment of a patient's vascular status and correction of any vascular problems in the affected limb if possible, optimization of nutritional status, optimization of glucose control, debridement by any means to remove devitalized tissue, maintenance of a clean, moist bed of granulation tissue with appropriate moist dressings, appropriate off-loading, and necessary treatment to resolve any infection that might be present. Failure to respond to standard wound care occurs when there are no measurable signs of healing for at least 30 consecutive days. Wounds must be evaluated at least every 30 days during administration of HBO therapy. Continued treatment with HBO therapy is not covered if measurable signs of healing have not been demonstrated within any 30-day period of treatment.

B. Noncovered Conditions.—All other indications not specified under §35-10 (A) are not covered under the Medicare program. No program payment may be made for any conditions other than those listed in §35-10(A).

No program payment may be made for HBO in the treatment of the following conditions:

1. Cutaneous, decubitus, and stasis ulcers.
2. Chronic peripheral vascular insufficiency.
3. Anaerobic septicemia and infection other than clostridial.
4. Skin burns (thermal).
5. Senility.
6. Myocardial infarction.
7. Cardiogenic shock.
8. Sickle cell anemia.
9. Acute thermal and chemical pulmonary damage, i.e., smoke inhalation with pulmonary insufficiency.
10. Acute or chronic cerebral vascular insufficiency.
11. Hepatic necrosis.
12. Aerobic septicemia.
13. Nonvascular causes of chronic brain syndrome (Pick's disease, Alzheimer's disease, Korsakoff's disease).
14. Tetanus.
15. Systemic aerobic infection.
16. Organ transplantation.
17. Organ storage.
18. Pulmonary emphysema.
19. Exceptional blood loss anemia.
20. Multiple Sclerosis.
21. Arthritic Diseases.
22. Acute cerebral edema.

C. Topical Application of Oxygen.—This method of administering oxygen does not meet the definition of HBO therapy as stated above. Also, its clinical efficacy has not been established. Therefore, no Medicare reimbursement may be made for the topical application of oxygen. (Cross reference: §35-31.)

D. Physician Supervision Requirement--For HBO therapy to be covered under the Medicare program, the physician must be in constant attendance during the entire treatment. This is a professional activity that cannot be delegated in that it requires independent medical judgement by the physician. The physician must be present, carefully monitoring the patient during the hyperbaric oxygen therapy session and be immediately available should a complication occur. This requirement applies in all settings: no payment will be made under Part A or Part B, unless the physician is in constant attendance during the HBO therapy procedure.

E. Credentials--A physician qualified in HBO therapy treatment is defined by Medicare for this purpose to be credentialed by the hospital in which HBO therapy is being performed specifically in hyperbaric medicine and the management of acute cardiopulmonary emergencies, including placement of chest tube. Credentialing includes, at a minimum, the following:

- Training, experience and privileges within the institution to manage acute cardiopulmonary emergencies, including advanced cardiac life support, and emergency myringotomy;
- Completion of a recognized hyperbaric medicine training program as established by either the American College of Hyperbaric Medicine or the Undersea and Hyperbaric Medical Society (UHMS) with a minimum of 60 hours of training and documented by a certificate of completion or an equivalent program; and
- Continuing medical education in hyperbaric medicine of a minimum of 16 hours every 2 years after initial credentialing.

An additional requirement that must be met for Medicare's payment for hyperbaric medical therapy is that cardiopulmonary resuscitation team coverage must be immediately available during the hours of the hyperbaric chamber operations.

35-13 PROLOTHERAPY, JOINT SCLEROTHERAPY, AND LIGAMENTOUS INJECTIONS WITH SCLEROSING AGENTS—NOT COVERED

The medical effectiveness of the above therapies has not been verified by scientifically controlled studies. Accordingly, reimbursement for these modalities should be denied on the ground that they are not reasonable and necessary as required by §1862(a)(1) of the law.

35-20 TREATMENT OF MOTOR FUNCTION DISORDERS WITH ELECTRIC NERVE STIMULATION—NOT COVERED

While electric nerve stimulation has been employed to control chronic intractable pain for some time, its use in the treatment of motor function disorders, such as multiple sclerosis, is a recent innovation, and the medical effectiveness of such therapy has not been verified by scientifically controlled studies. Therefore, where electric nerve stimulation is employed to treat motor function disorders, no reimbursement may be made for the stimulator or for the services related to its implantation since this treatment cannot be considered reasonable and necessary.

See §§35-27 and 65-8.

NOTE: For Medicare coverage of deep brain stimulation for essential tremor and Parkinson's disease, see §65-19.

35-27 BIOFEEDBACK THERAPY

Biofeedback therapy provides visual, auditory or other evidence of the status of certain body functions so that a person can exert voluntary control over the functions, and thereby alleviate an abnormal bodily condition. Biofeedback therapy often uses electrical devices to transform bodily signals indicative of such functions as heart rate, blood pressure, skin temperature, salivation, peripheral vasomotor activity, and gross muscle tone into a tone or light, the loudness or brightness of which shows the extent of activity in the function being measured.

Biofeedback therapy differs from electromyography, which is a diagnostic procedure used to record and study the electrical properties of skeletal muscle. An electromyography device may be used to provide feedback with certain types of biofeedback.

Biofeedback therapy is covered under Medicare only when it is reasonable and necessary for the individual patient for muscle re-education of specific muscle groups or for treating pathological muscle abnormalities of spasticity, incapacitating muscle spasm, or weakness, and more conventional treatments (heat, cold, massage, exercise, support) have not been successful. This therapy is not covered for treatment of ordinary muscle tension states or for psychosomatic conditions.

See HCFA-Pub. 14-3, §§2200ff, 2215, and 4161; HCFA-Pub. 13-3, §§3133.3, 3148, and 3149; HCFA-Pub. 10, §§242 and 242.5 for special physical therapy requirements. See also §35-20 and 65-8.)

35-34 FABRIC WRAPPING OF ABDOMINAL ANEURYSMS—NOT COVERED

Fabric wrapping of abdominal aneurysms is not a covered Medicare procedure. This is a treatment for abdominal aneurysms which involves wrapping aneurysms with cellophane or fascia lata. This procedure has not been shown to prevent eventual rupture. In extremely rare instances, external wall reinforcement may be indicated when the current accepted treatment (excision of the aneurysm and reconstruction with synthetic materials) is not a viable alternative, but external wall reinforcement is not fabric wrapping. Accordingly, fabric wrapping of abdominal aneurysms is not considered reasonable and necessary within the meaning of §1862(a)(1) of the Act.

35-46 ASSESSING PATIENT'S SUITABILITY FOR ELECTRICAL NERVE STIMULATION THERAPY

Electrical nerve stimulation is an accepted modality for assessing a patient's suitability for ongoing treatment with a transcutaneous or an implanted nerve stimulator. Accordingly, program payment may be made for the following techniques when used to determine the potential therapeutic usefulness of an electrical nerve stimulator:

A. Transcutaneous Electrical Nerve Stimulation (TENS).--This technique involves attachment of a transcutaneous nerve stimulator to the surface of the skin over the peripheral nerve to be stimulated. It is used by the patient on a trial basis and its effectiveness in modulating pain is monitored by the physician, or physical therapist. Generally, the physician or physical therapist is able to determine whether the patient is likely to derive a significant therapeutic benefit from continuous use of a transcutaneous stimulator within a trial period of 1 month; in a few cases this determination may take longer to make. Document the medical necessity for such services which are furnished beyond the first month. (See §45-25 for an explanation of coverage of medically necessary supplies for the effective use of TENS.)

   If TENS significantly alleviates pain, it may be considered as primary treatment; if it produces no relief or greater discomfort than the original pain electrical nerve stimulation therapy is ruled out.

However, where TENS produces incomplete relief, further evaluation with percutaneous electrical nerve stimulation may be considered to determine whether an implanted peripheral nerve stimulator would provide significant relief from pain. (See §35-46B.)

Usually, the physician or physical therapist providing the services will furnish the equipment necessary for assessment. Where the physician or physical therapist advises the patient to rent the TENS from a supplier during the trial period rather than supplying it himself/herself, program payment may be made for rental of the TENS as well as for the services of the physician or physical therapist who is evaluating its use. However, the combined program payment which is made for the physician's or physical therapist's services and the rental of the stimulator from a supplier should not exceed the amount which would be payable for the total service, including the stimulator, furnished by the physician or physical therapist alone.

B. Percutaneous Electrical Nerve Stimulation (PENS).--This diagnostic procedure which involves stimulation of peripheral nerves by a needle electrode inserted through the skin is performed only in a physician's office, clinic, or hospital outpatient department. Therefore, it is covered only when performed by a physician or incident to physician's service. If pain is effectively controlled by percutaneous stimulation, implantation of electrodes is warranted.

As in the case of TENS (described in subsection A), generally the physician should be able to determine whether the patient is likely to derive a significant therapeutic benefit from continuing use of an implanted nerve stimulator within a trial period of 1 month. In a few cases, this determination may take longer to make. The medical necessity for such diagnostic services which are furnished beyond the first month must be documented.

NOTE: Electrical nerve stimulators do not prevent pain but only alleviate pain as it occurs. A patient can be taught how to employ the stimulator, and once this is done, can use it safely and effectively without direct physician supervision. Consequently, it is inappropriate for a patient to visit his/her physician, physical therapist, or an outpatient clinic on a continuing basis for treatment of pain with electrical nerve stimulation. Once it is determined that electrical nerve stimulation should be continued as therapy and the patient has been trained to use the stimulator, it is expected that a stimulator will be implanted or the patient will employ the TENS on a continual basis in his/her home. Electrical nerve stimulation treatments furnished by a physician in his/her office, by a physical therapist or outpatient clinic are excluded from coverage by §1862(a)(1) of the Act. (See §65-8 for an explanation of coverage of the therapeutic use of implanted peripheral nerve stimulators under the prosthetic devices benefit. See §60-20 for an explanation of coverage of the therapeutic use of TENS under the durable medical equipment benefit.)

35-47 OSTEOGENIC STIMULATION

Electrical stimulation to augment bone repair can be attained either invasively or noninvasively. Invasive devices provide electrical stimulation directly at the fracture site either through percutaneously placed cathodes or by implantation of a coiled cathode wire into the fracture site. The power pack for the latter device is implanted into soft tissue near the fracture site and subcutaneously connected to the cathode, creating a self-contained system with no external components. The power supply for the former device is externally placed and the leads connected to the inserted cathodes. With the noninvasive device, opposing pads, wired to an external power supply, are placed over the cast. An electromagnetic field is created between the pads at the fracture site.

1. Noninvasive Stimulator.—The noninvasive stimulator device is covered only for the following indications:

   - Nonunion of long bone fractures;
   - Failed fusion, where a minimum of nine months has elapsed since the last surgery;
   - Congenital pseudarthroses; and
   - As an adjunct to spinal fusion surgery for patients at high risk of pseudarthrosis due to previously failed spinal fusion at the same site or for those undergoing multiple level fusion. A multiple level fusion involves 3 or more vertebrae (e.g., L3-L5, L4-S1, etc).

2. Invasive (Implantable) Stimulator.—The invasive stimulator device is covered only for the following indications:

   - Nonunion of long bone fractures; and
   - As an adjunct to spinal fusion surgery for patients at high risk of pseudarthrosis due to previously failed spinal fusion at the same site or for those undergoing multiple level fusion.

   A multiple level fusion involves 3 or more vertebrae (e.g., L3-L5, L4-S1, etc). Effective for services performed on or after September 15, 1980, nonunion of long bone fractures, for both noninvasive and invasive devices, is considered to exist only after 6 or more months have elapsed without healing of the fracture.

   Effective for services performed on or after April 1, 2000, nonunion of long bone fractures, for both noninvasive and invasive devices, is considered to exist only when serial radiographs have confirmed that fracture healing has ceased for three or more months prior to starting treatment with the electrical osteogenic stimulator. Serial radiographs must include a minimum of two sets of radiographs, each including multiple views of the fracture site, separated by a minimum of 90 days.

3. Ultrasonic Osteogenic Stimulators.—An ultrasonic osteogenic stimulator is a non-invasive device that emits low intensity, pulsed ultrasound. The ultrasound signal is applied to the skin surface at the fracture location via ultrasound, conductive gel in order to stimulate fracture healing.

   Effective for services performed on or after January 1, 2001, ultrasonic osteogenic stimulators are covered as medically reasonable and necessary for the treatment of non-union fractures. In demonstrating nonunion of fractures, we would expect:

   - A minimum of two sets of radiographs obtained prior to starting treatment with the osteogenic stimulator, separated by a minimum of 90 days. Each radiograph must include multiple views of the fracture site accompanied with a written interpretation by a physician stating that there has been no clinically significant evidence of fracture healing between the two sets of radiographs.
   - Indications that the patient failed at least one surgical intervention for the treatment of the fracture.

Non-unions of the skull, vertebrae, and those that are tumor-related are excluded from coverage. The ultrasonic osteogenic stimulator may not be used concurrently with other non-invasive osteogenic devices. The national non-coverage policy related to ultrasonic osteogenic stimulators for fresh fractures and delayed unions remains in place. This policy relates only to non-union as defined above.

35-50 COCHLEOSTOMY WITH NEUROVASCULAR TRANSPLANT FOR MENIERE'S DISEASE—NOT COVERED

Ménière's disease (or syndrome) is a common cause of paroxysmal vertigo. Ménière's syndrome is usually treated medically. When medical treatment fails, surgical treatment may be required.

While there are two recognized surgical procedures used in treating Ménière's disease (decompression of the endolymphatic hydrops and labyrinthectomy), there is no scientific evidence supporting the safety and effectiveness of cochleostomy with neurovascular transplant in treatment of Ménière's syndrome. Accordingly, Medicare does not cover cochleostomy with neurovascular transplant for treatment of Ménière's disease.

35-64 CHELATION THERAPY FOR TREATMENT OF ATHEROSCLEROSIS

Chelation therapy is the application of chelation techniques for the therapeutic or preventive effects of removing unwanted metal ions from the body. The application of chelation therapy using ethylenediamine-tetra-acetic acid (EDTA) for the treatment and prevention of atherosclerosis is controversial. There is no widely accepted rationale to explain the beneficial effects attributed to this therapy. Its safety is questioned and its clinical effectiveness has never been established by well designed, controlled clinical trials. It is not widely accepted and practiced by American physicians. EDTA chelation therapy for atherosclerosis is considered experimental. For these reasons, EDTA chelation therapy for the treatment or prevention of atherosclerosis is not covered.

Some practitioners refer to this therapy as chemoendarterectomy and may also show a diagnosis other than atherosclerosis, such as arteriosclerosis or calcinosis. Claims employing such variant terms should also be denied under this section.

Cross-reference: §45-20

35-74 EXTERNAL COUNTERPULSATION (ECP) FOR SEVERE ANGINA—COVERED

External counterpulsation (ECP), commonly referred to as enhanced external counterpulsation, is a non-invasive outpatient treatment for coronary artery disease refractory to medical and/or surgical therapy. Although ECP devices are cleared by the Food and Drug Administration (FDA) for use in treating a variety of cardiac conditions, including stable or unstable angina pectoris, acute myocardial infarction and cardiogenic shock, the use of this device to treat cardiac conditions other than stable angina pectoris is not covered, since only that use has developed sufficient evidence to demonstrate its medical effectiveness. Non-coverage of hydraulic versions of these types of devices remains in force.

Coverage is provided for the use of ECP for patients who have been diagnosed with disabling angina (Class III or Class IV, Canadian Cardiovascular Society Classification or equivalent classification) who, in the opinion of a cardiologist or cardiothoracic surgeon, are not readily amenable to surgical intervention, such as PTCA or cardiac bypass because: (1) their condition is inoperable, or at high risk of operative complications or post-operative failure; (2) their coronary anatomy is not readily amenable to such procedures; or (3) they have co-morbid states which create excessive risk.

A full course of therapy usually consists of 35 one-hour treatments, which may be offered once or twice daily, usually 5 days per week. The patient is placed on a treatment table where their lower trunk and lower extremities are wrapped in a series of three compressive air cuffs which inflate and deflate in synchronization with the patient's cardiac cycle.

During diastole the three sets of air cuffs are inflated sequentially (distal to proximal) compressing the vascular beds within the muscles of the calves, lower thighs and upper thighs. This action results in an increase in diastolic pressure, generation of retrograde arterial blood flow and an increase in venous return. The cuffs are deflated simultaneously just prior to systole, which produces a rapid drop in vascular impedance, a decrease in ventricular workload and an increase in cardiac output.

The augmented diastolic pressure and retrograde aortic flow appear to improve myocardial perfusion, while systolic unloading appears to reduce cardiac workload and oxygen requirements. The increased venous return coupled with enhanced systolic flow appears to increase cardiac output. As a result of this treatment, most patients experience increased time until onset of ischemia, increased exercise tolerance, and a reduction in the number and severity of anginal episodes. Evidence was presented that this effect lasted well beyond the immediate post-treatment phase, with patients symptom-free for several months to two years.

This procedure must be done under direct supervision of a physician.

35-77 NEUROMUSCULAR ELECTRICAL STIMULATION (NMES)

Neuromuscular electrical stimulation (NMES) involves the use of a device that transmits an electrical impulse to activate muscle groups by way of electrodes. There are two broad categories of NMES. One type of device stimulates the muscle when the patient is in a resting state to treat muscle atrophy. The second type is used to enhance functional activity of neurologically impaired patients.

Treatment of Muscle Atrophy

Coverage of NMES to treat muscle atrophy is limited to the treatment of patients with disuse atrophy where the nerve supply to the muscle is intact, including brain, spinal cord and peripheral nerves and other non-neurological reasons for disuse atrophy. Examples include casting or splinting of a limb, contracture due to scarring of soft tissue as in burn lesions, and hip orthotic training begins). (See CIM 45-25 for an explanation of coverage of medically necessary supplies for the effective use of NMES).

Use for Walking in Patients with Spinal Cord Injury (SCI)

The type of NMES that is used to enhance the ability to walk of SCI patients is commonly referred to as functional electrical stimulation (FES). These devices are surface units that use electrical impulses to activate paralyzed or weak muscles in precise sequence. Coverage for the use of NMES/FES is limited to SCI patients, for walking, who have completed a training program, which consists of at least 32 physical therapy sessions with the device over a period of 3 months. The trial period of physical therapy will enable the physician treating the patient for his or her spinal cord injury to properly evaluate the person's ability to use these devices frequently and for the long term. Physical therapy sessions are only covered in the inpatient hospital, outpatient hospital, comprehensive outpatient rehabilitation facilities, and outpatient rehabilitation facilities. The physical therapy necessary to perform this training must be directly performed by the physical therapist as part of a one-on-one training program; this service cannot be done unattended.

The goal of physical therapy must be to train SCI patients on the use of NMES/FES devices to achieve walking, not to reverse or retard muscle atrophy.

Coverage for NMES/FES for walking will be limited to SCI patients with all of the following characteristics:

1) persons with intact lower motor units (L1 and below) (both muscle and peripheral nerve);
2) persons with muscle and joint stability for weight bearing at upper and lower extremities that can demonstrate balance and control to maintain an upright support posture independently;
3) persons that demonstrate brisk muscle contraction to NMES and have sensory perception of electrical stimulation sufficient for muscle contraction;
4) persons that possess high motivation, commitment and cognitive ability to use such devices for walking;
5) persons that can transfer independently and can demonstrate independent standing tolerance for at least 3 minutes;
6) persons that can demonstrate hand and finger function to manipulate controls;
7) persons with at least 6-month post recovery spinal cord injury and restorative surgery;
8) persons without hip and knee degenerative disease and no history of long bone fracture secondary to osteoporosis; and
9) persons who have demonstrated a willingness to use the device long-term.

NMES/FES for walking will not be covered in SCI patients with any of the following:

1) persons with cardiac pacemakers;
2) severe scoliosis or severe osteoporosis;
3) skin disease or cancer at area of stimulation;
4) irreversible contracture; or
5) autonomic dysreflexia.

The only settings where therapists with the sufficient skills to provide these services are employed, are inpatient hospitals, outpatient hospitals, comprehensive outpatient rehabilitation facilities and outpatient rehabilitation facilities. The physical therapy necessary to perform this training must be part of a one-on-one training program.

Additional therapy after the purchase of the DME would be limited by our general policies on coverage of skilled physical therapy.

All other uses of NMES remain non-covered.

(Also reference Medicare Carriers' Manual, Part 3, Claims-§2210 and Medicare Intermediary Manual, Part 3, Claims-§3653 - See - Maintenance Program 271.1)

35-98 ELECTRICAL STIMULATION FOR THE TREATMENT OF WOUNDS

Electrical stimulation (ES) has been used or studied for many different applications, one of which is accelerating wound healing. The types of ES used for healing chronic venous and arterial wound and pressure ulcers are direct current (DC), alternating current (AC), pulsed current (PC), pulsed electromagnetic induction (PEMI), and spinal cord stimulation (SCS). An example of AC is transcutaneous electrical stimulation (TENS). The PEMI includes Pulsed Electromagnetic Field (PEMF) and Pulsed Electromagnetic Energy (PEE) using pulsed radio frequency energy, both of which are nonthermal i.e., they do not produce heat. Some ES use generators to create energy in the means such as coils, rather than by leads or surface electrodes.

There is insufficient evidence to determine any clinically significant differences in healing rates. Therefore, ES cannot be covered by Medicare because its effectiveness has not been adequately demonstrated.

35-102 ELECTRICAL STIMULATION FOR THE TREATMENT OF WOUNDS (Effective for services on and after April 1, 2003)

Electrical stimulation (ES) has been used or studied for many different applications, one of which is accelerating wound healing. Electrical stimulation for the treatment of wounds is the application of electrical current through electrodes placed directly on the skin in close proximity to the wound. Electrical stimulation for the treatment of wounds will only be covered for chronic Stage III or Stage IV pressure ulcers, arterial ulcers, diabetic ulcers and venous stasis ulcers. All other uses of electrical stimulation for the treatment of wounds are noncovered. Chronic ulcers are defined as ulcers that have not healed within 30 days of occurrence. Electrical stimulation will not be covered as an initial treatment modality.

The use of electrical stimulation for the treatment of wounds is considered an adjunctive therapy. Electrical stimulation will be covered only after appropriate standard wound therapy has been tried for at least 30-days and there are no measurable signs of healing. This 30-day period can begin while the wound is acute. Measurable signs of improved healing include a decrease in wound size, either surface area or volume, decrease in amount of exudates and decrease in amount of necrotic tissue. Standard wound care includes: optimization of nutritional status; debridement by any means to remove devitalized tissue; maintenance of a clean, moist bed of granulation tissue with appropriate moist dressings; and necessary treatment to resolve any infection that may be present. Standard wound care based on the specific type of wound includes: frequent repositioning of a patient with pressure ulcers (usually every 2 hours); off-loading of pressure and good glucose control for diabetic ulcers; establishment of adequate circulation for arterial ulcers; and the use of a compression system for patients with venous ulcers. Continued treatment with electrical stimulation is not covered if measurable signs of healing have not been demonstrated within any 30-day period of treatment. Electrical stimulation must be discontinued when the wound demonstrates 100 per-cent epithelialized wound bed. Any form of electromagnetic therapy for the treatment of chronic wounds will not be covered.

This service can only be covered when performed by a physician, physical therapist, or incident to a physician service. Evaluation of the wound is an integral part of wound therapy. When a physician, physical therapist, or a clinician incident to a physician, performs electrical stimulation, that practitioner must evaluate the wound and contact the treating physician if the wound worsens. If electrical stimulation is being used, wounds must be evaluated at least monthly by the treating physician.

Unsupervised use of electrical stimulation for wound therapy will not be covered, as this use has not been found to be medically reasonable and necessary.

45-3 INSULIN SYRINGE

Medical supplies are covered under §1861(s)(2)(A) of the Act only when they are furnished incident to a physician's professional services. To be covered under this provision an insulin syringe must have been used by the physician or under his/her direct personal supervision, and the insulin injection must have been given in an emergency situation (e.g., diabetic coma).

The use of an insulin syringe by a diabetic would not meet the requirements of §1861(s)(2)(A) of the Act.

See Intermediary Manual, §3112.4B and Carriers Manual, §2050.

45-4 VITAMIN B12 INJECTIONS TO STRENGTHEN TENDONS, LIGAMENTS, ETC., OF THE FOOT--NOT COVERED

Vitamin B12 injections to strengthen tendons, ligaments, etc., of the foot are not covered under Medicare because (1) there is no evidence that vitamin B12 injections are effective for the purpose of strengthening weakened tendons and ligaments, and (2) this is nonsurgical treatment under the subluxation exclusion. Accordingly, vitamin B12 injections are not considered reasonable and necessary within the meaning of §1862(a)(1) of the Act.

See Intermediary Manual, §§3101.3 and 3158 and Carriers Manual, §§2050.5 and 2323.

45-7 HYDROPHILIC CONTACT LENS FOR CORNEAL BANDAGE

Some hydrophilic contact lenses are used as moist corneal bandages for the treatment of acute or chronic corneal pathology, such as bullous keratopathy, dry eyes, corneal ulcers and erosion, keratitis, corneal edema, descemetocele, corneal ectasis, Mooren's ulcer, anterior corneal dystrophy, neurotrophic keratoconjunctivitis, and for other therapeutic reasons.

Payment may be made under §1861(s)(2) of the Act for a hydrophilic contact lens approved by the Food and Drug Administration (FDA) and used as a supply incident to a physician's service.

Payment for the lens is included in the payment for the physician's service to which the lens is incident. Contractors are authorized to accept an FDA letter of approval or other FDA published material as evidence of FDA approval. *(See §65-1 for coverage of a hydrophilic contact lens as a prosthetic device.) See Intermediary Manual, §3112.4 and Carriers Manual, §§2050.1 and 15010.*

45-12 PORCINE SKIN AND GRADIENT PRESSURE DRESSINGS

Porcine (pig) skin dressings are covered, if reasonable and necessary for the individual patient as an occlusive dressing for burns, donor sites of a homograft, and decubiti and other ulcers.

Gradient pressure dressings are Jobst elasticized heavy duty dressings used to reduce hypertrophic scarring and joint contractures following burn injury. They are covered when used for that purpose.

45-15 PHYSICIAN'S OFFICE WITHIN AN INSTITUTION--COVERAGE OF SERVICES AND SUPPLIES INCIDENT TO A PHYSICIAN'S SERVICES

Where a physician establishes an office within a nursing home or other institution, coverage of services and supplies furnished in the office must be determined in accordance with the "incident to a physician's professional service" provision (see Intermediary Manual, §3112.4A or Carriers Manual, §2050.1), as in any physician's office. A physician's office within an institution must be confined to a separately identified part of the facility which is used solely as the physician's office and cannot be construed to extend throughout the entire institution. Thus, services performed outside the "office" area would be subject to the coverage rules applicable to services furnished outside the office setting.

In order to accurately apply the criteria in §3112.4 or §2050.l, give consideration to the physical proximity of the institution and physician's office. When his office is located within a facility, a physician may not be reimbursed for services, supplies, and use of equipment which fall outside the scope of services "commonly furnished" in physician's offices generally, even though such services may be furnished in his institutional office. Additionally, make a distinction between the physician's office practice and the institution, especially when the physician is administrator or owner of the facility. Thus, for their services to be covered under the criteria in §3112.4A or §2050.l, the auxiliary medical personnel must be members of the office staff rather than of the institution's staff, and the cost of supplies must represent an expense to the physician's office practice. Finally, services performed by the employees of the physician outside the "office" area must be directly supervised by the physician; his presence in the facility as a whole would not suffice to meet this requirement. (In any setting, of course, supervision of auxiliary personnel in and of itself is not considered a "physician's professional service" to which the services of the auxiliary personnel could be an incidental part, i.e., in addition to supervision, the physician must perform or have performed a personal professional service to the patient to which the services of the auxiliary personnel could be considered an incidental part). Denials for failure to meet any of these requirements would be based on §l861(s)(2)(A) of the Act.

Establishment of an office within an institution would not modify rules otherwise applicable for determining coverage of the physician's personal professional services within the institution. However, in view of the opportunity afforded to a physician who maintains such an office for rendering services to a sizable number of patients in a short period of time or for performing frequent services for the same patient, claims for physicians. services rendered under such circumstances would require careful evaluation by the carrier to assure that payment is made only for services that are reasonable and necessary.

Cross-reference: Intermediary Manual, §3112.4A; Carriers Manual, §2050.1

45-16 CERTAIN DRUGS DISTRIBUTED BY THE NATIONAL CANCER INSTITUTE (Effective for services furnished on or after October 1, 1980.)

Under its Cancer Therapy Evaluation, the Division of Cancer Treatment of the National Cancer Institute (NCI), in cooperation with the Food and Drug Administration, approves and distributes certain drugs for use in treating terminally ill cancer patients. One group of these drugs, designated as Group C drugs, unlike other drugs distributed by the NCI, are not limited to use in clinical trials for the purpose of testing their efficacy. Drugs are classified as Group C drugs only if there is sufficient evidence demonstrating their efficacy within a tumor type and that they can be safely administered.
A physician is eligible to receive Group C drugs from the Division of Cancer Treatment only if the following requirements are met:

- A physician must be registered with the NCI as an investigator by having completed an FD-Form 1573;
- A written request for the drug, indicating the disease to be treated, must be submitted to the NCI;
- The use of the drug must be limited to indications outlined in the NCI's guidelines; and
- All adverse reactions must be reported to the Investigational Drug Branch of the Division of Cancer Treatment.

In view of these NCI controls on distribution and use of Group C drugs, intermediaries may assume, in the absence of evidence to the contrary, that a Group C drug and the related hospital stay are covered if all other applicable coverage requirements are satisfied.

If there is reason to question coverage in a particular case, the matter should be resolved with the assistance of the local PSRO, or if there is none, the assistance of your medical consultants.

Information regarding those drugs which are classified as Group C drugs may be obtained from:

Office of the Chief, Investigational Drug Branch Division of Cancer Treatment, CTEP, Landow Building Room 4C09, National Cancer Institute
Bethesda, Maryland 20205

45-19 TRANSCUTANEOUS ELECTRICAL NERVE STIMULATION (TENS) FOR ACUTE POST-OPERATIVE PAIN

The use of transcutaneous electrical nerve stimulation (TENS) for the relief of acute post-operative pain is covered under Medicare. TENS may be covered whether used as an adjunct to the use of drugs, or as an alternative to drugs, in the treatment of acute pain resulting from surgery.

TENS devices, whether durable or disposable, may be used in furnishing this service. When used for the purpose of treating acute post-operative pain, TENS devices are considered supplies. As such they may be hospital supplies furnished inpatients covered under Part A, or supplies incident to a physician's service when furnished in connection with surgery done on an outpatient basis, and covered under Part B.

It is expected that TENS, when used for acute post-operative pain, will be necessary for relatively short periods of time, usually 30 days or less. In cases when TENS is used for longer periods, contractors should attempt to ascertain whether TENS is no longer being used for acute pain but rather for chronic pain, in which case the TENS device may be covered as durable medical equipment as described in §60-20.

Cross-reference: HCFA Pub. 13-3, §§65-8, 3101.4, 3112.4, 3113; HCFA Pub. 14-3, §§65-8, 2050.1, 2100; HCFA Pub. 10, §§65-8, 210.4, 230, 235.

45-22 LYMPHOCYTE IMMUNE GLOBULIN, ANTI-THYMOCYTE GLOBULIN (EQUINE)

The lymphocyte immune globulin preparations are biologic drugs not previously approved or licensed for use in the management of renal allograft rejection. A number of other lymphocyte immune globulin products of equine, lapine, and murine origin are currently under investigation for their potential usefulness in controlling allograft rejections in human transplantation. These biologic drugs are viewed as adjunctive to traditional immunosuppressive products such as steroids and anti- metabolic drugs. At present, lymphocyte immune globulin preparations are not recommended to replace conventional immunosuppressive drugs, but to supplement them and to be used as alternatives to elevated or accelerated dosing with conventional immunosuppressive agents.

The FDA has approved one lymphocyte immune globulin preparation for marketing, lymphocyte immune globulin, anti-thymocyte globulin (equine). This drug is indicated for the management of allograft rejection episodes in renal transplantation. It is covered under Medicare when used for this purpose. Other forms of lymphocyte globulin preparation which the FDA approves for this indication in the future may be covered under Medicare.

45-22 DIMETHYL SULFOXIDE (DMSO)

DMSO is an industrial solvent produced as a chemical byproduct of paper production from wood pulp. The Food and Drug Administration has determined that the only purpose for which DMSO is safe and effective for humans is in the treatment of the bladder condition, interstitial cystitis. Therefore, the use of DMSO for all other indications is not considered to be reasonable and necessary. Payment may be made for its use only when reasonable and necessary for a patient in the treatment of interstitial cystitis.

45-23 ANTI-INHIBITOR COAGULANT COMPLEX (AICC)

Anti-inhibitor coagulant complex, AICC, is a drug used to treat hemophilia in patients with factor VIII inhibitor antibodies. AICC has been shown to be safe and effective and has Medicare coverage when furnished to patients with hemophilia A and inhibitor antibodies to factor VIII who have major bleeding episodes and who fail to respond to other, less expensive therapies.

45-25 SUPPLIES USED IN THE DELIVERY OF TRANSCUTANEOUS ELECTRICAL NERVE STIMULATION (TENS) AND NEURO-MUSCULAR ELECTRICAL STIMULATION (NMES)—(Effective for services rendered (i.e., items rented or purchased) on or after July 14, 1988.)

Transcutaneous Electrical Nerve Stimulation (TENS) and/or Neuromuscular Electrical Stimulation (NMES) can ordinarily be delivered to patients through the use of conventional electrodes, adhesive tapes and lead wires. There may be times, however, where it might be medically necessary for certain patients receiving TENS or NMES treatment to use, as an alternative to conventional electrodes, adhesive tapes and lead wires, a form-fitting conductive garment (i.e., a garment with conductive fibers which are separated from the patients' skin by layers of fabric).

A form-fitting conductive garment (and medically necessary related supplies) may be covered under the program only when:

1. It has received permission or approval for marketing by the Food and Drug Administration;
2. It has been prescribed by a physician for use in delivering covered TENS or NMES treatment; and
3. One of the medical indications outlined below is met:

   - The patient cannot manage without the conductive garment because there is such a large area or so many sites to be stimulated and the stimulation would have to be delivered so frequently that it is not feasible to use conventional electrodes, adhesive tapes and lead wires;
   - The patient cannot manage without the conductive garment for the treatment of chronic intractable pain because the areas or sites to be stimulated are inaccessible with the use of conventional electrodes, adhesive tapes and lead wires;
   - The patient has a documented medical condition such as skin problems that preclude the application of conventional electrodes, adhesive tapes and lead wires;
   - The patient requires electrical stimulation beneath a cast either to treat disuse atrophy, where the nerve supply to the muscle is intact, or to treat chronic intractable pain; or

- The patient has a medical need for rehabilitation strengthening (pursuant to a written plan of rehabilitation) following an injury where the nerve supply to the muscle is intact.

A conductive garment is not covered for use with a TENS device during the trial period specified in §35-46 unless:

4. The patient has a documented skin problem prior to the start of the trial period; and
5. The carrier's medical consultants are satisfied that use of such an item is medically necessary for the patient.

(See conditions for coverage of the use of TENS in the diagnosis and treatment of chronic intractable pain in §§35-46 and 60-20 and the use of NMES in the treatment of disuse atrophy in §35-77.)

45-29 INTRAVENOUS IRON THERAPY (EFFECTIVE FOR SERVICES PERFORMED ON OR AFTER12/01/00)

Iron deficiency is a common condition in end stage renal disease (ESRD) patients undergoing hemodialysis. Iron is a critical structural component of hemoglobin, a key protein found in normal red blood cells (RBCs) which transports oxygen. Without this important building block, anemic patients experience difficulty in restoring adequate, healthy RBCs that improve hematocrit levels. Clinical management of iron deficiency involves treating patients with iron replacement products while they undergo hemodialysis. Body iron stores can be supplemented with either oral or intravenous (IV) iron products.

The evidence suggests that there is little to distinguish various forms of IV iron therapy in terms of effectiveness. Rather, the medical literature indicates that the mode of intravenous administration is perhaps the most effective treatment for iron deficiency in hemodialysis patients. Unlike oral iron products which must be absorbed through the GI tract, IV iron products are infused directly into the bloodstream in a form that is readily available to the bone marrow for RBC synthesis, resulting in an earlier correction of iron deficiency and anemia. Review of medical literature indicated that the distinction among IV iron products lies within their safety profiles. The IV iron dextran products are associated with a small incidence of severe, life-threatening anaphylaxis. These type I hypersensitivity reactions, which are not dose-related, are immunoglobulin (Ig) E-mediated and are apparently exclusively associated with the dextran forms of injectable iron. In fact, clinical evidence indicates that the dextran component itself is what triggers the severe, life-threatening anaphylactic reactions. *Sodium ferric gluconate complex in sucrose injection* has demonstrated no life-threatening anaphylaxis and a less severe adverse-reaction rate when compared to iron dextran products.

Therefore, effective December 1, 2000, Medicare covers *sodium ferric gluconate complex in sucrose injection* when used as a first line treatment of iron deficiency anemia in patients undergoing chronic hemodialysis who are receiving supplemental erythropoietin therapy.

45-30 PHOTOSENSITIVE DRUGS

Photosensitive drugs are the light-sensitive agents used in photodynamic therapy. Once introduced into the body, these drugs selectively identify and adhere to diseased tissue. The drugs remain inactive until they are exposed to a specific wavelength of light, by means of a laser, that corresponds to their absorption peak. The activation of a photosensitive drug results in a photochemical reaction which treats the diseased tissue without affecting surrounding normal tissue.

Verteporfin

Verteporfin, a benzoporphyrin derivative, is an intravenous lipophilic photosensitive drug with an absorption peak of 690 nm. This drug was first approved by the Food and Drug Administration (FDA) on April 12, 2000, and subsequently, approved for inclusion in the United States Pharmacopoeia on July 18, 2000, meeting Medicare's definition of a drug as defined under §1861(t)(1) of the Social Security Act. Effective July 1, 2001, Verteporfin (Q3013 . Injection, Verteporfin, 15 mg) is only covered when used in conjunction with ocular photodynamic therapy (see §35-100 PHOTODYNAMIC THERAPY) when furnished intravenously incident to a physician's service. For patients with age-related macular degeneration, Verteporfin is only covered with a diagnosis of neovascular age-related macular degeneration (ICD-9-CM 362.52) with predominately classic subfoveal choroidal neovascular (CNV) lesions (where the area of classic CNV occupies ≥ 50% of the area of the entire lesion) at the initial visit as determined by a fluorescein angiogram (CPT code 92235). Subsequent follow-up visits will require a fluorescein angiogram prior to treatment. There are no requirements regarding visual acuity, lesion size, and number of retreatments.

50-4 GRAVLEE JET WASHER

The Gravlee Jet Washer is a sterile, disposable, diagnostic device for detecting endometrial cancer. The use of this device is indicated where the patient exhibits clinical symptoms or signs suggestive of endometrial disease, such as irregular or heavy vaginal bleeding.

Program payment cannot be made for the washer or the related diagnostic services when furnished in connection with the examination of an asymptomatic patient. Payment for routine physical checkups is precluded under the statute.

(See §1862(a)(7) of the Act.) (See Intermediary Manual, §3157 and Carriers Manual, §2320.)

50-10 VABRA ASPIRATOR

The VABRA aspirator is a sterile, disposable, vacuum aspirator which is used to collect uterine tissue for study to detect endometrial carcinoma. The use of this device is indicated where the patient exhibits clinical symptoms or signs suggestive of endometrial disease, such as irregular or heavy vaginal bleeding.

Program payment cannot be made for the aspirator or the related diagnostic services when furnished in connection with the examination of an asymptomatic patient. Payment for routine physical checkups is precluded under the statute (§1862(a)(7) of the Act).

Cross-reference: Intermediary Manual, §3157; Carriers Manual §2320; §50-4

50-15 ELECTROCARDIOGRAPHIC SERVICES

Reimbursement may be made under Part B for electrocardiographic (EKG) services rendered by a physician or incident to his/her services or by an approved laboratory or an approved supplier of portable X-ray services. Since there is no coverage for EKG services of any type rendered on a screening basis or as part of a routine examination, the claim must indicate the signs and symptoms or other clinical reason necessitating the services.

A separate charge by an attending or consulting physician for EKG interpretation is allowed only when it is the normal practice to make such charge in addition to the regular office visit charge. No payment is made for EKG interpretations by individuals other than physicians.

On a claim involving EKG services furnished by a laboratory or a portable X-ray supplier, identify the physician ordering the service and, when the charge includes both the taking of the tracing and its interpretation, include the identity of the physician making the interpretation. No separate bill for the services of a physician is paid unless it is clear that he/she was the patient's attending physician or was acting as a consulting physician. The taking of an EKG in an emergency, i.e., when the patient is or may be experiencing what is commonly referred to as a heart attack, is covered as a laboratory service or a diagnostic service by a portable X-ray supplier only when the evidence shows that a physician was in attendance at the time the service was performed or immediately thereafter.

Where EKG services are rendered in the patient's home and the laboratory's or portable X-ray supplier's charge is higher than that imposed for the same service when performed in the laboratory or portable X-ray supplier's office, the medical need for home service should be documented. In the absence of such justification, reimbursement for the service if otherwise medically necessary should be based on the reasonable charge applicable when performed in the laboratory or X-ray supplier's office.

The documentation required in the various situations mentioned above must be furnished not only when the laboratory or portable X-ray supplier bills the patient or carrier for its service, but also when such a facility bills the attending physician who, in turn, bills the patient or carrier for the EKG services. (In addition to the evidence required to document the claim, the laboratory or portable X-ray supplier must maintain in its records the referring physician's written order and the identity of the employee taking the tracing.)

Long Term EKG Monitoring, also referred to as long-term EKG recording, Holter recording, or dynamic electrocardiography, is a diagnostic procedure which provides a continuous record of the electrocardiographic activity of a patient's heart while he is engaged in his daily activities.

The basic components of the long-term EKG monitoring systems are a sensing element, the design of which may provide either for the recording of electrocardiographic information on magnetic tape or for detecting significant variations in rate or rhythm as they occur, and a component for either graphically recording the electrocardiographic data or for visual or computer assisted analysis of the information recorded on magnetic tape. The long-term EKG permits the examination in the ambulant or potentially ambulant patient of as many as 70,000 heartbeats in a 12-hour recording while the standard EKG which is obtained in the recumbent position, yields information on only 50 to 60 cardiac cycles and provides only a limited data base on which diagnostic judgments may be made.

Many patients with cardiac arrhythmias are unaware of the presence of an irregularity in heart rhythm. Due to the transient nature of many arrhythmias and the short intervals in which the rhythm of the heart is observed by conventional standard EKG techniques, the offending arrhythmias can go undetected. With the extended examination provided by the long-term EKG, the physician is able not only to detect but also to classify various types of rhythm disturbances and waveform abnormalities and note the frequency of their occurrence. The knowledge of the reaction of the heart to daily activities with respect to rhythm, rate, conduction disturbances, and changes are of great assistance in directing proper therapy and this modality is valuable in both inpatient and outpatient diagnosis and therapy. Long-term monitoring of ambulant or potentially ambulant inpatients provides significant potential for reducing the length of stay for post-coronary infarct patients in the intensive care setting and may result in earlier discharge from the hospital with greater assurance of safety to the patients. The indications for the use of this technique, noted below, are similar for both inpatients and outpatients.

The long-term EKG has proven effective in detecting transient episodes of cardiac dysrhythmia and in permitting the correlation of these episodes with cardiovascular symptomatology. It is also useful for patients who have symptoms of obscure etiology suggestive of cardiac arrhythmia. Examples of such symptoms include palpitations, chest pain, dizziness, light-headedness, near syncope, syncope, transient ischemic episodes, dyspnea, and shortness of breath.

This technique would also be appropriate at the time of institution of any arrhythmic drug therapy and may be performed during the course of therapy to evaluate response. It is also appropriate for evaluating a change of dosage and may be indicated shortly before and after the discontinuation of anti-arrhythmic medication. The therapeutic response to a drug whose duration of action and peak of effectiveness is defined in hours cannot be properly assessed by examining 30-40 cycles on a standard EKG rhythm strip. The knowledge that all patients placed on anti-arrhythmic medication do not respond to therapy and the known toxicity of anti-arrhythmic agents clearly indicate that proper assessment should be made on an individual basis to determine whether medication should be continued and at what dosage level.

The long-term EKG is also valuable in the assessment of patients with coronary artery disease. It enables the documentation of etiology of such symptoms as chest pain and shortness of breath. Since the standard EKG is often normal during the intervals between the episodes of precordial pain, it is essential to obtain EKG information while the symptoms are occurring. The long-term EKG has enabled the correlation of chest symptoms with the objective evidence of ST-segment abnormalities. It is appropriate for patients who are recovering from an acute myocardial infarction or coronary insufficiency before and after discharge from the hospital, since it is impossible to predict which of these patients is subject to ventricular arrhythmias on the basis of the presence or absence of rhythm disturbances during the period of initial coronary care. The long-term EKG enables the physician to identify patients who are at a higher risk of dying suddenly in the period following an acute myocardial infarction. It may also be reasonable and necessary where the high-risk patient with known cardiovascular disease advances to a substantially higher level of activity which might trigger increased or new types of arrhythmias necessitating treatment. Such a high-risk case would be one in which there is documentation that acute phase arrhythmias have not totally disappeared during the period of convalescence.

In view of recent developments in cardiac pacemaker monitoring techniques (see CIA 50-1), the use of the long-term EKG for routine assessment of pacemaker function can no longer be justified. Its use for the patient with an internal pacemaker would be covered only when he has symptoms suggestive of arrhythmia not revealed by the standard EKG or rhythm strip.

These guidelines are intended as a general outline of the circumstances under which the use of this diagnostic procedure would be warranted. Each patient receiving a long-term EKG should be evaluated completely, prior to performance of this diagnostic study. A complete history and physical examination should be obtained and the indications for use of the long-term EKG should be reviewed by the referring physician.

The performance of a long-term EKG does not necessarily require the prior performance of a standard EKG. Nor does the demonstration of a normal standard EKG preclude the need for a long- term EKG. Finally, the demonstration of an abnormal standard EKG does not obviate the need for a long-term EKG if there is suspicion that the dysrhythmia is transient in nature.

A period of recording of up to 24 hours would normally be adequate to detect most transient arrhythmias and provide essential diagnostic information. The medical necessity for longer periods of monitoring must be documented.

Medical documentation for adjudicating claims for the use of the long-term EKG should be similar to other EKG services, X-ray services, and laboratory procedures. Generally, a statement of the diagnostic impression of the referring physician with an indication of the patient's relevant signs and symptoms should be sufficient for purposes of making a determination regarding the reasonableness and medical necessity for the use of this procedure. However, the intermediaries or carriers should require whatever additional documentation their medical consultants deem necessary to properly adjudicate the individual claim where the information submitted is not adequate.

It should be noted that the recording device furnished to the patient is simply one component of the diagnostic system and a separate charge for it will not be recognized under the durable medical equipment benefit.

Patient-Activated EKG Recorders, distributed under a variety of brand names, permit the patient to record an EKG upon manifestation of symptoms, or in response to a physician's order (e.g., immediately following strong exertion).Most such devices also permit the patient to simultaneously voice-record in order to describe symptoms and/or activity. In addition, some of these devices permit transtelephonic transmission of the recording to a physician's office, clinic, hospital, etc., having a decoder/recorder for review and analysis, thus eliminating the need to physically transport the tape. Some of these devices also permit a "time sampling" mode of operation. However, the "time sampling" mode is not covered—only the patient-activated mode of operation, when used for the indications described below, is covered at this time.

Services in connection with patient-activated EKG recorders are covered when used as an alternative to the long-term EKG monitoring (described above) for similar indications--detecting and characterizing symptomatic arrhythmias, regulation of anti-arrhythmic drug therapy, etc. Like long- term EKG monitoring, use of these devices is covered for evaluating patients with symptoms of obscure etiology suggestive of cardiac arrhythmia such as palpitations, chest pain, dizziness, lightheadedness, near syncope, syncope, transient ischemic episodes, dyspnea and shortness of breath.

As with long-term EKG monitors, patient-activated EKG recorders may be useful for both inpatient and outpatient diagnosis and therapy. While useful for assessing some post-coronary infarct patients in the hospital setting, these devices should not, however, be covered for outpatient monitoring of recently discharged post-infarct patients.

Computer Analyzed Electrocardiograms.—Computer interpretation of EKG's is recognized as a valid and effective technique which will improve the quality and availability of cardiology services. Reimbursement may be made for such computer service when furnished in the setting and under the circumstances required for coverage of other electrocardiographic services. Where either a laboratory's or a portable x-ray supplier's charge for EKG services includes the physician review and certification of the printout as well as the computer interpretation, the certifying physician must be identified on the HCFA-1490 before the entire charge can be considered a reimbursable charge. Where the laboratory's (or portable x-ray supplier's) reviewing physician is not identified, the carrier should conclude that no professional component is involved and make its charge determination accordingly. If the supplying laboratory (or portable x-ray supplier when supplied by such a facility) does not include professional review and certification of the hard copy, a charge by the patient's physician may be recognized for the service. In any case the charge for the physician component should be substantially less than that for physician interpretation of the conventional EKG tracing in view of markedly reduced demand on the physician's time where computer interpretation is involved.

Considering the unit cost reduction expected of this innovation, the total charge for the complete EKG service (taking of tracing and interpretation) when computer interpretation is employed should never exceed that considered reasonable for the service when physician interpretation is involved.

Transtelephonic Electrocardiographic Transmissions (Formerly Referred to as EKG Telephone Reporter Systems).—Effective for services furnished on and after March 1, 1980, coverage is extended to include the use of transtelephonic electrocardiographic (EKG) transmissions as a diagnostic service for the indications described below, when performed with equipment meeting the standards described below, subject to the limitations and conditions specified below. Coverage is further limited to the amounts payable with respect to the physician's service in interpreting the results of such transmissions, including charges for rental of the equipment. The device used by the beneficiary is part of a total diagnostic system and is not considered durable medical equipment.

1. Covered Uses.—The use of transtelephonic EKGs is covered for the following uses:

    a. To detect, characterize, and document symptomatic transient arrhythmias;
    b. To overcome problems in regulating antiarrhythmic drug dosage;
    c. To carry out early posthospital monitoring of patients discharged after myocardial infarction; (only if 24-hour coverage is provided, see 4. below).

    Since cardiology is a rapidly changing field, some uses other than those specified above may be covered if, in the judgment of the contractor's medical consultants, such a use was justifiable in the particular case. The enumerated uses above represent uses for which a firm coverage determination has been made, and for which contractors may make payment without extensive claims development or review.

2. Specifications for Devices—The devices used by the patient are highly portable (usually pocket-sized) and detect and convert the normal EKG signal so that it can be transmitted via ordinary telephone apparatus to a receiving station. At the receiving end, the signal is decoded and transcribed into a conventional EKG. There are numerous devices available which transmit EKG readings in this fashion. For purposes of Medicare coverage, however, the transmitting devices must meet at least the following criteria:

    a. They must be capable of transmitting EKG Leads, I, II, or III;
    b. These lead transmissions must be sufficiently comparable to readings obtained by a conventional EKG to permit proper interpretation of abnormal cardiac rhythms.

3. Potential for Abuse - Need for Screening Guidelines.--While the use of these devices may often compare favorably with more costly alternatives, this is the case only where the information they contribute is actively utilized by a knowledgeable practitioner as part of overall medical management of the patient. Consequently, it is vital that contractors be aware of the potential for abuse of these devices, and adopt necessary screening and physician education policies to detect and halt potentially abusive situations. For example, use of these devices to diagnose and treat suspected arrhythmias as a routine substitute for more conventional methods of diagnosis, such as a careful history, physical

examination, and standard EKG and rhythm strip would not be appropriate. Moreover, contractors should require written justification for use of such devices in excess of 30 consecutive days in cases involving detection of transient arrhythmias.

Contractors may find it useful to review claims for these devices with a view toward detecting patterns of practice which may be useful in developing schedules which may be adopted for screening such claims in the future.

4. Twenty-four Hour Coverage.—No payment may be made for the use of these devices to carry out early posthospital monitoring of patients discharged after myocardial infarction unless provision is made for 24 hour coverage in the manner described below.

   Twenty-four hour coverage means that there must be, at the monitoring site (or sites) an experienced EKG technician receiving calls; tape recording devices do not meet this requirement. Further, such technicians should have immediate access to a physician, and have been instructed in when and how to contact available facilities to assist the patient in case of emergencies.

Cross-reference: HCFA-Pub. 13-3, §§3101.5, 3110, 3112.3, HCFA-Pub. 14-3, §§2070, 2255, 2050.1

50-20 DIAGNOSTIC PAP SMEARS (Effective for services performed on and after May 15, 1978)

A diagnostic pap smear and related medically necessary services are covered under Medicare Part B when ordered by a physician under one of the following conditions:

- Previous cancer of the cervix, uterus, or vagina that has been or is presently being treated;
- Previous abnormal pap smear;
- Any abnormal findings of the vagina, cervix, uterus, ovaries, or adnexa;
- Any significant complaint by the patient referable to the female reproductive system; or
- Any signs or symptoms that might in the physician's judgment reasonably be related to a gynecologic disorder.

In respect to the last bullet, the contractor's medical staff must determine whether in a particular case a previous malignancy at another site is an indication for a diagnostic pap smear or whether the test must be considered a screening pap smear as described in §50-20.1.

Use the following CPT codes for indicating diagnostic pap smears:

- 88150 Cytopathology, smears, cervical or vaginal (e.g., Papanicolaou), up to three smears; screening by technician under physician supervision; or
- 88151 Cytopathology, smears, cervical or vaginal (e.g., Papanicolaou), up to three smears; requiring interpretation by physician.

50-20.1 SCREENING PAP SMEARS AND PELVIC EXAMINATIONS FOR EARLY DETECTION OF CERVICAL OR VAGINAL CANCER

(For screening pap smears, effective for services performed on or after July 1, 1990. For pelvic examinations including clinical breast examination, effective for services furnished on or after January 1, 1998.)

A screening pap smear (use HCPCS code P3000 Screening Papanicolaou smear, cervical or vaginal, up to three smears; by technician under physician supervision or P3001 Screening Papanicolaou smear, cervical or vaginal, up to three smears requiring interpretation by physician). (Use HCPCS codes G0123 Screening Cytopathology, cervical or vaginal (any reporting system), collected in preservative fluid, automated thin layer preparation, screening by cytotechnologist under physician supervision or G0124 Screening Cytopathology, cervical or vaginal (any reporting system) collected in preservative fluid, automated thin layer preparation, requiring interpretation by physician) and related medically necessary services provided to a woman for the early detection of cervical cancer (including collection of the sample of cells and a physician's interpretation of the test results) and pelvic examination (including clinical breast examination) (use HCPCS code G0101 cervical or vaginal cancer screening; pelvic and clinical breast examination) are covered under Medicare Part B when ordered by a physician (or authorized practitioner) under one of the following conditions:

- She has not had such a test during the preceding 3 years or is a woman of childbearing age (§1861(nn) of the Act).
- There is evidence (on the basis of her medical history or other findings) that she is at high risk of developing cervical cancer and her physician (or authorized practitioner) recommends that she have the test performed more frequently than every 3 years.

High risk factors for cervical and vaginal cancer are:

- Early onset of sexual activity (under 16 years of age)
- Multiple sexual partners (five or more in a lifetime)
- History of sexually transmitted disease (including HIV infection)
- Fewer than three negative or any pap smears within the previous 7 years; and
- DES (diethylstilbestrol) - exposed daughters of women who took DES during pregnancy.

NOTE: Claims for pap smears must indicate the beneficiary's low or high risk status by including the appropriate ICD-9-CM on the line item (Item 24E of the HCFA-1500).

- V76.2, *special screening for malignant neoplasms of the cervix,* indicates low risk; and
- V15.89, *other specified personal history presenting hazards to health,* indicates high risk.

If pap smear or pelvic exam claims do not point to one of these diagnosis codes, the claim will reject in the Common Working File. Claims can contain up to four diagnosis codes, but the one pointed to on the line item must be either V76.2 or V15.89.

Definitions:

A woman as described in §1861(nn) of the Act is a woman who is of childbearing age and has had a pap smear test during any of the preceding 3 years that indicated the presence of cervical or vaginal cancer or other abnormality, or is at high risk of developing cervical or vaginal cancer.

A woman of childbearing age is one who is premenopausal and has been determined by a physician or other qualified practitioner to be of childbearing age, based upon the medical history or other findings.

Other qualified practitioner", as defined in 42 CFR 410.56(a) includes a certified nurse midwife (as defined in §1861(gg) of the Act), or a physician assistant, nurse practitioner, or clinical nurse specialist (as defined in §1861(aa) of the Act) who is authorized under State law to perform the examination.

Screening Pelvic Examination:

Section 4102 of the Balanced Budget Act of 1997 provides for coverage of screening pelvic examinations (including a clinical breast examination) for all female beneficiaries, effective January 1, 1998, subject to certain frequency and other limitations. A screening pelvic examination (including a clinical breast examination) should include at least seven of the following eleven elements:

- Inspection and palpation of breasts for masses or lumps, tenderness, symmetry, or nipple discharge.
- Digital rectal examination including sphincter tone, presence of hemorrhoids, and rectal masses.

Pelvic examination (with or without specimen collection for smears and cultures) including:

- External genitalia (for example, general appearance, hair distribution, or lesions).
- Urethral meatus (for example, size, location, lesions, or prolapse).
- Urethra (for example, masses, tenderness, or scarring).
- Bladder (for example, fullness, masses, or tenderness).
- Vagina (for example, general appearance, estrogen effect, discharge lesions, pelvic support, cystocele, or rectocele).
- Cervix (for example, general appearance, lesions, or discharge).
- Uterus (for example, size, contour, position, mobility, tenderness, consistency, descent, or support).
- Adnexa/parametria (for example, masses, tenderness, organomegaly, or nodularity).
- Anus and perineum.

This description is from *Documentation Guidelines for Evaluation and Management Services*, published in May 1997 and was developed by the Health Care Financing Administration and the American Medical Association.

50-42 AMBULATORY BLOOD PRESSURE MONITORING

Ambulatory blood pressure monitoring (ABPM) involves the use of a non-invasive device which is used to measure blood pressure in 24-hour cycles. These 24-hour measurements are stored in the device and are later interpreted by the physician. ABPM must be performed for at least 24 hours to meet coverage criteria.

ABPM is only covered for those patients with suspected white coat hypertension. Suspected white coat hypertension is defined as 1) office blood pressure >140/90 mm Hg on at least three separate clinic/office visits with two separate measurements made at each visit; 2) at least two documented blood pressure measurements taken outside the office which are <140/90 mm Hg; and 3) no evidence of end-organ damage. The information obtained by ABPM is necessary in order to determine the appropriate management of the patient. ABPM is not covered for any other uses. In the rare circumstance that ABPM needs to be performed more than once in a patient, the qualifying criteria described above must be met for each subsequent ABPM test.

For those patients that undergo ABPM and have an ambulatory blood pressure of <135/85 with no evidence of end-organ damage, it is likely that their cardiovascular risk is similar to that of normotensives. They should be followed over time. Patients for which ABPM demonstrates a blood pressure of >135/85 may be at increased cardiovascular risk, and a physician may wish to consider antihypertensive therapy.

50-56 HOME PROTHROMBIN TIME INTERNATIONAL NORMALIZED RATIO (INR) MONITORING FOR ANTICOAGULATION MANAGEMENT

Use of the International Normalized Ratio (INR) allows physicians to determine the level of anticoagulation in a patient independent of the laboratory reagents used. The INR is the ratio of the patient's prothrombin time compared to the mean prothrombin time for a group of normal individuals. Maintaining patients within the therapeutic range minimizes adverse events associated with inadequate or excessive anticoagulation such as serious bleeding or thromboembolic events.

Patient self-testing and self-management through the use of a home INR monitor may be used to improve the time in therapeutic rate (TTR) for select groups of patients. Increased TTR leads to improved clinical outcomes and reductions in thromboembolic and hemorrhagic events. Home prothrombin monitoring with the use of INR devices is covered only for patients with mechanical heart valves. The monitor and the home testing must be prescribed by a treating physician as provided at 42 C.F.R. 410.32 (a) and the following requirements must be met:

1. The patient must have been anticoagulated for at least three months prior to use of the home INR device;

2. The patient must undergo an educational program on anticoagulation management and the use of the device prior to its use in the home; and

3. Self-testing with the device should not occur more frequently than once a week.

55-1 WATER PURIFICATION AND SOFTENING SYSTEMS USED IN CONJUNCTION WITH HOME DIALYSIS

Water Purification Systems—Water used for home dialysis should be chemically free of heavy trace metals and/or organic contaminants which could be hazardous to the patient. It should also be as free of bacteria as possible but need not be biologically sterile. Since the characteristics of natural water supplies in most areas of the country are such that some type of water purification system is needed, such a system used in conjunction with a home dialysis (either peritoneal or hemodialysis) unit is covered under Medicare.

There are two types of water purification systems which will satisfy these requirements:

- Deionization-The removal of organic substances, mineral salts of magnesium and calcium (causing hardness), compounds of fluoride and chloride from tap water using the process of filtration and ion exchange; or
- Reverse Osmosis-The process used to remove impurities from tap water utilizing pressure to force water through a porous membrane.

Use of both a deionization unit and reverse osmosis unit in series, theoretically to provide the advantages of both systems, has been determined medically unnecessary since either system can provide water which is both chemically and bacteriologically pure enough for acceptable use in home dialysis. In addition, spare deionization tanks are not covered since they are essentially a precautionary supply rather than a current requirement for treatment of the patient. Activated carbon filters used as a component of water purification systems to remove unsafe concentrations of chlorine and chloramines are covered when prescribed by a physician.

Water Softening System.-Except as indicated below, a water softening system used in conjunction with home dialysis is excluded from coverage under Medicare as not being reasonable and necessary within the meaning of S1862(a)(1) of the law. Such a system, in conjunction with a home dialysis unit, does not adequately remove the hazardous heavy metal contaminants (such as arsenic) which may be present in trace amounts.

A water softening system may be covered when used to pretreat water to be purified by a reverse osmosis (RO) unit for home dialysis where:

- The manufacturer of the RO unit has set standards for the quality of water entering the RO (e.g., the water to be purified by the RO must be of a certain quality if the unit is to perform as intended);

- The patients water is demonstrated to be of a lesser quality than required; and

- The softener is used only to soften water entering the RO unit, and thus, used only for dialysis. (The softener need not actually be built into the RO unit, but must be an integral part of the dialysis system.)

- Developing Need When a Water Softening System is Replaced with a Water Purification Unit in an Existing Home Dialysis System.-The medical necessity of water purification units must be care fully developed when they replace water softening systems in existing home dialysis systems. A purification system may be ordered under these circumstances for a number of reasons. For example, changes in the medical community's opinions regarding the quality of water necessary for safe dialysis may lead the physician to decide the quality of water previously used should be improved, or the water quality itself may have deteriorated. Patients may have dialyzed using only an existing water softener previous to Medicare ESRD coverage because of inability to pay for a purification system. On the other hand, in some cases, the installation of a purification system is not medically necessary. Thus, when such a case comes to your attention, ask the physician to furnish the reason for the changes. Supporting documentation, such as the supplier's recommendations or water analysis, may be required. All such cases should be reviewed by your medical consultants.

  Cross-reference: Intermediary Manual, SS3113, 3643 (item ic); Carriers Manual, SS2100, 2100.2 2130, 2105 (item ic); Hospital Manual, S235.

55-2 PERIDEX CAPD FILTER SET -- NOT COVERED

The Peridex Filter Set is used by home continuous ambulatory peritoneal dialysis (CAPD) patients. The Peridex Filter Set is designed to provide sterile filtration during infusion of the dialysis solution in a beneficiary's peritoneal cavity; included in the filter set is a bacterial filter designed to block peritonitis-causing organisms and thus reduce the incidence of peritonitis.

Based upon advice of our medical consultants, we have determined that the Peridex CAPD Filter Set cannot be covered at this time by Medicare because it has not yet been shown to be safe and effective in preventing peritonitis.

60-3 WHITE CANE FOR USE BY A BLIND PERSON—NOT COVERED

A white cane for use by a blind person is more an identifying and self-help device rather than an item which makes a meaningful contribution in the treatment of an illness or injury.

60-4 HOME USE OF OXYGEN

A. General.—Medicare coverage of home oxygen and oxygen equipment under the durable medical equipment (DME) benefit (see §1861(s)(6)of the Act) is considered reasonable and necessary only for patients with significant hypoxemia who meet the medical documentation, laboratory evidence, and health conditions specified in subsections B, C, and D. This section also includes special coverage criteria for portable oxygen systems. Finally, a statement on the absence of coverage of the professional services of a respiratory therapist under the DME benefit is included in subsection F.

B. Medical documentation.—Initial claims for oxygen services must include a completed Form HCFA-484 (Certificate of Medical Necessity: Oxygen)to establish whether coverage criteria are met and to ensure that the oxygen services provided are consistent with the physician's prescription or other medical documentation. The treating physician's prescription or other medical documentation must indicate that other forms of treatment (e.g., medical and physical therapy directed at secretions, bronchospasm and infection) have been tried, have not been sufficiently successful, and oxygen therapy is still required. While there is no substitute for oxygen therapy, each patient must receive optimum therapy before long-term home oxygen therapy is ordered. Use Form HCFA-484 for recertifications. (See Medicare Carriers Manual §3312 for completion of Form HCFA-484.)

The medical and prescription information in section B of Form HCFA-484 can be completed only by the treating physician, the physician's employee, or another clinician (e.g., nurse, respiratory therapist, etc.) as long as that person is not the DME supplier. Although hospital discharge coordinators and medical social workers may assist in arranging for physician-prescribed home oxygen, they do not have the authority to prescribe the services. Suppliers may not enter this information. While this section may be completed by nonphysician clinician or a physician employee, it must be reviewed and the form HCFA-484 signed by the attending physician.

A physician's certification of medical necessity for oxygen equipment must include the results of specific testing before coverage can be determined.

Claims for oxygen must also be supported by medical documentation in the patient's record. Separate documentation is used with electronic billing. (See Medicare Carriers Manual, Part 3, §4105.5.) This documentation may be in the form of a prescription written by the patient's attending physician who has recently examined the patient (normally within a month of the start of therapy) and must specify:

- A diagnosis of the disease requiring home use of oxygen;
- The oxygen flow rate; and

An estimate of the frequency, duration of use (e.g., 2 liters per minute, 10 minutes per hour, 12 hours per day), and duration of need (e.g., 6 months or lifetime).
NOTE: A prescription for "Oxygen PRN" or "Oxygen as needed" does not meet this last requirement. Neither provides any basis for determining if the amount of oxygen is reasonable and necessary for the patient.

A member of the carrier's medical staff should review all claims with oxygen flow rates of more than 4 liters per minute before payment can be made.

The attending physician specifies the type of oxygen delivery system to be used (i.e., gas, liquid, or concentrator) by signing the completed form HCFA-484. In addition the supplier or physician may use the space in section C for written confirmation of additional details of the physician's order. The additional order information contained in section C may include the means of oxygen delivery (mask, nasal, cannula, etc.), the specifics of varying flow rates, and/or the noncontinuous use of oxygen as appropriate. The physician confirms this order information with their signature in section D.

New medical documentation written by the patient's attending physician must be submitted to the carrier in support of revised oxygen requirements when there has been a change in the patient's condition and need for oxygen therapy.

Carriers are required to conduct periodic, continuing medical necessity reviews on patients whose conditions warrant these reviews and on patients with indefinite or extended periods of necessity as described in Medicare Carriers Manual, Part 3, §4105.5. When indicated, carriers may also request documentation of the results of a repeat arterial blood gas or oximetry study.

NOTE: Section 4152 of OBRA 1990 requires earlier recertification and retesting of oxygen patients who begin coverage with an arterial blood gas result at or above a partial pressure of 55 or an arterial oxygen saturation percentage at or above 89. (See Medicare Carriers Manual §4105.5 for certification and retesting schedules.)

C. Laboratory Evidence.—Initial claims for oxygen therapy must also include the results of a blood gas study that has been ordered and evaluated by the attending physician. This is usually in the form of a measurement of the partial pressure of oxygen (PO2) in arterial blood. (See Medicare Carriers Manual, Part 3, §2070.1 for instructions on clinical laboratory tests.) A measurement of arterial oxygen saturation obtained by ear or pulse oximetry, however, is also acceptable when ordered and evaluated by the attending physician and performed under his or her supervision or when performed by a qualified provider or supplier of laboratory services. When the arterial blood gas and the oximetry studies are both used to document the need for home oxygen therapy and the results are conflicting, the arterial blood gas study is the preferred source of documenting medical need. A DME supplier is not considered a qualified provider or supplier of laboratory services for purposes of these guidelines. This prohibition does not extend to the results of blood gas test conducted by a hospital certified to do such tests. The conditions under which the laboratory tests are performed must be specified in writing and submitted with the initial claim, i.e., at rest, during exercise, or during sleep.

The preferred sources of laboratory evidence are existing physician and/or hospital records that reflect the patient's medical condition. Since it is expected that virtually all patients who qualify for home oxygen coverage for the first time under these guidelines have recently been discharged from a hospital where they submitted to arterial blood gas tests, the carrier needs to request that such test results be submitted in support of their initial claims for home oxygen. If more than one arterial blood gas test is performed during the patient's hospital stay, the test result obtained closest to, but no earlier than 2 days prior to the hospital discharge date is required as evidence of the need for home oxygen therapy.

For those patients whose initial oxygen prescription did not originate during a hospital stay, blood gas studies should be done while the patient is in the chronic stable state, i.e., not during a period of an acute illness or an exacerbation of their underlying disease."

Carriers may accept a attending physician's statement of recent hospital test results for a particular patient, when appropriate, in lieu of copies of actual hospital records.

A repeat arterial blood gas study is appropriate when evidence indicates that an oxygen recipient has undergone a major change in their condition relevant to home use of oxygen. If the carrier has reason to believe that there has been a major change in the patient's physical condition, it may ask for documentation of the results of another blood gas or oximetry study.

D. Health Conditions.—Coverage is available for patients with significant hypoxemia in the chronic stable state if: (1) the attending physician has determined that the patient has a health condition outlined in subsection D.1, (2) the patient meets the blood gas evidence requirements specified in subsection D.3, and (3) the patient has appropriately tried other alternative treatment measures without complete success. (See subsection B.)

1. Conditions for Which Oxygen Therapy May Be Covered.—

   - A severe lung disease, such as chronic obstructive pulmonary disease, diffuse interstitial lung disease, whether of known or unknown etiology; cystic fibrosis bronchiectasis; widespread pulmonary neoplasm; or
   - Hypoxia-related symptoms or findings that might be expected to improve with oxygen therapy. Examples of these symptoms and findings are pulmonary hypertension, recurring congestive heart failure due to chronic cor pulmonale, erythrocytosis, impairment of the cognitive process, nocturnal restlessness, and morning headache.

2. Conditions for Which Oxygen Therapy Is Not Covered.—

   - Angina pectoris in the absence of hypoxemia. This condition is generally not the result of a low oxygen level in the blood, and there are other preferred treatments;
   - Breathlessness without cor pulmonale or evidence of hypoxemia. Although intermittent oxygen use is sometimes prescribed to relieve this condition, it is potentially harmful and psychologically addicting;
   - Severe peripheral vascular disease resulting in clinically evident desaturation in one or more extremities. There is no evidence that increased PO2 improves the oxygenation of tissues with impaired circulation; or
   - Terminal illnesses that do not affect the lungs.

3. Covered Blood Gas Values.—If the patient has a condition specified in subsection D.1, the carrier must review the medical documentation and laboratory evidence that has been submitted for a particular patient (see subsections B and C) and determine if coverage is available under one of the three group categories outlined below.

   a. Group I.—Except as modified in subsection d, coverage is provided for patients with significant hypoxemia evidenced by any of the following:

      (1) An arterial PO2 at or below 55 mm Hg, or an arterial oxygen saturation at or below 88 percent, taken at rest, breathing room air.

      (2) An arterial PO2 at or below 55 mm Hg, or an arterial oxygen saturation at or below 88 percent, taken during sleep for a patient who demonstrates an arterial PO2 at or above 56 mm Hg, or an arterial oxygen saturation at or above 89 percent, while awake; or a greater than normal fall in oxygen level during sleep (a decrease in arterial PO2 more than 10 mm Hg, or decrease in arterial oxygen saturation more than 5 percent) associated with symptoms or signs reasonably attributable to hypoxemia (e.g., impairment of cognitive

processes and nocturnal restlessness or insomnia). In either of these cases, coverage is provided only for use of oxygen during sleep, and then only one type of unit will be covered. Portable oxygen, therefore, would not be covered in this situation.

(3) An arterial PO2 at or below 55 mm Hg or an arterial oxygen saturation at or below 88 percent, taken during exercise for a patient who demonstrates an arterial PO2 at or above 56 mm Hg, or an arterial oxygen saturation at or above 89 percent, during the day while at rest. In this case, supplemental oxygen is provided for during exercise if there is evidence the use of oxygen improves the hypoxemia that was demonstrated during exercise when the patient was breathing room air.

b. Group II.—Except as modified in subsection d, coverage is available for patients whose arterial PO2 is 56-59 mm Hg or whose arterial blood oxygen saturation is 89 percent, if there is evidence of:

(1) Dependent edema suggesting congestive heart failure;
(2) Pulmonary hypertension or cor pulmonale, determined by measurement of pulmonary artery pressure, gated blood pool scan, echocardiogram, or "P" pulmonale on EKG (P wave greater than 3 mm in standard leads II, III, or AVFL; or
(3) Erythrocythemia with a hematocrit greater than 56 percent.

c. Group III.—Except as modified in subsection d, carriers must apply a rebuttable presumption that a home program of oxygen use is not medically necessary for patients with arterial PO2 levels at or above 60 mm Hg, or arterial blood oxygen saturation at or above 90 percent. In order for claims in this category to be reimbursed, the carrier's reviewing physician needs to review any documentation submitted in rebuttal of this presumption and grant specific approval of the claims. HCFA expects few claims to be approved for coverage in this category.

d. Variable Factors That May Affect Blood Gas Values.—In reviewing the arterial PO2 levels and the arterial oxygen saturation percentages specified in subsections D. 3. a, b and c, the carrier's medical staff must take into account variations in oxygen measurements that may result from such factors as the patient's age, the altitude level, or the patient's decreased oxygen carrying capacity.

E. Portable Oxygen Systems.—A patient meeting the requirements specified below may qualify for coverage of a portable oxygen system either (1) by itself or (2) to use in addition to a stationary oxygen system. A portable oxygen system is covered for a particular patient if:

- The claim meets the requirements specified in subsections A-D, as appropriate; and
- The medical documentation indicates that the patient is mobile in the home and would benefit from the use of a portable oxygen system in the home. Portable oxygen systems are not covered for patients who qualify for oxygen solely based on blood gas studies obtained during sleep.

F. Respiratory Therapists.—Respiratory therapists' services are not covered under the provisions for coverage of oxygen services under the Part B durable medical equipment benefit as outlined above. This benefit provides for coverage of home use of oxygen and oxygen equipment, but does not include a professional component in the delivery of such services.

(See §60-9; Intermediary Manual, Part 3, §3113ff; and Medicare Carriers Manual, Part 3, §2100ff.)

60-5 POWER-OPERATED VEHICLES THAT MAY BE USED AS WHEELCHAIRS

Power-operated vehicles that may be appropriately used as wheelchairs are covered under the durable medical equipment provision.

These vehicles have been appropriately used in the home setting for vocational rehabilitation and to improve the ability of chronically disabled persons to cope with normal domestic, vocational and social activities. They may be covered if a wheelchair is medically necessary and the patient is unable to operate a wheelchair manually.

A specialist in physical medicine, orthopedic surgery, neurology, or rheumatology must provide an evaluation of the patient's medical and physical condition and a prescription for the vehicle to assure that the patient requires the vehicle and is capable of using it safely. When an intermediary determines that such a specialist is not reasonably accessible, e.g., more than 1 day's round trip from the beneficiary's home, or the patient's condition precludes such travel, a prescription from the beneficiary's physician is acceptable.

The intermediary's medical staff reviews all claims for a power-operated vehicle, including the specialists' or other physicians' prescriptions and evaluations of the patient's medical and physical conditions, to insure that all coverage requirements are met. (See §60-9 and Intermediary Manual, Part 3, §3629.)

60-6 SPECIALLY SIZED WHEELCHAIRS

Payment may be made for a specially sized wheelchair even though it is more expensive than a standard wheelchair. For example, a narrow wheelchair may be required because of the narrow doorways of a patient's home or because of a patient's slender build. Such difference in the size of the wheelchair from the standard model is not considered a deluxe feature.

A physician's certification or prescription that a special size is needed is not required where you can determine from the information in file or other sources that a specially sized wheelchair (rather than a standard one) is needed to accommodate the wheelchair to the place of use or the physical size of the patient.

To determine the reasonable charge in these cases, use the criteria set out in Carriers Manual, §§5022, 5022.1, 5200, and 5205, as necessary.

Cross-reference: Intermediary Manual, §§3113.2C, 3642.1, 3643 (item 3); Carriers Manual, §§2100.2c, 2105, 4105.2, 5107; Hospital Manual, §§235.2c, 420.1 (item 13).

60-7 SELF-CONTAINED PACEMAKER MONITORS

Self-contained pacemaker monitors are accepted devices for monitoring cardiac pacemakers. Accordingly, program payment may be made for the rental or purchase of either of the following pacemaker monitors when it is prescribed by a physician for a patient with a cardiac pacemaker:

A. Digital Electronic Pacemaker Monitor.—This device provides the patient with an instantaneous digital readout of his pacemaker pulse rate. Use of this device does not involve professional services until there has been a change of five pulses (or more) per minute above or below the initial rate of the pacemaker; when such change occurs, the patient contacts his physician.

B. Audible/Visible Signal Pacemaker Monitor.—This device produces an audible and visible signal which indicates the pacemaker rate. Use of this device does not involve professional services until a change occurs in these signals; at such time, the patient contacts his physician.

NOTE: The design of the self-contained pacemaker monitor makes it possible for the patient to monitor his pacemaker periodically and minimizes the need for regular visits to the outpatient department of the provider.

Therefore, documentation of the medical necessity for pacemaker evaluation in the outpatient department of the provider should be obtained where such evaluation is employed in addition to the self-contained pacemaker monitor used by the patient in his home.

Cross-reference: §50-1

60-8 SEAT LIFT

Reimbursement may be made for the rental or purchase of a medically necessary seat lift when prescribed by a physician for a patient with severe arthritis of the hip or knee and patients with muscular dystrophy or other neuromuscular diseases when it has been determined the patient can benefit therapeutically from use of the device. In establishing medical necessity for the seat lift, the evidence must show that the item is included in the physician's course of treatment, that it is likely to effect improvement, or arrest or retard deterioration in the patient's condition, and that the severity of the condition is such that the alternative would be chair or bed confinement.

Coverage of seat lifts is limited to those types which operate smoothly, can be controlled by the patient, and effectively assist a patient in standing up and sitting down without other assistance. Excluded from coverage is the type of lift which operates by a spring release mechanism with a sudden, catapult-like motion and jolts the patient from a seated to a standing position. Limit the payment for units which incorporate a recliner feature along with the seat lift to the amount payable for a seat lift without this feature.

Cross-reference: Carriers Manual, § 5107

60-8 DURABLE MEDICAL EQUIPMENT REFERENCE LIST

The durable medical equipment (DME) list which follows is designed to facilitate your processing of DME claims. This section is designed to be used as a quick reference tool for determining the coverage status of certain pieces of DME and especially for those items which are commonly referred to by both brand and generic names. The information contained herein is applicable (where appropriate) to all DME coverage determinations discussed in the DME portion of this manual. The list is organized into two columns. The first column lists alphabetically various generic categories of equipment on which national coverage decisions have been made by HCFA; and the second column notes the coverage status of each equipment category.

In the case of equipment categories that have been determined by HCFA to be covered under the DME benefit, the list outlines the conditions of coverage that must be met if payment is to be allowed for the rental or purchase of the DME by a particular patient, or cross-refers to another section of the manual where the applicable coverage criteria are described in more detail. With respect to equipment categories that cannot be covered as DME, the list includes a brief explanation of why the equipment is not covered. This DME list will be updated periodically to reflect any additional national coverage decisions that HCFA may make with regard to other categories of equipment.

When you receive a claim for an item of equipment which does not appear to fall logically into any of the generic categories listed, you have the authority and responsibility for deciding whether those items are covered under the DME benefit. These decisions must be made by each contractor based on the advice of its medical consultants, taking into account:

- The general DME coverage instructions in the Carriers Manual, §2100ff and Intermediary Manual, §3113ff (see below for brief summary);
- Whether the item has been approved for marketing by the Food and Drug Administration (FDA) (see Carriers Manual, §2303.1 and Intermediary Manual, §3151.1) and is otherwise generally considered to be safe and effective for the purpose intended; and
- Whether the item is reasonable and necessary for the individual patient.
- As provided in the Carriers Manual, § 2100.1, and Intermediary Manual,
- §3113.1, the term DME is defined as equipment which
- Can withstand repeated use; i.e., could normally be rented, and used by successive patients;
- Is primarily and customarily used to serve a medical purpose;
- Generally is not useful to a person in the absence of illness or injury; and
- Is appropriate for use in a patient's home.

Durable Medical Equipment Reference List:

Item	Coverage Status
Air Cleaners	deny--environmental control equipment; not primarily medical in nature (§l86l(n) of the Act)
Air Conditioners	deny--environmental control equipment; not primarily medical in nature (§l861(n) of the Act)
Air-Fluidized Bed	(See §60-19.)
Alternating Pressure Pads, and Mattresses and Lambs Wool Pads	covered if patient has, or is highly susceptible to, decubitus ulcers and patient's physician has specified that he will be supervising its use in connection with his course of treatment.
Audible/Visible Signal Pacemaker Monitor	(See Self-Contained Pacemaker Monitor.)
Augmentative Communication Device	(See Speech Generating Devices, §60-23.)
Bathtub Lifts	deny--convenience item; not primarily medical in nature (§l861(n) of the Act)
Bathtub Seats	deny--comfort or convenience item; hygienic equipment; not primarily medical in nature (§l861(n) of the Act)
Bead Bed	(See §60-19.)
Bed Baths (home type)	deny--hygienic equipment; not primarily medical in nature (§l861(n) of the Act)
Bed Lifter (bed elevator)	deny--not primarily medical in nature (§1861(n) of the Act.

Item	Coverage Status
Bed boards	deny--not primarily medical in nature (§1861(n) of the Act)
Bed Pans (autoclavable hospital type)	covered if patient is bed confined
Bed Side Rails	(See Hospital Beds, §60-18.)
Beds-Lounge (power or manual)	deny--not a hospital bed; comfort or convenience item; not primarily medical in nature (§186l(n) of the Act)
Beds--Oscillating	deny--institutional equipment; inappropriate for home use
Bidet Toilet Seat	(See Toilet Seats.)
Blood Glucose Analyzer Reflectance Colorimeter	deny--unsuitable for home use (See §60-11.)
Blood Glucose Monitor	covered if patient meets certain conditions (See §60-11.)
Braille Teaching Texts	deny--educational equipment; not primarily medical in nature (§1861(n) of the Act)
Canes	covered if patient's condition impairs ambulation (See §60-3.)
Carafes	deny--convenience item; not primarily medical in nature (§l861(n) of the Act)
Catheters	deny--nonreusable disposable supply (§l861(n) of the Act)
Commodes	covered if patient is confined to bed or room. NOTE: The term "room confined" means that the patient's condition is such that leaving the room is medically contraindicated. The accessibility of bathroom facilities generally would not be a factor in this determination. However, confinement of a patient to his home in a case where there are no toilet facilities in the home may be equated to room confinement. Moreover, payment may also be made if a patient's medical condition confines him to a floor of his home and there is no bathroom located on that floor (See hospital beds in §60-18 for definition of "bed confinement".)
Communicator	(See §60-23, Speech Generating Device
Continuous Passive Motion	Continuous passive motion devices are devices covered for patients who have received a total knee replacement. To qualify for coverage, use of the device must commence within 2 days following surgery. In addition, coverage is limited to that portion of the three week period following surgery during which the device is used in the patient's home. There is insufficient evidence to justify coverage of these devices for longer periods of time or for other applications.
Continuous Positive Airway Pressure (CPAP)	(See §60-17.)
Crutches	covered if patient's condition impairs Ambulation
Cushion Lift Power Seat	(See Seat Lifts.)
Dehumidifiers (room or central heating system type)	deny--environmental control equipment; not primarily medical in nature (§l861(n) of the Act
Diathermy Machines (standard pulses wave types)	deny--inappropriate for home use (See and §35-41.)
Digital Electronic Pacemaker Monitor	(See Self-Contained Pacemaker Monitor.)
Disposable Sheets and Bags	deny--nonreusable disposable supplies (§l861(n) of the Act)

Item	Coverage Status
Elastic Stockings	deny--nonreusable supply; not rental-type items (§l861(n) of the Act)
Electric Air Cleaners	deny--(See Air Cleaners.) (§l861(n) of the Act)
Electric Hospital Beds	(See Hospital Beds §60-18.)
Electrical Stimulation for Wounds	deny--inappropriate for home use
Electrostatic Machines	deny--(See Air Cleaners and Air Conditioners.) (§l861(n) of the Act)
Elevators	deny--convenience item; not primarily medical in nature (§l861(n) of the Act)
Emesis Basins	deny--convenience item; not primarily medical in nature (§l861(n) of the Act)
Esophageal Dilator	deny--physician instrument; inappropriate for patient use
Exercise Equipment	deny--not primarily medical in nature (§l861(n) of the Act)
Fabric Supports	deny--nonreusable supplies; not rental-type it (§l861(n) of the Act)
Face Masks (oxygen)	covered if oxygen is covered (See § 60-4.)
Face Masks (surgical)	deny--nonreusable disposable items (§l861(n) of the Act)
Flowmeter	(See Medical Oxygen Regulators)
Fluidic Breathing Assister	(See IPPB Machines.)
Fomentation Device	(See Heating Pads.)
Gel Flotation Pads and Mattresses	(See Alternating Pressure Pads and Mattresses.)
Grab Bars	deny--self-help device; not primarily medical in nature (§l861(n) of the Act)
Heat and Massage Foam Cushion Pad	deny--not primarily medical in nature; personal comfort item (§§ l861(n) and l862(a)(6) of the Act)
Heating and Cooling Plants	deny--environmental control equipment; not primarily medical in nature(§l861(n) of the Act)
Heating Pads	covered if the contractor's medical staff determines patient's medical condition is one for which the application of heat in the form of a heating pad is therapeutically effective.
Heat Lamps	covered if the contractor's medical staff determines patient's medical condition is one for which the application of heat in the form of a heat lamp is therapeutically effective.
Hospital Beds	(See § 60-18.)
Hot Packs	(See Heating Pads.)
Humidifiers (oxygen)	(See Oxygen Humidifiers.)
Humidifiers (room or central heating system types)	deny--environmental control equipment; not medical in nature (§l861(n) of the Act)
Hydraulic Lift	(See Patient Lifts.)
Incontinent Pads	deny--nonreusable supply; hygienic item (§ l861(n) of the Act.)
Infusion Pumps	For external and implantable pumps, see §60-14. If the pump is used with an enteral or parenteral malnutritional therapy system, see §§65-10 - 65.10.2 0.2 for special coverage rules.
Injectors (hypodermic jet devices for injection of insulin	deny-- noncovered self-administered drug supply, §1861(s)(2)(A) of the Act)
IPPB Machines	covered if patient's ability to breathe is severely impaired

Item	Coverage Status
Iron Lungs	(See Ventilators.)
Irrigating Kit	deny--nonreusable supply; hygienic equipment (§l861(n) of the Act)
Lambs Wool Pads	covered under same conditions as alternating pressure pads and mattresses
Leotards	deny--(See Pressure Leotards.) (§l861(n)of the Act)
Lymphedema Pumps	covered (See §60-16.)(segmental and non-segmental therapy types)
Massage Devices	deny--personal comfort items; not primarily medical in nature (§§l861(n) and l862(a)(6) of the Act)
Mattress	covered only where hospital bed is medically necessary (Separate Charge for replacement mattresses should not be allowed where hospital bed with mattress is rented.) (See §60-18.)
Medical Oxygen Regulators	covered if patient's ability to breathe is severely impaired (See §60-4.)
Mobile Geriatric Chair	(See Rolling Chairs.)
Motorized Wheelchairs	(See Wheelchairs (power operated).)
Muscle Stimulators	Covered for certain conditions (See §35-77.)
Nebulizers	covered if patient's ability to breathe is severely impaired
Oscillating Beds	deny--institutional equipment--inappropriate for home use
Over bed Tables	deny--convenience item; not primarily medical in nature (§l861(n) of the Act)
Oxygen	covered if the oxygen has been prescribed for use in connection with medically necessary durable medical equipment (See §60-4.)
Oxygen Humidifiers	covered if a medical humidifier has been prescribed for use in connection with medically necessary durable medical equipment for purposes of moisturizing oxygen (See §60-4.)
Oxygen Regulators (Medical)	(See Medical Oxygen Regulators.)
Oxygen Tents	(See § 60-4.)
Paraffin Bath Units (Portable)	(See Portable Paraffin Bath Units.)
Paraffin Bath Units (Standard)	deny--institutional equipment; inappropriate for home use
Parallel Bars	deny--support exercise equipment; primarily for institutional use; in the home setting other devices (e.g., a walker) satisfy the patient's need
Patient Lifts	covered if contractor's medical staff determines patient's condition is such that periodic movement is necessary to effect improvement or to arrest or retard deterioration in his condition.
Percussors	covered for mobilizing respiratory tract secretions in patients with chronic obstructive lung disease, chronic bronchitis, or emphysema, when patient or operator of powered percussor has received appropriate training by a physician or therapist, and no one competent to administer manual therapy is available.
Portable Oxygen Systems	1. Regulated (adjustable --covered under conditions specified in flow rate)§60-4. Refer all claims to medical staff for this determination. 2. Preset (flow rate --deny--emergency, first-aid, or not

Item	Coverage Status
	adjustable) precautionary equipment; essentially not therapeutic in nature
Portable Paraffin Bath Units	covered when the patient has undergone a successful trial period of paraffin therapy ordered by a physician and the patient's condition is expected to be relieved by long term use of this modality.
Portable Room Heaters	deny--environmental control equipment; not primarily medical in nature (§l861(n) of the Act)
Portable Whirlpool Pumps	deny--not primarily medical in nature; personal comfort items (§§l861(n) and l862(a)(6) of the Act)
Postural Drainage Boards	covered if patient has a chronic pulmonary condition
Preset Portable Oxygen Units	deny--emergency, first-aid, or precautionary equipment; essentially not therapeutic in nature
Pressure Leotards	deny--nonreusable supply, not rental-type item (§l861(n) of the Act)
Pulse Tachometer	deny--not reasonable or necessary for monitoring pulse of homebound patient with or without a cardiac pacemaker
Quad-Canes	(See Walkers.)
Raised Toilet Seats	deny--convenience item; hygienic equipment; not primarily medical in nature (§l861(n) of the Act)
Reflectance Colorimeters	(See Blood Glucose Analyzers.)
Respirators	(See Ventilators.)
Rolling Chairs	covered if the contractor's medical staff determines that the patient's condition is such that there is a medical need for this item and it has been prescribed by the patient's physician in lieu of a wheelchair. Coverage is limited to those rollabout chairs having casters of at least 5 inches in diameter and specifically designed to meet the needs of ill, injured, or otherwise impaired individuals. Coverage is denied for the wide range of chairs with smaller casters as are found in general use in homes, offices, and institutions for many purposes not related to the care or treatment of ill or injured persons. This type is not primarily medical in nature. (§l861(n) of the Act)
Safety Roller	(See §60-15.)
Sauna Baths	deny--not primarily medical in nature; personal comfort items (§§l861(n) and (l862(a)(6) of the Act)
Seat Lift	covered under the conditions specified in §60-8. Refer all to medical staff for this determination.
Self-Contained Pacemaker Monitor	covered when prescribed by a physician for a patient with a cardiac pacemaker (See §§50-1C and 60-7.)
Sitz Bath	covered if the contractor's medical staff determines patient has an infection or injury of the perineal area and the item has been prescribed by the patient's physician as a part of his planned regimen of treatment in the patient's home.
Spare Tanks of Oxygen	deny--convenience or precautionary supply
Speech Teaching Machine	deny--education equipment; not primarily medical in nature (§l861(n) of the Act)
Stairway Elevators	deny--(See Elevators.) (§l861(n) of the Act)

Item	Coverage Status
Standing Table	deny--convenience item; not primarily medical in nature (§1861(n) of the Act)
Steam Packs	these packs are covered under the same condition as a heating pad (See Heating Pads.)
Suction Machine	covered if the contractor's medical staff determines that the machine specified in the claim is medically required and appropriate for home use without technical or professional supervision.
Support Hose	deny (See Fabric Supports.) (§l861(n) of the Act)
Surgical Leggings	deny--nonreusable supply; not rental-type item (§l861(n) of the Act)
Telephone Alert Systems	deny--these are emergency communications systems and do not serve a diagnostic or therapeutic purpose
Telephone Arms	deny--convenience item; not medical in nature (§l861(n) of the Act)
Toilet Seats	deny--not medical equipment (§l861(n)of the Act)
Traction Equipment	covered if patient has orthopedic impairment requiring traction equipment which prevents ambulation during the period of use (Consider covering devices usable during ambulation; e.g., cervical traction collar, under the brace provision)
Trapeze Bars	covered if patient is bed confined and the patient needs a trapeze bar to sit up because of respiratory condition, to change body position for other medical reasons, or to get in and out of bed.
Treadmill Exerciser	deny--exercise equipment; not primarily medical in nature(§l861(n) of the Act)
Ultraviolet Cabinet	covered for selected patients with generalized intractable psoriasis. Using appropriate consultation, the contractor should determine whether medical and other factors justify treatment at home rather than at alternative sites, e.g., outpatient department of a hospital.
Urinals (autoclavable hospital type)	covered if patient is bed confined
Vaporizers	covered if patient has a respiratory illness
Ventilators	covered for treatment of neuromuscular diseases, thoracic restrictive diseases, and chronic respiratory failure consequent to chronic obstructive pulmonary disease. Includes both positive and negative pressure types.
Walkers	covered if patient's condition impairs ambulation (See also §60-15.)
Water and Pressure Pads and Mattresses	(See Alternating Pressure Pads and Mattresses.)
Wheelchairs	covered if patient's condition is such that without the use of a wheelchair he would otherwise be bed or chair confined. An individual may qualify for a wheelchair and still be considered bed confined.
Wheelchairs (power operated) and wheelchairs with other special features	covered if patient's condition is such and that a wheelchair is medically necessary and the patient is unable to operate the wheelchair manually. Any claim involving a power wheelchair or a wheelchair with other special features should be referred for medical consultation since payment for the special features is

Item	Coverage Status
	limited to those which are medically required because of the patient's condition. (See §60-5 for power operated and §60-6 for specially sized wheelchairs.) NOTE: A power-operated vehicle that may appropriately be used as a wheelchair can be covered. (See §60-5 for coverage details.)
Whirlpool Bath Equipment	covered if patient is homebound and has a (standard) condition for which the whirlpool bath can be expected to provide substantial therapeutic benefit justifying its cost. Where patient is not homebound but has such a condition, payment is restricted to the cost of providing the services elsewhere; e.g., an outpatient department of a participating hospital, if that alternative is less costly. In all cases, refer claim to medical staff for a determination.
Whirlpool Pumps	deny--(See Portable Whirlpool Pumps.) (§1861(n) of the Act)

60-11 HOME BLOOD GLUCOSE MONITORS

There are several different types of blood glucose monitors that use reflectance meters to determine blood glucose levels. Medicare coverage of these devices varies, both with respect to the type of device and the medical condition of the patient for whom the device is prescribed.

Reflectance colorimeter devices used for measuring blood glucose levels in clinical settings are not covered as durable medical equipment for use in the home because their need for frequent professional re-calibration makes them unsuitable for home use. However, some types of blood glucose monitors which use a reflectance meter specifically designed for home use by diabetic patients may be covered as durable medical equipment, subject to the conditions and limitations described below.

Blood glucose monitors are meter devices that read color changes produced on specially treated reagent strips by glucose concentrations in the patient's blood. The patient, using a disposable sterile lancet, draws a drop of blood, places it on a reagent strip and, following instructions which may vary with the device used, inserts it into the device to obtain a reading. Lancets, reagent strips, and other supplies necessary for the proper functioning of the device are also covered for patients for whom the device is indicated. Home blood glucose monitors enable certain patients to better control their blood glucose levels by frequently checking and appropriately contacting their attending physician for advice and treatment. Studies indicate that the patient's ability to carefully follow proper procedures is critical to obtaining satisfactory results with these devices. In addition, the cost of the devices, with their supplies, limits economical use to patients who must make frequent checks of their blood glucose levels. Accordingly, coverage of home blood glucose monitors is limited to patients meeting the following conditions:

- The patient has been diagnosed as having diabetes;
- The patient's physician states that the patient is capable of being trained to use the particular device prescribed in an appropriate manner. In some cases, the patient may not be able to perform this function, but a responsible individual can be trained to use the equipment and monitor the patient to assure that the intended effect is achieved. This is permissible if the record is properly documented by the patient's physician; and
- The device is designed for home rather than clinical use.

There is also a blood glucose monitoring system designed especially for use by those with visual impairments. The monitors used in such systems are identical in terms of reliability and sensitivity to the standard blood glucose monitors described above. They differ by having such features as voice synthesizers, automatic timers, and specially designed arrangements of supplies and materials to enable the visually impaired to use the equipment without assistance.

These special blood glucose monitoring systems are covered under Medicare if the following conditions are met:

- The patient and device meet the three conditions listed above for coverage of standard home blood glucose monitors; and
- The patient's physician certifies that he or she has a visual impairment severe enough to require use of this special monitoring system.

The additional features and equipment of these special systems justify a higher reimbursement amount than allowed for standard blood glucose monitors. Separately identify claims for such devices and establish a separate reimbursement amount for them. For those carriers using HCPCS, the procedure code and definition is: E0609--Blood Glucose Monitor--with special features (e.g., voice synthesizers, automatic timer).

60-14 INFUSION PUMPS

The following indications for treatment using infusion pumps are covered under Medicare:

A. External Infusion Pumps.—

1. Iron Poisoning (Effective for Services Performed On or After 9/26/84).—When used in the administration of deferoxamine for the treatment of acute iron poisoning and iron overload, only external infusion pumps are covered.
2. Thromboembolic Disease (Effective for Services Performed On or After 9/26/84).—When used in the administration of heparin for the treatment of thromboembolic disease and/or pulmonary embolism, only external infusion pumps used in an institutional setting are covered.
3. Chemotherapy for Liver Cancer (Effective for Services Performed On or After 1/29/85).—The external chemotherapy infusion pump is covered when used in the treatment of primary hepatocellular carcinoma or colorectal cancer where this disease is unresectable or where the patient refuses surgical excision of the tumor.
4. Morphine for Intractable Cancer Pain (Effective for Services Performed On or After 4/22/85).—Morphine infusion via an external infusion pump is covered when used in the treatment of intractable pain caused by cancer (in either an inpatient or outpatient setting, including a hospice).
5. Continuous subcutaneous insulin infusion pumps (CSII) (Effective for Services Performed On or After 4/1/2000).—

An external infusion pump and related drugs/supplies are covered as medically necessary in the home setting in the following situation:

Treatment of Diabetes

In order to be covered, patients must meet criterion A or B:

(A) The patient has completed a comprehensive diabetes education program, and has been on a program of multiple daily injections of insulin (i.e. at least 3 injections per day), with frequent self-adjustments of insulin dose for at least 6 months prior to initiation of the insulin pump, and has documented frequency of glucose self-testing an average of at least 4 times per day during the 2 months prior to initiation of the insulin pump, and meets one or more of the following criteria while on the multiple daily injection regimen:

(1) Glycosylated hemoglobin level (HbAlc) > 7.0 percent
(2) History of recurring hypoglycemia
(3) Wide fluctuations in blood glucose before mealtime
(4) Dawn phenomenon with fasting blood sugars frequently Exceeding 200 mg/dl
(5) History of severe glycemic excursions

(B) The patient with diabetes has been on a pump prior to enrollment in Medicare and has documented frequency of glucose self-testing an average of at least 4 times per day during the month prior to Medicare enrollment.

Diabetes needs to be documented by a fasting C-peptide level that is less than or equal to 110 percent of the lower limit of normal of the laboratory's measurement method. (Effective for Services Performed on or after January 1, 2002.)

Continued coverage of the insulin pump would require that the patient has been seen and evaluated the treating physician at least every 3 months.

The pump must be ordered by and follow-up care of the patient must be managed by a physician who manages multiple patients with CSII and who works closely with a team including nurses, diabetes educators, and dietitians who are knowledgeable in the use of CSII.

6. Other uses of external infusion pumps are covered if the contractor's medical staff verifies the appropriateness of the therapy and of the prescribed pump for the individual patient.

   NOTE: Payment may also be made for drugs necessary for the effective use of an external infusion pump as long as the drug being used with the pump is itself reasonable and necessary for the patient's treatment.

B. Implantable Infusion Pumps.—

1. Chemotherapy for Liver Cancer (Effective for Services Performed On or After 9/26/84).—The implantable infusion pump is covered for intra-arterial infusion of 5-FUdR for the treatment of liver cancer for patients with primary hepatocellular carcinoma or Duke's Class D colorectal cancer, in whom the metastases are limited to the liver, and where (1) the disease is unresectable or (2) where the patient refuses surgical excision of the tumor.

2. Anti-Spasmodic Drugs for Severe Spasticity.—An implantable infusion pump is covered when used to administer anti-spasmodic drugs intrathecally (e.g., baclofen) to treat chronic intractable spasticity in patients who have proven unresponsive to less invasive medical therapy as determined by the following criteria:

- As indicated by at least a 6-week trial, the patient cannot be maintained on noninvasive methods of spasm control, such as oral anti-spasmodic drugs, either because these methods fail to control adequately the spasticity or produce intolerable side effects, and
- Prior to pump implantation, the patient must have responded favorably to a trial intrathecal dose of the anti-spasmodic drug.

3. Opioid Drugs for Treatment of Chronic Intractable Pain.—An implantable infusion pump is covered when used to administer opioid drugs (e.g., morphine) intrathecally or epidurally for treatment of severe chronic intractable pain of malignant or nonmalignant origin in patients who have a life expectancy of at least 3 months and who have proven unresponsive to less invasive medical therapy as determined by the following criteria:

   - The patient's history must indicate that he/she would not respond adequately to non-invasive methods of pain control, such as systemic opioids (including attempts to eliminate physical and behavioral abnormalities which may cause an exaggerated reaction to pain); and
   - A preliminary trial of intraspinal opioid drug administration must be undertaken with a temporary intrathecal/epidural catheter to substantiate adequately acceptable pain relief and degree of side effects (including effects on the activities of daily living) and patient acceptance.

4. Coverage of Other Uses of Implanted Infusion Pumps .—Determinations may be made on coverage of other uses of implanted infusion pumps if the contractor's medical staff verifies that:

   The drug is reasonable and necessary for the treatment of the individual patient;

   - It is medically necessary that the drug be administered by an implanted infusion pump; and
   - The FDA approved labeling for the pump must specify that the drug being administered and the purpose for which it is administered is an indicated use for the pump.

5. Implantation of Infusion Pump Is Contraindicated.—The implantation of an infusion pump is contraindicated in the following patients:

   - Patients with a known allergy or hypersensitivity to the drug being used (e.g., oral baclofen, morphine, etc.);
   - Patients who have an infection;
   - Patients whose body size is insufficient to support the weight and bulk of the device; and
   - Patients with other implanted programmable devices since crosstalk between devices may inadvertently change the prescription.

   NOTE: Payment may also be made for drugs necessary for the effective use of an implantable infusion pump as long as the drug being used with the pump is itself reasonable and necessary for the patient's treatment.

The following indications for treatment using infusion pumps are not covered under Medicare:

A. External Infusion Pumps.—

   1. Vancomycin (Effective for Services Beginning On or After September 1, 1996).—Medicare coverage of vancomycin as a durable medical equipment infusion pump benefit is not covered.

There is insufficient evidence to support the necessity of using an external infusion pump, instead of a disposable elastomeric pump or the gravity drip method, to administer vancomycin in a safe and appropriate manner.

B. Implantable Infusion Pump.—

1. Thromboembolic Disease (Effective for Services Performed On or After 9/26/84).—According to the Public Health Service, there is insufficient published clinical data to support the safety and effectiveness of the heparin implantable pump. Therefore, the use of an implantable infusion pump for infusion of heparin in the treatment of recurrent thromboembolic disease is not covered.
2. Diabetes—Implanted infusion pumps for the infusion of insulin to treat diabetes is not covered. The data do not demonstrate that the pump provides effective administration of insulin.

60-15 SAFETY ROLLER (Effective for Claims Adjudicated On or After 6/3/85)

"Safety roller" is the generic name applied to devices for patients who cannot use standard wheeled walkers. They may be appropriate, and therefore covered, for some patients who are obese, have severe neurological disorders, or restricted use of one hand, which makes it impossible to use a wheeled walker that does not have the sophisticated braking system found on safety rollers.

In order to assure that payment is not made for a safety roller when a less expensive standard wheeled walker would satisfy the patient's medical needs, carriers refer safety roller claims to their medical consultants. The medical consultant determines whether some or all of the features provided in a safety roller are necessary, and therefore covered and reimbursable. If it is determined that the patient could use a standard wheeled walker, the charge for the safety roller is reduced to the charge of a standard wheeled walker.
Some obese patients who could use a standard wheeled walker if their weight did not exceed the walker's strength and stability limits can have it reinforced and its wheel base expanded. Such modifications are routine mechanical adjustments and justify a moderate surcharge. In these cases the carrier reduces the charge for the safety roller to the charge for the standard wheeled walker plus the surcharge for modifications.

In the case of patients with medical documentation showing severe neurological disorders or restricted use of one hand which makes it impossible for them to use a wheeled walker that does not have a sophisticated braking system, a reasonable charge for the safety roller may be determined without relating it to the reasonable charge for a standard wheeled walker. (Such reasonable charge should be developed in accordance with the instructions in Medicare Carriers Manual §§5010 and 5205.)

Cross-reference: Carriers Manual §§2100ff., §60-9.

60-16 PNEUMATIC COMPRESSION DEVICES

Pneumatic compression devices consist of an inflatable garment for the arm or leg and an electrical pneumatic pump that fills the garment with compressed air. The garment is intermittently inflated and deflated with cycle times and pressures that vary between devices. Pneumatic devices are covered for the treatment of lymphedema or for the treatment of chronic venous insufficiency with venous stasis ulcers.

Lymphedema

Lymphedema is the swelling of subcutaneous tissues due to the accumulation of excessive lymph fluid. The accumulation of lymph fluid results from impairment to the normal clearing function of the lymphatic system and/or from an excessive production of lymph. Lymphedema is divided into two broad classes according to etiology. Primary lymphedema is a relatively uncommon, chronic condition which may be due to such causes as Milroy's Disease or congenital anomalies. Secondary lymphedema, which is much more common, results from the destruction of or damage to formerly functioning lymphatic channels, such as surgical removal of lymph nodes or post radiation fibrosis, among other causes.

Pneumatic compression devices are covered in the home setting for the treatment of lymphedema if the patient has undergone a four-week trial of conservative therapy and the treating physician determines that there has been no significant improvement or if significant symptoms remain after the trial. The trial of conservative therapy must include use of an appropriate compression bandage system or compression garment, exercise, and elevation of the limb. The garment may be prefabricated or custom-fabricated but must provide adequate graduated compression.

Chronic Venous Insufficiency with Venous Stasis Ulcers

Chronic venous insufficiency (CVI) of the lower extremities is a condition caused by abnormalities of the venous wall and valves, leading to obstruction or reflux of blood flow in the veins. Signs of CVI include hyperpigmentation, stasis dermatitis, chronic edema, and venous ulcers.

Pneumatic compression devices are covered in the home setting for the treatment of CVI of the lower extremities only if the patient has one or more venous stasis ulcer(s) which have failed to heal after a 6 month trial of conservative therapy directed by the treating physician. The trial of conservative therapy must include a compression bandage system or compression garment, appropriate dressings for the wound, exercise, and elevation of the limb.

General Coverage Criteria

Pneumatic compression devices are covered only when prescribed by a physician and when they are used with appropriate physician oversight, i.e., physician evaluation of the patient's condition to determine medical necessity of the device, assuring suitable instruction in the operation of the machine, a treatment plan defining the pressure to be used and the frequency and duration of use, and ongoing monitoring of use and response to treatment.

The determination by the physician of the medical necessity of a pneumatic compression device must include (1) the patient's diagnosis and prognosis; (2) symptoms and objective findings, including measurements which establish the severity of the condition; (3) the reason the device is required, including the treatments which have been tried and failed; and (4) the clinical response to an initial treatment with the device. The clinical response includes the change in pre-treatment measurements, ability to tolerate the treatment session and parameters, and ability of the patient (or caregiver) to apply the device for continued use in the home.

The only time that a segmented, calibrated gradient pneumatic compression device (HCPCS code E0652) would be covered is when the individual has unique characteristics that prevent them from receiving satisfactory pneumatic compression treatment using a nonsegmented device in conjunction with a segmented appliance or a segmented compression device without manual control of pressure in each chamber.

Cross-reference: §60-9.

60-17 CONTINUOUS POSITIVE AIRWAY PRESSURE (CPAP)

CPAP is a non-invasive technique for providing single levels of air pressure from a flow generator, via a nose mask, through the nares. The purpose is to prevent the collapse of the oropharyngeal walls and the obstruction of airflow during sleep, which occurs in obstructive sleep apnea (OSA).

Effective for services furnished between and including January 12, 1987 and March 31, 2002:

The diagnosis of OSA requires documentation of at least 30 episodes of apnea, each lasting a minimum of 10 seconds, during 6-7 hours of recorded sleep. The use of CPAP is covered under Medicare when used in adult patients with moderate or severe OSA for whom surgery is a likely alternative to CPAP.

Initial claims must be supported by medical documentation (separate documentation where electronic billing is used), such as a prescription written by the patient's attending physician, that specifies:

- a diagnosis of moderate or severe obstructive sleep apnea, and
- surgery is a likely alternative.

The claim must also certify that the documentation supporting a diagnosis of OSA (described above) is available.

Effective for services furnished on or after April 1, 2002:

The use of CPAP devices are covered under Medicare when ordered and prescribed by the licensed treating physician to be used in adult patients with OSA if either of the following criteria using the Apnea-Hypopnea Index (AHI) are met:

- AHI = 15 events per hour, or
- AHI = 5 and = 14 events per hour with documented symptoms of excessive daytime sleepiness, impaired cognition, mood disorders or insomnia, or documented hypertension, ischemic heart disease or history of stroke.

The AHI is equal to the average number of episodes of apnea and hypopnea per hour and must be based on a minimum of 2 hours of sleep recorded by polysomnography using actual recorded hours of sleep (i.e., the AHI may not be extrapolated or projected).

Apnea is defined as a cessation of airflow for at least 10 seconds. Hypopnea is defined as an abnormal respiratory event lasting at least 10 seconds with at least a 30% reduction in thoracoabdominal movement or airflow as compared to baseline, and with at least a 4% oxygen desaturation.

The polysomnography must be performed in a facility - based sleep study laboratory, and not in the home or in a mobile facility.

Initial claims for CPAP devices must be supported by information contained in the medical record indicating that the patient meets Medicare's stated coverage criteria.

Cross-reference: §60-9.

60-18 HOSPITAL BEDS

A. General Requirements for Coverage of Hospital Beds.—A physician's prescription, and such additional documentation as the contractors' medical staffs may consider necessary, including medical records and physicians' reports, must establish the medical necessity for a hospital bed due to one of the following reasons:

- The patient's condition requires positioning of the body; e.g., to alleviate pain, promote good body alignment, prevent contractures, avoid respiratory infections, in ways not feasible in an ordinary bed; or
- The patient's condition requires special attachments that cannot be fixed and used on an ordinary bed.

B. Physician's Prescription.—The physician's prescription, which must accompany the initial claim, and supplementing documentation when required, must establish that a hospital bed is medically necessary. If the stated reason for the need for a hospital bed is the patient's condition requires positioning, the prescription or other documentation must describe the medical condition, e.g., cardiac disease, chronic obstructive pulmonary disease, quadriplegia or paraplegia, and also the severity and frequency of the symptoms of the condition, that necessitates a hospital bed for positioning.

If the stated reason for requiring a hospital bed is the patient's condition requires special attachments, the prescription must describe the patient's condition and specify the attachments that require a hospital bed.

C. Variable Height Feature.—In well documented cases, the contractors' medical staffs may determine that a variable height feature of a hospital bed, approved for coverage under subsection A above, is medically necessary and, therefore, covered, for one of the following conditions:

- Severe arthritis and other injuries to lower extremities; e.g., fractured hip. The condition requires the variable height feature to assist the patient to ambulate by enabling the patient to place his or her feet on the floor while sitting on the edge of the bed;
- Severe cardiac conditions. For those cardiac patients who are able to leave bed, but who must avoid the strain of "jumping" up or down;
- Spinal cord injuries, including quadriplegic and paraplegic patients, multiple limb amputee and stroke patients. For those patients who are able to transfer from bed to a wheelchair, with or without help; or
- Other severely debilitating diseases and conditions, if the variable height feature is required to assist the patient to ambulate.

D. Electric Powered Hospital Bed Adjustments.—Electric powered adjustments to lower and raise head and foot may be covered when the contractor's medical staff determines that the patient's condition requires frequent change in body position and/or there may be an immediate need for a change in body position (i.e., no delay can be tolerated) and the patient can operate the controls and cause the adjustments. Exceptions may be made to this last requirement in cases of spinal cord injury and brain damaged patients.

E. Side Rails.—If the patient's condition requires bed side rails, they can be covered when an integral part of, or an accessory to, a hospital bed.

Cross-reference: Carriers Manual, §5015.4

60-19 AIR-FLUIDIZED BED (Effective for services rendered on or after: 07/30/90)

An air-fluidized bed uses warm air under pressure to set small ceramic beads in motion which simulate the movement of fluid. When the patient is placed in the bed, his body weight is evenly distributed over a large surface area which creates a sensation of "floating." Medicare payment for home use of the air-fluidized bed for treatment of pressure sores can be made if such use is reasonable and necessary for the individual patient.

A decision that use of an air-fluidized bed is reasonable and necessary requires that:

- The patient has a stage 3 (full thickness tissue loss) or stage 4 (deep tissue destruction) pressure sore;
- The patient is bedridden or chair bound as a result of severely limited mobility;
- In the absence of an air-fluidized bed, the patient would require institutionalization;
- The air-fluidized bed is ordered in writing by the patient's attending physician based upon a comprehensive assessment and evaluation of the patient after completion of a course of conservative treatment designed to optimize conditions that promote wound healing. This course of treatment must have been at least one month in duration without progression toward wound healing. This month of prerequisite conservative treatment may include some period in an institution as long as there is documentation available to verify that the necessary conservative treatment has been rendered.
- Use of wet-to-dry dressings for wound debridement, begun during the period of conservative treatment and which continue beyond 30 days, will not preclude coverage of air-fluidized bed. Should additional debridement again become necessary, while a patient is using an air-fluidized bed (after the first 30-day course of conservative treatment) that will not cause the air-fluidized bed to become non-covered. In all instances documentation verifying the continued need for the bed must be available.
- Conservative treatment must include:

  - Frequent repositioning of the patient with particular attention to relief of pressure over bony prominences (usually every 2 hours);
  - Use of a specialized support surface (Group II) designed to reduce pressure and shear forces on healing ulcers and to prevent new ulcer formation;
  - Necessary treatment to resolve any wound infection;
  - Optimization of nutrition status to promote wound healing;
  - Debridement by any means (including wet to dry dressings-which does not require an occlusive covering) to remove devitalized tissue from the wound bed;
  - Maintenance of a clean, moist bed of granulation tissue with appropriate moist dressings protected by an occlusive covering, while the wound heals.

- A trained adult caregiver is available to assist the patient with activities of daily living, fluid balance, dry skin care, repositioning, recognition and management of altered mental status, dietary needs, prescribed treatments, and management and support of the air-fluidized bed system and its problems such as leakage;
- A physician directs the home treatment regimen, and reevaluates and recertifies the need for the air-fluidized bed on a monthly basis; and
- All other alternative equipment has been considered and ruled out.

Home use of the air-fluidized bed is not covered under any of the following circumstances:

- The patient has coexisting pulmonary disease (the lack of firm back support makes coughing ineffective and dry air inhalation thickens pulmonary secretions);
- The patient requires treatment with wet soaks or moist wound dressings that are not protected with an impervious covering such as plastic wrap or other occlusive material; an air-fluidized bed;
- The caregiver is unwilling or unable to provide the type of care required by the patient on an air-fluidized bed;
- Structural support is inadequate to support the weight of the air-fluidized bed system (it generally weighs 1600 pounds or more);
- Electrical system is insufficient for the anticipated increase in energy consumption; or
- Other known contraindications exist.

Coverage of an air-fluidized bed is limited to the equipment itself. Payment for this covered item may only be made if the written order from the attending physician is furnished to the supplier prior to the delivery of the equipment. Payment is not included for the caregiver or for architectural adjustments such as electrical or structural improvement.

Cross-reference: Carriers Manual, §5102.2.

60-20 TRANSCUTANEOUS ELECTRICAL NERVE STIMULATORS (TENS)

TENS is a type of electrical nerve stimulator that is employed to treat chronic intractable pain. This stimulator is attached to the surface of the patient's skin over the peripheral nerve to be stimulated. It may be applied in a variety of settings (in the patient's home, a physician's office, or in an outpatient clinic). Payment for TENS may be made under the durable medical equipment benefit. (See §45-25 for an explanation of coverage of medically necessary supplies for the effective use of TENS and §45-19 for an explanation of coverage of TENS for acute post-operative pain.)

60-23 SPEECH GENERATING DEVICES

Effective January 1, 2001, augmentative and alternative communication devices or communicators, which are hereafter referred to as "speech generating devices" are now considered to fall within the DME benefit category established by §1861(n) of the Social Security Act. They may be covered if the contractor's medical staff determines that the patient suffers from a severe speech impairment and that the medical condition warrants the use of a device based on the following definitions.

Definition of Speech Generating Devices

Speech generating devices are defined as speech aids that provide an individual who has a severe speech impairment with the ability to meet his functional speaking needs. Speech generating are characterized by:

- Being a dedicated speech device, used solely by the individual who has a severe speech impairment;
- May have digitized speech output, using pre-recorded messages, less than or equal to 8 minutes recording time;
- May have digitized speech output, using pre-recorded messages, greater than 8 minutes recording time;

- May have synthesized speech output, which requires message formulation by spelling and device access by physical contact with the device-direct selection techniques;
- May have synthesized speech output, which permits multiple methods of message formulation and multiple methods of device access; or
- May be software that allows a laptop computer, desktop computer or personal digital assistant (PDA) to function as a speech generating device.

Devices that would not meet the definition of speech generating devices and therefore, do not fall within the scope of §1861(n) are characterized by:

- Devices that are not dedicated speech devices, but are devices that are capable of running software for purposes other than for speech generation, e.g., devices that can also run a word processing package, an accounting program, or perform other non-medical function.
- Laptop computers, desktop computers, or PDAs, which may be programmed to perform the same function as a speech generating device, are non-covered since they are not primarily medical in nature and do not meet the definition of DME. For this reason, they cannot be considered speech generating devices for Medicare coverage purposes.
- A device that is useful to someone without severe speech impairment is not considered a speech generating device for Medicare coverage purposes.

60-24 NON-IMPLANTABLE PELVIC FLOOR ELECTRICAL STIMULATOR

Non-implantable pelvic floor electrical stimulators provide neuromuscular electrical stimulation through the pelvic floor with the intent of strengthening and exercising pelvic floor musculature. Stimulation is generally delivered by vaginal or anal probes connected to an external pulse generator.

The methods of pelvic floor electrical stimulation vary in location, stimulus frequency (Hz), stimulus intensity or amplitude (mA), pulse duration (duty cycle), treatments per day, number of treatment days per week, length of time for each treatment session, overall time period for device use and between clinic and home settings. In general, the stimulus frequency and other parameters are chosen based on the patient's clinical diagnosis.
Pelvic floor electrical stimulation with a non-implantable stimulator is covered for the treatment of stress and/or urge urinary incontinence in cognitively intact patients who have failed a documented trial of pelvic muscle exercise (PME) training.

A failed trial of PME training is defined as no clinically significant improvement in urinary continence after completing 4 weeks of an ordered plan of pelvic muscle exercises designed to increase periurethral muscle strength.

65-1 HYDROPHILIC CONTACT LENSES

Hydrophilic contact lenses are eyeglasses within the meaning of the exclusion in §l862(a)(7) of the law and are not covered when used in the treatment of nondiseased eyes with spherical ametropia, refractive astigmatism, and/or corneal astigmatism. Payment may be made under the prosthetic device benefit, however, for hydrophilic contact lenses when prescribed for an aphakic patient.

Contractors are authorized to accept an FDA letter of approval or other FDA published material as evidence of FDA approval.

(See §45-7 for coverage of a hydrophilic lens as a corneal bandage.)

Cross-reference: Intermediary Manual, §§3110.3, 3110.4, 3151, and 3157; Carriers Manual, §§2130, 2320; Hospital Manual, §§228.3, 228.4, 260.1 and 260.7.

65-2 ELECTRICAL CONTINENCE AID--NOT COVERED

An electrical continence aid is a device consisting of a plastic plug, molded into the shape of the patient's anal canal, which contains two implanted electrodes that are connected by a wire to a small portable generator. An electrical current is produced which stimulates the anal musculature to cause a contraction sufficient to hold the plug in while allowing the patient to ambulate without incontinence.

Electrical continence aids are in the experimental stage of development and there is no valid scientific documentation of their effectiveness and safety. Therefore, they are not covered under Medicare since they cannot be considered to be reasonable and necessary for the treatment of an illness or injury or to improve the functioning of a malformed body member as required by §1862(a)(1) of the law.

65-3 SCLERAL SHELL

Scleral shell (or shield) is a catchall term for different types of hard scleral contact lenses.

A scleral shell fits over the entire exposed surface of the eye as opposed to a corneal contact lens which covers only the central non-white area encompassing the pupil and iris. Where an eye has been rendered sightless and shrunken by inflammatory disease, a scleral shell may, among other things, obviate the need for surgical enucleation and prosthetic implant and act to support the surrounding orbital tissue.

In such a case, the device serves essentially as an artificial eye. In this situation, payment may be made for a scleral shell under §1861(s)(8) of the law.

Scleral shells are occasionally used in combination with artificial tears in the treatment of "dry eye" of diverse etiology. Tears ordinarily dry at a rapid rate, and are continually replaced by the lacrimal gland. When the lacrimal gland fails, the half-life of artificial tears may be greatly prolonged by the use of the scleral contact lens as a protective barrier against the drying action of the atmosphere. Thus, the difficult and sometimes hazardous process of frequent installation of artificial tears may be avoided. The lens acts in this instance to substitute, in part, for the functioning of the diseased lacrimal gland and would be covered as a prosthetic device in the rare case when it is used in the treatment of "dry eye."

Cross-reference: HCFA-Pub. 13-3, §§3110.4, 3110.5; HCFA-Pub. 14-3, §§2130, 2133; HCFA- Pub. 10, §§210.4, 211

65-5 ELECTRONIC SPEECH AIDS

Electronic speech aids are covered under Part B as prosthetic devices when the patient has had a laryngectomy or his larynx is permanently inoperative. There are two types of speech aids. One operates by placing a vibrating head against the throat; the other amplifies sound waves through a tube which is inserted into the user's mouth. A patient who has had radical neck surgery and/or extensive radiation to the anterior part of the neck would generally be able to use only the "oral tube" model or one of the more sensitive and more expensive "throat contact" devices.

Cross-reference: HCFA-Pub. 13-3, §3110.4; HCFA-Pub. 14-3, §2130; HCFA-Pub. 10, §228.4

65-7 INTRAOCULAR LENSES (IOLs)

An intraocular lens, or pseudophakos, is an artificial lens which may be implanted to replace the natural lens after cataract surgery. Intraocular lens implantation services, as well as the lens itself, may be covered if reasonable and necessary for the individual. Implantation services may include hospital, surgical, and other medical services, including pre-implantation ultrasound (A-can) eye measurement of one or both eyes.

Cross-reference: HCFA Pub. 13-3, §§3110.4, 3151, and 3157; HCFA Pub.14-3, §2130; HCFA Pub. 10, §228.4

65-8 ELECTRICAL NERVE STIMULATORS

Two general classifications of electrical nerve stimulators are employed to treat chronic intractable pain: peripheral nerve stimulators and central nervous system stimulators.

A. Implanted Peripheral Nerve Stimulators.—Payment may be made under the prosthetic device benefit for implanted peripheral nerve stimulators. Use of this stimulator involves implantation of electrodes around a selected peripheral nerve. The stimulating electrode is connected by an insulated lead to a receiver unit which is implanted under the skin at a depth not greater than 1/2 inch. Stimulation is induced by a generator connected to an antenna unit which is attached to the skin surface over the receiver unit. Implantation of electrodes requires surgery and usually necessitates an operating room.

   NOTE: Peripheral nerve stimulators may also be employed to assess a patient's suitability for continued treatment with an electric nerve stimulator. As explained in §35-46, such use of the stimulator is covered as part of the total diagnostic service furnished to the beneficiary rather than as a prosthesis.

B. Central Nervous System Stimulators (Dorsal Column and Depth Brain Stimulators).—The implantation of central nervous system stimulators may be covered as therapies for the relief of chronic intractable pain, subject to the following conditions:

   1. Types of Implantations.—There are two types of implantations covered by this instruction:

      a. Dorsal Column (Spinal Cord) Neurostimulation.—The surgical implantation of neurostimulator electrodes within the dura mater (endodural) or the percutaneous insertion of electrodes in the epidural space is covered.
      b. Depth Brain Neurostimulation.—The stereotactic implantation of electrodes in the deep brain (e.g., thalamus and periaqueductal gray matter) is covered.

   2. Conditions for Coverage.—No payment may be made for the implantation of dorsal column or depth brain stimulators or services and supplies related to such implantation, unless all of the conditions listed below have been met:

      a. The implantation of the stimulator is used only as a late resort (if not a last resort) for patients with chronic intractable pain;

b. With respect to item a, other treatment modalities (pharmacological, surgical, physical, or psychological therapies) have been tried and did not prove satisfactory, or are judged to be unsuitable or contraindicated for the given patient;
c. Patients have undergone careful screening, evaluation and diagnosis by a multidisciplinary team prior to implantation. (Such screening must include psychological, as well as physical evaluation);
d. All the facilities, equipment, and professional and support personnel required for the proper diagnosis, treatment training, and followup of the patient (including that required to satisfy item c) must be available; and
e. Demonstration of pain relief with a temporarily implanted electrode precedes permanent implantation.

Contractors may find it helpful to work with PROs to obtain the information needed to apply these conditions to claims.

See Intermediary Manual, §3110.4 and §§35-20 and 35-27.

65-9 INCONTINENCE CONTROL DEVICE

A. Mechanical/Hydraulic Incontinence Control Devices. Mechanical/ hydraulic incontinence control devices are accepted as safe and effective in the management of urinary incontinence in patients with permanent anatomic and neurologic dysfunctions of the bladder. This class of devices achieves control of urination by compression of the urethra. The materials used and the success rate may vary somewhat from device to device. Such a device is covered when its use is reasonable and necessary for the individual patient.

B. Collagen Implant.—A collagen implant, which is injected into the submucosal tissues of the urethra and/or the bladder neck and into tissues adjacent to the urethra, is a prosthetic device used in the treatment of stress urinary incontinence resulting from intrinsic sphincter deficiency (ISD). ISD is a cause of stress urinary incontinence in which the urethral sphincter is unable to contract and generate sufficient resistance in the bladder, especially during stress maneuvers.

Prior to collagen implant therapy, a skin test for collagen sensitivity must be administered and evaluated over a 4 week period.

In male patients, the evaluation must include a complete history and physical examination and a simple cystometrogram to determine that the bladder fills and stores properly. The patient then is asked to stand upright with a full bladder and to cough or otherwise exert abdominal pressure on his bladder. If the patient leaks, the diagnosis of ISD is established.

In female patients, the evaluation must include a complete history and physical examination (including a pelvic exam) and a simple cystometrogram to rule out abnormalities of bladder compliance and abnormalities of urethral support. Following that determination, an abdominal leak point pressure (ALLP) test is performed. Leak point pressure, stated in cm H2O, is defined as the intra-abdominal pressure at which leakage occurs from the bladder (around a catheter) when the bladder has been filled with a minimum of 150 cc fluid. If the patient has an ALLP of less than 100 cm H2O, the diagnosis of ISD is established.

To use a collagen implant, physicians must have urology training in the use of a cystoscope and must complete a collagen implant training program.

Coverage of a collagen implant, and the procedure to inject it, is limited to the following types of patients with stress urinary incontinence due to ISD:

- Male or female patients with congenital sphincter weakness secondary to conditions such as myelomeningocele or epispadias;
- Male or female patients with acquired sphincter weakness secondary to spinal cord lesions;
- Male patients following trauma, including prostatectomy and/or radiation; and
- Female patients without urethral hypermobility and with abdominal leak point pressures of 100 cm H2O or less.

Patients whose incontinence does not improve with 5 injection procedures (5 separate treatment sessions) are considered treatment failures, and no further treatment of urinary incontinence by collagen implant is covered. Patients who have a reoccurrence of incontinence following successful treatment with collagen implants in the past (e.g., 6-12 months previously) may benefit from additional treatment sessions. Coverage of additional sessions may be allowed but must be supported by medical justification.

See Intermediary Manual, §3110.4.

65-10 ENTERAL AND PARENTERAL NUTRITIONAL THERAPY COVERED AS PROSTHETIC DEVICE
(Effective for items and services furnished on or after 07-11-84.)

There are patients who, because of chronic illness or trauma, cannot be sustained through oral feeding. These people must rely on either enteral or parenteral nutritional therapy, depending upon the particular nature of their medical condition.

Coverage of nutritional therapy as a Part B benefit is provided under the prosthetic device benefit provision, which requires that the patient must have a permanently inoperative internal body organ or function thereof. (See Intermediary Manual, §3110.4.) Therefore, enteral and parenteral nutritional therapy are not covered under Part B in situations involving temporary impairments. Coverage of such therapy, however, does not require a medical judgment that the impairment giving rise to the therapy will persist throughout the patient's remaining years. If the medical record, including the judgment of the attending physician, indicates that the impairment will be of long and indefinite duration, the test of permanence is considered met.

If the coverage requirements for enteral or parenteral nutritional therapy are met under the prosthetic device benefit provision, related supplies, equipment and nutrients are also covered under the conditions in the following paragraphs and the Intermediary Manual, §3110.4.

65-10.1 Parenteral Nutrition Therapy.—Daily parenteral nutrition is considered reasonable and necessary for a patient with severe pathology of the alimentary tract which does not allow absorption of sufficient nutrients to maintain weight and strength commensurate with the patient's general condition.

Since the alimentary tract of such a patient does not function adequately, an indwelling catheter is placed percutaneously in the subclavian vein and then advanced into the superior vena cava where intravenous infusion of nutrients is given for part of the day. The catheter is then plugged by the patient until the next infusion. Following a period of hospitalization, which is required to initiate parenteral nutrition and to train the patient in catheter care, solution preparation, and infusion technique, the parenteral nutrition can be provided safely and effectively in the patient's home by nonprofessional persons who have undergone special training. However, such persons cannot be paid for their services, nor is payment available for any services furnished by nonphysician professionals except as services furnished incident to a physician's service.

For parenteral nutrition therapy to be covered under Part B, the claim must contain a physician's written order or prescription and sufficient medical documentation to permit an independent conclusion that the requirements of the prosthetic device benefit are met and that parenteral nutrition therapy is medically necessary. An example of a condition that typically qualifies for coverage is a massive small bowel resection resulting in severe nutritional deficiency in spite of adequate oral intake. However, coverage of parenteral nutrition therapy for this and any other condition must be approved on an individual, case-by-case basis initially and at periodic intervals of no more than 3 months by the carrier's medical consultant or specially trained staff, relying on such medical and other documentation as the carrier may require. If the claim involves an infusion pump, sufficient evidence must be provided to support a determination of medical necessity for the pump. Program payment for the pump is based on the reasonable charge for the simplest model that meets the medical needs of the patient as established by medical documentation.

Nutrient solutions for parenteral therapy are routinely covered. However, Medicare pays for no more than one month's supply of nutrients at any one time. Payment for the nutrients is based on the reasonable charge for the solution components unless the medical record, including a signed statement from the attending physician, establishes that the beneficiary, due to his/her physical or mental state, is unable to safely or effectively mix the solution and there is no family member or other person who can do so. Payment will be on the basis of the reasonable charge for more expensive pre-mixed solutions only under the latter circumstances.

65-10.2 Enteral Nutrition Therapy.—Enteral nutrition is considered reasonable and necessary for a patient with a functioning gastrointestinal tract who, due to pathology to or nonfunction of the structures that normally permit food to reach the digestive tract, cannot maintain weight and strength commensurate with his or her general condition. Enteral therapy may be given by nasogastric, jejunostomy, or gastrostomy tubes and can be provided safely and effectively in the home by nonprofessional persons who have undergone special training. However, such persons cannot be paid for their services, nor is payment available for any services furnished by nonphysician professionals except as services furnished incident to a physician's service.

Typical examples of conditions that qualify for coverage are head and neck cancer with reconstructive surgery and central nervous system disease leading to interference with the neuromuscular mechanisms of ingestion of such severity that the beneficiary cannot be maintained with oral feeding. However, claims for Part B coverage of enteral nutrition therapy for these and any other conditions must be approved on an individual, case-by-case basis. Each claim must contain a physician's written order or prescription and sufficient medical documentation (e.g., hospital records, clinical findings from the attending physician) to permit an independent conclusion that the patient's condition meets the requirements of the prosthetic device benefit and that enteral nutrition therapy is medically necessary. Allowed claims are to be reviewed at periodic intervals of no more than 3 months by the contractor's medical consultant or specially trained staff, and additional medical documentation considered necessary is to be obtained as part of this review.

Medicare pays for no more than one month's supply of enteral nutrients at any one time.

If the claim involves a pump, it must be supported by sufficient medical documentation to establish that the pump is medically necessary, i.e., gravity feeding is not satisfactory due to aspiration, diarrhea, dumping syndrome. Program payment for the pump is based on the reasonable charge for the simplest model that meets the medical needs of the patient as established by medical documentation.

65-10.3 Nutritional Supplementation.—Some patients require supplementation of their daily protein and caloric intake. Nutritional supplements are often given as a medicine between meals to boost protein-caloric intake or the mainstay of a daily nutritional plan. Nutritional supplementation is not covered under Medicare Part B.

65-14 COCHLEAR IMPLANTATION

A cochlear implant device is an electronic instrument, part of which is implanted surgically to stimulate auditory nerve fibers, and part of which is worn or carried by the individual to capture, analyze and code sound. Cochlear implant devices are available in single channel and multi-channel models. The purpose of implanting the device is to provide an awareness and identification of sounds and to facilitate communication for persons who are profoundly hearing impaired.

Medicare coverage is provided only for those patients who meet all of the following selection guidelines.

A. General.—

- Diagnosis of bilateral severe-to-profound sensorineural hearing impairment with limited benefit from appropriate hearing (or vibrotactile) aids;
- Cognitive ability to use auditory clues and a willingness to undergo an extended program of rehabilitation;
- Freedom from middle ear infection, an accessible cochlear lumen that is structurally suited to implantation, and freedom from lesions in the auditory nerve and acoustic areas of the central nervous system;
- No contraindications to surgery; and
- The device must be used in accordance with the FDA-approved labeling.

B. Adults.—Cochlear implants may be covered for adults (over age 18) for prelinguistically, perilinguistically, and post linguistically deafened adults. Post linguistically deafened adults must demonstrate test scores of 30 percent or less on sentence recognition scores from tape recorded tests in the patient's best listening condition.

C. Children.—Cochlear implants may be covered for prelinguistically and post linguistically deafened children aged 2 through 17. Bilateral profound sensorineural deafness must be demonstrated by the inability to improve on age appropriate closed-set word identification tasks with amplification.

65-16 TRACHEOSTOMY SPEAKING VALVE

A trachea tube has been determined to satisfy the definition of a prosthetic device, and the tracheostomy speaking valve is an add on to the trachea tube which may be considered a medically necessary accessory that enhances the function of the tube. In other words, it makes the system a better prosthesis. As such, a tracheostomy speaking valve is covered as an element of the trachea tube which makes the tube more effective.

65-17 URINARY DRAINAGE BAGS

Urinary collection and retention system are covered as prosthetic devices that replace bladder function in the case of permanent urinary incontinence. Urinary drainage bags that can be used either as bedside or leg drainage bags may be either multi-use or single use systems. Both the multi-use and the single use bags have a system that prevents urine backflow. However, the single use system is non-drainable. There is insufficient evidence to support the medical necessity of a single use system bag rather than the multi-use bag. Therefore, a single use drainage system is subject to the same coverage parameters as the multi-use drainage bags.

70-1 CORSET USED AS HERNIA SUPPORT

A hernia support (whether in the form of a corset or truss) which meets the definition of a brace is covered under Part B under §1861(s)(9) of the Act.

See Intermediary Manual, §3110.5; Medicare Carriers Manual, §2133; and Hospital Manual, §228.5.

70-2 SYKES HERNIA CONTROL

Based on professional advice, it has been determined that the Sykes hernia control (a spring-type, U-shaped, strapless truss) is not functionally more beneficial than a conventional truss. Make program reimbursement for this device only when an ordinary truss would be covered. (Like all trusses, it is only of benefit when dealing with a reducible hernia). Thus, when a charge for this item is substantially in excess of that which would be reasonable for a conventional truss used for the same condition, base reimbursement on the reasonable charges for the conventional truss.

See Intermediary Manual, §3110.5; Medicare Carriers Manual, §2133; and Hospital Manual, §228.5.

MEDICARE CARRIERS MANUAL (MCM) REFERENCES

The following Medicare references refer to policy issues identified in the main body of the HCPCS code section. Medicare Carriers Manual references are identified with the term MCM: followed by the reference number(s). .

2000 COVERED MEDICAL AND OTHER HEALTH SERVICES

The supplementary medical insurance plan covers expenses incurred for the following medical and other health services:

1. Physician's services, including surgery, consultation, and office, and institutional calls, and services and supplies furnished incident to a physician's professional service;
2. Outpatient hospital services furnished incident to physicians services;
3. Outpatient diagnostic services furnished by a hospital;
4. Outpatient physical therapy; outpatient speech pathology services;
5. Diagnostic X-ray tests, laboratory tests, and other diagnostic tests;
6. X-ray, radium, and radioactive isotope therapy;

7. Surgical dressings, and splints, casts, and other devices used for reduction of fractures and dislocations;
8. Rental or purchase of durable medical equipment for use in the patient's home;
9. Ambulance service;
10. Prosthetic devices which replace all or part of an internal body organ;
11. Leg, arm, back and neck braces and artificial legs, arms, and eyes;
12. Certain medical supplies used in connection with home dialysis delivery systems;
13. Rural health clinic (RHC) services.
14. Ambulatory surgical center (ASC) services.

(See §2255 for provisions regarding supplementary medical insurance coverage of certain of these services when furnished to hospital and SNF inpatients.)

Supplementary medical insurance also provides coverage for home health visits for which the intermediary makes payment on the basis of the reasonable cost. Outpatient hospital services are also reimbursed by the intermediary.

Some medical services may be considered for coverage under more than one of the above enumerated categories. For example, EKGs can be covered as physician's services, services incident to a physician's service or as other diagnostic tests. It is sufficient to determine that the requirements for coverage under one category are met to permit payment.

Payment for physician services and medical and other health services rendered to beneficiaries is made on a reasonable charge basis. Make payment to the beneficiary, or the physician or supplier who renders the service, depending on whether the itemized bill or assignment method is used. Payment for medical services performed by a provider-based physician is made to the physician or beneficiary or, when the physician authorizes it, to the provider. When covered medical and other health services are furnished by a nonparticipating skilled nursing facility, make payment to the SNF or to the beneficiary on the basis of the reasonable charge.

An organization which furnishes medical and other health services on a prepayment basis may elect to be paid on the basis of reasonable costs in lieu of reasonable charges.

Payment may not be made under Part B for services furnished an individual if he is entitled to have payment made for those services under Part A. An individual is considered entitled to have payment made under Part A if the expenses incurred were used to satisfy a Part A deductible or coinsurance amount, or if payment would be made under Part A except for the lack of a request for payment or physician certification.

When covered Part B services are furnished by a participating hospital, skilled nursing facility, or home health agency, the intermediary makes payment on a reasonable cost basis to the provider only. Outpatient physical therapy or speech pathology providers are reimbursed on a reasonable cost basis by the designated intermediary or carrier.

Where covered Part B services are furnished by a nonparticipating hospital, the emergency intermediary makes payment on the basis of reasonable charges to the hospital or to the patient.

Membership dues, subscription fees, charges for service policies, insurance premium and other payments analogous to premiums which entitle enrollees to services or to repairs or replacement of devices or equipment or parts therefore without charge or at a reduced charge, are not considered expenses incurred for covered items or services furnished under such contracts or undertakings. Examples of such arrangements are memberships in ambulance companies, insurance for replacement of prosthetic lenses, and service contracts for durable medical equipment.

2005.1 Physicians' Expense for Surgery, Childbirth, and Treatment for Infertility

A. Surgery and Childbirth.—Skilled medical management is appropriate throughout the events of pregnancy, beginning with diagnosis, continuing through delivery and ending after the necessary postnatal care. Similarly, in the event of termination of pregnancy, regardless of whether terminated spontaneously or for therapeutic reasons (i.e., where the life of the mother would be endangered if the fetus were brought to term), the need for skilled medical management and/or medical services is equally important as in those cases carried to full term. After the infant is delivered and is a separate individual, items and services furnished to the infant are not covered on the basis of the mother's eligibility.

Most surgeons and obstetricians bill patients an all inclusive package charge intended to cover all services associated with the surgical procedure or delivery of the child. All expenses for surgical and obstetrical care, including preoperative/prenatal examinations and tests and postoperative/postnatal services are considered incurred on the date of surgery or delivery, as appropriate. This policy applies whether the physician bills on a package charge basis, or itemizes his/her bill separately for these items.

Occasionally, a physician's bill may include charges for additional services not directly related to the surgical procedure or the delivery. Such charges are considered incurred on the date the additional services are furnished.

The above policy applies only where the charges are imposed by one physician or by a clinic on behalf of a group of physicians. Where charges are imposed by more than one physician for surgical or obstetrical services, all preoperative/prenatal and postoperative/postnatal services performed by the physician who performed the surgery or delivery are considered incurred on the date of the surgery or delivery. Expenses for services rendered by other physicians are considered incurred on the date they were performed. for services rendered by other physicians are considered incurred on the date they were performed.

B. Treatment for Infertility.—Reasonable and necessary services associated with treatment for infertility are covered under Medicare. Infertility is a condition sufficiently at variance with the usual state of health to make it appropriate for a person who normally is expected to be fertile to seek medical consultation and treatment. Coordinate with PROs to see that utilization guidelines are established for this treatment if inappropriate utilization or abuse is suspected.

2049 DRUGS AND BIOLOGICALS

The Medicare program provides limited benefits for outpatient drugs. The program covers drugs that are furnished "incident to" a physician's service provided that the drugs are not usually self-administered by the patients who take them.

Generally, drugs and biologicals are covered only if all of the following requirements are met:

- They meet the definition of drugs or biologicals (see §2049.1);

- They are of the type that are not usually self-administered by the patients who take them. (See §2049.2);
- They meet all the general requirements for coverage of items as incident to a physician's services (see § §2050.1 and 2050.3);
- They are reasonable and necessary for the diagnosis or treatment of the illness or injury for which they are administered according to accepted standards of medical practice (see §2049.4);
- They are not excluded as immunizations (see §2049.4.B); and
- They have not been determined by the FDA to be less than effective. (See §2049.4 D.)

Drugs that are usually self-administered by the patient, such as those in pill form, or are used for self-injection, are generally not covered by Part B. However, there are a limited number of self-administered drugs that are covered because the Medicare statute explicitly provides coverage. Examples of self-administered drugs that are covered include blood clotting factors, drugs used in immunosuppressive therapy, erythropoietin for dialysis patients, osteoporosis drugs for certain homebound patients, and certain oral cancer drugs.

(See §§2100.5 and 2130.D for coverage of drugs which are necessary to the effective use of DME or prosthetic devices.)

Definition of Drug or Biological.--Drugs and biologicals must be determined to meet the statutory definition.

Section 1861(t)(1) provides that the terms "drugs" and "biologicals" "include only such drugs (including contrast agents) and biologicals, respectively, as are included (or approved for inclusion) in one of several pharmacopoeias (except for any drugs and biologicals unfavorably evaluated therein), or as are approved by the pharmacy and drug therapeutics committee (or equivalent committee) of the medical staff of the hospital furnishing such drugs and biologicals for use in such hospital." One such pharmacopeia is the United States Pharmacopeia, Drug Indications (USP DI). The inclusion of an item in the USP DI does not necessarily mean that the item is a drug or biological. The USP DI is a database of drug information developed by the U.S. Pharmacopeia but maintained by Micromedex, which contains medically accepted uses for generic and brand name drug products. Inclusion in such reference (or approval by a hospital committee) is a necessary condition for a product to be considered a drug or biological under the Medicare program, however, it is not enough. Rather, the product must also meet all other program requirements to be determined to be a drug or biological.

Determining Self-Administration of Drug or Biological.—Whether a drug or biological is of a type which cannot be self-administered is based on the usual method of administration of the form of that drug or biological as furnished by the physician.

Whole blood is a biological which cannot be self-administered and is covered when furnished incident to a physician's services. Payment may also be made for blood fractions if all coverage requirements are satisfied. (See §2455 on Part B blood deductible.)

Medicare carriers have discretion in applying the criteria in this instruction in determining whether drugs are subject to this exclusion in their local areas. Carriers are to follow the instructions below when applying the exclusion for drugs that are usually self-administered by the patient. Each individual contractor must make its own individual determination on each drug. Contractors must continue to apply the policy that not only the drug is medically reasonable and necessary for any individual claim, but also that the route of administration is medically reasonable and necessary. That is, if a drug is available in both oral and injectable forms, the injectable form of the drug must be medically reasonable and necessary as compared to using the oral form. (See §2049.4.2)

For certain injectable drugs, it will be apparent due to the nature of the condition(s) for which they are administered or the usual course of treatment for those conditions, they are, or are not, usually self-administered. For example, an injectable drug used to treat migraine headaches is usually self-administered. On the other hand, an injectable drug, administered at the same time as chemotherapy, used to treat anemia secondary to chemotherapy is not usually self-administered.

Administered—The term "administered" refers only to the physical process by which the drug enters the patient's body. It does not refer to whether the process is supervised by a medical professional (for example, to observe proper technique or side-effects of the drug). Only injectable (including intravenous) drugs are eligible for inclusion under the "incident to" benefit. Other routes of administration including, but not limited to, oral drugs, suppositories, topical medications are all considered to be usually self-administered by the patient.

Usually—In arriving at a single determination as to whether a drug is usually self-administered, contractors should make a separate determination for each indication for a drug as to whether that drug is usually self-administered.

After determining whether a drug is usually self-administered for each indication, contractors should determine the relative contribution of each indication to total use of the drug (i.e., weighted average) in order to make an overall determination as to whether the drug is usually self-administered. For example, if a drug has three indications, is not self-administered for the first indication, but is self-administered for the second and third indications, and the first indication makes up 40% of total usage, the second indication makes up 30% of total usage, and the third indication makes up 30% of total usage, then the drug would be considered usually self-administered.

Reliable statistical information on the extent of self-administration by the patient may not always be available. Consequently, we offer the following guidance for each contractor's consideration in making this determination in the absence of such data:

1. Absent evidence to the contrary, drugs delivered intravenously should be presumed to be not usually self-administered by the patient.

2. Absent evidence to the contrary, drugs delivered by intramuscular injection should be presumed to be not usually self-administered by the patient. (For example, interferon beta-1a, trade name Avonex, when delivered by intramuscular injection is not usually self administered by the patient.) The contractor may consider the depth and nature of the particular intramuscular injection in applying this presumption.

3. Absent evidence to the contrary, drugs delivered by subcutaneous injection should be presumed to be self-administered by the patient.

In applying these presumptions, contractors should examine the use of the particular drug and consider the following factors:

A. Acute condition.—For the purposes of determining whether a drug is usually self-administered, an acute condition means a condition that begins over a short time period, is likely to be of short duration and/or the expected course of treatment is for a short, finite interval. A course of treatment consisting of scheduled injections lasting less than two weeks, regardless of frequency or route of administration, is considered acute. Evidence to support this may include Food and Drug administration (FDA) approval language, package inserts, drug compendia, and other information.

B. Frequency of administration.—How often is the injection given? For example, if the drug is administered once per month, it is less likely to be self-administered by the patient. However, if it is administered once or more per week, it is likely that the drug is self-administered by the patient.

C. By the patient—The term "by the patient" means Medicare beneficiaries as a collective whole. Include only the patients themselves and not other individuals (that is, do not include spouses, friends, or other care-givers). Base your determination on whether the drug is self-administered by the patient a majority of the time that the drug is used on an outpatient basis by Medicare beneficiaries for medically necessary indications. Ignore all instances when the drug is administered on an inpatient basis. Make this determination on a drug-by-drug basis, not on a beneficiary-by-beneficiary basis. In evaluating whether beneficiaries as a collective whole self-administer, do not consider individual beneficiaries who do not have the capacity to self-administer any drug due to a condition other than the condition for which they are taking the drug in question. For example, an individual afflicted with paraplegia or advanced dementia would not have the capacity to self-administer any injectable drug, so such individuals would not be included in the population upon which the determination for self-administration by the patient was based. Note that some individuals afflicted with a less severe stage of an otherwise debilitating condition would be included in the population upon which the determination for "self-administered by the patient" was based; for example, an early onset of dementia.

D. Evidentiary Criteria —In making a self-administration determination, contractors are only required to consider the following types of evidence: peer reviewed medical literature, standards of medical practice, evidence-based practice guidelines, FDA approved label, and package inserts. Contractors may also consider other evidence submitted by interested individuals or groups subject to their judgment.

   Contractors should also use these evidentiary criteria when reviewing requests for making a determination as to whether a drug is usually self-administered, and requests for reconsideration of a pending or published determination.

   Please note that prior to August 1, 2002, one of the principal factors used to determine whether a drug was subject to the self-administered exclusion was whether the FDA label contained instructions for self-administration. However, we note that under the standard in effect after August 1, 2002, the fact that the FDA label includes instructions for self-administration is not, by itself, a determining factor that a drug is subject to this exclusion.

E. Provider Notice of Non-Covered Drugs—Contractors must describe the process they will use to determine whether a drug is usually self-administered and thus does not meet the "incident to" benefit category. Contractors must place a description of the process on their Web site. Contractors must publish a list of the injectable drugs that are subject to the self-administered exclusion on their Web site, including the data and rationale that led to the determination. Contractors will report the workload associated with developing new coverage statements in CAFM 21208.

Contractors must provide notice 45 days prior to the date that these drugs will not be covered. During the 45-day time period, contractors will maintain existing medical review and payment procedures. After the 45-day notice, contractors may deny payment for the drugs subject to the notice.

Contractors must not develop local medical review policies (LMRPs) for this purpose because further elaboration to describe drugs that do not meet the 'incident to' and the 'not usually self-administered' provisions of the statute are unnecessary. Current LMRPs based solely on these provisions must be withdrawn. LMRPs that address the self-administered exclusion and other information may be reissued absent the self-administered drug exclusion material. Contractors will report this workload in CAFM 21206. However, contractors may continue to use and write LMRPs to describe reasonable and necessary uses of drugs that are not usually self-administered.

F. Conferences Between Contractors—Contractors' Medical Directors may meet and discuss whether a drug is usually self-administered without reaching a formal consensus. Each contractor uses its discretion as to whether or not it will participate in such discussions. Each contractor must make its own individual determinations, except that fiscal intermediaries may, at their discretion, follow the determinations of the local carrier with respect to the self-administered exclusion.

G. Beneficiary Appeals—If a beneficiary's claim for a particular drug is denied because the drug is subject to the "self-administered drug" exclusion, the beneficiary may appeal the denial. Because it is a "benefit category" denial and not a denial based on medical necessity, an Advance Beneficiary Notice (ABN) is not applicable. A "benefit category" denial (i.e., a denial based on the fact that there is no benefit category under which the drug may be covered) does not trigger the financial liability protection provisions of Limitation On Liability [under §1879 of the Act]. Therefore, physicians or providers may charge the beneficiary for an excluded drug. See Chapter XV of the Medicare Carrier Manual for more detail on the appeals process.

H. Provider and Physician Appeals—A physician accepting assignment may appeal a denial under the provisions found in §12000 of the Medicare Carriers Manual. See Chapter XV of the Medicare Carrier Manual for more detail on the appeals process.

Reporting Requirements—Each carrier must report to CMS, every September 1 and March 1, its complete list of injectable drugs that the contractor has determined are excluded when furnished incident to a physician's service on the basis that the drug is usually self-administered. We anticipate that contractors will review injectable drugs on a rolling basis and publish their list of excluded drugs as it is developed. For example, contractors should not wait to publish this list until every drug has been reviewed.

Incident-to Requirements.—In order for Medicare payment to be made for a drug, the "incident to" requirements are met. "Incident to" a physician's professional service means that the services are furnished as an integral, although incidental, part of the physician's personal professional services in the course of diagnosis or treatment of an illness or injury. See §2050.1 for more detail on incident-to requirements.

In order to meet all the general requirements for coverage under the incident-to provision, an FDA approved drug or biological must be furnished by a physician and administered by him/her or by auxiliary personnel employed by him/her under his/her personal supervision. The charge, if any, for the drug or biological must be included in the physician's bill, and the cost of the drug or biological must represent an expense to the physician. Drugs and biologicals furnished by other health professionals may also meet these requirements. (See §§2154, 2156, 2158 and 2160 for specific instructions.)

Reasonableness and Necessity.—Use of the drug or biological must be safe and effective and otherwise reasonable and necessary. (See §2303.) Drugs or biologicals approved for marketing by the Food and Drug Administration (FDA) are considered safe and effective for purposes of this requirement when used for indications specified on the labeling. Therefore, you may pay for the use of an FDA approved drug or biological, if:

- It was injected on or after the date of the FDA's approval;
- It is reasonable and necessary for the individual patient; and
- All other applicable coverage requirements are met.

Deny coverage for drugs and biologicals which have not received final marketing approval by the FDA unless you receive instructions from CMS to the contrary. For specific guidelines on coverage of Group C cancer drugs, see the Coverage Issues Manual.

If there is reason to question whether the FDA has approved a drug or biological for marketing, obtain satisfactory evidence of FDA's approval. Acceptable evidence includes a copy of the FDA's letter to the drug's manufacturer approving the new drug application (NDA); or listing of the drug or biological in the FDA's Approved Drug Products or FDA Drug and Device Product Approvals; or a copy of the manufacturer's package insert, approved by the FDA as part of the labeling of the drug, containing its recommended uses and dosage, as well as possible adverse reactions and recommended precautions in using it. When necessary, the RO may be able to help in obtaining information.

An unlabeled use of a drug is a use that is not included as an indication on the drug's label as approved by the FDA. FDA approved drugs used for indications other than what is indicated on the official label may be covered under Medicare if the carrier determines the use to be medically accepted, taking into consideration the major drug compendia, authoritative medical literature and/or accepted standards of medical practice. In the case of drugs used in an anti-cancer chemotherapeutic regimen, unlabeled uses are covered for a medically accepted indication as defined in §2049.4.C.

Determinations as to whether medication is reasonable and necessary for an individual patient should be made on the same basis as all other such determinations (i.e., with the advice of medical consultants and with reference to accepted standards of medical practice and the medical circumstances of the individual case). The following guidelines identify three categories with specific examples of situations in which medications would not be reasonable and necessary according to accepted standards of medical practice.

1. Not for Particular Illness.—Medications given for a purpose other than the treatment of a particular condition, illness, or injury are not covered (except for certain immunizations).

   Exclude the charge for medications, e.g., vitamins, given simply for the general good and welfare of the patient and not as accepted therapy for a particular illness.

2. Medication given by injection (parenterally) is not covered if standard medical practice indicates that the administration of the medication by mouth(orally) is effective and is an accepted or preferred method of administration. For example, the accepted standards of medical practice for the treatment of certain diseases is to initiate therapy with parenteral penicillin and to complete therapy with oral penicillin.

Exclude the entire charge for penicillin injections given after the initiation of therapy if oral penicillin is indicated unless there are special medical circumstances which justify additional injections.

3. Excessive Medications.—Medications administered for treatment of a disease which exceed the frequency or duration of injections indicated by accepted standards of medical practice are not covered. For example, the accepted standard of medical practice in the maintenance treatment of pernicious anemia is one vitamin B-12 injection per month. Exclude the entire charge for injections given in excess of this frequency unless there are special medical circumstances which justify additional injections.

Supplement the guidelines as necessary with guidelines concerning appropriate use of specific injections in other situations. Use the guidelines to screen out questionable cases for special review, further development or denial when the injection billed for would not be reasonable and necessary. Coordinate any type of drug treatment review with the PRO.

If a medication is determined not to be reasonable and necessary for diagnosis or treatment of an illness or injury according to these guidelines, exclude the entire charge (i.e., for both the drug and its administration). Also exclude from payment any charges for other services (such as office visits) which were primarily for the purpose of administering a noncovered injection (i.e., an injection that is not reasonable and necessary for the diagnosis or treatment of an illness or injury).

A. Antigens.—Payment may be made for a reasonable supply of antigens that have been prepared for a particular patient if: (1) the antigens are prepared by a physician who is a doctor of medicine or osteopathy, and (2) the physician who prepared the antigens has examined the patient and has determined a plan of treatment and a dosage regimen. Antigens must be administered in accordance with the plan of treatment and by a doctor of medicine or osteopathy or by a properly instructed person (who could be the patient) under the supervision of the doctor. he associations of allergists that HCFA consulted advised that a reasonable supply of antigens is considered to be not more than a 12-week supply of antigens that has been prepared for a particular patient at any one time. The purpose of the reasonable supply limitation is to assure that the antigens retain their potency and effectiveness over the period in which they are to be administered to the patient. (See §§2005.2 and 2050.2.)

B. Immunizations.—Vaccinations or inoculations are excluded as immunizations unless they are directly related to the treatment of an injury or direct exposure to a disease or condition, such as anti-rabies treatment, tetanus antitoxin or booster vaccine, botulin antitoxin, antivenin sera, or immune globulin. In the absence of injury or direct exposure, preventive immunization (vaccination or inoculation) against such diseases as smallpox, polio, diphtheria, etc., is not covered. However, pneumococcal, hepatitis B, and influenza virus vaccines are exceptions to this rule. (See items 1, 2, and 3.) In cases where a vaccination or inoculation is excluded from coverage, deny the entire charge.

   1. Pneumococcal Pneumonia Vaccinations.—Furnished on or after May 1, 1981, the Medicare Part B program covers pneumococcal pneumonia vaccine and its administration when furnished in compliance with any applicable State law by any provider of services or any entity or individual with a supplier number. This includes revaccination of patients at highest risk of pneumococcal infection. Typically, these vaccines are administered once in a lifetime except for persons at highest risk. Effective July 1, 2000, Medicare does not require for coverage purposes that the vaccine must be ordered by a doctor of medicine or osteopathy. Therefore, the beneficiary may receive the vaccine upon request without a physician's order and without physician supervision.

An initial vaccine may be administered only to persons at high risk (see below) of pneumococcal disease. Revaccination may be administered only to persons at highest risk of serious Pneumococcal Pneumonia Vaccinations.—Effective for services pneumococcal infection and those likely to have a rapid decline in pneumococcal antibody levels, provided that at least 5 years have passed since receipt of a previous dose of pneumococcal vaccine.

Persons at high risk for whom an initial vaccine may be administered include all people age 65 and older; immunocompetent adults who are at increased risk of pneumococcal disease or its complications because of chronic illness (e.g., cardiovascular disease, pulmonary disease, diabetes mellitus, alcoholism, cirrhosis, or cerebrospinal fluid leaks); and individuals with compromised immune systems (e.g., splenic dysfunction or anatomic asplenia, Hodgkin's disease, lymphoma, multiple myeloma, chronic renal failure, HIV infection, nephrotic syndrome, sickle cell disease, or organ transplantation).

Persons at highest risk and those most likely to have rapid declines in antibody levels are those for whom revaccination may be appropriate. This group includes persons with functional or anatomic asplenia (e.g., sickle cell disease, splenectomy), HIV infection, leukemia, lymphoma, Hodgkin's disease, multiple myeloma, generalized malignancy, chronic renal failure, nephrotic syndrome, or other conditions associated with immunosuppression such as organ or bone marrow transplantation, and those receiving immuno-suppressive chemotherapy. Routine revaccination of people age 65 or older who are not at highest risk is not appropriate.

Those administering the vaccine should not require the patient to present an immunization record prior to administering the pneumococcal vaccine, nor should they feel compelled to review the patient's complete medical record if it is not available. Instead, provided that the patient is competent, it is acceptable for them to rely on the patient's verbal history to determine prior vaccination status. If the patient is uncertain about their vaccination history in the past 5 years, the vaccine should be given. However, if the patient is certain he/she was vaccinated in the last 5 years, the vaccine should not be given. If the patient is certain that the vaccine was given and that more than 5 years have passed since receipt of the previous dose, revaccination is not appropriate unless the patient is at highest risk.

2. Hepatitis B Vaccine.—With the enactment of P.L. 98-369, coverage under Part B was extended to hepatitis B vaccine and its administration, furnished to a Medicare beneficiary who is at high or intermediate risk of contracting hepatitis B. This coverage is effective for services furnished on or after September 1, 1984.

   High-risk groups currently identified include (see exception below):

   - End stage renal disease (ESRD) patients;
   - Hemophiliacs who receive Factor VIII or IX concentrates; Clients of institutions for the mentally retarded;
   - Persons who live in the same household as an Hepatitis B Virus (HBV) carrier; Homosexual men; and
   - Illicit injectable drug abusers.
   - Intermediate risk groups currently identified include:
   - Staff in institutions for the mentally retarded; and

- Workers in health care professions who have frequent contact with blood or blood-derived body fluids during routine work.

EXCEPTION: Persons in the above-listed groups would not be considered at high or intermediate risk of contracting hepatitis B, however, if there is laboratory evidence positive for antibodies to hepatitis B. (ESRD patients are routinely tested for hepatitis B antibodies as part of their continuing monitoring and therapy.)

For Medicare program purposes, the vaccine may be administered upon the order of a doctor of medicine or osteopathy by home health agencies, skilled nursing facilities, ESRD facilities, hospital outpatient departments, persons recognized under the incident to physicians' services provision of law, and doctors of medicine and osteopathy.

A charge separate from the ESRD composite rate will be recognized and paid for administration of the vaccine to ESRD patients.

For ESRD laboratory tests, see Coverage Issues Manual, §50-17.

3. Influenza Virus Vaccine.—Effective for services furnished on or after May 1, 1993, the Medicare Part B program covers influenza virus vaccine and its administration when furnished in compliance with any applicable State law by any provider of services or any entity or individual with a supplier number. Typically, these vaccines are administered once a year in the fall or winter. Medicare does not require for coverage purposes that the vaccine must be ordered by a doctor of medicine or osteopathy. Therefore, the beneficiary may receive the vaccine upon request without a physician's order and without physician supervision.

C. Unlabeled Use For Anti-Cancer Drugs.—Effective January 1, 1994, unlabeled uses of FDA approved drugs and biologicals used in an anti-cancer chemotherapeutic regimen for a medically accepted indication are evaluated under the conditions described in this paragraph. A regimen is a combination of anti-cancer agents which has been clinically recognized for the treatment of a specific type of cancer. An example of a drug regimen is: Cyclophosphamide + vincristine + prednisone (CVP) for non-Hodgkin's lymphoma.

In addition to listing the combination of drugs for a type of cancer, there may be a different regimen or combinations which are used at different times in the history of the cancer (induction, prophylaxis of CNS involvement, post remission, and relapsed or refractory disease). A protocol may specify the combination of drugs, doses, and schedules for administration of the drugs. For purposes of this provision, a cancer treatment regimen includes drugs used to treat toxicities or side effects of the cancer treatment regimen when the drug is administered incident to a chemotherapy treatment. Contractors must not deny coverage based solely on the absence of FDA approved labeling for the use, if the use is supported by one of the following and the use is not listed as "not indicated" in any of the three compendia. (See note at the end of this subsection.)

1. American Hospital Formulary Service Drug Information.—Drug monographs are arranged in alphabetical order within therapeutic classifications. Within the text of the monograph, information concerning indications is provided, including both labeled and unlabeled uses. Unlabeled uses are identified with daggers. The text must be analyzed to make a determination whether a particular use is supported.

2. American Medical Association Drug Evaluations.—Drug evaluations are organized into sections and chapters that are based on therapeutic classifications. The evaluation of a drug provides information concerning indications, including both labeled and unlabeled uses. Unlabeled uses are not specifically identified as such. The text must be analyzed to make a determination whether a particular use is supported. In making these determinations, also refer to the AMA Drug Evaluations Subscription, Volume III, section 17 (Oncolytic Drugs), chapter 1 (Principles of Cancer Chemotherapy), tables 1 and 2.

   Table 1, Specific Agents Used In Cancer Chemotherapy, lists the anti-neoplastic agents which are currently available for use in various cancers. The indications presented in this table for a particular anti- cancer drug include labeled and unlabeled uses (although they are not identified as such). Any indication appearing in this table is considered to be a medically accepted use.

   Table 2, Clinical Responses To Chemotherapy, lists some of the currently preferred regimens for various cancers. The table headings include (1) type of cancer, (2) drugs or regimens currently preferred, (3) alternative or secondary drugs or regimens, and (4) other drugs or regimens with reported activity.

   A regimen appearing under the preferred or alternative/secondary headings is considered to be a medically accepted use.

   A regimen appearing under the heading "Other Drugs or Regimens With Reported Activity" is considered to be for a medically accepted use provided:

   - The preferred and alternative/secondary drugs or regimens are contraindicated; or
   - A preferred and/or alternative/secondary drug or regimen was used but was not tolerated or was ineffective; or
   - here was tumor progression or recurrence after an initial response.

3. United States Pharmacopoeia Drug Information (USPDI).— Monographs are arranged in alphabetic order by generic or family name. Indications for use appear as accepted, unaccepted, or insufficient data. An indication is considered to be a medically accepted use only if the indication is listed as accepted. Unlabeled uses are identified with brackets. A separate indications index lists all indications included in USPDI along with the medically accepted drugs used in treatment or diagnosis.

4. A Use Supported by Clinical Research That Appears in Peer Reviewed Medical Literature.—This applies only when an unlabeled use does not appear in any of the compendia or is listed as insufficient data or investigational. If an unlabeled use of a drug meets these criteria, contact the compendia to see if a report regarding this use is forthcoming. If a report is forthcoming, use this information as a basis for your decision making. The compendium process for making decisions concerning unlabeled uses is very thorough and continuously updated. Peer reviewed medical literature includes scientific, medical, and pharmaceutical publications in which original manuscripts are published, only after having been critically reviewed for scientific accuracy, validity, and reliability by unbiased independent experts. This does not include in-house publications of pharmaceutical manufacturing companies or abstracts (including meeting abstracts)

In determining whether there is supportive clinical evidence for a particular use of a drug, your medical staff (in consultation with local medical specialty groups) must evaluate the quality of the evidence in published peer reviewed medical literature. When evaluating this literature, consider (among other things) the following:

- The prevalence and life history of the disease when evaluating the adequacy of the number of subjects and the response rate. While a 20 percent response rate may be adequate for highly prevalent disease states, a lower rate may be adequate for rare diseases or highly unresponsive conditions.
- The effect on the patient's well-being and other responses to therapy that indicate effectiveness, e.g., a significant increase in survival rate or life expectancy or an objective and significant decrease in the size of the tumor or a reduction in symptoms related to the tumor. Stabilization is not considered a response to therapy.
- The appropriateness of the study design. Consider:

  1. Whether the experimental design in light of the drugs and conditions under investigation is appropriate to address the investigative question. (For example, in some clinical studies, it may be unnecessary or not feasible to use randomization, double blind trials, placebos, or crossover.);
  2. That nonrandomized clinical trials with a significant number of subjects may be a basis for supportive clinical evidence for determining accepted uses of drugs; and
  3. That case reports are generally considered uncontrolled and anecdotal information and do not provide adequate supportive clinical evidence for determining accepted uses of drugs.

  Use peer reviewed medical literature appearing in the following publications:

  - *American Journal of Medicine;*
  - *Annals of Internal Medicine;*
  - *The Journal of the American Medical Association;*
  - *Journal of Clinical Oncology;*
  - *Blood;*
  - *Journal of the National Cancer Institute;*
  - *The New England Journal of Medicine;*
  - *British Journal of Cancer;*
  - *British Journal of Hematology;*
  - *British Medical Journal;*
  - *Cancer*;
  - *Drugs*;
  - *European Journal of Cancer* (formerly *European Journal of Cancer and Clinical Oncology)*;
  - *Lancet*; or
  - *Leukemia.*

  You are not required to maintain copies of these publications. If a claim raises a question about the use of a drug for a purpose not included in the FDA approved labeling or the compendia, ask the physician to submit copies of relevant supporting literature

4. Unlabeled uses may also be considered medically accepted if determined by you to be medically accepted generally as safe and effective for the particular use.

   NOTE: If a use is identified as not indicated by HCFA or the FDA or if a use is specifically identified as not indicated in one or more of the three compendia mentioned or if you determine based on peer reviewed medical literature that a particular use of a drug is not safe and effective, the off- label usage is not supported and, therefore, the drug is not covered.

5. Less Than Effective Drug.—This is a drug that has been determined by the Food and Drug Administration (FDA) to lack substantial evidence of effectiveness for all labeled indications.

   Also, a drug that has been the subject of a Notice of an Opportunity for a Hearing (NOOH) published in the Federal Register before being withdrawn from the market, and for which the Secretary has not determined there is a compelling justification for its medical need, is considered less than effective. This includes any other drug product that is identical, similar, or related. Payment may not be made for a less than effective drug.

   Because the FDA has not yet completed its identification of drug products that are still on the market, existing FDA efficacy decisions must be applied to all similar products once they are identified.

6. Denial of Medicare Payment for Compounded Drugs Produced in Violation of Federal Food, Drug, and Cosmetic Act.—The Food and Drug Administration (FDA) has found that, from time to time, firms established as retail pharmacies engage in mass production of compounded drugs, beyond the normal scope of pharmaceutical practice, in violation of the Federal Food, Drug, and Cosmetic Act (FFDCA). By compounding drugs on a large scale, a company may be operating as a drug manufacturer within the meaning of the FFDCA, without complying with requirements of that law. Such companies may be manufacturing drugs which are subject to the new drug application (NDA) requirements of the FFDCA, but for which FDA has not approved an NDA or which are misbranded or adulterated. If the manufacturing and processing procedures used by these facilities have not been approved by the FDA, the FDA has no assurance that the drugs these companies are producing are safe and effective. The safety and effectiveness issues pertain to such factors as chemical stability, purity, strength, bioequivalency, and bioavailability.

   Section 1862(a)(1)(A) of the Act requires that drugs must be reasonable and necessary in order to by covered under Medicare. This means, in the case of drugs, they must have been approved for marketing by the FDA. Section 2049.4 instructs carriers to deny coverage for drugs that have not received final marketing approval by the FDA, unless instructed otherwise by HCFA. Section 2300.1 instructs carriers to deny coverage of services related to the use of noncovered drugs as well. Hence, if DME or a prosthetic device is used to administer a noncovered drug, coverage is denied for both the nonapproved drug and the DME or prosthetic device.

   In those cases in which the FDA has determined that a company is producing compounded drugs in violation of the FFDCA, Medicare does not pay for the drugs because they do not meet the FDA approval requirements of the Medicare program. In addition, Medicare does not pay for the DME or prosthetic device used to administer such a drug if FDA determines that a required NDA has not been approved or that the drug is misbranded or adulterated.

HCFA will notify you when the FDA has determined that compounded drugs are being produced in violation of the FFDCA. Do not stop Medicare payment for such a drug unless you are notified that it is appropriate to do so through a subsequent instruction. In addition, if you or ROs become aware that other companies are possibly operating in violation of the FFDCA, notify:

Health Care Financing Administration Bureau of Policy Development Office of Physician and Ambulatory Care Policy Baltimore, MD 21244-1850

Self-Administered Drugs and Biologicals.—Drugs that are self-administered are not covered by Medicare Part B unless the statute provides for such coverage. This includes blood clotting factors, drugs used in immunosuppressive therapy, erythropoietin for dialysis patients, certain oral anti-cancer drugs, and oral anti-nausea drugs when used in certain situations.

A. Until January 1, 1995, immunosuppressive drugs are covered under Part B for a period of one year following discharge from a hospital for a Medicare covered organ transplant. HCFA interprets the 1-year period after the date of the transplant procedure to mean 365 days from the day on which an inpatient is discharged from the hospital. Beneficiaries are eligible to receive additional Part B coverage within 18 months after the discharge date for drugs furnished in 1995; within 24 months for drugs furnished in 1996; within 30 months for drugs furnished in 1997; and within 36 months for drugs furnished after 1997.

   Covered drugs include those immunosuppressive drugs that have been specifically labeled as such and approved for marketing by the FDA, as well as those prescription drugs, such as prednisone, that are used in conjunction with immunosuppressive drugs as part of a therapeutic regimen reflected in FDA approved labeling for immunosuppressive drugs. Therefore, antibiotics, hypertensives, and other drugs that are not directly related to rejection are not covered. The FDA had identified and approved for marketing five specifically labeled immunosuppressive drugs. They are Sandimmune (cyclosporine),Sandoz Pharmaceutical; Imuran (azathioprine), Burroughs Wellcome; Atgam (antithymocyte globulin), Upjohn; and Orthoclone OKT3 (Muromonab-CD3), Ortho Pharmaceutical and, Prograf (tacrolimus), Fujisawa USA, Inc. You are expected to keep informed of FDA additions to the list of the immunosuppressive drugs.

B. Erythropoietin (EPO).—The statute provides that EPO is covered for the treatment of anemia for patients with chronic renal failure who are on dialysis. Coverage is available regardless of whether the drug is administered by the patient or the patient's caregiver. EPO is a biologically engineered protein which stimulates the bone marrow to make new red blood cells.

   NOTE: Non-ESRD patients who are receiving EPO to treat anemia induced by other conditions such as chemotherapy or the drug zidovudine (commonly called AZT) must meet the coverage requirements in §2049.

   EPO is covered for the treatment of anemia for patients with chronic renal failure who are on dialysis when:

- It is administered in the renal dialysis facility; or
- It is self-administered in the home by any dialysis patient (or patient caregiver) who is determined competent to use the drug and meets the other conditions detailed below.

NOTE: Payment may not be made for EPO under the incident to provision when EPO is administered in the renal dialysis facility. (See §5202.4.)

Medicare covers EPO and items related to its administration for dialysis patients who use EPO in the home when the following conditions are met.

1. Patient Care Plan.—A dialysis patient who uses EPO in the home must have a current care plan (a copy of which must be maintained by the designated back-up facility for Method II patients) for monitoring home use of EPO which includes the following:

   a. Review of diet and fluid intake for aberrations as indicated by hyperkalemia and elevated blood pressure secondary to volume overload;
   b. Review of medications to ensure adequate provision of supplemental iron;
   c. Ongoing evaluations of hematocrit and iron stores;
   d. Reevaluation of the dialysis prescription taking into account the patient's increased appetite and red blood cell volume;
   e. Method for physician and facility (including back-up facility for Method II patients) follow-up on blood tests and a mechanism (such as a patient log) for keeping the physician informed of the results;
   f. Training of the patient to identify the signs and symptoms of hypotension and hypertension; and
   g. The decrease or discontinuance of EPO if hypertension is uncontrollable.

2. Patient Selection.—The dialysis facility, or the physician responsible for all dialysis-related services furnished to the patient, must make a comprehensive assessment that includes the following:

   a. Pre-selection monitoring. The patient's hematocrit (or hemoglobin), serum iron, transferrin saturation, serum ferritin, and blood pressure must be measured.
   b. Conditions the patient must meet. The assessment must find that the patient meets the following conditions:

      (1) Is a dialysis patient;
      (2) Has a hematocrit (or comparable hemoglobin level) that is as follows:
         (a) For a patient who is initiating EPO treatment, no higher than 30 percent unless there is medical documentation showing the need for EPO despite a hematocrit (or comparable hemoglobin level) higher than 30 percent. Patients with severe angina, severe pulmonary distress, or severe hypotension may require EPO to prevent adverse symptoms even if they have higher hematocrit or hemoglobin levels.
         (b) For a patient who has been receiving EPO from the facility or the physician, between 30 and 36 percent; and

3. Is under the care of:

   a. A physician who is responsible for all dialysis-related services and who prescribes the EPO and follows the drug labeling instructions when monitoring the EPO home therapy; and

b. A renal dialysis facility that establishes the plan of care and monitors the progress of the home EPO therapy.
c. The assessment must find that the patient or a caregiver meets the following conditions:

(1) Is trained by the facility to inject EPO and is capable of carrying out the procedure;
(2) Is capable of reading and understanding the drug labeling; and
(3) Is trained in, and capable of observing, aseptic techniques.

d. Care and storage of drug. The assessment must find that EPO can be stored in the patient's residence under refrigeration and that the patient is aware of the potential hazard of a child's having access to the drug and syringes.

4. Responsibilities of Physician or Dialysis Facility.—The patient's physician or dialysis facility must:

a. Develop a protocol that follows the drug label instructions;
b. Make the protocol available to the patient to ensure safe and effective home use of EPO;
c. Through the amounts prescribed, ensure that the drug on hand at any time does not exceed a 2-month supply; and
d. Maintain adequate records to allow quality assurance for review by the network and State survey agencies. For Method II patients, current records must be provided to and maintained by the designated back-up facility.

See §5202.4 for information on EPO payment.

Submit claims for EPO in accordance with §§4273.1 and 4273.2.

C. Oral Anti-Cancer Drugs.—Effective January 1, 1994, Medicare Part B coverage is extended to include oral anti-cancer drugs that are prescribed as anti-cancer chemotherapeutic agents providing they have the same active ingredients and are used for the same indications as anti-cancer chemotherapeutic agents which would be covered if they were not self administered and they were furnished incident to a physician's service as drugs and biologicals.

This provision applies only to the coverage of anti-neoplastic chemotherapeutic agents. It does not apply to oral drugs and/or biologicals used to treat toxicity or side effects such as nausea or bone marrow depression. Medicare will cover anti-neoplastic chemotherapeutic agents, the primary drugs which directly fight the cancer, and self-administered antiemetics which are necessary for the administration and absorption of the anti-neoplastic chemotherapeutic agents when a high likelihood of vomiting exists. The substitution of an oral form of an anti-neoplastic drug requires that the drug be retained for absorption. The antiemetics drug is covered as a necessary means for administration of the oral drug (similar to a syringe and needle necessary for injectable administration).

Oral drugs prescribed for use with the primary drug which enhance the anti-neoplastic effect of the primary drug or permit the patient to tolerate the primary anti-neoplastic drug in higher doses for longer periods are not covered. Self-administered antiemetics to reduce the side effects of nausea and vomiting brought on by the primary drug are not included beyond the administration necessary to achieve drug absorption.

In order to assure uniform coverage policy, regional carriers and FIs must be apprised of local carriers' anti-cancer drug medical review policies which may impact on future medical review policy development. Local carrier's current and proposed anti-cancer drug medical review polices should be provided by local carrier medical directors to regional carrier or FI medical directors, upon request.

For an oral anti-cancer drug to be covered under Part B, it must:

- Be prescribed by a physician or other practitioner licensed under State law to prescribe such drugs as anti-cancer chemotherapeutic agents;
- Be a drug or biological that has been approved by the Food and Drug Administration (FDA);
- Have the same active ingredients as a non-self-administrable anti-cancer chemotherapeutic drug or biological that is covered when furnished incident to a physician's service. The oral anti-cancer drug and the non-self-administrable drug must have the same chemical/generic name as indicated by the FDA's Approved Drug Products (Orange Book), Physician's Desk Reference (PDR), or an authoritative drug compendium; —or, effective January 1, 1999, be a prodrug—an oral drug ingested into the body that metabolizes into the same active ingredient that is found in the non-self-administrable form of the drug;
- Be used for the same indications, including unlabeled uses, as the non-self-administrable version of the drug; and
- Be reasonable and necessary for the individual patient.

D. Oral Anti-Nausea Drugs—Section 4557 of the Balanced Budget Act of 1997 amends §1861(s)(2) by extending the coverage of oral anti-emetic drugs under the following conditions:

- Coverage is provided only for oral drugs approved by FDA for use as anti-emetics; the oral anti-emetic(s) must either be administered by the treating physician or in accordance with a written order from the physician as part of a cancer chemotherapy regimen;
- Oral anti-emetic drug(s) administered with a particular chemotherapy treatment must be initiated within 2 hours of the administration of the chemotherapeutic agent and may be continued for a period not to exceed 48 hours from that time.
- The oral anti-emetic drug(s) provided must be used as a full therapeutic replacement for the intravenous anti-emetic drugs that would have otherwise been administered at the time of the chemotherapy treatment.

Only drugs pursuant to a physician's order at the time of the chemotherapy treatment qualify for this benefit. The dispensed number of dosage units may not exceed a loading dose administered within 2 hours of that treatment, plus a supply of additional dosage units not to exceed 48 hours of therapy. However, more than one oral anti-emetic drug may be prescribed and will be covered for concurrent usage within these parameters if more than one oral drug is needed to fully replace the intravenous drugs that would otherwise have been given.

Oral drugs that are not approved by the FDA for use as anti-emetics and which are used by treating physicians adjunctively in a manner incidental to cancer chemotherapy are not covered by this benefit and are not reimbursable within the scope of this benefit.

It is recognized that a limited number of patients will fail on oral anti-emetic drugs. Intravenous anti-emetics may be covered (subject to the rules of medical necessity) when furnished to patients who fail on oral anti-emetic therapy.

This coverage, effective for services on or after January 1, 1998, is subject to regular Medicare Part B coinsurance and deductible provisions.

NOTE: Existing coverage policies authorizing the administration of suppositories to prevent vomiting when oral cancer drugs are used are unchanged by this new coverage.

E. Hemophilia Clotting Factors.—Section 1861(s)(2)(I) of the Act provides Medicare coverage of blood clotting factors for hemophilia patients competent to use such factors to control bleeding without medical supervision, and items related to the administration of such factors. Hemophilia, a blood disorder characterized by prolonged coagulation time, Is caused by deficiency of a factor in plasma necessary for blood to clot. (The discovery in 1964 of a cryoprecipitate rich in antihemophilic factor activity facilitated management of acute bleeding episodes.) For purposes of Medicare Part B coverage, hemophilia encompasses the following conditions:

- Factor VIII deficiency (classic hemophilia);
- Factor IX deficiency (also termed plasma thromboplastin component (PTC) or Christmas factor deficiency); and
- Von Willebrand's disease.

Claims for blood clotting factors for hemophilia patients with these diagnoses may be covered if the patient is competent to use such factors without medical supervision.

The amount of clotting factors determined to be necessary to have on hand and thus covered under this provision is based on the historical utilization pattern or profile developed by the carrier for each patient. It is expected that the treating source; e.g., a family physician or comprehensive hemophilia diagnostic and treatment center, has such information. From this data, the contractor is able to make reasonable projections concerning the quantity of clotting factors anticipated to be needed by the patient over a specific period of time. Unanticipated occurrences involving extraordinary events, such as automobile accidents of inpatient hospital stays, will change this base line data and should be appropriately considered. In addition, changes in a patient's medical needs over a period of time require adjustments in the profile. (See §5245 for payment policies.)

2070.4 Coverage of Portable X-ray Services Not Under the Direct Supervision of a Physician.-

A. Diagnostic X-ray Tests.—Diagnostic x-ray services furnished by a portable x-ray supplier are covered under Part B when furnished in a place or residence used as the patient's home and in nonparticipating institutions. These services must be performed under the general supervision of a physician and certain conditions relating to health and safety (as prescribed by the Secretary) must be met.

Diagnostic portable x-ray services are also covered under Part B when provided in participating SNFs and hospitals, under circumstances in which they cannot be covered under hospital insurance, i.e., the services are not furnished by the participating institution either directly or under arrangements that provide for the institution to bill for the services. (See §2255 for reimbursement for Part B services furnished to inpatients of participating and nonparticipating institutions.)

B. Applicability of Health and Safety Standards.—The health and safety standards apply to all suppliers of portable x-ray services, except physicians who provide immediate personal supervision during the administration of diagnostic x-ray services. Payment is made only for services of approved suppliers who have been found to meet the standards. Notice of the coverage dates for services of approved suppliers are given to carriers by the RO.

When the services of a supplier of portable x-ray services no longer meet the conditions of coverage, physicians having an interest in the supplier's certification status must be notified. The notification action regarding suppliers of portable x-ray equipment is the same as required for decertification of independent laboratories, and the procedures explained in §2070.lC should be followed.

C. Scope of Portable X-Ray Benefit.—In order to avoid payment for services which are inadequate or hazardous to the patient, the scope of the covered portable x-ray benefit is defined as:

- Skeletal films involving arms and legs, pelvis, vertebral column, and skull;
- Chest films which do not involve the use of contrast media (except routine screening procedures and tests in connection with routine physical examinations); and
- Abdominal films which do not involve the use of contrast media.

D. Exclusions From Coverage as Portable X-Ray Services.— Procedures and examinations which are not covered under the portable x-ray provision include the following:

- Procedures involving fluoroscopy;
- Procedures involving the use of contrast media;
- Procedures requiring the administration of a substance to the patient or injection of a substance into the patient and/or special manipulation of the patient;
- Procedures which require special medical skill or knowledge possessed by a doctor of medicine or doctor of osteopathy or which require that medical judgment be exercised;
- Procedures requiring special technical competency and/or special equipment or materials;
- Routine screening procedures; and
- Procedures which are not of a diagnostic nature.

E. Reimbursement Procedure.

1. Name of Ordering Physician. — Assure that portable x-ray tests have been provided on the written order of a physician. Accordingly, if a bill does not include the name of the physician who ordered the service, that information must be obtained before payment may be made.

2. Reason Chest X-Ray Ordered. — Because all routine screening procedures and tests in connection with routine physical examinations are excluded from coverage under Medicare, all bills for portable x-ray services involving the chest contain, in addition to the name of the physician who ordered the service, the reason an x-ray test was required.

   If this information is not shown, it is obtained from either the supplier or the physician. If the test was for an excluded routine service, no payment may be made.

See also §§4110 ff. for additional instructions on reviewing bills involving portable x-ray.

F. Electrocardiograms.—The taking of an electrocardiogram tracing by an approved supplier of portable x-ray services may be covered as an "other diagnostic test." The health and safety standards referred to in §2070.4B are thus also applicable to such diagnostic EKG services, e.g., the technician must meet the personnel qualification requirements in the Conditions for Coverage of Portable x-ray Services. (See §50-15 (Electrocardiographic Services) in the Coverage Issues Manual.)

2079 SURGICAL DRESSINGS, AND SPLINTS, CASTS, AND OTHER DEVICES USED FOR REDUCTIONS OF FRACTURES AND DISLOCATIONS

Surgical dressings are limited to primary and secondary dressings required for the treatment of a wound caused by, or treated by, a surgical procedure that has been performed by a physician or other health care professional to the extent permissible under State law. In addition, surgical dressings required after debridement of a wound are also covered, irrespective of the type of debridement, as long as the debridement was reasonable and necessary and was performed by a health care professional who was acting within the scope of his or her legal authority when performing this function. Surgical dressings are covered for as long as they are medically necessary.

Primary dressings are therapeutic or protective coverings applied directly to wounds or lesions either on the skin or caused by an opening to the skin. Secondary dressing materials that serve a therapeutic or protective function and that are needed to secure a primary dressing are also covered. Items such as adhesive tape, roll gauze, bandages, and disposable compression material are examples of secondary dressings. Elastic stockings, support hose, foot coverings, leotards, knee supports, surgical leggings, gauntlets, and pressure garments for the arms and hands are examples of items that are not ordinarily covered as surgical dressings. Some items, such as transparent film, may be used as a primary or secondary dressing.

If a physician, certified nurse midwife, physician assistant, nurse practitioner, or clinical nurse specialist applies surgical dressings as part of a professional service that is billed to Medicare, the surgical dressings are considered incident to the professional services of the health care practitioner. (See sections 2050.1, 2154, 2156, 2158, and 2160.) When surgical dressings are not covered incident to the services of a health care practitioner and are obtained by the patient from a supplier (e.g., a drugstore, physician, or other health care practitioner that qualifies as a supplier) on an order from a physician or other health care professional authorized under State law or regulation to make such an order, the surgical dressings are covered separately under Part B.

2100 DURABLE MEDICAL EQUIPMENT - GENERAL

Expenses incurred by a beneficiary for the rental or purchase of durable medical equipment (DME) are reimbursable if the following three requirements are met. The decision whether to rent or purchase an item of equipment resides with the beneficiary.

A. The equipment meets the definition of DME (§2100.1); and
B. The equipment is necessary and reasonable for the treatment of the patient's illness or injury or to improve the functioning of his malformed body member (§2100.2); and
C. The equipment is used in the patient's home (§2100.3).

Payment may also be made under this provision for repairs, maintenance, and delivery of equipment as well as for expendable and nonreusable items essential to the effective use of the equipment subject to the conditions in §2100.4.

See §2105 and its appendix for coverage guidelines and screening list of DME. See §4105.3 for models of payment: decisions as to rental or purchase, lump sum and periodic payments, etc. Where covered DME is furnished to a beneficiary by a supplier of services other than a provider of services, reimbursement is made by the carrier on the basis of the reasonable charge. If the equipment is furnished by a provider of services, reimbursement is made to the provider by the intermediary on a reasonable cost basis; see Coverage Issues Appendix 25-1 for hemodialysis equipment and supplies.

2100.1 Definition of Durable Medical Equipment.—Durable medical equipment is equipment which a) can withstand repeated use, and b) is primarily and customarily used to serve a medical purpose, and c) generally is not useful to a person in the absence of an illness or injury; and d) is appropriate for use in the home.

All requirements of the definition must be met before an item can be considered to be durable medical equipment.

A. Durability.—An item is considered durable if it can withstand repeated use, i.e., the type of item which could normally be rented. Medical supplies of an expendable nature such as, incontinent pads, lambs wool pads, catheters, ace bandages, elastic stockings, surgical face masks, irrigating kits, sheets and bags are not considered "durable" within the meaning of the definition. There are other items which, although durable in nature, may fall into other coverage categories such as braces, prosthetic devices, artificial arms, legs, and eyes.

B. Medical Equipment.—Medical equipment is equipment which is primarily and customarily used for medical purposes and is not generally useful in the absence of illness or injury. In most instances, no development will be needed to determine whether a specific item of equipment is medical in nature. However, some cases will require development to determine whether the item constitutes medical equipment. This development would include the advice of local medical organizations (hospitals, medical schools, medical societies) and specialists in the field of physical medicine and rehabilitation. If the equipment is new on the market, it may be necessary, prior to seeking professional advice, to obtain information from the supplier or manufacturer explaining the design, purpose, effectiveness and method of using the equipment in the home as well as the results of any tests or clinical studies that have been conducted.

   1. Equipment Presumptively Medical.—Items such as hospital beds, wheelchairs, hemodialysis equipment, iron lungs, respirators, intermittent positive pressure breathing machines, medical regulators, oxygen tents, crutches, canes, trapeze bars, walkers, inhalators, nebulizers, commodes, suction machines and traction equipment presumptively constitute medical equipment. (Although hemodialysis equipment is a prosthetic device (§ 2130), it also meets the definition of DME, and reimbursement for the rental or purchase of such equipment for use in the beneficiary's home will be made only under the provisions for payment applicable to DME. See 25-1 and 25-2 of the Coverage Issues Appendix for coverage of home use of hemodialysis.)

      NOTE: There is a wide variety in type of respirators and suction machines. The carrier's medical staff should determine whether the apparatus specified in the claim is appropriate for home use.

2. Equipment Presumptively Nonmedical.—Equipment which is primarily and customarily used for a nonmedical purpose may not be considered "medical" equipment for which payment can be made under the medical insurance program. This is true even though the item has some remote medically related use. For example, in the case of a cardiac patient, an air conditioner might possibly be used to lower room temperature to reduce fluid loss in the patient and to restore an environment conducive to maintenance of the proper fluid balance. Nevertheless, because the primary and customary use of an air conditioner is a nonmedical one, the air conditioner cannot be deemed to be medical equipment for which payment can be made.

   Other devices and equipment used for environmental control or to enhance the environmental setting in which the beneficiary is placed are not considered covered DME. These include, for example, room heaters, humidifiers, dehumidifiers, and electric air cleaners. Equipment which basically serves comfort or convenience functions or is primarily for the convenience of a person caring for the patient, such as elevators, stairway elevators, and posture chairs do not constitute medical equipment. Similarly, physical fitness equipment, e.g., an exercycle; first-aid or precautionary-type equipment, e.g., present portable oxygen units; self-help devices, e.g., safety grab bars; and training equipment, e.g., speech teaching machines and braille training texts, are considered nonmedical in nature.

3. Special Exception Items.—Specified items of equipment may be covered under certain conditions even though they do not meet the definition of DME because they are not primarily and customarily used to serve a medical purpose and/or are generally useful in the absence of illness or injury. These items would be covered when it is clearly established that they serve a therapeutic purpose in an individual case and would include:

   a. Gel pads and pressure and water mattresses (which generally serve a preventive purpose) when prescribed for a patient who had bed sores or there is medical evidence indicating that he is highly susceptible to such ulceration; and
   b. Heat lamps for a medical rather than a soothing or cosmetic purpose, e.g., where the need for heat therapy has been established.

   In establishing medical necessity (§2100.2) for the above items, the evidence must show that the item is included in the physician's course of treatment and a physician is supervising its use. (See also Appendix to § 2105.)

   NOTE: The above items represent special exceptions and no extension of coverage to other items should be inferred.

Repairs, Maintenance, Replacement, and Delivery.—Under the circumstances specified below, payment may be made for repair, maintenance, and replacement of medically required DME, including equipment which had been in use before the user enrolled in Part B of the program. However, do not pay for repair, maintenance, or replacement of equipment in the frequent and substantial servicing or oxygen equipment payment categories. In addition, payments for repair and maintenance may not include payment for parts and labor covered under a manufacturer's or supplier's warranty.

A. Repairs.— To repair means to fix or mend and to put the equipment back in good condition after damage or wear. Repairs to equipment which a beneficiary owns are covered when necessary to make the equipment serviceable. However, do not pay for repair of previously denied equipment or equipment in the frequent and substantial servicing or oxygen equipment payment categories. If the expense for repairs exceeds the estimated expense of purchasing or renting another item of equipment for the remaining period of medical need, no payment can be made for the amount of the excess. (See subsection C where claims for repairs suggest malicious damage or culpable neglect.)

Since renters of equipment recover from the rental charge the expenses they incur in maintaining in working order the equipment they rent out, separately itemized charges for repair of rented equipment are not covered. This includes items in the frequent and substantial servicing, oxygen equipment, capped rental, and inexpensive or routinely purchased payment categories which are being rented.

A new Certificate of Medical Necessity (CMN) and/or physician's order is not needed for repairs. For replacement items, see Subsection C below.

B. Maintenance.—Routine periodic maintenance, such as testing, cleaning, regulating and checking of the beneficiary's equipment is not covered. Such routine maintenance is generally expected to be done by the owner rather than by a retailer or some other person who charges the beneficiary. Normally, purchasers of DME are given operating manuals which describe the type of servicing an owner may perform to properly maintain the equipment. It is reasonable to expect that beneficiaries will perform this maintenance. Thus, hiring a third party to do such work is for the convenience of the beneficiary and is not covered.

However, more extensive maintenance which, based on the manufacturers' recommendations, is to be performed by authorized technicians, is covered as repairs for medically necessary equipment which a beneficiary owns. This might include, for example, breaking down sealed components and performing tests which require specialized testing equipment not available to the beneficiary. Do not pay for maintenance of purchased items that require frequent and substantial servicing or oxygen equipment. See §5102.2.G.

Since renters of equipment recover from the rental charge the expenses they incur in maintaining in working order the equipment they rent out, separately itemized charges for maintenance of rented equipment are generally not covered. Payment may not be made for maintenance of rented equipment other than the maintenance and servicing fee established for capped rental items in §5102.1.E.4.

A new CMN and/or physician's order is not needed for covered maintenance.

C. Replacement.—Replacement refers to the provision of an identical or nearly identical item. Situations involving the provision of a different item because of a change in medical condition are not addressed in this section.

Equipment which the beneficiary owns or is a capped rental item may be replaced in cases of loss or irreparable damage. Irreparable damage refers to a specific accident or to a natural disaster (e.g., fire, flood, etc.). A physician's order and/or new Certificate of Medical Necessity (CMN), when required, is needed to reaffirm the medical necessity of the item.

Irreparable wear refers to deterioration sustained from day-to-day usage over time and a specific event cannot be identified. Replacement of equipment due to irreparable wear takes into consideration the reasonable useful lifetime of the equipment. If the item of equipment has been in continuous use by the patient on either a rental or purchase basis for the equipment's useful lifetime, the beneficiary may elect to obtain a new piece of equipment. Replacement may be reimbursed when a new physician order and/or new CMN, when required, is needed to reaffirm the medical necessity of the item.

The reasonable useful lifetime of durable medical equipment is determined through program instructions. In the absence of program instructions, carriers may determine the reasonable useful lifetime of equipment, but in no case can it be less than 5 years. Computation of the useful lifetime is based on when the equipment is delivered to the beneficiary, not the age of the equipment. Replacement due to wear is not covered during the reasonable useful lifetime of the equipment. During the reasonable useful lifetime, Medicare does cover repair up to the cost of replacement (but not actual replacement) for medically necessary equipment owned by the beneficiary. (See subsection A.)

Charges for the replacement of oxygen equipment, items that require frequent and substantial servicing or inexpensive or routinely purchased items which are being rented are not covered.

Cases suggesting malicious damage, culpable neglect or wrongful disposition of equipment as discussed in §2100.6 should be investigated and denied where the DMERC/Carrier determines that it is unreasonable to make program payment under the circumstances.

D. Delivery.—Payment for delivery of DME whether rented or purchased is generally included in the fee schedule allowance for the item. See §5105 for the rules that apply to making reimbursement for exceptional cases.

E. Leased Renal Dialysis Equipment.—Generally, where renal dialysis equipment is leased directly from the manufacturer, the rental charge is closely related to the manufacturer's cost of the equipment which means it does not include a margin for recovering the cost of repairs beyond the initial warranty period.

In view of physical distance and other factors which may make it impractical for the manufacturer to perform repairs, it is not feasible to make the manufacturer responsible for all repairs and include a margin for the additional costs. Therefore, reimbursement may be made for the repair and maintenance of home dialysis equipment leased directly from the manufacturer (or other party acting essentially as an intermediary between the patient and the manufacturer for the purpose of assuming the financial risk) if the rental charge does not include a margin to recover these costs, and then only when the patient is free to secure repairs locally in the most economical manner.

Where, on the other hand, a third party is in the business of medical equipment retail supply and rental, the presumption that there is a margin in the rental charge for dialysis equipment to cover the costs of repair services will be retained. The exclusion from coverage of separately itemized repair charges will, therefore, continue to be applied in these situations, and the patient must look to the supplier to perform (or cover the cost of) necessary repairs, maintenance, and replacement of the home dialysis equipment.

In all cases, whether the dialysis equipment is being purchased, is owned outright, or is being leased, Medicare payment is to be made only after the initial warranty period has expired. Generally, reimbursement for repairs, maintenance, and replacement parts for medically necessary home dialysis equipment may be made in a lump sum payment. However, where extensive repairs are required and the charge for repairing the item represents a substantial proportion of the purchase price of a replacement system, exercise judgment with respect to a possible need to make periodic payments, instead of a lump-sum payment, for repair of such equipment.

As in the case of the maintenance of purchased DME, routine periodic servicing of leased dialysis equipment, including most testing and cleaning, is not covered. While reimbursement will be made for more extensive maintenance and necessary repairs of leased dialysis equipment, the patient or family member is expected to perform those services for which the training for home or self-dialysis would have qualified them, e.g., replacement of a light bulb.

Reasonable charges for travel expenses related to the repair of leased dialysis equipment are covered if the repairman customarily charges for travel and this is a common practice among other repairman in the area. When a repair charge includes an element for travel, however, the location of other suitably qualified repairmen will be considered in determining the allowance for travel.

NOTE: The above coverage instructions pertain to a special case and no extension of such coverage with respect to other items should be inferred.

Coverage of Supplies and Accessories.— Reimbursement may be made for supplies, e.g., oxygen (see §60-4 in the Coverage Issues Manual for the coverage of oxygen in the home), that are necessary for the effective use of durable medical equipment. Such supplies include those drugs and biologicals which must be put directly into the equipment in order to achieve the therapeutic benefit of the durable medical equipment or to assure the proper functioning of the equipment, e.g., tumor chemotherapy agents used with an infusion pump or heparin used with a home dialysis system. However, the coverage of such drugs or biologicals does not preclude the need for a determination that the drug or biological itself is reasonable and necessary for treatment of the illness or injury or to improve the functioning of a malformed body member.

In the case of prescription drugs, other than oxygen, used in conjunction with durable medical equipment, prosthetic, orthotics, and supplies (DMEPOS) or prosthetic devices, the entity that dispenses the drug must furnish it directly to the patient for whom a prescription is written. The entity that dispenses the drugs must have a Medicare supplier number, must possess a current license to dispense prescription drugs in the State in which the drug is dispensed, and must bill and receive payment in its own name.

A supplier that is not the entity that dispenses the drugs cannot purchase the drugs used in conjunction with DME for resale to the beneficiary. Payments made for drugs provided on or after December 1, 1996 to suppliers not having a valid pharmacy license to dispense prescription drugs must be recouped.

2120.1 Vehicle and Crew Requirement

A. The Vehicle.—The vehicle must be a specially designed and equipped automobile or other vehicle (in some areas of the United States this might be a boat or plane) for transporting the sick or injured. It must have customary patient care equipment including a stretcher, clean linens, first aid supplies, oxygen equipment, and it must also have such other safety and lifesaving equipment as is required by State or local authorities.

B. The Crew.—The ambulance crew must consist of at least two members. Those crew members charged with the care or handling of the patient must include one individual with adequate first aid training, i.e., training at least equivalent to that provided by the standard and advanced Red Cross first aid courses. Training "equivalent" to the standard and advanced Red Cross first aid training courses included ambulance service training and experience acquired in military service, successful completion by the individual of a comparable first aid course furnished by or under the sponsorship of State or local authorities, an educational institution, a fire department, a hospital, a professional organization, or other such qualified organization. On-the-job training involving the administration of first aid under the supervision of or in conjunction with trained first aid personnel for a period of time sufficient to assure the trainee's proficiency in handling the wide range of patient care services that may have to be performed by a qualified attendant can also be considered as "equivalent training."

C. Verification of Compliance.—In determining whether the vehicles and personnel of each supplier meet all of the above requirements, carriers may accept the supplier's statement (absent information to the contrary) that its vehicles and personnel meet all of the requirements if (l) the statement describes the first aid, safety, and other patient care items with which the vehicles are equipped, (2) the statement shows the extent of first aid training acquired by the personnel assigned to those vehicles, (3) the statement contains the supplier's agreement to notify the carrier of any change in operation which could affect the coverage of his ambulance services, and (4) the information provided indicates that the requirements are met. The statement must be accompanied by documentary evidence that the ambulance has the equipment required by State and local authorities. Documentary evidence could include a letter from such authorities, a copy of a license, permit certificate, etc., issued by the authorities. The statement and supporting documentation would be kept on file by the carrier.

   When a supplier does not submit such a statement or whenever there is a question about a supplier's compliance with any of the above requirements for vehicle and crew (including suppliers who have completed the statement), carriers should take appropriate action including, where necessary, on-site inspection of the vehicles and verification of the qualifications of personnel to determine whether the ambulance service qualifies for reimbursement under Medicare. Since the requirements described above for coverage of ambulance services are applicable to the overall operation of the ambulance supplier's service, it is not required that information regarding personnel and vehicles be obtained on an individual trip basis.

D. Ambulance of Providers of Services.—The Part A intermediary is responsible for the processing of claims for ambulance service furnished by participating hospitals, skilled nursing facilities and home health agencies and has the responsibility to determine the compliance of provider's ambulance and crew. Since provider ambulance services furnished "under arrangements" with suppliers can be covered only if the supplier meets the above requirements, the Part A intermediary may ask the carrier to identify those suppliers who meet the requirements.

E. Equipment and Supplies.—As mentioned above, the ambulance must have customary patient care equipment and first aid supplies. Reusable devices and equipment such as backboards, neck boards and inflatable leg and arm splints are considered part of the general ambulance service and would be included in the charge for the trip. On the other hand, separate reasonable charge based on actual quantities used may be recognized for nonreusable items and disposable supplies such as oxygen, gauze and dressings required in the care of the patient during his trip.

2125 COVERAGE GUIDELINES FOR AMBULANCE SERVICE CLAIMS

Reimbursement may be made for expenses incurred by a patient for ambulance service provided the following conditions have been met:

A. Patient was transported by an approved supplier of ambulance services.
B. The patient was suffering from an illness or injury which contraindicated transportation by other means. (section 2120.2A)
C. The patient was transported from and to points listed below.(section 2120.3)

1. From patient's residence (or other place where need arose) to hospital or skilled nursing home.
2. Skilled nursing home to a hospital or hospital to a skilled nursing home.
3. Hospital to hospital or skilled nursing home to skilled nursing home.
4. From a hospital or skilled nursing home to patient's residence.
5. Round trip for hospital or participating skilled nursing facility inpatients to the nearest hospital or nonhospital treatment facility

A patient's residence is the place where he makes his home and dwells permanently, or for an extended period of time. A skilled nursing home is one which is listed in the Directory of Medical Facilities as a participating SNF or as an institution which meets section 1861(j)(1) of the law. Ambulance service to a physician's office or a physician-directed clinic is not covered. (See section 2120.3G where a stop is made at a physician's office enroute to a hospital and 2120.3C for additional exceptions.)

2130 PROSTHETIC DEVICES

A. General.—Prosthetic devices (other than dental) which replace all or part of an internal body organ (including contiguous tissue), or replace all or part of the function of a permanently inoperative or malfunctioning internal body organ are covered when furnished on a physician's order. This does not require a determination that there is no possibility that the patient's condition may improve sometime in the future. If the medical record, including the judgment of the attending physician, indicates the condition is of long and indefinite duration, the test of permanence is considered met. (Such a device may also be covered under §2050.l as a supply when furnished incident to a physician's service.)

Examples of prosthetic devices include cardiac pacemakers, prosthetic lenses (see subsection B), breast prostheses (including a surgical brassiere) for postmastectomy patients, maxillofacial devices and devices which replace all or part of the ear or nose. A urinary collection and retention system with or without a tube is a prosthetic device replacing bladder function in case of permanent urinary incontinence. The Foley catheter is also considered a prosthetic device when ordered for a patient with permanent urinary incontinence. However, chucks, diapers, rubber sheets, etc., are supplies that are not covered under this provision. (Although hemodialysis equipment is a prosthetic device, payment for the rental or purchase of such equipment for use in the home is made only under the provisions for payment applicable to durable medical equipment (see §4105ff) or the special rules that apply to the ESRD program.)

NOTE: Medicare does not cover a prosthetic device dispensed to a patient prior to the time at which the patient undergoes the procedure that makes necessary the use of the device. For example, do not make a separate Part B payment for an intraocular lens (IOL) or pacemaker that a physician, during an office visit prior to the actual surgery, dispenses to the patient for his/her use. Dispensing a prosthetic device in this manner raises health and safety issues. Moreover, the need for the device cannot be clearly established until the procedure that makes its use possible is successfully performed.

Therefore, dispensing a prosthetic device in this manner is not considered reasonable and necessary for the treatment of the patient's condition.

Colostomy (and other ostomy) bags and necessary accouterments required for attachment are covered as prosthetic devices. This coverage also includes irrigation and flushing equipment and other items and supplies directly related to ostomy care, whether the attachment of a bag is required.

Accessories and/or supplies which are used directly with an enteral or parenteral device to achieve the therapeutic benefit of the prosthesis or to assure the proper functioning of the device are covered under the prosthetic device benefit subject to the additional guidelines in the Coverage Issues Manual §§65-10 - 65-10.3.

Covered items include catheters, filters, extension tubing, infusion bottles, pumps (either food or infusion), intravenous (I.V) pole, needles, syringes, dressings, tape, Heparin Sodium (parenteral only), volumetric monitors (parenteral only), and parenteral and enteral nutrient solutions. Baby food and other regular grocery products that can be blenderized and used with the enteral system are not covered. Note that some of these items, e.g., a food pump and an I.V. pole, qualify as DME. Although coverage of the enteral and parenteral nutritional therapy systems is provided on the basis of the prosthetic device benefit, the payment rules relating to rental or purchase of DME apply of such items. (See §4105.3.) Code claims in accordance with the HCFA Common procedure Coding System (HCPCS).

The coverage of prosthetic devices includes replacement of and repairs to such devices as explained in subsection D.

B. Prosthetic Lenses.—The term "internal body organ" includes the lens of an eye. Prostheses replacing the lens of an eye include post-surgical lenses customarily used during convalescence from eye surgery in which the lens of the eye was removed. In addition, permanent lenses are also covered when required by an individual lacking the organic lens of the eye because of surgical removal or congenital absence. Prosthetic lenses obtained on or after the beneficiary's date of entitlement to supplementary medical insurance benefits may be covered even though the surgical removal of the crystalline lens occurred before entitlement.

1. Prosthetic Cataract Lenses.—Make payment for one of the following prosthetic lenses or combinations of prosthetic lenses when determined to be medically necessary by a physician (see §2020.25 for coverage of prosthetic lenses prescribed by a doctor of optometry) to restore essentially the vision provided by the crystalline lens of the eye:

   - prosthetic bifocal lenses in frames;
   - prosthetic lenses in frames for far vision, and prosthetic lenses in frames for near vision; or
   - when a prosthetic contact lens(es) for far vision is prescribed (including cases of binocular and monocular aphakia), make payment for the contact lens(es) and prosthetic lenses in frames for near vision to be worn at the same time as the contact lens(es), and prosthetic lenses in frames to be worn when the contacts have been removed.

   Make payment for lenses which have ultraviolet absorbing or reflecting properties, in lieu of payment for regular (untinted) lenses, if it has been determined that such lenses are medically reasonable and necessary for the individual patient.

Do not make payment for cataract sunglasses obtained in addition to the regular (untinted) prosthetic lenses since the sunglasses duplicate the restoration of vision function performed by the regular prosthetic lenses.

2. Payment for IOLs Furnished in Ambulatory Surgical Centers (ASCs). Effective for services furnished on or after March 12, 1990, payment for IOLs inserted during or subsequent to cataract surgery in a Medicare certified ASC is included with the payment for facility services that are furnished in connection with the covered surgery. Section 5243.3 explains payment procedures for ASC facility services and the IOL allowance.

3. Limitation on Coverage of Conventional Lenses.—Make payment for no more than one pair of conventional eyeglasses or conventional contact lenses furnished after each cataract surgery with insertion of an IOL.

C. Dentures.—Dentures are excluded from coverage. However, when a denture or a portion thereof is an integral part (built-in) of a covered prosthesis (e.g., an obturator to fill an opening in the palate), it is covered as part of that prosthesis.

D. Supplies, Repairs, Adjustments, and Replacement.—Make payment for supplies that are necessary for the effective use of a prosthetic device (e.g., the batteries needed to operate an artificial larynx). Adjustment of prosthetic devices required by wear or by a change in the patient's condition is covered when ordered by a physician. To the extent applicable, follow the provisions relating to the repair and replacement of durable medical equipment in §2100.4 for the repair and replacement of prosthetic devices. (See §2306.D in regard to payment for devices replaced under a warranty.) Regardless of the date that the original eyewear was furnished (i.e., whether before, on, or after January 1, 1991), do not pay for replacement of conventional eyeglasses or contact lenses covered under subsection B.3.

Necessary supplies, adjustments, repairs, and replacements are covered even when the device had been in use before the user enrolled in Part B of the program, so long as the device continues to be medically required.

2133 LEG, ARM, BACK, AND NECK BRACES, TRUSSES, AND ARTIFICIAL LEGS, ARMS, AND EYES

These appliances are covered when furnished incident to physicians' services or on a physician's order. A brace includes rigid and semi-rigid devices which are used for the purpose of supporting a weak or deformed body member or restricting or eliminating motion in a diseased or injured part of the body. Elastic stockings, garter belts, and similar devices do not come within the scope of the definition of a brace. Back braces include, but are not limited to, special corsets, e.g., sacroiliac, sacrolumbar, dorsolumbar corsets and belts. A terminal device (e.g., hand or hook) is covered under this provision whether an artificial limb is required by the patient. (See §2323.) Stump stockings and harnesses (including replacements) are also covered when these appliances are essential to the effective use of the artificial limb.

Adjustments to an artificial limb or other appliance required by wear or by a change in the patient's condition are covered when ordered by a physician. To the extent applicable, follow the provisions in §2100.4 relating to the repair and replacement of durable medical equipment for the repair and replacement of artificial limbs, braces, etc. Adjustments, repairs and replacements are covered even when the item had been in use before the user enrolled in Part B of the program so long as the device continues to be medically required.

2134 THERAPEUTIC SHOES FOR INDIVIDUALS WITH DIABETES

Coverage of therapeutic shoes (depth or custom-molded) along with inserts for individuals with diabetes is available as of May 1, 1993.These diabetic shoes are covered if the requirements as specified in this section concerning certification and prescription are fulfilled. In addition, this benefit provides for a pair of diabetic shoes even if only one foot suffers from diabetic foot disease. Each shoe is equally equipped so that the affected limb, as well as the remaining limb, is protected.

Claims for therapeutic shoes for diabetics are processed by the Durable Medical Equipment Regional Carriers (DMERCs.)

A. Definitions.—The following items may be covered under the diabetic shoe benefit:

1. Custom-Molded Shoes.—Custom-molded shoes are shoes that are:

    - Constructed over a positive model of the patient's foot; Made from leather or other suitable material of equal quality;
    - Have removable inserts that can be altered or replaced as the patient's condition warrants; and
    - Have some form of shoe closure.

2. Depth Shoes.—Depth shoes are shoes that:

    - Have a full length, heel-to-toe filler that, when removed, provides a minimum of 3/16 inch of additional depth used to accommodate custom-molded or customized inserts;
    - Are made from leather or other suitable material of equal quality;
    - Have some form of shoe closure; and
    - Are available in full and half sizes with a minimum of 3 widths so that the sole is graded to the size and width of the upper portions of the shoes according to the American standard last sizing schedule or its equivalent. (The American standard last sizing schedule is the numerical shoe sizing system used for shoes sold in the United States.)

3. Inserts.—Inserts are total contact, multiple density, removable inlays that are directly molded to the patient's foot or a model of the patient's foot and that are made of a suitable material with regard to the patient's condition.

B. Coverage.—

1. Limitations.—For each individual, coverage of the footwear and inserts is limited to one of the following within one calendar year:

    - No more than one pair of custom-molded shoes (including inserts provided with such shoes) and two additional pairs of inserts; or
    - No more than one pair of depth shoes and three pairs of inserts (not including the non-customized removable inserts provided with such shoes).

2. Coverage of Diabetic Shoes and Brace.—Orthopedic shoes, as stated in §2323.D, generally are not covered. This exclusion does not apply to orthopedic shoes that are an integral part of a leg brace. In situations in which an individual qualifies for both diabetic shoes and a leg brace, these items are covered separately. Thus, the diabetic shoes may be covered if the requirements for this section are met, while the brace may be covered if the requirements of section 2133 are met.

3. Substitution of Modifications for Inserts.—An individual may substitute modification(s) of custom-molded or depth shoes instead of obtaining a pair(s) of inserts in any combination. Payment for the modification(s) may not exceed the limit set for the inserts for which the individual is entitled. The following is a list of the most common shoe modifications available, but it is not meant as an exhaustive list of the modifications available for diabetic shoes:

   - Rigid Rocker Bottoms. These are exterior elevations with apex positions for 51 percent to 75 percent distance measured from the back end of the heel. The apex is a narrowed or pointed end of an anatomical structure. The apex must be positioned behind the metatarsal heads and tapering off sharply to the front tip of the sole. Apex height helps to eliminate pressure at the metatarsal heads.

     Rigidity is ensured by the steel in the shoe. The heel of the shoe tapers off in the back in order to cause the heel to strike in the middle of the heel.

   - Roller Bottoms (Sole or Bar). These are the same as rocker bottoms, but the heel is tapered from the apex to the front tip of the sole.
   - Metatarsal Bars.—An exterior bar is placed behind the metatarsal heads in order to remove pressure from the metatarsal heads. The bars are of various shapes, heights, and construction depending on the exact purpose.
   - Wedges (Posting). Wedges are either of hind foot, fore foot, or both and may be in the middle or to the side. The function is to shift or transfer weight bearing upon standing or during ambulation to the opposite side for added support, stabilization, equalized weight distribution, or balance.
   - Offset Heels. This is a heel flanged at its base either in the middle, to the side, or a combination, that is then extended upward to the shoe in order to stabilize extreme positions of the hind foot.
   - Other modifications to diabetic shoes include, but are not limited to:

     - Flared heels;
     - Velcro closures; and Inserts for missing toes.

4. Separate Inserts. Inserts may be covered and dispensed independently of diabetic shoes if the supplier of the shoes verifies in writing that the patient has appropriate footwear into which the insert can be placed. This footwear must meet the definitions found above for depth shoes and custom-molded shoes.

C. Certification. The need for diabetic shoes must be certified by a physician who is a doctor of medicine or a doctor of osteopathy and who is responsible for diagnosing and treating the patient's diabetic systemic condition through a comprehensive plan of care. This managing physician must:

- Document in the patient's medical record that the patient has diabetes;

- Certify that the patient is being treated under a comprehensive plan of care for his or her diabetes, and that he or she needs diabetic shoes; and
- Document in the patient's record that the patient has one or more of the following conditions:

  - Peripheral neuropathy with evidence of callus formation;
  - History of pre-ulcerative calluses;
  - History of previous ulceration;
  - Foot deformity;
  - Previous amputation of the foot or part of the foot; or
  - Poor circulation.

D. Prescription. Following certification by the physician managing the patient's systemic diabetic condition, a podiatrist or other qualified physician who is knowledgeable in the fitting of diabetic shoes and inserts may prescribe the particular type of footwear necessary.

E. Furnishing Footwear. The footwear must be fitted and furnished by a podiatrist or other qualified individual such as a pedorthist, an orthotist, or a prosthetist. The certifying physician may not furnish the diabetic shoes unless he or she is the only qualified individual in the area. It is left to the discretion of each carrier to determine the meaning of "in the area."

F. Payment. For 1994, payment for diabetic shoes and inserts is limited to 80 percent of the reasonable charge, up to a limit of $348 for one pair of custom-molded shoes including any initial inserts, $59 for each additional pair of custom-molded shoe inserts, $116 for one pair of depth shoes, and $59 for each pair of depth shoe inserts. These limits are based on 1988 amounts that were set forth in §1833(o) of the Act and then adjusted by the same percentage increases allowed for DME for fee screen limits by applying the same update factor that is applied to DME fees, except that if the updated limit is not a multiple of $1, it is rounded to the nearest multiple of $1.

   Although percentage increase in payment for diabetic shoes are the same percentage increases that are used for payment of DME through the DME fee schedule, the shoes are not subject to DME coverage rules or the DME fee schedule. In addition, diabetic shoes are neither considered DME nor orthotics, but a separate category of coverage under Medicare Part B. (See §1861(s)(12) and §1833(o) of the Act.)

   Payment for the certification of diabetic shoes and for the prescription of the shoes is considered to be included in the payment for the visit or consultation during which these services are provided. If the sole purpose of an encounter with the beneficiary is to dispense or fit the shoes, then no payment may be made for a visit or consultation provided on the same day by the same physician. Thus, a separate payment is not made for certification of the need for diabetic shoes, the prescribing of diabetic shoes, or the fitting of diabetic shoes unless the physician documents that these services were not the sole purpose of the visit or consultation.

2303 SERVICES NOT REASONABLE AND NECESSARY

Items and services which are not reasonable and necessary for the diagnosis or treatment of illness or injury, or to improve the functioning of a malformed body member; e.g., payment cannot be made for the rental of a special hospital bed to be used by the patient in his home unless it was a reasonable and necessary part of the patient's treatment. See also §2318.

2320 ROUTINE SERVICES AND APPLIANCES

Routine physical checkups; eyeglasses, contact lenses, and eye examinations for the purpose of prescribing, fitting or changing eyeglasses; eye refractions; hearing aids and examinations for hearing aids; and immunizations are not covered.

The routine physical checkup exclusion applies to (a) examinations performed without relationship to treatment or diagnosis for a specific illness, symptom, complaint, or injury, and (b) examinations required by third parties such as insurance companies, business establishments, or Government agencies.

(If the claim is for a diagnostic test or examination performed solely for the purpose of establishing a claim under title IV of Public Law 91-173 (Black Lung Benefits), advise the claimant to contact his/her Social Security office regarding the filing of a claim for reimbursement under that program.)

The exclusions apply to eyeglasses or contact lenses and eye examinations for the purpose of prescribing, fitting, or changing eyeglasses or contact lenses for refractive errors. The exclusions do not apply to physician services (and services incident to a physician's service) performed in conjunction with an eye disease (e.g., glaucoma or cataracts) or to postsurgical prosthetic lenses which are customarily used during convalescence from eye surgery in which the lens of the eye was removed or to permanent prosthetic lenses required by an individual lacking the organic lens of the eye, whether by surgical removal or congenital disease. Such prosthetic lens is a replacement for an internal body organ (the lens of the eye). (See §2130.)

The coverage of services rendered by an ophthalmologist is dependent on the purpose of the examination rather than on the ultimate diagnosis of the patient's condition. When a beneficiary goes to an ophthalmologist with a complaint or symptoms of an eye disease or injury, the ophthalmologist's services (except for eye refractions) are covered regardless of the fact that only eyeglasses were prescribed. However, when a beneficiary goes to his/her ophthalmologist for an eye examination with no specific complaint, the expenses for the examination are not covered even though as a result of such examination the doctor discovered a pathologic condition.

In the absence of evidence to the contrary, you may carrier may assume that an eye examination performed by an ophthalmologist on the basis of a complaint by the beneficiary or symptoms of an eye disease was not for the purpose of prescribing, fitting, or changing eyeglasses.

Expenses for all refractive procedures, whether performed by an ophthalmologist (or any other physician) or an optometrist and without regard to the reason for performance of the refraction, are excluded from coverage. (See
§§4125 and 5217 for claims review and reimbursement instructions concerning refractive services.)

With the exception of vaccinations for pneumococcal pneumonia, hepatitis B, and influenza, which are specifically covered under the law, vaccinations or inoculations are generally excluded as immunizations unless they are directly related to the treatment of an injury or direct exposure such as antirabies treatment, tetanus antitoxin or booster vaccine, botulin antitoxin, antivenin, or immune globulin.

2323 FOOT CARE AND SUPPORTIVE DEVICES FOR FEET

NOTE: See §4281 for the relationship between foot care and the coverage and billing of the diagnosis and treatment of peripheral neuropathy with loss of protective sensation (LOPS) in people with diabetes.

A. Exclusion of Coverage.—The following foot care services are generally excluded from coverage under both Part A and Part B. Exceptions to this general exclusion for limited treatment of routine foot care services are described in subsections A.2 and B. (See §4120 for procedural instructions in applying foot care exclusions.)

1. Treatment of Flat Foot.—The term "flat foot" is defined as a condition in which one or more arches of the foot have flattened out. Services or devices directed toward the care or correction of such conditions, including the prescription of supportive devices, are not covered.

2. Treatment of Subluxation of Foot.—Subluxations of the foot are defined as partial dislocations or displacements of joint surfaces, tendons ligaments, or muscles of the foot. Surgical or nonsurgical treatments undertaken for the sole purpose of correcting a subluxated structure in the foot as an isolated entity are not covered.

   This exclusion does not apply to medical or surgical treatment of subluxation of the ankle joint (talo-crural joint). In addition, reasonable and necessary medical or surgical services, diagnosis, or treatment for medical conditions that have resulted from or are associated with partial displacement of structures is covered. For example, if a patient has osteoarthritis that has resulted in a partial displacement of joints in the foot, and the primary treatment is for the osteoarthritis, coverage is provided.

3. Routine Foot Care.—Except as provided in subsection B, routine foot care is excluded from coverage. Services that normally are considered routine and not covered by Medicare include the following:

   - The cutting or removal of corns and calluses;
   - The trimming, cutting, clipping, or debriding of nails; and
   - Other hygienic and preventive maintenance care, such as cleaning and soaking the feet, the use of skin creams to maintain skin tone of either ambulatory or bedfast patients, and any other service performed in the absence of localized illness, injury, or symptoms involving the foot.

B. Exceptions to Routine Foot Care Exclusion.—

1. Necessary and Integral Part of Otherwise Covered Services.—In certain circumstances, services ordinarily considered to be routine may be covered if they are performed as a necessary and integral part of otherwise covered services, such as diagnosis and treatment of ulcers, wounds, or infections.

2. Treatment of Warts on Foot.—The treatment of warts (including plantar warts) on the foot is covered to the same extent as services provided for the treatment of warts located elsewhere on the body.

3. Presence of Systemic Condition.—The presence of a systemic condition such ametabolic, neurologic, or peripheral vascular disease may require scrupulous foot care by a professional that in the absence of such condition(s) would be considered routine (and, therefore, excluded from coverage). Accordingly, foot care that would otherwise be considered routine may be covered

when systemic condition(s) result in severe circulatory embarrassment or areas of diminished sensation in the individual's legs or feet. (See subsection C.)

In these instances, certain foot care procedures that otherwise are considered routine (e.g., cutting or removing corns and calluses, or trimming, cutting, clipping, or debriding nails) may pose a hazard when performed by a nonprofessional person on patients with such systemic conditions. (See §4120 for procedural instructions.)

4. Mycotic Nails.—In the absence of a systemic condition, treatment of mycotic nails may be covered.

   The treatment of mycotic nails for an ambulatory patient is covered only when the physician attending the patient's mycotic condition documents that (1) there is clinical evidence of mycosis of the toenail, and (2) the patient has marked limitation of ambulation, pain, or secondary infection resulting from the thickening and dystrophy of the infected toenail plate.

   The treatment of mycotic nails for a nonambulatory patient is covered only when the physician attending the patient's mycotic condition documents that (1) there is clinical evidence of mycosis of the toenail, and (2) the patient suffers from pain or secondary infection resulting from the thickening and dystrophy of the infected toenail plate.

   For the purpose of these requirements, documentation means any written information that is required by the carrier in order for services to be covered. Thus, the information submitted with claims must be substantiated by information found in the patient's medical record. Any information, including that contained in a form letter, used for documentation purposes is subject to carrier verification in order to ensure that the information adequately justifies coverage of the treatment of mycotic nails. (See §4120 for claims processing criteria.)

C. Systemic Conditions.—Although not intended as a comprehensive list, the following metabolic, neurologic, and peripheral vascular diseases (with synonyms in parentheses) most commonly represent the underlying conditions that might justify coverage for routine foot care.

- Diabetes mellitus
- Arteriosclerosis obliterans (A.S.O., arteriosclerosis of the extremities, occlusive peripheral arteriosclerosis)
- Buerger's disease (thromboangiitis obliterans)
- Chronic thrombophlebitis
- Peripheral neuropathies involving the feet
- Associated with malnutrition and vitamin deficiency
- Malnutrition (general, pellagra)
- Alcoholism
- Malabsorption (celiac disease, tropical sprue)
- Pernicious anemia
- Associated with carcinoma
- Associated with diabetes mellitus
- Associated with drugs and toxins
- Associated with multiple sclerosis
- Associated with uremia (chronic renal disease)
- Associated with traumatic injury

- Associated with leprosy or neurosyphilis
- Associated with hereditary disorders
- Hereditary sensory radicular neuropathy
- Angiokeratoma corporis diffusum (Fabry's)
- Amyloid neuropathy

When the patient's condition is one of those designated by an asterisk (*), routine procedures are covered only if the patient is under the active care of a doctor of medicine or osteopathy who documents the condition.

D. Supportive Devices for Feet.—Orthopedic shoes and other supportive devices for the feet generally are not covered. However, this exclusion does not apply to such a shoe if it is an integral part of a leg brace (see §2133), and its expense is included as part of the cost of the brace. Also, this exclusion does not apply to therapeutic shoes furnished to diabetics. (See §2134.)

E. Coding.—You are responsible for informing all medical specialties that codes and policies for routine foot care and supportive devices for the feet are not exclusively for the use of podiatrists. These codes must be used to report foot care services regardless of the specialty of the physician who furnishes the services. Instruct physicians to use the most appropriate code available when billing for routine foot care.

4107 DURABLE MEDICAL EQUIPMENT - BILLING AND PAYMENT CONSIDERATIONS UNDER THE FEE SCHEDULE

The Omnibus Budget Reconciliation Act of 1987 requires that payment for DME, prosthetics and orthotics be made under fee schedules effective January 1, 1989. The allowable charge is limited to the lower of the actual charge for the equipment, or the fee schedule amount. The equipment is categorized into one of six classes:

- Inexpensive or other routinely purchased DME;
- Items requiring frequent and substantial servicing;
- Customized items;
- Prosthetic and orthotic devices;
- Capped rental items; or
- Oxygen and oxygen equipment.

The fee schedule allowances for each class are determined in accord with
§§5102ff

4107.6 Written Order Prior to Delivery.--Ensure that your system will pay for the equipment listed below only when the supplier has a written order in hand prior to delivery. Otherwise, do not pay for that item even if a written order is subsequently furnished. However, you can pay for a similar item if it is subsequently provided by an unrelated supplier which has a written order in hand prior to delivery. The HCPCS codes for the equipment requiring a written order are:

B0180 B0181 B0182 B0183 B0184 B0185 B0188 B0189 B0190 B0192 B0195 B0620 B0720 B0730 B1230

EOMB Messages.--The following EOMB messages are suggested: (See §§7012ff. for other applicable messages.)

A. General.—

- "This is the maximum approved amount for this item." (Use when payment is reduced for a line item.)

B. Inexpensive/Frequently Purchased Equipment.—

- "The total approved amount for this item is____________whether this item is purchased or rented." (Use in first month.)
- "This is your next to last rental payment."
- "This is your last rental payment."
- "This item has been rented up to the Medicare payment limit."
- "The approved amount has been reduced by the previously approved rental amounts."

C. Items Requiring Frequent and Substantial Servicing.—Use the general rental messages in §4107.8A, if applicable. If the beneficiary has purchased the item prior to June 1, 1989, follow §7014.6. If the beneficiary purchase an item in this category on or after June 1, 1989, use the following message:

- "This equipment can only be paid for on a rental basis."

D. Customized Items and Other Prosthetic and Orthotic Devices.—

- "The total approved amount for this item is__________."

E. Capped Rental Items.—

- "Under a provision of Medicare law, monthly rental payments for this item can continue for up to 15 months from the first rental month or until the equipment is no longer needed, whichever comes first."
- "If you no longer are using this equipment or have recently moved and will rent this item from a different supplier, please contact our office." (Use on beneficiary's EOMB.)
- "This is your next to last rental payment."
- "This is your last rental payment."
- "This item has been rented up to the 15 month Medicare payment limit."
- "Your equipment supplier must supply and service this item for as long as you continue to need it."
- "Medicare cannot pay for maintenance and/or servicing of this item until 6 months have elapsed since the end of the 15th paid rental month."
- If the beneficiary purchased a capped rental item prior to June 1, 1989, follow §7014.6.

If the beneficiary purchased a capped rental item on or after June 1, 1989, use the following denial message:

- "This equipment can only be paid for on a rental basis."

F. Oxygen and Oxygen Equipment.—

- "The monthly allowance includes payment for all covered oxygen contents and supplies." "Payment for the amount of oxygen supplied has been reduced or denied based on the patient's medical condition." (To supplier after medical review.)
- "The approved amount has been reduced to the amount allowable for medically necessary oxygen therapy." (To beneficiary.)
- "Payment denied because the allowance for this item is included in the monthly payment amount."
- "Payment denied because Medicare oxygen coverage requirements are not met." If the beneficiary purchased an oxygen system prior to June 1, 1989, follow §7014.6. If the beneficiary purchased an oxygen system on or after June 1, 1989, use the following denial message:
- "This item can only be paid for on a rental basis."

G. Items Requiring a Written Order Prior to Delivery.—

- "Payment is denied because the supplier did not obtain a written order from your doctor prior to the delivery of this item."

Oxygen HCPCS Codes Effective 1/1/89.--

NEW	OLD	DEFINITION
Q0036 notes (1) and (8)	E1377-E1385, E1397	Oxygen concentrator, See High humidity
Q0038 See note (2)	E0400, E0405	Oxygen contents, gaseous, per unit (for use with owned gaseous stationary systems or when both a stationary and portable gaseous system are owned; 1 unit = 50 cubic ft.)
Q0039 See note (2)	E0410, E0415O	Oxygen contents, liquid, per unit, (for use with owned stationary liquid systems or when both a stationary and portable liquid system are owned; 1 unit = 10 lbs.)
Q0040 See note (2)	E0416	Portable oxygen contents, per unit (for use only with portable gaseous systems when no stationary gas system is used; 1 unit = 5 cubic ft.)
Q0041 See note (2)	None	Portable oxygen contents, liquid, per unit (for use only with portable liquid systems when no stationary liquid system is used; 1 unit = 1 lb.)

NEW	OLD	DEFINITION
Q0042	E0425	Stationary compressed See note (3)gas system rental, includes contents (per unit), regulator with flow gauge, humidifier, nebulizer, cannula or mask & tubing; 1 unit = 50 cubic ft.
E0425 See notes (4) and (8)	Same	No change
E0430 See notes (8) and (9)	Same	No change
E0435 See notes (7) and 8	Same	No change in terminology, but and (8)see note (7).
Q0043	E0440	Stationary liquid (see note (3) oxygen system rental), includes contents (per unit), use of reservoir, contents indicator, flowmeter, humidifier, nebulizer, cannula or mask and tubing; 1 unit of contents = 10 lbs.
B0440 See note (4)	Same	No change
E0455	Same	No change See note (6)
E0555 See note (6)	Same	No change
E0580	Same	No change See note (6)
E1351	Same	No change See note (6)
E1352 See note (6)	Same	No change
E1353	Same See notes (6) and (8)	No change
E1354 See note (6)	Same	No change
E1371	Same See note (6)	No change
E1374 See note (6)	Same	No change
E1400 See note (1) and (8)	E1388-E1396	Same as Q0014
E1401 See notes (1) and (8)	E1388-E1396	Same as Q0015
E1402	Same	No change
E1403	Same	No change
E1404	Same	No change
E1405	Q0037	Combine the fee See note (10)schedule amounts for the stationary oxygen system and the nebulizer with a compressor and heater (code E0585) to determine the fee schedule amount to apply to oxygen enrichers with a heater (code E1405)

NEW	OLD	DEFINITION
E1406	Q0037	Combine the fee schedule amounts for the stationary oxygen system and the nebulizer with only a compressor (i.e., without a heater, code E0570) to determine the fee schedule amount to apply to oxygen enrichers without a heater (code E1406)

4120 FOOT CARE

NOTE: See §4281 for the relationship between foot care and the coverage and billing of the diagnosis and treatment of peripheral neuropathy with loss of protective sensation (LOPS) in people with diabetes.

4120.1 Application of Foot Care Exclusions to Physicians' Services.--The exclusion of foot care is determined by the nature of the service (§2323). Thus, reimbursement for an excluded service should be denied whether performed by a podiatrist, osteopath, or a doctor of medicine, and without regard to the difficulty or complexity of the procedure.

When an itemized bill shows both covered services and noncovered services not integrally related to the covered service, the portion of charges attributable to the noncovered services should be denied. (For example, if an itemized bill shows surgery for an ingrown toenail and also removal of calluses not necessary for the performance of toe surgery, any additional charge attributable to removal of the calluses should be denied.)

In reviewing claims involving foot care, the carrier should be alert to the following exceptional situations:

1. Payment may be made for incidental noncovered services performed as a necessary and integral part of, and secondary to, a covered procedure. For example, if trimming of toenails is required for application of a cast to a fractured foot, the carrier need not allocate and deny a portion of the charge for the trimming of the nails. However, a separately itemized charge for such excluded service should be disallowed. When the primary procedure is covered the administration of anesthesia necessary for the performance of such procedure is also covered.

2. Payment may be made for initial diagnostic services performed in connection with a specific symptom or complaint if it seems likely that its treatment would be covered even though the resulting diagnosis may be one requiring only noncovered care.

4273 CLAIMS FOR PAYMENT FOR EPOETIN ALFA (EPO)

Effective June 1, 1989, the drug EPO is covered under Part B if administered incident to a physician's services. EPO is used to treat anemia associated with chronic renal failure, including patients on dialysis and those who are not on dialysis.

Completion of Initial Claim for EPO.—The following information is required. Due to space limitations, some items must be documented on a separate form. Therefore, initial claims are generally submitted on

paper unless your electronic billers are able to submit supplemental documentation with EMC claims. Return incomplete assigned claims in accordance with §3311.
Develop incomplete unassigned claims.

A. Diagnoses.—The diagnoses must be submitted according to ICD-9-CM and correlated to the procedure. This information is in Items 23A and 24D, of the Form HCFA-1500.

B. Hematocrit (HCT)/Hemoglobin (Hgb).—There are special HCPCS codes for reporting the injection of EPO. These allow the simultaneous reporting of the patient's latest HCT or Hgb reading before administration of EPO.

   Instruct the physician and/or staff to enter a separate line item for injections of EPO at different HCT/Hgb levels. The Q code for each line items is entered in Item 24C.

   1. Code Q9920 - Injection of EPO, per l,000 units, at patient HCT of 20 or less/Hgb of 6.8 or less.

   2. Codes Q9921 through Q9939 - Injection of EPO, per 1,000 units, at patient HCT of 2l to 39/Hgb of 6.9 to 13.1.

      For HCT levels of 2l or more, up to a HCT of 39/Hgb of 6.9 to 13.1, a Q code that includes the actual HCT levels is used. To convert actual Hgb to corresponding HCT values for Q code reporting, multiply the Hgb value by 3 and round to the nearest whole number. Use the whole number to determine the appropriate Q code.

      EXAMPLES: If the patient's HCT is 25/Hgb is 8.2-8.4, Q9925 must be entered on the claim. If the patient's HCT is 39/Hgb is 12.9-13.1, Q9939 is entered.

   3. Code Q9940 - Injection of EPO, per l,000 units at patient HCT of 40 or above. A single line item may include multiple doses of EPO administered while th patient's HCT level remained the same.

C. Units Administered.—The standard unit of EPO is 1,000. The number of 1,000 units administered per line item is included on the claim. The physician's office enters 1 in the units field for each multiple of 1,000 units. For example, if 12,000 units are administered, 12 is entered. This information is shown in Item 24F (Days/Units) on Form HCFA-1500.

   In some cases, the dosage for a single line item does not total an even multiple of 1,000. If this occurs, the physician's office rounds down supplemental dosages of 0 to 499 units to the prior 1,000 units. Supplemental dosages of 500 to 999 are rounded up to the next 1,000 units.

   EXAMPLES: A patient's HCT reading on August 6 was 22/Hgb was 7.3.The patient received 5,000 units of EPO on August 7, August 9 and August 11, for a total of 15,000 units. The first line of Item 24 of Form HCFA-1500 shows:

Dates of Service	Procedure Code	Days or Units
8/7-8/11	Q9922	15

   On September 13, the patient's HCT reading increased to 27/Hgb increased to 9. The patient received 5,100 units of EPO on September 13, September 15, and September 17, for a total of 15,300 units.

Since less than 15,500 units were given, the figure is rounded down to 15,000. This line on the claim form shows:

Dates of Service	Procedure Code	Days or Units
9/13-9/17	Q9927	15

On October 16, the HCT level increased to 33/Hgb increased to 11.The patient received doses of 4,850 units on October 16, October 18, and October 20 for a total of 14,550 units. Since more than 14,500 units were administered, the figure is rounded up to 15,000. Form HCFA-1500 shows:

Dates of Service	Procedure Code	Days or Units
10/16-10/20	Q9933	15

D. Date of the patient's most recent HCT or Hgb.

E. Most recent HCT or Hgb level prior to initiation of EPO therapy.

F. Date of most recent HCT or Hgb level prior to initiation of EPO therapy.

G Patient's most recent serum creatinine, within the last month, prior to initiation of EPO therapy.
H. Date of most recent serum creatinine prior to initiation of EPO therapy.

I. Patient's weight in kilograms.

J. Patient's starting dose per kilogram. (The usual starting dose is 50-100 units per kilogram.) When a claim is submitted on Form HCFA-1500, these items are submitted on a separate document. It is not necessary to enter them into your claims processing system. This information is used in utilization review.

Completion of Subsequent Claims for EPO.--Subsequent claims include the following:

A. Diagnoses.

B. Hematocrit or Hemoglobin.—This is indicated by the appropriate Q code. Claims include a EJ modifier to the Q code. This allows you to identify subsequent claims which do not require as much information as initial claims and prevent unnecessary development.

C. Number of units administered.—See §4273.1 for a description of these items. Subsequent claims may be submitted electronically. See §3023.7 for including the number of units in standard format EMC claims.

4450. PARENTERAL AND ENTERAL NUTRITION (PEN)

PEN coverage is determined by information provided by the attending physician and the PEN supplier. A certification of medical necessity (CMN) contains pertinent information needed to ensure consistent coverage and payment determinations nationally. A completed CMN must accompany and support the claims for PEN to establish whether coverage criteria are met and to ensure that the PEN provided is consistent with the attending physician's prescription.

The medical and prescription information on a PEN CMN can be completed most appropriately by the attending physician, or from information in the patient's records by an employee of the physician for the physician's review and signature. Although PEN suppliers may assist in providing PEN items they cannot complete the CMN since they do not have the same access to patient information needed to properly enter medical or prescription information.

A. Scheduling and Documenting Certifications and Recertifications of Medical Necessity for PEN.--A PEN CMN must accompany the initial claim submitted. The initial certification is valid for three months. Establish the schedule on a case-by-case basis for recertifying the need for PEN therapy. A change in prescription for a beneficiary past the initial certification period does not restart the certification process. A period of medical necessity ends when PEN is not medically required for two consecutive months. The entire certification process, if required, begins after the period of two consecutive months have elapsed.

B. Initial Certifications.--In reviewing the claim and the supporting data on the CMN, compare certain items, especially pertinent dates of treatment. For example, the start date of PEN coverage cannot precede the date of physician certification. The estimated duration of therapy must be contained on the CMN. Use this information to verify that the test of permanence is met. Once coverage is established, the estimated length of need at the start of PEN services will determine the recertification schedule. (See §4450 A.)

   Verify that the information shown on the certification supports the need for PEN supplies as billed. A diagnosis must show a functional impairment that precludes the enteral patient from swallowing and the parenteral patient from absorbing nutrients.
   The attending physician and/or his/her designated employee are in a position to accurately complete the patient's medical information including:

   - The patient's general condition, estimated duration of therapy, and other treatments or therapies (see §3329 B.2.);
   - The patient's clinical assessment relating to the need for PEN therapy (see §3329 B.3.); and
   - The nutritional support therapy (i.e., the enteral or parenteral formulation). (See §3329 B.4.)

   Initial assigned claims with the following conditions can be denied without development:

   - Inappropriate or missing diagnosis or functional impairment;
   - Estimated duration of therapy is less than 90 consecutive days;
   - Duration of therapy is not listed;
   - Supplies have not been provided;
   - Supplies were provided prior to onset date of therapy; and
   - Stamped physician's signature.

   Develop unassigned claims for missing or incomplete information. (See §3329 C.)

   Review all claims with initial certifications and recertifications before payment is authorized.

C. Revised Certifications/Change in Prescription.--Remind suppliers to submit revised certifications if the attending physician changes the PEN prescription. A revised certification is appropriate when:

- There is a change in the attending physician's orders in the category of nutrients and/or calories prescribed;
- There is a change by more than one liter in the daily volume of parenteral solutions;
- There is a change from home-mix to pre-mix or pre-mix to home-mix parenteral solutions;
- There is a change from enteral to parenteral or parenteral to enteral therapy; or
- There is a change in the method of infusion (e.g., from gravity-fed to pump-fed).

Do not adjust payments on PEN claims unless a revised or renewed certification documents the necessity for the change. Adjust payments timely, if necessary, for supplies since the PEN prescription was changed.

Do not exceed payment levels for the most current certification or recertification if a prescription change is not documented by a new recertification.

Adjust your diary for scheduled recertifications. When the revised certification has been considered, reschedule the next recertification according to the recertification schedule. (See § 4450 A.)

D. Items Requiring Special Attention.--

1. Nutrients.--Category IB of enteral nutrients contains products that are natural intact protein/protein isolates commonly known as blenderized nutrients. Additional documentation is required to justify the necessity of Category IB nutrients. The attending physician must provide sufficient information to indicate that the patient:

   - Has an intolerance to nutritionally equivalent (semi-synthetic) products;
   - Had a severe allergic reaction to a nutritionally equivalent (semi-synthetic) product; or
   - Was changed to a blenderized nutrient to alleviate adverse symptoms expected to be of permanent duration with continued use of semi-synthetic products.

   Also, enteral nutrient categories III through VI require additional medical justification for coverage.

   Parenteral nutrition may be either "self-mixed" (i.e., the patient is taught to prepare the nutrient solution aseptically) or "pre-mixed" (i.e., the nutrient solution is prepared by trained professionals employed or contracted by the PEN supplier). The attending physician must provide information to justify the reason for "pre-mixed" parenteral nutrient solutions.

2. Prospective Billing.--Pay for no more than a one-month supply of parenteral or enteral nutrients for any one prospective billing period. Claims submitted retroactively may include multiple months.

3. Pumps.--Enteral nutrition may be administered by syringe, gravity, or pump. The attending physician must specify the reason that necessitates the use of an enteral feeding pump. Ensure that the equipment for which payment is claimed is consistent with that prescribed (e.g., expect a claim for an I.V. pole, if a pump is used).

   Effective April 1, 1990, claims for parenteral and enteral pumps are limited to rental payments for a total of 15 months during a period of medical need. A period of medical need ends when enteral or parenteral nutrients are not medically necessary for two consecutive months.

Do not allow additional rental payments once the 15-month limit is reached, unless the attending physician changes the prescription between parenteral and enteral nutrients.

Do not continue rental payments after a pump is purchased unless the attending physician changes the prescription between parenteral and enteral nutrients.

Do not begin a new 15-month rental period when a patient changes suppliers. The new supplier is entitled to the balance remaining on the 15-month rental period.

Effective October 1, 1990, necessary maintenance and servicing of pumps after the 15-month rental limit is reached, includes repairs and extensive maintenance that involves the breaking down of sealed components or performing tests that require specialized testing equipment not available to the beneficiary or nursing home.

4. Supplies.--Enteral care kits contain all the necessary supplies for the enteral patient using the syringe, gravity, or pump method of nutrient administration. Parenteral nutrition care kits and their components are considered all inclusive items necessary to administer therapy during a monthly period.

   Compare the enteral feeding care kits on the claim with the method of administration indicated on the CMN.

   - Reduce the allowance to the amount paid for a gravity-fed care kit when billed for a pump feeding kit in the absence of documentation or unacceptable documentation for a pump.
   - Limit payment to a one-month supply.
   - Deny payment for additional components included as part of the PEN supply kit.

5. Attending Physician Identification.--A CMN must contain the attending physician's Unique Physician Identification Number (UPIN) and be signed and dated by the attending physician. A stamped signature is unacceptable.

   Deny certifications and recertifications altered by "whiting out" or "pasting over" and entering new data. Consider suppliers that show a pattern of altering CMNs for educational contact and/or audit.

   Be alert to certifications from suppliers who have questionable utilization or billing practices or who are under sanction. Consider an audit of any such situations.

4471 PAYMENT FOR IMMUNOSUPPRESSIVE DRUGS

Beginning January 1, 1987, Medicare pays for FDA approved immunosuppressive drugs and for drugs used in immunosuppressive therapy.(See §2050.5.)Generally, pay for self-administered immunosuppressive drugs that are specifically labeled and approved for marketing as such by the FDA, or identified in FDA-approved labeling for use in conjunction with immunosuppressive drug therapy. This benefit is subject to the Part B deductible and coinsurance provision and is limited to the 1-year period after the date of the transplant. Pay for immunosuppressive drugs which are provided outside the 1-year period if they are covered under another provision of the law (e.g., as inpatient hospital services or are furnished incident to a physician's service).

"One-year period after the date of the transplant" means 365 days from the day on which an inpatient is discharged from the hospital. From surgery until hospital discharge, payment for these drugs is included in Medicare's Part A payment to the hospital. If the same patient receives a subsequent transplant operation within 365 days, the period begins anew.

Prescriptions generally should be nonrefillable and limited to a 30 day supply. The 30 day guideline is necessary because dosage frequently diminishes over a period of time, and further, it is not uncommon for the physician to change the prescription from one drug to another. Also, these drugs are expensive and the coinsurance liability on unused drugs could be a financial burden to the beneficiary. Unless there are special circumstances, do not consider a supply of drugs in excess of 30 days to be reasonable and necessary.

Routing Claims

Route claims for immunosuppressive drugs and any supporting documentation to one of two specialty carriers. Process your part of the claim and notify the beneficiary, and if needed, the physician and supplier of the transfer. The specialty carrier to which to route the claim is based upon the drug supplier's home office.

If the supplier's home office is west of the Mississippi river or in Minnesota:

Transamerica Occidental Life Insurance Company
Medicare Immuno Drug Claims
P.O. Box 60549
Los Angeles, CA 90060-0549

If the supplier's home office is east of the Mississippi river, excluding Minnesota:

Blue Cross and Blue Shield of South Carolina Medicare Immunosuppressive Drug Unit PEN Claims
P.O. Box 102401
Columbia, SC29224

Notify all suppliers regularly of the billing address for the specialty carriers for submission of immunosuppressive drug claims.

Determination of Eligibility

Benefit eligibility is limited to the l-year period following the date of the beneficiary's discharge from a hospital or transplant center after a Medicare covered kidney, heart or liver transplant.(See §5249.)The specialty carrier consults one of three alternative sources of information to determine the date of kidney transplant:

HCFA compiles and furnishes in hardcopy or tape format to specialty carriers a monthly listing of beneficiaries who have received kidney transplants. HCFA's system is not yet equipped to handle heart and liver transplant data. The initial listing included all beneficiaries who had received a kidney transplant since January 1, 1986.It is updated monthly. The listing includes:

- HICN under which benefits are paid.
- Last name, first name, and middle initial of person receiving benefits.

- Month, day, and year of beneficiary's most recent kidney transplant (MMDDYY).
- Month, day, and year that beneficiary died (MMDDYY)
- Month, day, and year of kidney transplant failure (MMDDYY).
- Intermediaries send copies of the Part A Medicare Benefit Notice which contains the date of transplant to the specialty carriers. The specialty carriers maintain the data and release it to area carriers upon request.

If you are unable to locate the beneficiary's transplant information above, refer to the discharge date listed on the prescription form. The prescription form, or facsimile thereof, should accompany the initial claim and indicate the date of discharge. You may contact the prescribing physician for substantiation of the discharge date. If you do not have any eligibility information other than the prescription regarding the discharge date, you may pay for 1 month's supply of immunosuppressive drugs based upon the discharge date listed. If the information obtained indicates transplant failure, do not approve payment for drugs in subsequent periods.

Reasonable Charge Determinations

For purposes of establishing customary and prevailing charges, the United States is considered a single locality structure.

Since immunosuppressive drugs have not been previously covered, there is no existing charge data base for determining customary or prevailing charges. Therefore, the normal gap filling techniques in §5022 are not appropriate.

To establish reimbursement for the initial 3 month coverage period; i.e., January 1, 1987 through March 31, 1987, use available drug pricing data. Sources for pricing ingredient costs may include the Drug Topics Red Book, the American Druggist Blue Book, or manufacturers price lists. Also consider the appropriateness of an additional charge for administration.

During the initial 3 month interim coverage period, gather charge data and use it to establish customary and prevailing charges. Establish and maintain reasonable charge screens until a general revision is made to the reasonable charge screens at the beginning of the new fee screen year, i.e., January 1, 1988.Then use the charge data for the period January 1 through June 30, 1987 as the base year to calculate reasonable charges.

Adjust prevailing charges if they are grossly deficient or excessive in comparison to data from other sources.(See §5246 for determining appropriateness of charges.)For example, prevailing charges may be adjusted where they appear grossly excessive in relation to charge data from mail order pharmacies reflecting substantial discounts over published prices.

HCPCS Codes

The following HCPCS codes are assigned:

Code	Definition
Q0004	Azathioprine (e.g., Imuran) - oral, tab, 50 mg., 100s ea.
Q0005	Azathioprine (e.g., Imuran) - parenteral, vial, 100 mg., 20 ml. ea.
Q0006	Cyclosporine (e.g., Sandimmune) - oral, sol; 100 mg/ml., 50 ml., ea.
Q0007	Cyclosporine (e.g., Sandimmune) - parenteral amp, I.V, 250 mg., 5 ml., 10s ea UD

Q0008	Lymphocyte Immune Globulin, Antithymocyte Globulin (e.g., Atgam) - parenteral, amp, 50 mg./ml., 5 lea.
Q0009	Monoclonal Antibodies (eg Muromonab C D3; Orthoclone) -parenteral, amp, 5 mg./5 ml., 5 ml. ea.

5102.3 Transition to Fee Schedule-Relationship to Prior Rules.—

A. Comparability and Inherent Reasonableness Limitations.—Effective January 1, 1989, until further notice, you may no longer apply the comparable circumstances provision contained in §5026. Between January 1, 1989 and December 31, 1990, you may not apply the special limitations provision contained in §5246.

B. Purchase of Items Requiring Frequent and Substantial Servicing or Capped Rental Items.-

1. Purchase Prior to January 1, 1989.—If the beneficiary purchased an item of equipment in either of these two categories (see §5102.1.B or E) prior to January 1, 1989, pay the reasonable and necessary charges for maintenance and servicing of this equipment. In the event the item of equipment needs to be replaced on or after June 1, 1989, pay on a rental basis according to the instructions in §5102.1.B. or E.

   If the beneficiary purchased the equipment even though you determined that rental was more economical under the rent/purchase guidelines, or if the beneficiary made an approved purchase on an installment plan, make payment on an installment basis until the purchase price has been reached or medical necessity terminated. If the purchase price has not been reached by January 1, 1989, continue paying on an installment basis but at the monthly fee schedule amount until the purchase price is reached, the purchase price fee schedule calculated under prior instructions is reached, or the medical necessity ends, whichever occurs first. The limitation on total payments to 15 months rental (as described in §5102.1.E) does not apply.

2. Purchase On Or After June 1, 1989.—If a beneficiary purchased an item of equipment that requires frequent and substantial servicing on or after June 1, 1989, do not make payment. Also, do not make payment for maintenance and servicing or for replacement of items in either category that are purchased on or after June 1, 1989.

   If a beneficiary purchased an item of equipment in the capped rental category between June 1, 1989 and April 30, 1991, do not make payment. Also, do not make payment for maintenance and servicing. However, see §5102.1.E.5 or 6 for payment of purchase options after April 30, 1991 and for payment of replacement of items purchased between June 1, 1989 and April 30, 1991.

3. Purchase Between January 1, 1989 and June 1, 1989.—If a beneficiary purchased an item of equipment in either category after December 31, 1988, but before June 1, 1989, pay monthly installments equivalent to the rental fee schedule amounts until the medical necessity ends, the purchase price fee schedule calculated under prior instructions is reached, or the actual purchase charge has been reached, whichever occurs first. Pay the reasonable and necessary charges for maintenance and servicing of this equipment. In the event the item of equipment needs to be replaced on or after June 1, 1989, pay on a rental basis according to the instructions in §5102.1.B. or E. Payment may be made for purchase even if the purchase was preceded by a period of rental.

However, total payments for rental plus purchase of capped rental items may not exceed the amount that would have been paid had the equipment been continuously rented for 15 months. (Therefore, if a purchase occurs during a period of continuous use after 15 months of rentals have been paid, no payment may be made other than the reasonable and necessary charges for servicing as described in §5102.1.E.4.)

C. Purchase of Oxygen Equipment.—

1. Purchase Prior to June 1, 1989.—If the beneficiary purchased stationary or portable oxygen equipment (see §5102.1.F) prior to June 1, 1989, pay the reasonable and necessary charges for maintenance and servicing of this equipment. In the event the item of equipment needs to be replaced on or after June 1, 1989, pay on a rental basis according to the instructions in §5102.1.F. If the beneficiary purchased the equipment even though you determined that rental was more economical under the rent/purchase guidelines, or if the beneficiary made an approved purchase on an installment plan, make payment on an installment basis until the purchase price had been reached or medical necessity terminated. If the purchase price has not been reached by June 1, 1989, continue paying on an installment basis (see §5102.1.F.9) but at the monthly fee schedule amount until the purchase price is reached or the medical necessity ends, whichever occurs first.

2. Purchase On Or After June 1, 1989.—If a beneficiary purchased stationary or portable oxygen equipment on or after June 1, 1989, do not make payment for the equipment. However, make payment for the contents in accordance with §5102.1.F.4 or 5. Also, do not make payment for maintenance and servicing or for replacement of oxygen equipment that is purchased on or after June 1, 1989.

D. 15-Month Ceiling.—For purposes of computing the 10-month purchase option or the 15-month period for capped rental items, begin counting the first month that the beneficiary continuously rented the equipment. For example, if the beneficiary began renting the equipment in July 1988, the rental month which begins in January 1989 is counted as the beneficiary's 7th month of rental. Therefore, if the equipment has been continuously rented prior to October 2, 1987, no further rental payments are made since the 15-month period is terminated before January 1, 1989. The maintenance and service provision in §5102.1.E.4 begins July l, 1989.

If the beneficiary has reached (on a date of service prior to January 1989) the purchase price limitation on a rental claim, do not make any further purchase or rental payments until the useful life has elapsed according to the instructions in §5102.1.E.7. However, for capped rental items previously rented that have reached the purchase cap under the rent/purchase rules, pay claims for maintenance and servicing fees in accordance with §5102.1.E.4 effective July 1, 1989.

E. Oxygen.—Claims for oxygen contents provided after May 31, 1989, but prior to the start of the June equipment rental month, may be paid in either of the following two ways. Either continue paying the reasonable charge payment amount for contents through the end of the May monthly rental period; or pay the reasonable charge payment amount for contents through the end of May and pay the actual charge for contents up to the fee schedule allowance for oxygen contents only, as prorated for the period June 1 through the end of the May rental period. Begin paying the appropriate full fee schedule amount at the beginning of the new rental period. For example, a beneficiary's rental period began May 15, 1989. Pay on a reasonable charge basis from May 15 through June 14; or pay on a reasonable charge basis from May 15 through May 31, 1989 and pay the actual charge up to 14/31 of the oxygen contents fee (established in §5102.1.F.4) from June 1 through June 14, 1989. Pay the lesser of the full fee schedule amount or actual charge beginning June 15, 1989.

F. Purchase Options For Capped Rental Items.—

1. Electric Wheelchairs.—If the beneficiary purchases an electric wheelchair prior to May 1, 1991, pay for the wheelchair as a routinely purchased item in accordance with §5102.1.A. If the beneficiary elects to rent an electric wheelchair prior to May 1, 1991, pay the rental fee schedule amount not to exceed the purchase price in accordance with §5102.1.A. If, on May 1,1991, the purchase price has not been reached, convert the monthly fee schedule amount from routinely purchased to capped rental. As such, each month's rental before and after conversion must be counted toward the 10 month purchase option in §5102.1.E.6 and the 15 month rental cap in §5102.1.E.2.

2. All Other Capped Rental Items.—If the beneficiary purchased a capped rental item prior to May 1, 1991, do not make payment. If the beneficiary rented a capped rental item prior to May 1, 1991, pay the rental fee schedule amount not to exceed the 15 month rental cap in accordance with §5102.1.E.2.Each month's rental must be counted toward the 10 month purchase option in §5102.1.E.6 and the 15 month rental cap in §5102.1.E.2.

15030 SUPPLIES

Make a separate payment for supplies furnished in connection with a procedure only when one of the two following conditions exists:

A. HCPCS codes A4550, A4200, and A4263 are billed in conjunction with the appropriate procedure in the Medicare Physician Fee Schedule Data Base (place of service is physician's office); or

B. The supply is a pharmaceutical or radiopharmaceutical diagnostic imaging agent (including codes A4641 through A4647); pharmacologic stressing agent (code J1245); or therapeutic radionuclide (CPT code 79900). The procedures performed are:

- Diagnostic radiologic procedures (including diagnostic nuclear medicine) requiring pharmaceutical or radiopharmaceutical contrast media and/or pharmacological stressing agent,
- Other diagnostic tests requiring a pharmacological stressing agent,
- Clinical brachytherapy procedures (other than remote afterloading high intensity brachytherapy procedures (CPT codes 77781 through 77784) for which the expendable source is included in the TC RVUs), or
- Therapeutic nuclear medicine procedures.

15360 ECHOCARDIOGRAPHY SERVICES (CODES 93303 - 93350)

Separate Payment for Contrast Media.—Effective October 1, 2000, physicians may separately bill for contrast agents used in echocardiography. Physicians should use HCPCS Code A9700 (Supply of injectable contrast material for use in echocardiography, per study). The type of service code is 9. This code will be carrier-priced.

APPENDIX E: PQRS CROSS-REFERENCES

The measure specifications contained in this section are intended for claims-based and registry reporting of individual measures for the Physician Quality Reporting System (PQRS—formerly known as Physician Quality Reporting Initiative or PQRI). Each measure is assigned a unique number. This section contains only those PQRS measures that specifically include HCPCS codes.

WHAT IS PQRS?

PQRS is a quality reporting program that uses negative payment adjustments to promote reporting of quality information by individual EPs and group practices. Those who do not satisfactorily report data on quality measures for covered Medicare Physician Fee Schedule (MPFS) services furnished to Medicare Part B beneficiaries (including Railroad Retirement Board, Medicare Secondary Payer, and Critical Access Hospitals [CAH] method II) will be subject to a negative payment adjustment under PQRS. Medicare Part C–Medicare Advantage beneficiaries are not included. Reporters may choose from the following reporting mechanisms to submit their quality data:

- Reporting electronically using an electronic health record (EHR)
- Qualified Registry
- Qualified Clinical Data Registry (QCDR)
- PQRS group practice via GPRO Web Interface
- CMS-Certified Survey Vendor Claims

WHO IS ELIGIBLE TO PARTICIPATE IN PQRS?

Medicare physicians, practitioners, and therapists providing covered professional services paid under or based on the MPFS are EPs under PQRS. To the extent that EPs are providing services which get paid under or based on the MPFS, those services are eligible for PQRS negative payment adjustments. Individual EPs, EPs in group practices participating via GPRO (PQRS group practices), Accountable Care Organizations (ACOs) reporting PQRS via the GPRO Web Interface, and Comprehensive Primary Care (CPC) practice sites are eligible to participate in PQRS. View the complete list of EPs (identified on claims by their individual National Provider Identifier [NPI] and Tax Identification Number [TIN]). EPs or group practices participating via GPRO, using their individual rendering NPI or TIN, may report the quality clinical action for measures within PQRS. Most services payable under fee schedules or methodologies other than the MPFS are not included in 2015 PQRS (for example, services provided under federally qualified health center or rural health clinics methodologies, portable X-ray suppliers, independent laboratories including place-of-service code "81," hospitals, , skilled nursing facilities, ambulance providers, and ambulatory surgery center facilities). Suppliers of durable medical equipment (DME) are not eligible to report measures via PQRS since DME is not paid under the MPFS.

WHAT ARE QUALITY MEASURES?

Quality measures are indicators of the quality of care provided by physicians. They are tools that help us measure or quantify health care processes, outcomes, patient perceptions, and organizational structure and/or systems that are associated with the ability to provide high-quality health care and/or that relate to one or more quality goals for health care. These goals include: effective, safe, efficient, patient-centered, equitable, and timely care. Refer to page 7 for more information on quality measures. It is important to review and understand each measure specification especially as it pertains to a specific reporting mechanism. The measure specification specific to the reporting mechanism will provide definitions and specific instructions for satisfactorily reporting the measure.

HCPCS CODES INCLUDED IN THE PQRS MEASURES

The following list includes all HCPCS 2016 codes listed in the 2016 Physician Quality Report System (PQRS) as published by CMS (2017 PQRS has not yet been published). The list is in HCPCS code order and includes the PQRS measure numbers where the HCPCS code is referenced, modifier codes where included, age and/or age ranges, and gender. Refer to the 2016 Physician Quality Reporting System (PQRS) Measures Group Specifications Manual published by CMS for complete instructions in the use of HCPCS codes in the PQRS measures.

HCPCS	MEASURE	MODIFIER	AGE	GENDER
G0101	**128**		≥18	M, F
	130		≥18	M, F
	131		≥18	M, F
	134		≥12	M, F
	181		≥65	M, F
	317		≥18	M, F
G0105	**185**	≠ 52, 53, 73 or 74	≥18	M, F
	425	≠73, 74	≥0	M, F
G0106	**145**		≥0	M, F
G0108	**128**		≥18	M, F
	130		≥18	M, F
G0120	**145**		≥0	M, F
G0121	**320**	≠ 52, 53, 73 or 74	50-75	M, F
	343	≠ 52, 53, 73 or 75	≥50	M, F
	439		>85	M, F
	425	≠73, 74	≥0	M, F
G0122	**145**		≥0	M, F
G0177	**383**		≥18	M, F
G0202	**146**		≥0	M, F
	225		≥0	M, F
G0270	**1**		18-75	M, F
	128		≥18	M, F
	130		≥18	M, F
	181		≥65	M, F
	431		≥18	M, F
G0271	**1**		18-75	M, F
	128		≥18	M, F
	431		≥18	M, F
G0278	**145**		≥0	M, F
G0402	**1**		18-75	M, F
	24		≥50	M, F
	41		≥50	M, F
	46		18-64	M, F

HCPCS	MEASURE	MODIFIER	AGE	GENDER
	46.01		≥65	M, F
	46.02		≥18	M, F
	47		≥65	M, F
	48		≥65	F
	50		≥65	F
	65		3mo-18yrs	M, F
	66		18-Mar	M, F
	111		≥65	M, F
	112		50-74	F
	113		50-75	M, F
	116		18-64	M, F
	117		18-75	M, F
	119		18-75	M, F
	128		≥18	M, F
	130		≥18	M, F
	131		≥18	M, F
	134		≥12	M, F
	154		≥65	M, F
	155		≥65	M, F
	178		≥18	M, F
	181		≥65	M, F
	204		≥18	M, F
	205		≥13	M, F
	236		18-85	M, F
	317		≥18	M, F
	337		≥0	M, F
	370		≥18	M, F
	394		13	M, F
	411		≥18	M, F
	418		50-85	F
G0409	**383**		≥18	M, F
G0410	**383**		≥18	M, F
G0411	**383**		≥18	M, F
G0438	**1**		18-75	M, F
	46		18-64	M, F
	46.01		≥65	M, F
	46.02		≥18	M, F
	47		≥65	M, F
	110		≥6mo	M, F
	111		≥65	M, F
	112		50-74	F
	113		50-75	M, F

	116		18-64	M, F
	117		18-75	M, F
	119		18-75	M, F
	128		≥18	M, F
	130		≥18	M, F
	131		≥18	M, F
	134		≥12	M, F
	154		≥65	M, F
	155		≥65	M, F
	181		≥65	M, F
	204		≥18	M, F
	226		≥18	M, F
	236		18-85	M, F
	238		≥66	M, F
	238.01		≥66	M, F
	243		≥18	M, F
	317		≥18	M, F
	370		≥18	M, F
	387		≥0	M, F
	400		≥18	M, F
	402		20-Dec	M, F
	410		≥0	M, F
	411		≥18	M, F
	431		≥18	M, F
	438		≥21	M, F
	438.01		≥21	M, F
	438.02		40-75	M, F
G0439	**1**		18-75	M, F
	46		18-64	M, F
	46.01		≥65	M, F
	46.02		≥18	M, F
	47		≥65	M, F
	110		≥6mo	M, F
	111		≥65	M, F
	112		50-74	F
	113		50-75	M, F
	116		18-64	M, F
	117		18-75	M, F
	119		18-75	M, F
	128		≥18	M, F
	130		≥18	M, F
	131		≥18	M, F
	134		≥12	M, F
	154		≥65	M, F

HCPCS	MEASURE	MODIFIER	AGE	GENDER
	155		≥65	M, F
	181		≥65	M, F
	204		≥18	M, F
	226		≥18	M, F
	236		18-85	M, F
	238		≥66	M, F
	238.01		≥66	M, F
	243		≥18	M, F
	317		≥18	M, F
	370		≥18	M, F
	387		≥0	M, F
	400		≥18	M, F
	402		20-Dec	M, F
	410		≥0	M, F
	411		≥18	M, F
	431		≥18	M, F
	438		≥21	M, F
	438.01		≥21	M, F
	438.02		40-75	M, F
G0444	**134**		≥12	M, F
G0447	**128**		≥18	M, F
G0463	**116**		18-64	M, F
	383		≥18	M, F
G0913	**303**		≥18	M, F
G0914	**303**		≥18	M, F
G0915	**303**		≥18	M, F
G0916	**304**		≥18	M, F
G0917	**304**		≥18	M, F
G0918	**304**		≥18	M, F
G8397	**19**		≥18	M, F
G8398	**19**		≥18	M, F
G8399	**39**		65-85	F
G8400	**39**		65-85	F
G8401	**39**		65-85	F
G8404	**126**		≥18	M, F
G8405	**126**		≥18	M, F
G8410	**127**		≥18	M, F
G8415	**127**		≥18	M, F
G8416	**127**		≥18	M, F
G8417	**128**		≥18	M, F
G8418	**128**		≥18	M, F
G8419	**128**		≥18	M, F

G8420	**128**		≥18	M, F
G8421	**128**		≥18	M, F
G8422	**128**		≥18	M, F
G8427	**130**		≥18	M, F
G8428	**130**		≥18	M, F
G8430	**130**		≥18	M, F
G8431	**134**		≥12	M, F
G8432	**134**		≥12	M, F
G8433	**134**		≥12	M, F
G8442	**131**		≥18	M, F
G8450	**8**		≥18	M, F
	8.01		≥18	M, F
G8451	**8**		≥18	M, F
	8.01		≥18	M, F
G8452	**8**		≥18	M, F
	8.01		≥18	M, F
G8465	**104**		≥0	M
G8473	**118.01**		≥18	M, F
G8474	**118.01**		≥18	M, F
G8475	**118.01**		≥18	M, F
G8476	**122**		≥18	M, F
G8477	**122**		≥18	M, F
G8478	**122**		≥18	M, F
G8482	**110**		≥6mo	M, F
G8483	**110**		≥6mo	M, F
G8484	**110**		≥6mo	M, F
G8506	**119**		18-75	M, F
G8509	**131**		≥18	M, F
G8510	**134**		≥12	M, F
G8511	**134**		≥12	M, F
G8535	**181**		≥65	M, F
G8536	**181**		≥65	M, F
G8539	**182**		≥18	M, F
G8540	**182**		≥18	M, F
G8541	**182**		≥18	M, F
G8542	**182**		≥18	M, F
G8543	**182**		≥18	M, F
G8569	**164**		≥18	M, F
G8570	**164**		≥18	M, F
G8598	**204**		≥18	M, F
G8599	**204**		≥18	M, F
G8600	**187**		≥18	M, F
G8601	**187**		≥18	M, F
G8602	**187**		≥18	M, F

HCPCS	MEASURE	MODIFIER	AGE	GENDER
G8627	192		≥18	M, F
G8628	192		≥18	M, F
G8633	418		50-85	F
	418.01		50-85	F
G8634	418		50-85	F
	418.01		50-85	F
G8635	418		50-85	F
	418.01		50-85	F
G8647	217		≥18	M, F
	217.01		≥18	M, F
G8648	217		≥18	M, F
	217.01		≥18	M, F
G8649	217		≥18	M, F
	217.01		≥18	M, F
G8650	217		≥18	M, F
	217.01		≥18	M, F
G8651	218		≥18	M, F
	218.01		≥18	M, F
G8652	218		≥18	M, F
	218.01		≥18	M, F
G8653	218		≥18	M, F
	218.01		≥18	M, F
G8654	218		≥18	M, F
	218.01		≥18	M, F
G8655	219		≥18	M, F
	219.01		≥18	M, F
G8656	219		≥18	M, F
	219.01		≥18	M, F
G8657	219		≥18	M, F
	219.01		≥18	M, F
G8658	219		≥18	M, F
	219.01		≥18	M, F
G8659	220		≥18	M, F
	220.01		≥18	M, F
G8660	220		≥18	M, F
	220.01		≥18	M, F
G8661	220		≥18	M, F
	220.01		≥18	M, F
G8662	220		≥18	M, F
	220.01		≥18	M, F
G8663	221		≥18	M, F
	221.01		≥18	M, F

G8664	**221**		≥18	M, F
	221.01		≥18	M, F
G8665	**221**		≥18	M, F
	221.01		≥18	M, F
G8666	**221**		≥18	M, F
	221.01		≥18	M, F
G8667	**222**		≥18	M, F
	222.01		≥18	M, F
G8668	**222**		≥18	M, F
	222.01		≥18	M, F
G8669	**222**		≥18	M, F
	222.01		≥18	M, F
G8670	**222**		≥18	M, F
	222.01		≥18	M, F
G8671	**223**		≥18	M, F
	223.01		≥18	M, F
G8672	**223**		≥18	M, F
	223.01		≥18	M, F
G8673	**223**		≥18	M, F
	223.01		≥18	M, F
G8674	**223**		≥18	M, F
	223.01		≥18	M, F
G8694	**7**		≥18	M, F
G8696	**32**		≥18	M, F
G8697	**32**		≥18	M, F
G8698	**32**		≥18	M, F
G8708	**65**		3mo-18yrs	M, F
G8709	**65**		3mo-18yrs	M, F
G8710	**65**		3mo-18yrs	M, F
G8711	**66**		18-Mar	M, F
G8721	**100**		≥0	M, F
G8722	**100**		≥0	M, F
G8723	**100**		≥0	M, F
G8724	**100**		≥0	M, F
G8725	**121**		≥18	M, F
G8726	**121**		≥18	M, F
G8728	**121**		≥18	M, F
G8730	**131**		≥18	M, F
	131		≥18	M, F
G8731	**131**		≥18	M, F
G8732	**131**		≥18	M, F
G8733	**181**		≥65	M, F
G8734	**181**		≥65	M, F
G8735	**181**		≥65	M, F

HCPCS	MEASURE	MODIFIER	AGE	GENDER
G8749	224		≥0	M, F
	224.01		≥0	M, F
G8752	236		18-85	M, F
G8753	236		18-85	M, F
G8754	236		18-85	M, F
G8755	236		18-85	M, F
G8756	236		18-85	M, F
G8783	317		≥18	M, F
G8784	317		≥18	M, F
G8785	317		≥18	M, F
G8797	249		≥0	M, F
G8798	250		≥0	M
G8806	254		14-50	F
G8807	254		14-50	F
G8808	254		14-50	F
	254		14-50	F
G8809	255		14-50	F
G8810	255		14-50	F
G8811	255		14-50	F
G8815	257		≥18	M, F
G8816	257		≥18	M, F
G8817	257		≥18	M, F
G8818	258		≥18	M, F
G8825	258		≥18	M, F
G8826	259		≥18	M, F
G8833	259		≥18	M, F
G8834	260		≥18	M, F
G8838	260		≥18	M, F
G8856	261		≥0	M, F
G8857	261		≥0	M, F
G8858	261		≥0	M, F
G8861	271		≥18	M, F
G8868	274		≥18	M, F
G8869	275		≥18	M, F
G8872	262		≥18	M, F
G8873	262		≥18	M, F
G8874	262		≥18	M, F
G8875	263		≥18	M, F
G8876	263		≥18	M, F
G8877	263		≥18	M, F
G8878	264		≥18	M, F
G8879	264		≥18	M, F

G8880	**264**		≥18	M, F
G8882	**264**		≥18	M, F
G8883	**265**		≥0	M, F
G8884	**265**		≥0	M, F
G8885	**265**		≥0	M, F
G8923	**8**		≥18	M, F
	8.01		≥18	M, F
G8924	**52**		≥18	M, F
G8925	**52**		≥18	M, F
G8926	**52**		≥18	M, F
G8927	**72**		18-80	M, F
G8928	**72**		18-80	M, F
G8929	**72**		18-80	M, F
G8934	**118**		≥18	M, F
G8935	**118**		≥18	M, F
G8936	**118**		≥18	M, F
G8937	**118**		≥18	M, F
G8938	**128**		≥18	M, F
G8939	**131**		≥18	M, F
G8940	**134**		≥12	M, F
G8941	**181**		≥65	M, F
G8942	**182**		≥18	M, F
G8944	**224**		≥0	M, F
G8946	**263**		≥18	M, F
G8950	**317**		≥18	M, F
G8952	**317**		≥18	M, F
G8955	**327**		0-17	M, F
G8956	**327**		0-17	M, F
G8958	**327**		0-17	M, F
G8959	**325**		≥18	M, F
G8960	**325**		≥18	M, F
G8961	**322**		≥18	M, F
G8962	**322**		≥18	M, F
G8963	**323**		≥18	M, F
G8964	**323**		≥18	M, F
G8965	**324**		≥18	M, F
G8966	**324**		≥18	M, F
G8967	**326**		≥18	M, F
G8968	**326**		≥18	M, F
G8969	**326**		≥18	M, F
G8970	**326**		≥18	M, F
G8971	**326**		≥18	M, F
G8972	**326**		≥18	M, F
G8973	**328**		0-17	M, F

HCPCS	MEASURE	MODIFIER	AGE	GENDER
G8974	**328**		0-17	M, F
G8975	**328**		0-17	M, F
G8976	**328**		0-17	M, F
G8980	**217**		≥18	M, F
	217.01		≥18	M, F
	218		≥18	M, F
	218.01		≥18	M, F
	219		≥18	M, F
	219.01		≥18	M, F
	220		≥18	M, F
	220.01		≥18	M, F
	221		≥18	M, F
	221.01		≥18	M, F
	222		≥18	M, F
	222.01		≥18	M, F
	223		≥18	M, F
	223.01		≥18	M, F
G8983	**217**		≥18	M, F
	217.01		≥18	M, F
	218		≥18	M, F
	218.01		≥18	M, F
	219		≥18	M, F
	219.01		≥18	M, F
	220		≥18	M, F
	220.01		≥18	M, F
	221		≥18	M, F
	221.01		≥18	M, F
	222		≥18	M, F
	222.01		≥18	M, F
	223		≥18	M, F
	223.01		≥18	M, F
G8986	**217**		≥18	M, F
	217.01		≥18	M, F
	218		≥18	M, F
	218.01		≥18	M, F
	219		≥18	M, F
	219.01		≥18	M, F
	220		≥18	M, F
	220.01		≥18	M, F
	221		≥18	M, F
	221.01		≥18	M, F
	222		≥18	M, F

	222.01		≥18	M, F
	223		≥18	M, F
	223.01		≥18	M, F
G8989	**217**		≥18	M, F
	217.01		≥18	M, F
	218		≥18	M, F
	218.01		≥18	M, F
	219		≥18	M, F
	219.01		≥18	M, F
	220		≥18	M, F
	220.01		≥18	M, F
	221		≥18	M, F
	221.01		≥18	M, F
	222		≥18	M, F
	222.01		≥18	M, F
	223		≥18	M, F
	223.01		≥18	M, F
G8992	**217**		≥18	M, F
	217.01		≥18	M, F
	218		≥18	M, F
	218.01		≥18	M, F
	219		≥18	M, F
	219.01		≥18	M, F
	220		≥18	M, F
	220.01		≥18	M, F
	221		≥18	M, F
	221.01		≥18	M, F
	222		≥18	M, F
	222.01		≥18	M, F
	223		≥18	M, F
	223.01		≥18	M, F
G8995	**217**		≥18	M, F
	217.01		≥18	M, F
	218		≥18	M, F
	218.01		≥18	M, F
	219		≥18	M, F
	219.01		≥18	M, F
	220		≥18	M, F
	220.01		≥18	M, F
	221		≥18	M, F
	221.01		≥18	M, F
	222		≥18	M, F
	222.01		≥18	M, F
	223		≥18	M, F

HCPCS	MEASURE	MODIFIER	AGE	GENDER
	223.01		≥18	M, F
G9188	7		≥18	M, F
G9189	7		≥18	M, F
G9190	7		≥18	M, F
G9191	7		≥18	M, F
G9192	7		≥18	M, F
G9196	21		≥18	M, F
G9197	21		≥18	M, F
G9198	21		≥18	M, F
G9227	182		≥18	M, F
G9228	205		≥13	M, F
G9229	205		≥13	M, F
G9230	205		≥13	M, F
G9231	236		18-85	M, F
G9232	325		≥18	M, F
G9239	329		≥18	M, F
G9240	329		≥18	M, F
	330		≥18	M, F
G9241	329		≥18	M, F
G9250	342		≥18	M, F
G9251	342		≥18	M, F
G9254	344		≥18	M, F
G9255	344		≥18	M, F
G9256	345		≥18	M, F
G9257	345		≥18	M, F
G9258	346		≥18	M, F
G9259	345		≥18	M, F
G9260	346		≥18	M, F
G9261	346		≥18	M, F
G9262	347		≥18	M, F
G9263	347		≥18	M, F
G9264	330		≥18	M, F
G9265	330		≥18	M, F
G9266	330		≥18	M, F
G9267	348		≥65	M, F
G9268	348.1		≥65	M, F
G9269	348		≥65	M, F
G9270	348.1		≥65	M, F
G9286	331		≥18	M, F
G9287	331		≥18	M, F
G9313	332		≥18	M, F
G9314	332		≥18	M, F

G9315	332		≥18	M, F
G9316	358		≥18	M, F
G9317	358		≥18	M, F
G9348	333		≥18	M, F
G9349	333		≥18	M, F
G9350	333		≥18	M, F
G9352	334		≥18	M, F
G9353	334		≥18	M, F
G9354	334		≥18	M, F
G9355	335		≥0	M, F
G9356	335		≥0	M, F
G9357	336		≥0	M, F
G9358	336		≥0	M, F
G9359	337		≥0	M, F
G9360	337		≥0	M, F
G9361	335		≥0	M, F
G9364	332		≥18	M, F
G9365	238		≥66	M, F
G9366	238		≥66	M, F
G9367	238.01		≥66	M, F
G9368	238.01		≥66	M, F
G9380	386		≥0	M, F
G9381	386		≥0	M, F
G9382	386		≥0	M, F
G9383	387		≥0	M, F
G9384	387		≥0	M, F
G9385	387		≥0	M, F
G9386	387		≥0	M, F
G9389	388		≥18	M, F
G9390	388		≥18	M, F
G9399	390		≥18	M, F
G9400	390		≥18	M, F
G9401	390		≥18	M, F
G9402	391		≥6	M, F
G9403	391		≥6	M, F
G9404	391		≥6	M, F
G9405	391.01		≥6	M, F
G9406	391.01		≥6	M, F
G9407	391.01		≥6	M, F
G9408	392		≥18	M, F
G9409	392		≥18	M, F
G9410	393		≥0	M, F
G9411	393		≥0	M, F
G9412	393.01		≥0	M, F

HCPCS	MEASURE	MODIFIER	AGE	GENDER
G9413	**393.01**		≥0	M, F
G9414	**394**		13	M, F
G9415	**394**		13	M, F
G9416	**394**		13	M, F
G9417	**394**		13	M, F
G9418	**395**		≥18	M, F
G9419	**395**		≥18	M, F
G9420	**395**		≥18	M, F
G9421	**395**		≥18	M, F
G9422	**396**		≥18	M, F
G9423	**396**		≥18	M, F
G9424	**396**		≥18	M, F
G9425	**396**		≥18	M, F
G9428	**397**		≥18	M, F
G9429	**397**		≥18	M, F
G9430	**397**		≥18	M, F
G9431	**397**		≥18	M, F
G9432	**398**		17-May	M, F
	398.01		18-50	M, F
G9434	**398**		17-May	M, F
	398.01		18-50	M, F
G9435	**399**		≥18	M, F
G9436	**399**		≥18	M, F
G9437	**399**		≥18	M, F
G9438	**399**		≥18	M, F
G9439	**399**		≥18	M, F
G9440	**399**		≥18	M, F
G9441	**399**		≥18	M, F
G9442	**399**		≥18	M, F
G9443	**399**		≥18	M, F
G9448	**400**		≥18	M, F
G9449	**400**		≥18	M, F
G9450	**400**		≥18	M, F
G9451	**400**		≥18	M, F
G9452	**400**		≥18	M, F
G9453	**400**		≥18	M, F
G9454	**400**		≥18	M, F
G9455	**401**		≥18	M, F
G9456	**401**		≥18	M, F
G9457	**401**		≥18	M, F
G9458	**402**		20-Dec	M, F
G9459	**402**		20-Dec	M, F

G9460	**402**		20-Dec	M, F
G9467	**270**		≥18	M, F
G9469	**271**		≥18	M, F
G9472	**271**		≥18	M, F
G9497	**404**		≥18	M, F
G9498	**332**		≥18	M, F
G9503	**192**		≥18	M, F
G9504	**275**		≥18	M, F
G9505	**331**		≥18	M, F
G9506	**337**		≥0	M, F
G9509	**370**		≥18	M, F
G9510	**370**		≥18	M, F
G9511	**370**		≥18	M, F
G9512	**383**		≥18	M, F
G9513	**383**		≥18	M, F
G9514	**384**		≥18	M, F
G9515	**384**		≥18	M, F
G9516	**385**		≥18	M, F
G9517	**385**		≥18	M, F
G9519	**389**		≥18	M, F
G9520	**389**		≥18	M, F
G9521	**398**		17-May	M, F
	398.01		18-50	M, F
G9522	**398**		17-May	M, F
	398.01		18-50	M, F
G9523	**403**		≥18	M, F
G9524	**403**		≥18	M, F
G9525	**403**		≥18	M, F
G9526	**403**		≥18	M, F
G9529	**415**		≥18	M, F
G9530	**415**		≥18	M, F
G9531	**415**		≥18	M, F
G9532	**415**		≥18	M, F
G9533	**415**		≥18	M, F
G9534	**419**		≥0	M, F
G9535	**419**		≥0	M, F
G9536	**419**		≥0	M, F
G9537	**419**		≥0	M, F
G9538	**419**		≥0	M, F
G9539	**421**		≥0	M, F
G9540	**421**		≥0	M, F
G9541	**421**		≥0	M, F
G9542	**421**		≥0	M, F
G9543	**421**		≥0	M, F

HCPCS	MEASURE	MODIFIER	AGE	GENDER
G9544	421		≥0	M, F
G9547	405		≥18	M, F
G9548	405		≥18	M, F
G9549	405		≥18	M, F
G9550	405		≥18	M, F
G9551	405		≥18	M, F
G9552	406		≥18	M, F
G9554	406		≥18	M, F
G9555	406		≥18	M, F
G9556	406		≥18	M, F
G9557	406		≥18	M, F
G9558	407		≥18	M, F
G9559	407		≥18	M, F
G9560	407		≥18	M, F
G9561	408		≥18	M, F
G9562	408		≥18	M, F
G9563	408		≥18	M, F
G9572	411		≥18	M, F
G9573	411		≥18	M, F
G9574	411		≥18	M, F
G9577	412		≥18	M, F
G9578	412		≥18	M, F
G9579	412		≥18	M, F
G9580	413		≥0	M, F
G9581	413		≥0	M, F
G9582	413		≥0	M, F
G9583	414		≥18	M, F
G9584	414		≥18	M, F
G9585	414		≥18	M, F
G9593	416		17-Feb	M, F
G9594	416		17-Feb	M, F
G9595	416		17-Feb	M, F
G9596	416		17-Feb	M, F
G9597	416		17-Feb	M, F
G9600	417		≥18	M, F
G9601	417		≥18	M, F
G9602	417		≥18	M, F
G9603	420		≥0	M, F
G9604	420		≥0	M, F
G9605	420		≥0	M, F
G9606	422		≥0	M, F
G9607	422		≥0	M, F

G9608	**422**		≥0	M, F
G9609	**423**		≥18	M, F
G9610	**423**		≥18	M, F
G9611	**423**		≥18	M, F
G9612	**425**		≥0	M, F
G9613	**425**		≥0	M, F
G9614	**425**		≥0	M, F
G9615	**428**		≥0	M, F
G9616	**428**		≥0	M, F
G9617	**428**		≥0	M, F
G9618	**429**		≥0	M, F
G9619	**429**		≥0	M, F
G9620	**429**		≥0	M, F
G9621	**431**		≥18	M, F
G9622	**431**		≥18	M, F
G9623	**431**		≥18	M, F
G9624	**431**		≥18	M, F
G9625	**432**		≥0	M, F
G9626	**432**		≥0	M, F
G9627	**432**		≥0	M, F
G9628	**433**		≥0	M, F
G9629	**433**		≥0	M, F
G9630	**433**		≥0	M, F
G9631	**434**		≥0	M, F
G9632	**434**		≥0	M, F
G9633	**434**		≥0	M, F
G9634	**435**		≥0	M, F
G9635	**435**		≥0	M, F
G9636	**435**		≥0	M, F
G9637	**436**		≥18	M, F
G9638	**436**		≥18	M, F
G9639	**437**		≥0	M, F
G9640	**437**		≥0	M, F
G9641	**437**		≥0	M, F
G9642	**404**		≥18	M, F
G9643	**404**		≥18	M, F
G9644	**404**		≥18	M, F
G9645	**404**		≥18	M, F
G9646	**409**		≥0	M, F
G9647	**409**		≥0	M, F
G9648	**409**		≥0	M, F
G9649	**410**		≥18	M, F
G9650	**410**		≥18	M, F
G9651	**410**		≥18	M, F

HCPCS	MEASURE	MODIFIER	AGE	GENDER
G9652	410		≥18	M, F
G9653	410		≥18	M, F
G9654	424		≥0	M, F
G9655	426		≥0	M, F
G9656	426		≥0	M, F
G9657	426		≥0	M, F
G9658	426		≥0	M, F
G9659	439		>85	M, F
G9660	439		>85	M, F
G9661	439		>85	M, F
G9662	438		≥21	M, F
G9663	438.01		≥21	M, F
G9664	438		≥21	M, F
	438.01		≥21	M, F
	438.02		40-75	M, F
G9665	438		≥21	M, F
	438.01		≥21	M, F
	438.02		40-75	M, F
G9667	438		≥21	M, F
	438.01		≥21	M, F
	438.02		40-75	M, F

APPENDIX F: HCPCS CROSS-REFERENCE TO NDC

HCPCS	HCPCS DESCRIPTION	NDC LABEL
A4216	Sterile water, saline and/or dextrose, diluent/flush, 10 ml	Monoject prefill advanced
		Normal saline flush
		Saline solution
		Sodium chloride
		Sodium chloride (LifeCare)
		Sodium chloride (Luer lock)
		Sodium chloride/respiratory therapy
		Sterile water bacteriostatic
		Syrex
		Vasceze sodium chloride (Luer slip nozzle)
		Water for injection
		Water for injection bacteriostatic
A4217	Sterile water/saline, 500 ml	Curity sterile saline
		Sodium chloride
		Water for injection
		Water for irrigation
A4218	Sterile saline or water, metered dose dispenser, 10 ml	Sodium chloride
G9017	Amantadine hydrochloride, oral, per 100 mg (for use in a Medicare approved demonstration project)	Amantadine HCL
J0129	Injection, abatacept, 10 mg	Orencia clickject
J0130	Injection, abciximab, 10 mg	ReoPro
J0132	Injection, acetylcysteine, 100 mg	Acetylcysteine
J0133	Injection, acyclovir, 5 mg	Acyclovir
		Acyclovir sodium
J0135	Injection, adalimumab, 20 mg	Humira
J0153	Injection, adenosine, 1 mg (not to be used to report any adenosine phosphate compounds)	Adenocard
		Adenosine
J0171	Injection, adrenalin, epinephrine, 0.1 mg	Epinephrine
J0178	Injection, aflibercept, 1 mg	Eylea
J0180	Injection, agalsidase beta, 1 mg	Fabrazyme
J0207	Injection, amifostine, 500 mg	Amifostine
J0210	Injection, methyldopate HCl, up to 250 mg	Methyldopate HCL

HCPCS	HCPCS DESCRIPTION	NDC LABEL
J0256	Injection, alpha 1 proteinase inhibitor (human), not otherwise specified, 10 mg	Aralast Np
		Prolastin-c
J0257	Injection, alpha 1 proteinase inhibitor (human), (glassia), 10 mg	Glassia
J0270	Injection, alprostadil, 1.25 mcg (code may be used for Medicare when drug administered under the direct supervision of a physician, not for use when drug is self administered)	Alprostadil
		Caverject
		Prostaglandin e1
		Prostin vr pediatric
J0278	Injection, amikacin sulfate, 100 mg	Amikacin sulfate
J0280	Injection, Aminophyllin, up to 250 mg	Aminophylline
J0282	Injection, amiodarone hydrochloride, 30 mg	Amiodarone
J0285	Injection, amphotericin b, 50 mg	Amphotericin b
J0287	Injection, amphotericin b lipid complex, 10 mg	Abelcet
J0289	Injection, amphotericin b liposome, 10 mg	AmBisome
J0290	Injection, ampicillin sodium, 500 mg	Ampicillin
		Ampicillin sodium
		Novaplus ampicillin
		Premierpro rx ampicillin
J0295	Injection, ampicillin sodium/ sulbactam sodium, per 1.5 gm	Amerinet choice ampicillin and sulbactam
		Ampicillin and sulbactam
		Ampicillin-sulbactam
		Novaplus ampicillin and sulbactam
		Unasyn
J0330	Injection, succinylcholine chloride, up to 20 mg	Amerinet choice succinylcholine chloride
		Anectine
		Quelicin
J0360	Injection, hydralazine HCl, up to 20 mg	Hydralazine HCL
		Novaplus hydralazine HCL
J0364	Injection, apomorphine hydrochloride, 1 mg	Apomorphine HCL
J0456	Injection, azithromycin, 500 mg	Azithromycin
		Azithromycin dihydrate

HCPCS	HCPCS DESCRIPTION	NDC LABEL
		Novaplus azithromycin
		Zithromax
J0475	Injection, baclofen, 10 mg	Baclofen
		Lioresal intrathecal refill kit
J0476	Injection, baclofen, 50 mcg for intrathecal trial	Lioresal intrathecal screening kit
J0480	Injection, basiliximab, 20 mg	Simulect
J0500	Injection, dicyclomine HCl, up to 20 mg	Bentyl
		Dicyclocot
		Dicyclomine
J0515	Injection, benztropine mesylate, per 1 mg	Benztropine mesylate
		Cogentin
J0520	Injection, bethanechol chloride, Myotonachol or urecholine, up to 5 mg	Bethanechol chloride
J0561	Injection, penicillin g benzathine, 100,000 units	Bicillin l-a
J0583	Injection, bivalirudin, 1 mg	Angiomax
		Bivalirudin
J0585	Injection, onabotulinumtoxinA, 1 unit	Botox
J0587	Injection, rimabotulinumtoxinB, 100 units	Myobloc
J0588	Injection, incobotulinumtoxin a, 1 unit	Xeomin
J0592	Injection, buprenorphine hydrochloride, 0.1 mg	Buprenex
		Buprenorphine HCL
J0595	Injection, butorphanol tartrate, 1 mg	Butorphanol tartrate
		Novaplus butorphanol tartrate
J0600	Injection, edetate calcium disodium, up to 1000 mg	Edetate calcium disodium
J0610	Injection, calcium gluconate, per 10 ml	Calcium gluconate
J0630	Injection, calcitonin salmon, up to 400 units	Miacalcin
J0636	Injection, calcitriol, 0.1 mcg	Calcitriol
		Calcitriol in almond oil
J0637	Injection, caspofungin acetate, 5 mg	Cancidas
J0640	Injection, leucovorin calcium, per 50 mg	Leucovorin calcium
J0641	Injection, levoleucovorin calcium, 0.5 mg	Levoleucovorin calcium
J0670	Injection, mepivacaine hydrochloride,	Carbocaine

HCPCS	HCPCS DESCRIPTION	NDC LABEL
	per 10 ml	
		Mepivacaine HCL
		Polocaine-mpf
J0690	Injection, cefazolin sodium, 500 mg	Cefazolin
		Novaplus cefazolin
J0692	Injection, cefepime hydrochloride, 500 mg	Cefepime
		Cefepime HCL
J0694	Injection, cefoxitin sodium, 1 gm	Cefoxitin
		Novaplus cefoxitin
J0696	Injection, ceftriaxone sodium, per 250 mg	Ceftriaxone
J0697	Injection, sterile cefuroxime sodium, per 750 mg	Cefuroxime sodium
J0698	Injection, cefotaxime sodium, per gm	Amerinet Claforan
		Cefotaxime
		Claforan
		Novaplus Claforan
J0702	Injection, betamethasone acetate 3mg and betamethasone sodium phosphate 3mg	Celestone sol USP an
J0706	Injection, caffeine citrate, 5mg	Cafcit
		Caffeine citrate
J0713	Injection, ceftazidime, per 500 mg	Ceftazidime
		Novaplus Tazicef
		Tazicef
J0720	Injection, chloramphenicol sodium succinate, up to 1 gm	Chloramphenicol sodium succinate
J0725	Injection, chorionic gonadotropin, per 1,000 USP units	Chorionic gonadotropin
		Novarel
		Pregnyl
J0735	Injection, clonidine hydrochloride, 1 mg	Clonidine HCL
		Duraclon
J0740	Injection, cidofovir, 375 mg	Vistide
J0743	Injection, cilastatin sodium; imipenem, per 250 mg	Primaxin iv
J0744	Injection, ciprofloxacin for intravenous infusion, 200 mg	Amerinet choice ciprofloxacin
		Ciprofloxacin
J0745	Injection, codeine phosphate, per 30 mg	Codeine phosphate
J0760	Injection, colchicine, per 1mg	Colchicine

HCPCS	HCPCS DESCRIPTION	NDC LABEL
J0770	Injection, colistimethate sodium, up to 150 mg	Colistimethate
J0780	Injection, prochlorperazine, up to 10 mg	Prochlorperazine edisylate
J0795	Injection, corticorelin ovine triflutate, 1 microgram	Acthrel
J0878	Injection, daptomycin, 1 mg	Cubicin
J0881	Injection, darbepoetin alfa, 1 microgram (non-ESRD use)	Aranesp
J0885	Injection, epoetin alfa, (for non-ESRD use), 1000 units	Epogen
		Procrit
J0894	Injection, decitabine, 1 mg	Dacogen
		Decitabine
J0895	Injection, deferoxamine mesylate, 500 mg	Deferoxamine mesylate
		Desferal
J0897	Injection, denosumab, 1 mg	Prolia
		Xgeva
J0945	Injection, brompheniramine maleate, per 10 mg	Brompheniramine maleate
J1000	Injection, depo-estradiol cypionate, up to 5 mg	Depo-estradiol
		Estradiol cypionate
J1030	Injection, methylprednisolone acetate, 40 mg	Depo-Medrol
		Methylprednisolone
		Methylprednisolone acetate
		Methylprednisolone acetate micronized
J1040	Injection, methylprednisolone acetate, 80 mg	Methylprednisolone acetate
J1050	Injection, medroxyprogesterone acetate, 1 mg	Depo-Provera contraceptive
		Medroxyprogesterone acetate
J1071	Injection, testosterone cypionate, 1 mg	Depo-testosterone
		Testosterone cypionate
J1094	Injection, dexamethasone acetate, 1 mg	Dexamethasone acetate
		Dexasone l.a.
J1100	Injection, dexamethasone sodium phosphate, 1 mg	Dexamethasone sodium phosphate
J1110	Injection, dihydroergotamine mesylate, per 1 mg	DHE.
		Dihydroergotamine mesylate

HCPCS	HCPCS DESCRIPTION	NDC LABEL
J1160	Injection, digoxin, up to 0.5 mg	Digoxin
J1165	Injection, phenytoin sodium, per 50 mg	Phenytoin sodium
J1170	Injection, hydromorphone, up to 4 mg	Hydromorphone HCL
J1180	Injection, dyphylline, up to 500 mg	Dyphylline
J1200	Injection, diphenhydramine HCl, up to 50 mg	Banaril
		Diphenhydramine HCL
		Diphenhydramine HCL (Luer lock, Carpuject)
J1205	Injection, chlorothiazide sodium, per 500 mg	Chlorothiazide sodium
J1212	Injection, DMSO, dimethyl sulfoxide, 50%, 50 ml	Dimethyl sulfoxide
		Rimso-50
J1230	Injection, methadone HCl, up to 10 mg	Methadone HCL
J1240	Injection, dimenhydrinate, up to 50 mg	Dimenhydrinate
J1245	Injection, dipyridamole, per 10 mg	Dipyridamole
J1250	Injection, dobutamine hydrochloride, per 250 mg	Dextrose/dobutamine
		Dobutamine
J1260	Injection, dolasetron mesylate, 10 mg	Anzemet
J1265	Injection, dopamine HCl, 40 mg	Dextrose/dopamine HCL
		Dopamine HCL
J1270	Injection, doxercalciferol, 1 mcg	Doxercalciferol
		Hectorol
J1300	Injection, eculizumab, 10 mg	Soliris
J1320	Injection, amitriptyline HCl, up to 20 mg	Amitriptyline HCL
J1324	Injection, enfuvirtide, 1 mg	Fuzeon
J1325	Injection, epoprostenol, 0.5 mg	Epoprostenol
		Flolan
		Veletri
J1327	Injection, eptifibatide, 5 mg	Eptifibatide
		Integrilin
J1335	Injection, ertapenem sodium, 500 mg	Invanz
J1364	Injection, erythromycin lactobionate, per 500 mg	Erythrocin lactobionate
J1380	Injection, estradiol valerate, up to 10 mg	Delestrogen
		Estradiol valerate
J1410	Injection, estrogen conjugated, per 25 mg	Premarin intravenous

HCPCS	HCPCS DESCRIPTION	NDC LABEL
J1430	Injection, ethanolamine oleate, 100 mg	Ethamolin
J1435	Injection, estrone, per 1 mg	Estrone
J1438	Injection, etanercept, 25 mg (code may be used for Medicare when drug administered under the direct supervision of a physician, not for use when drug is self administered)	Enbrel
J1442	Injection, filgrastim (g-csf), excludes biosimilars, 1 microgram	Neupogen
J1450	Injection fluconazole, 200 mg	Amerinet choice fluconazole
		Fluconazole
J1451	Injection, fomepizole, 15 mg	Fomepizole
J1455	Injection, foscarnet sodium, per 1000 mg	Foscarnet sodium
J1458	Injection, galsulfase, 1 mg	Naglazyme
J1459	Injection, immune globulin (Privigen), intravenous, non-lyophilized (e.g. liquid), 500 mg	Privigen
J1460	Injection, gamma globulin, intramuscular, 1 cc	GamaSTAN
J1556	Injection, immune globulin (Bivigam), 500 mg	Bivigam
J1557	Injection, immune globulin (Gammaplex), intravenous, non-lyophilized (e.g., liquid) 500 mg	Gammaplex
J1559	Injection, immune globulin (Hizentra), 100 mg	Hizentra
J1561	Injection, immune globulin, (Gamunex/Gamunex-c/gammaked), non-lyophilized (e.g. liquid), 500 mg	Gammaked
		Gamunex-c
J1566	Injection, immune globulin, intravenous, lyophilized (e.g. powder), not otherwise specified, 500 mg	Carimune nf
		Gammagard
		Polygam
J1568	Injection, immune globulin, (Octagam), intravenous, non-lyophilized (e.g. liquid), 500 mg	Octagam
J1569	Injection, immune globulin, (Gammagard liquid), non-lyophilized,(e.g. liquid), 500 mg	Gammagard liquid
J1570	Injection, ganciclovir sodium, 500 mg	Cytovene iv

HCPCS	HCPCS DESCRIPTION	NDC LABEL
J1572	Injection, immune globulin, (Flebogamma/Flebogamma dif), intravenous, non-lyophilized (e.g. liquid), 500 mg	Flebogamma
J1573	Injection, hepatitis b immune globulin (HepaGam b), intravenous, 0.5 ml	HepaGam b
		Novaplus HepaGam b
J1575	Injection, immune globulin/hyaluronidase, (hyqvia), 100 mg immune globulin	Hyqvia
J1580	Injection, Garamycin, gentamicin, up to 80 mg	Gentamicin sulfate
J1595	Injection, glatiramer acetate, 20 mg	Copaxone
J1600	Injection, gold sodium thiomalate, up to 50 mg	Gold sodium thiomalate
J1610	Injection, glucagon hydrochloride, per 1 mg	GlucaGen
J1626	Injection, granisetron hydrochloride, 100 mcg	Granisetron HCL
J1630	Injection, haloperidol, up to 5 mg	Haloperidol
		Haloperidol lactate
J1631	Injection, haloperidol decanoate, per 50 mg	Haloperidol Amerinet choice
		Haloperidol decanoate
		Novaplus haloperidol decanoate
J1642	Injection, heparin sodium, (heparin lock flush), per 10 units	Heparin lock flush
		Hepflush-10
		Monoject prefill heparin lock flush
		Vasceze heparin lock flush (Luer slip nozzle)
J1644	Injection, heparin sodium, per 1000 units	Dextrose/heparin sodium
		Heparin sodium
J1645	Injection, dalteparin sodium, per 2500 iu	Fragmin
J1650	Injection, enoxaparin sodium, 10 mg	Enoxaparin sodium
		Lovenox
J1652	Injection, fondaparinux sodium, 0.5 mg	Arixtra
		Fondaparinux sodium
J1670	Injection, tetanus immune globulin, human, up to 250 units	Hypertet
J1700	Injection, hydrocortisone acetate, up to 25 mg	Hydrocortisone acetate

HCPCS	HCPCS DESCRIPTION	NDC LABEL
J1720	Injection, hydrocortisone sodium succinate, up to 100 mg	A-hydroCort
		Solu-Cortef
J1725	Injection, hydroxyprogesterone caproate, 1 mg	Hydroxyprogesterone caproate
		Makena
J1730	Injection, diazoxide, up to 300 mg	Diazoxide
J1740	Injection, ibandronate sodium, 1 mg	Ibandronate sodium
J1742	Injection, ibutilide fumarate, 1 mg	Corvert
J1743	Injection, idursulfase, 1 mg	Elaprase
J1745	Injection infliximab, 10 mg	Remicade
J1750	Injection, iron dextran, 50 mg	INFeD
J1756	Injection, iron sucrose, 1 mg	Venofer
J1790	Injection, droperidol, up to 5 mg	Droperidol
J1800	Injection, propranolol HCl, up to 1 mg	Propranolol
J1815	Injection, insulin, per 5 units	Humalog
		Humulin
		Lantus
		Novolin
		NovoLog (PenFill cartridge)
J1817	Insulin for administration through DME (i.e., insulin pump) per 50 units	Apidra
		Humalog
		Humulin r u-500
		Insulin-Humalog
		NovoLog
J1826	Injection, interferon beta-1a, 30 mcg	Avonex
J1830	Injection interferon beta-1b, 0.25 mg (code may be used for Medicare when drug administered under the direct supervision of a physician, not for use when drug is self administered)	Betaseron
J1835	Injection, itraconazole, 50 mg	Itraconazole
J1885	Injection, ketorolac tromethamine, per 15 mg	Ketorolac tromethamine
J1930	Injection, lanreotide, 1 mg	Somatuline depot
J1931	Injection, laronidase, 0.1 mg	Aldurazyme
J1940	Injection, furosemide, up to 20 mg	Furosemide
		Premierpro rx furosemide
J1950	Injection, leuprolide acetate (for depot suspension), per 3.75 mg	Lupron depot
J1953	Injection, levetiracetam, 10 mg	Levetiracetam
J1955	Injection, levocarnitine, per 1 gm	Carnitor

HCPCS	HCPCS DESCRIPTION	NDC LABEL
		L-carnitine free base
		L-carnitine HCL
		Levocarnitine
J1956	Injection, levofloxacin, 250 mg	Levofloxacin
J1960	Injection, levorphanol tartrate, up to 2 mg	Levorphanol tartrate
J1980	Injection, hyoscyamine sulfate, up to 0.25 mg	Hyoscyamine sulfate
J2001	Injection, lidocaine HCl for intravenous infusion, 10 mg	Dextrose/lidocaine HCL
		Lidocaine
		Xylocaine
J2010	Injection, lincomycin HCl, up to 300 mg	Lincocin
		Lincomycin HCL
J2020	Injection, linezolid, 200mg	Linezolid
		Zyvox
J2060	Injection, lorazepam, 2 mg	Ativan
		Lorazepam
J2150	Injection, mannitol, 25% in 50 ml	Mannitol
J2170	Injection, mecasermin, 1 mg	Increlex
J2175	Injection, meperidine hydrochloride, per 100 mg	Demerol
		Meperidine HCL
J2185	Injection, meropenem, 100 mg	Meropenem
		Merrem iv
J2248	Injection, micafungin sodium, 1 mg	Mycamine
J2250	Injection, midazolam hydrochloride, per 1 mg	Midazolam
		Novaplus midazolam HCL
J2260	Injection, milrinone lactate, 5 mg	Dextrose/milrinone lactate
		Milrinone lactate
J2270	Injection, morphine sulfate, up to 10 mg	Dextrose/morphine sulfate
		Morphine sulfate
J2274	Injection, morphine sulfate, preservative-free for epidural or intrathecal use, 10mg	Duramorph
		Infumorph
		Morphine sulfate
J2278	Injection, ziconotide, 1 microgram	Prialt
J2280	Injection, moxifloxacin, 100 mg	Avelox i.v.
		Moxifloxacin HCL

HCPCS	HCPCS DESCRIPTION	NDC LABEL
J2300	Injection, nalbuphine hydrochloride, per 10 mg	Nalbuphine HCL
J2310	Injection, naloxone hydrochloride, per 1 mg	Naloxone HCL
J2325	Injection, nesiritide, 0.1 mg	Natrecor
J2353	Injection, octreotide, depot form for intramuscular injection, 1 mg	Sandostatin lar depot
J2354	Injection, octreotide, non-depot form for subcutaneous or intravenous injection, 25 mcg	Octreotide acetate
		Sandostatin
J2357	Injection, omalizumab, 5 mg	Xolair
J2360	Injection, orphenadrine citrate, up to 60 mg	Antiflex
		Orphenadrine citrate
J2370	Injection, phenylephrine HCl, up to 1 ml	Neo-synephrine HCL
		Phenylephrine HCL
J2405	Injection, ondansetron hydrochloride, per 1 mg	Amerinet choice ondansetron
		Ondansetron
		Ondansetron HCL
		Zofran
J2410	Injection, oxymorphone HCl, up to 1 mg	Opana
J2430	Injection, pamidronate disodium, per 30 mg	Pamidronate disodium
J2440	Injection, papaverine HCl, up to 60 mg	Papaverine HCL
J2460	Injection, oxytetracycline HCl, up to 50 mg	Oxytetracycline HCL
J2501	Injection, paricalcitol, 1 mcg	Paricalcitol
		Zemplar
J2502	Injection, Pasireotide long acting, 1 mg	Signifor lar
J2504	Injection, pegademase bovine, 25 iu	Adagen
J2505	Injection, pegfilgrastim, 6 mg	Neulasta
J2510	Injection, penicillin g procaine, aqueous, up to 600,000 units	Penicillin g procaine
J2515	Injection, pentobarbital sodium, per 50 mg	Pentobarbital sodium
J2540	Injection, penicillin g potassium, up to 600,000 units	Penicillin g potassium
		Pfizerpen

HCPCS	HCPCS DESCRIPTION	NDC LABEL
J2543	Injection, piperacillin sodium/ tazobactam sodium, 1 gram/0.125 grams (1.125 grams)	Piperacillin and tazobactam
		Zosyn
J2545	Pentamidine isethionate, inhalation solution, compounded product, administered through DME, unit dose form, per 300 mg	NebuPent
J2550	Injection, promethazine HCl, up to 50 mg	Phenergan
		Promethazine HCL
		Promethazine HCL (Luer lock, Carpuject)
J2560	Injection, phenobarbital sodium, up to 120 mg	Phenobarbital sodium
J2590	Injection, oxytocin, up to 10 units	Novaplus oxytocin
		Oxytocin
		Oxytocin-sodium chloride
		Pitocin
J2597	Injection, desmopressin acetate, per 1 mcg	DDAVP
		Desmopressin acetate
J2650	Injection, prednisolone acetate, up to 1 ml	Prednisolone acetate micronized
J2675	Injection, progesterone, per 50 mg	Progesterone
		Progesterone in sesame oil
		Progesterone micronized
J2680	Injection, fluphenazine decanoate, up to 25 mg	Fluphenazine decanoate
J2690	Injection, procainamide HCl, up to 1 gm	Procainamide HCL
J2700	Injection, oxacillin sodium, up to 250 mg	Novaplus oxacillin
		Oxacillin
J2710	Injection, neostigmine methylsulfate, up to 0.5 mg	Neostigmine methylsulfate
J2720	Injection, protamine sulfate, per 10 mg	Novaplus protamine sulfate
		Protamine sulfate
J2724	Injection, protein c concentrate, intravenous, human, 10 iu	Ceprotin
J2725	Injection, protirelin, per 250 mcg	Protirelin
J2730	Injection, pralidoxime chloride, up to 1 gm	Pralidoxime chloride
		Protopam chloride
J2760	Injection, phentolamine mesylate, up to 5 mg	Phentolamine mesylate

HCPCS	HCPCS DESCRIPTION	NDC LABEL
J2765	Injection, metoclopramide HCl, up to 10 mg	Metoclopramide HCL
J2770	Injection, quinupristin/dalfopristin, 500 mg (150/350)	Synercid
J2778	Injection, ranibizumab, 0.1 mg	Lucentis
J2780	Injection, ranitidine hydrochloride, 25 mg	Ranitidine HCL
		Zantac
J2783	Injection, rasburicase, 0.5 mg	Elitek
J2788	Injection, rho d immune globulin, human, minidose, 50 micrograms (250 i.u.)	HyperRHO
		MICRhoGAM ultra-filtered plus
J2790	Injection, rho d immune globulin, human, full dose, 300 micrograms (1500 i.u.)	HyperRHO
		RhoGAM ultra-filtered plus
J2791	Injection, rho(d) immune globulin (human), (Rhophylac), intramuscular or intravenous, 100 iu	Rhophylac
J2792	Injection, rho d immune globulin, intravenous, human, solvent detergent, 100 iu	HyperRHO
		WinRho sdf
J2794	Injection, risperidone, long acting, 0.5 mg	Risperdal consta
J2795	Injection, ropivacaine hydrochloride, 1 mg	Naropin
		Ropivacaine HCL
J2796	Injection, romiplostim, 10 micrograms	Nplate
J2800	Injection, methocarbamol, up to 10 ml	Methocarbamol
		Robaxin
J2805	Injection, sincalide, 5 micrograms	Kinevac
J2810	Injection, theophylline, per 40 mg	Dextrose/theophylline
		Theophylline
J2916	Injection, sodium ferric gluconate complex in sucrose injection, 12.5 mg	Sodium ferric gluconate complex in sucrose
J2920	Injection, methylprednisolone sodium succinate, up to 40 mg	A-methaPred
		Methylprednisolone sodium succinate
J2930	Injection, methylprednisolone sodium succinate, up to 125 mg	A-methaPred
		Methylprednisolone sodium succinate
		Solu-Medrol
J2941	Injection, somatropin, 1 mg	Genotropin

HCPCS	HCPCS DESCRIPTION	NDC LABEL
		Humatrope
		Norditropin flexpro (prefilled purple pen)
		Nutropin aq pen cartridge
		Omnitrope
		Saizen
		Serostim
		Zomacton
		Zorbtive
J2997	Injection, alteplase recombinant, 1 mg	Activase
		Cathflo Activase
J3000	Injection, streptomycin, up to 1 gm	Streptomycin sulfate
J3010	Injection, fentanyl citrate, 0.1 mg	Fentanyl citrate
J3030	Injection, sumatriptan succinate, 6 mg (code may be used for Medicare when drug administered under the direct supervision of a physician, not for use when drug is self administered)	Imitrex
		Sumatriptan succinate
		Sumavel DosePro
		Zembrace symtouch
J3070	Injection, pentazocine, 30 mg	Talwin lactate
J3095	Injection, telavancin, 10 mg	Vibativ
J3105	Injection, terbutaline sulfate, up to 1 mg	Terbutaline sulfate
J3121	Injection, testosterone enanthate,1 mg	Delatestryl
		Testosterone enanthate
J3230	Injection, chlorpromazine HCl, up to 50 mg	Chlorpromazine HCL
J3240	Injection, thyrotropin alpha, 0.9 mg, provided in 1.1 mg vial	Thyrogen
J3243	Injection, tigecycline, 1 mg	Tygacil
J3246	Injection, tirofiban HCl, 0.25mg	Aggrastat
J3250	Injection, trimethobenzamide HCl, up to 200 mg	Benzacot
		Tigan
		Trimethobenzamide HCL
J3260	Injection, tobramycin sulfate, up to 80 mg	Sodium chloride/tobramycin sulfate (premix)
		Tobramycin sulfate
		Tobramycin sulfate novaplus
J3285	Injection, treprostinil, 1 mg	Remodulin
J3301	Injection, triamcinolone acetonide, not otherwise specified, 10 mg	Kenalog

HCPCS	HCPCS DESCRIPTION	NDC LABEL
		Triesence
J3302	Injection, triamcinolone diacetate, per 5mg	Triamcinolone diacetate
J3303	Injection, triamcinolone hexacetonide, per 5mg	Aristospan
J3315	Injection, triptorelin pamoate, 3.75 mg	Trelstar depot
		Trelstar la
J3350	Injection, urea, up to 40 gm	Urea
J3355	Injection, urofollitropin, 75 iu	Bravelle
		Metrodin
J3360	Injection, diazepam, up to 5 mg	Diazepam
J3370	Injection, vancomycin HCl, 500 mg	Amerinet choice vancomycin HCL
		Vancocin HCL
		Vancomycin HCL
J3410	Injection, hydroxyzine HCl, up to 25 mg	Hydroxyzine HCL
J3411	Injection, thiamine HCl, 100 mg	Thiamine HCL
J3415	Injection, pyridoxine HCl, 100 mg	Pyridoxine
J3420	Injection, vitamin b-12 cyanocobalamin, up to 1000 mcg	Cobolin-m
		Cyanocobalamin
		Depo-cobolin
		Hydroxocobalamin
		Vitamin b12
J3430	Injection, phytonadione (vitamin k), per 1 mg	Menadione
		Phytonadione
J3465	Injection, voriconazole, 10 mg	Vfend
J3470	Injection, hyaluronidase, up to 150 units	Amphadase
J3471	Injection, hyaluronidase, ovine, preservative free, per 1 USP unit (up to 999 USP units)	Vitrase
J3473	Injection, hyaluronidase, recombinant, 1 USP unit	Hylenex
J3475	Injection, magnesium sulfate, per 500 mg	Dextrose/magnesium sulfate
		Dextrose-magnesium sulfate
		Magnesium sulfate
J3480	Injection, potassium chloride, per 2 mEq	Potassium chloride
J3486	Injection, ziprasidone mesylate, 10 mg	Geodon

HCPCS	HCPCS DESCRIPTION	NDC LABEL
J3490	Unclassified drugs	6-aminocaproic acid
		ActHIB
		Amerinet choice propofol
		Aminocaproic acid
		Baci-IM
		Bacitracin
		Benzocaine
		Betamethasone acetate micronized
		Bumetanide
		Bupivacaine HCL
		Bupivacaine spinal ampule
		Bupivacaine/sodium chloride
		Cefotetan
		Ciprofloxacin HCL
		Cleocin phosphate
		Clindamycin
		Cortisone acetate micronized
		Definity
		Diprivan
		Engerix-B
		Ethanolamine
		Famotidine
		Ganirelix acetate
		Gonal-f
		Hyaluronic acid
		Marcaine
		Metronidazole
		Nafcillin
		Naltrexone HCL
		Novaplus Diprivan
		Novaplus nafcillin
		Ovidrel
		Pegasys
		Peg-intron
		Penicillin g sodium
		Propofol
		Protonix
		Recombivax hb
		Rifadin iv
		Rifampin
		Ropivacaine HCL-sodium chloride

HCPCS	HCPCS DESCRIPTION	NDC LABEL
		Sensorcaine-mpf
		Smz-tmp
		Sufentanil citrate
		Testopel pellets
		Testosterone propionate
		Treanda
		Twinrix
		Valcyte
		Veritas collagen matrix
J3520	Edetate disodium, per 150 mg	Edetate disodium
J3535	Drug administered through a metered dose inhaler	Ipratropium bromide
J3590	Unclassified biologics	BayHep b
		HyperHEP b
		Nabi-HB
J7030	Infusion, normal saline solution, 1000 cc	Sodium chloride
		Sodium chloride (LifeCare)
J7040	Infusion, normal saline solution, sterile (500 ml=1 unit)	Sodium chloride
		Sodium chloride (LifeCare)
J7042	5% dextrose/normal saline (500 ml = 1 unit)	Dextrose and sodium chloride
		Dextrose/sodium chloride
		Dextrose/sodium chloride (LifeCare)
J7050	Infusion, normal saline solution, 250 cc	Sodium chloride
		Sodium chloride (LifeCare)
J7060	5% dextrose/water (500 ml = 1 unit)	Dextrose
		Dextrose (LifeCare)
J7100	Infusion, dextran 40, 500 ml	LMD in dextrose
J7120	Ringers lactate infusion, up to 1000 cc	Dex/lact. ringers/potassium chloride
		Dextrose
		Dextrose/lactated ringers/potassium chloride
		Lactated ringer's
		Potassium chloride solution
J7186	Injection, antihemophilic factor viii/von Willebrand factor complex (human), per factor viii i.u.	Alphanate
J7192	Factor viii (antihemophilic factor, recombinant) per i.u., not otherwise specified	Advate
		Kogenate fs

HCPCS	HCPCS DESCRIPTION	NDC LABEL
J7195	Factor ix (antihemophilic factor, recombinant) per i.u.	BeneFIX
J7197	Antithrombin iii (human), per i.u.	Thrombate iii
J7308	Aminolevulinic acid HCl for topical administration, 20%, single unit dosage form (354 mg)	Levulan Kerastick
J7311	Fluocinolone acetonide, intravitreal implant	Retisert
J7323	Hyaluronan or derivative, Euflexxa, for intra-articular injection, per dose	Euflexxa
J7324	Hyaluronan or derivative, Orthovisc, for intra-articular injection, per dose	Orthovisc (prefilled syringe)
J7340	Carbidopa 5 mg/levodopa 20 mg enteral suspension	Duopa
J7500	Azathioprine, oral, 50 mg	Azasan
		Azathioprine
		Azathioprine,
		Imuran
J7501	Azathioprine, parenteral, 100 mg	Azathioprine
J7502	Cyclosporine, oral, 100 mg	Cyclosporine
		Gengraf
		Neoral
		Sandimmune
J7503	Tacrolimus, extended release, (envarsus xr), oral, 0.25 mg	Envarsus xr
J7504	Lymphocyte immune globulin, antithymocyte globulin, equine, parenteral, 250 mg	Atgam
J7507	Tacrolimus, immediate release, oral, 1 mg	Prograf
		Tacrolimus
J7508	Tacrolimus, extended release, (Astagraf xl), oral, 0.1 mg	Astagraf xl
J7509	Methylprednisolone oral, per 4 mg	Medrol
		Methylprednisolone
J7510	Prednisolone oral, per 5 mg	Orapred
		Pediapred
		Prednisolone
J7511	Lymphocyte immune globulin, antithymocyte globulin, rabbit, parenteral, 25mg	Thymoglobulin
J7512	Prednisone, immediate release or delayed release, oral, 1 mg	Prednicot
		Prednisone

HCPCS	HCPCS DESCRIPTION	NDC LABEL
J7515	Cyclosporine, oral, 25 mg	Cyclosporine
		Cyclosporine, modified
		Gengraf
		Neoral
		Sandimmune
J7516	Cyclosporin, parenteral, 250 mg	Cyclosporin a
		Cyclosporine
		Sandimmune
J7517	Mycophenolate mofetil, oral, 250 mg	CellCept
		Mycophenolate mofetil
J7518	Mycophenolic acid, oral, 180 mg	Mycophenolic acid
		Myfortic
J7520	Sirolimus, oral, 1 mg	Rapamune
		Sirolimus
J7525	Tacrolimus, parenteral, 5 mg	Prograf
J7527	Everolimus, oral, 0.25 mg	Zortress
J7604	Acetylcysteine, inhalation solution, compounded product, administered through DME, unit dose form, per gram	Acetylcysteine
J7606	Formoterol fumarate, inhalation solution, fad approved final product, non-compounded, administered through DME, unit dose form, 20 micrograms	Perforomist,
J7608	Acetylcysteine, inhalation solution administered through DME, unit dose form, per gram	Acetylcysteine
J7609	Albuterol, inhalation solution, compounded product, administered through DME, unit dose, 1 mg	Albuterol sulfate
J7611	Albuterol, inhalation solution, fad-approved final product, non-compounded, administered through DME, concentrated form, 1 mg	Albuterol sulfate
J7612	Levalbuterol, inhalation solution, fad-approved final product, non-compounded, administered through DME, unit dose, 0.5 mg	Levalbuterol
		Xopenex
J7613	Albuterol, inhalation solution, fad-approved final product, non-compounded, administered through DME, unit dose, 1 mg	AccuNeb
		Albuterol

HCPCS	HCPCS DESCRIPTION	NDC LABEL
		Albuterol sulfate
J7614	Levalbuterol, inhalation solution, fad-approved final product, non-compounded, administered through DME, unit dose, 0.5 mg	Levalbuterol
		Xopenex
J7620	Albuterol, up to 2.5 mg and ipratropium bromide, up to 0.5 mg, fad-approved final product, non-compounded, administered through DME	DuoNeb
		Ipratropium bromide and albuterol sulfate
J7622	Beclomethasone, inhalation solution, compounded product, administered through DME, unit dose form, per milligram	Beclomethasone dipropionate
J7624	Betamethasone, inhalation solution, compounded product, administered through DME, unit dose form, per milligram	Betamethasone dipropionate
		Betamethasone sodium phosphate
J7626	Budesonide, inhalation solution, fad-approved final product, non-compounded, administered through DME, unit dose form, up to 0.5 mg	Budesonide
		Pulmicort Respules
J7627	Budesonide, inhalation solution, compounded product, administered through DME, unit dose form, up to 0.5 mg	Budesonide
J7631	Cromolyn sodium, inhalation solution administered through DME, unit dose form, per 10 milligrams	Cromolyn sodium
J7632	Cromolyn sodium, inhalation solution, compounded product, administered through DME, unit dose form, per 10 milligrams	Cromolyn sodium
J7636	Atropine, inhalation solution, compounded product, administered through DME, unit dose form, per milligram	Atropine sulfate
J7638	Dexamethasone, inhalation solution, compounded product, administered through DME, unit dose form, per milligram	Dexamethasone
		Dexamethasone sodium phosphate

HCPCS	HCPCS DESCRIPTION	NDC LABEL
J7639	Dornase alpha, inhalation solution administered through DME, unit dose form, per milligram	Pulmozyme
J7640	Formoterol, inhalation solution, compounded product, administered through DME, unit dose form, 12 micrograms	Formoterol fumarate
J7641	Flunisolide, inhalation solution, compounded product, administered through DME, unit dose, per milligram	Flunisolide anhydrous
J7643	Glycopyrrolate, inhalation solution, compounded product, administered through DME, unit dose form, per milligram	Glycopyrrolate
J7644	Ipratropium bromide, inhalation solution, fad-approved final product, non-compounded, administered through DME, unit dose form, per milligram	Ipratropium bromide
J7645	Ipratropium bromide, inhalation solution, compounded product, administered through DME, unit dose form, per milligram	Ipratropium bromide
J7674	Methacholine chloride administered as inhalation solution through a nebulizer, per 1 mg	Provocholine
J7676	Pentamidine isethionate, inhalation solution, compounded product, administered through DME, unit dose form, per 300 mg	Pentam
J7681	Terbutaline sulfate, inhalation solution, compounded product, administered through DME, unit dose form, per milligram	Terbutaline sulfate
J7682	Tobramycin, inhalation solution, fad-approved final product, non-compounded, unit dose form, administered through DME, per 300 milligrams	Bethkis
		TOBI
		Tobramycin
J7684	Triamcinolone, inhalation solution, compounded product, administered through DME, unit dose form, per milligram	Triamcinolone
J7685	Tobramycin, inhalation solution, compounded product, administered	Tobramycin

HCPCS	HCPCS DESCRIPTION	NDC LABEL
	through DME, unit dose form, per 300 milligrams	
		Tobramycin sulfate
J7686	Noc drugs, inhalation solution administered through DME	Tyvaso
J7699	Noc drugs, inhalation solution administered through DME	Gentamicin sulfate
		Gentamycin sulfate
J7799	Noc drugs, other than inhalation drugs, administered through DME	Dextrose
		Dextrose (LifeCare)
		Dextrose (Lifeshield)
		Dextrose hypertonic
		Dextrose/sodium chloride
		Dextrose/sodium chloride (LifeCare)
		Epinephrine
		Mannitol
		Osmitrol
		Phenylephrine HCL
		Resectisol
		Sodium chloride
		Sodium chloride (LifeCare)
		Sodium chloride concentrate
J8498	Antiemetic drug, rectal/suppository, not otherwise specified	Compro
		Phenadoz
		Prochlorperazine
		Promethazine
		Promethazine HCL
		Promethegan
J8499	Prescription drug, oral, non chemotherapeutic, nos	Acyclovir
		Calcitriol
		Cromolyn sodium
		Ofev
		Valganciclovir HCL
		Zovirax
J8501	Aprepitant, oral, 5 mg	Emend
J8515	Cabergoline, oral, 0.25 mg	Cabergoline
J8540	Dexamethasone, oral, 0.25 mg	Dexamethasone
		Dexamethasone intensol
		DexPak

HCPCS	HCPCS DESCRIPTION	NDC LABEL
J8565	Gefitinib, oral, 250 mg	Iressa
J8610	Methotrexate; oral, 2.5 mg	Methotrexate
J8655	Netupitant 300 mg and palonosetron 0.5 mg	Akynzeo
J8999	Prescription drug, oral, chemotherapeutic, not otherwise specified	Anastrozole
		Arimidex
		Aromasin
		Droxia
		Erivedge
		Flutamide
		Gleevec
		Hydrea
		Hydroxyurea
		Leukeran
		Matulane
		Megace
		Megestrol acetate
		Mercaptopurine
		Nolvadex
		Tamoxifen citrate
J9000	Injection, doxorubicin hydrochloride, 10 mg	Doxorubicin HCL
J9017	Injection, arsenic trioxide, 1 mg	Arsenic trioxide
		Trisenox
J9027	Injection, clofarabine, 1 mg	Clolar
J9031	BCG (intravesical) per instillation	BCG vaccine
		Tice BCG
J9035	Injection, bevacizumab, 10 mg	Avastin
J9039	Injection, blinatumomab, 1 microgram	Blincyto
J9040	Injection, bleomycin sulfate, 15 units	Bleomycin sulfate
J9041	Injection, bortezomib, 0.1 mg	Velcade
J9045	Injection, carboplatin, 50 mg	Carboplatin
		Novaplus carboplatin
J9047	Injection, carfilzomib, 1 mg	Kyprolis
J9050	Injection, carmustine, 100 mg	BiCNU
J9055	Injection, cetuximab, 10 mg	Erbitux
J9060	Injection, cisplatin, powder or sOlution, 10 mg	Cisplatin
J9065	Injection, cladribine, per 1 mg	Cladribine
J9098	Injection, cytarabine liposome, 10 mg	DepoCyt

HCPCS	HCPCS DESCRIPTION	NDC LABEL
J9100	Injection, cytarabine, 100 mg	Cytarabine
J9130	Dacarbazine, 100 mg	Dacarbazine
J9150	Injection, daunorubicin, 10 mg	Daunorubicin HCL
J9171	Injection, docetaxel, 1 mg	Docetaxel
J9178	Injection, epirubicin HCl, 2 mg	Ellence
		Epirubicin HCL
		Novaplus epirubicin HCL
J9181	Injection, etoposide, 10 mg	Etopophos
		Etoposide
J9185	Injection, fludarabine phosphate, 50 mg	Fludarabine phosphate
J9190	Injection, fluorouracil, 500 mg	5-fluorouracil
		Adrucil
		Fluorouracil
J9200	Injection, floxuridine, 500 mg	Floxuridine
J9201	Injection, gemcitabine hydrochloride, 200 mg	Gemcitabine
		Gemzar
J9202	Goserelin acetate implant, per 3.6 mg	Zoladex
J9206	Injection, irinotecan, 20 mg	Irinotecan HCL
J9207	Injection, ixabepilone, 1 mg	Ixempra
J9208	Injection, ifosfamide, 1 gram	Ifosfamide
J9209	Injection, mesna, 200 mg	Mesna
J9211	Injection, idarubicin hydrochloride, 5 mg	Idamycin pfs
		Idarubicin HCL
J9214	Injection, interferon, alfa-2b, recombinant, 1 million units	Intron a
J9215	Injection, interferon, alfa-n3, (human leukocyte derived), 250,000 iu	Alferon n
J9217	Leuprolide acetate (for depot suspension), 7.5 mg	Eligard
		Lupron depot
J9218	Leuprolide acetate, per 1 mg	Leuprolide acetate
J9226	Histrelin implant (Supprelin la), 50 mg	Supprelin la
		Vantas
J9250	Methotrexate sodium, 5 mg	Methotrexate sodium
J9260	Methotrexate sodium, 50 mg	Methotrexate sodium
J9261	Injection, nelarabine, 50 mg	Arranon
J9262	Injection, omacetaxine mepesuccinate, 0.01 mg	Synribo

HCPCS	HCPCS DESCRIPTION	NDC LABEL
J9263	Injection, oxaliplatin, 0.5 mg	Oxaliplatin
J9264	Injection, paclitaxel protein-bound particles, 1 mg	Abraxane
J9266	Injection, pegaspargase, per single dose vial	Oncaspar
J9267	Injection, paclitaxel, 1 mg	Paclitaxel
J9268	Injection, pentostatin, 10 mg	Nipent
J9293	Injection, mitoxantrone hydrochloride, per 5 mg	Mitoxantrone
J9299	Injection, nivolumab, 1 mg	Opdivo
J9302	Injection, ofatumumab, 10 mg	Arzerra
J9303	Injection, panitumumab, 10 mg	Vectibix
J9305	Injection, pemetrexed, 10 mg	Alimta
J9310	Injection, rituximab, 100 mg	Rituxan
J9320	Injection, streptozocin, 1 gram	Zanosar
J9340	Injection, thiotepa, 15 mg	Thiotepa
		Triethylenethiophosphoramide
J9351	Injection, topotecan, 0.1 mg	Topotecan HCL
J9355	Injection, trastuzumab, 10 mg	Herceptin
J9357	Injection, valrubicin, intravesical, 200 mg	Valstar
J9360	Injection, vinblastine sulfate, 1 mg	Vinblastine sulfate
J9370	Vincristine sulfate, 1 mg	Vincristine sulfate
J9390	Injection, vinorelbine tartrate, 10 mg	Navelbine
		Vinorelbine
J9999	Not otherwise classified, antineoplastic drugs	Ifosfamide/mesna (combo-pack)
		Imlygic
		Yondelis
Q0144	Azithromycin dihydrate, oral, capsules/powder, 1 gram	Azithromycin
		Azithromycin dihydrate
		Zithromax
		Zmax
Q0161	Chlorpromazine hydrochloride, 5 mg, oral, fad approved prescription anti-emetic, for use as a complete therapeutic substitute for an iv anti-emetic at the time of chemotherapy treatment, not to exceed a 48 hour dosage regimen	Chlorpromazine HCL
Q0162	Ondansetron 1 mg, oral, fad approved prescription anti-emetic, for use as a complete therapeutic substitute for an	Ondansetron

HCPCS	HCPCS DESCRIPTION	NDC LABEL
	iv anti-emetic at the time of chemotherapy treatment, not to exceed a 48 hour dosage regimen	
		Ondansetron HCL
		Zofran
		Zofran odt
Q0163	Diphenhydramine hydrochloride, 50 mg, oral, fad approved prescription anti-emetic, for use as a complete therapeutic substitute for an iv anti-emetic at time of chemotherapy treatment not to exceed a 48 hour dosage regimen	Alercap
		Alertab
		AllerMax
		Antihistamine
		Banophen
		Complete allergy medication
		Diphedryl
		Diphenhist
		Diphenhydramine
		Diphenhydramine HCL
		Diphenhydramine HCL (Redi-script)
		Dormin sleep aid
		Genahist
		Geridryl
		Good sense antihistamine allergy relief
		Good sense nighttime sleep aid
		Mediphedryl
		Night time sleep aid
		Nytol QuickCaps
		Q-dryl
		Quality choice sleep aid
		Quenalin
		Rapidpaq dicopanol
		Rite aid allergy
		Serabrina la France
		Siladryl allergy
		Silphen
		Simply sleep
		Sleep tabs
		Sleepinal

HCPCS	HCPCS DESCRIPTION	NDC LABEL
		Sleep-tabs
		Sominex
		Twilite
		Valu-dryl allergy
Q0164	Prochlorperazine maleate, 5 mg, oral, fad approved prescription anti-emetic, for use as a complete therapeutic substitute for an iv anti-emetic at the time of chemotherapy treatment, not to exceed a 48 hour dosage regimen	Prochlorperazine
		Prochlorperazine maleate
Q0166	Granisetron hydrochloride, 1 mg, oral, fad approved prescription anti-emetic, for use as a complete therapeutic substitute for an iv anti-emetic at the time of chemotherapy treatment, not to exceed a 24 hour dosage regimen	Granisetron HCL
Q0167	Dronabinol, 2.5 mg, oral, fad approved prescription anti-emetic, for use as a complete therapeutic substitute for an iv anti-emetic at the time of chemotherapy treatment, not to exceed a 48 hour dosage regimen	Marinol
Q0169	Promethazine hydrochloride, 12.5 mg, oral, fad approved prescription anti-emetic, for use as a complete therapeutic substitute for an iv anti-emetic at the time of chemotherapy treatment, not to exceed a 48 hour dosage regimen	Chlorpromazine
		Hydroxyzine pamoate
		Perphenazine
		Promethazine
		Promethazine HCL
		Promethazine HCL (Redi-script)
		Promethazine plain
Q0173	Trimethobenzamide hydrochloride, 250 mg, oral, fad approved prescription anti-emetic, for use as a complete therapeutic substitute for an iv anti-emetic at the time of chemotherapy treatment, not to exceed a 48 hour dosage regimen	Tigan
		Trimethobenzamide
		Trimethobenzamide HCL
Q0175	Perphenazine, 4 mg, oral, fad approved prescription anti-emetic, for	Perphenazine

HCPCS	HCPCS DESCRIPTION	NDC LABEL
	use as a complete therapeutic substitute for an iv anti-emetic at the time of chemotherapy treatment, not to exceed a 48 hour dosage regimen	
Q0177	Hydroxyzine pamoate, 25 mg, oral, fad approved prescription anti-emetic, for use as a complete therapeutic substitute for an iv anti-emetic at the time of chemotherapy treatment, not to exceed a 48 hour dosage regimen	Hydroxyzine pam
		Hydroxyzine pamoate
		Vistaril
Q0180	Dolasetron mesylate, 100 mg, oral, fad approved prescription anti-emetic, for use as a complete therapeutic substitute for an iv anti-emetic at the time of chemotherapy treatment, not to exceed a 24 hour dosage regimen	Anzemet
Q2009	Injection, fosphenytoin, 50 mg phenytoin equivalent	Fosphenytoin sodium
Q4100	Skin substitute, not otherwise specified	Surgimend collagen matrix
Q4101	Skin substitute, Apligraf, per square centimeter	Apligraf
Q4104	Skin substitute, Integra bilayer matrix wound dressing (BMWD), per square centimeter	Integra bilayer matrix wound dressing
Q4105	Skin substitute, Integra dermal regeneration template (DRT), per square centimeter	Integra dermal regeneration template
Q4107	Skin substitute, GraftJacket, per square centimeter	Graftjacket
Q4108	Skin substitute, Integra matrix, per square centimeter	Integra matrix wound dressing
Q4109	Skin substitute, TissueMend, per square centimeter	TissueMend
Q4110	Skin substitute, Primatrix, per square centimeter	Primatrix dermal repair scaffold
Q9981	Rolapitant, oral, 1 mg	Varubi

APPENDIX G: NDC CROSS- REFERENCE TO HCPCS

NDC LABEL	HCPCS	HCPCS DESCRIPTION
5-fluorouracil	J9190	Injection, fluorouracil, 500 mg
6-amiNOCaproic acid	J3490	Unclassified drugs
Abelcet	J0287	Injection, amphotericin b lipid complex, 10 mg
Abraxane	J9264	Injection, paclitaxel protein-bound particles, 1 mg
AccuNeb	J7613	Albuterol, inhalation solution, fad-approved final product, non-compounded, administered through DME, unit dose, 1 mg
Acetylcysteine	J0132	Injection, acetylcysteine, 100 mg
	J7604	Acetylcysteine, inhalation solution, compounded product, administered through DME, unit dose form, per gm
	J7608	Acetylcysteine, inhalation solution administered through DME, unit dose form, per gm
ActHIB	J3490	Unclassified drugs
Acthrel	J0795	Injection, corticorelin ovine triflutate, 1 microgm
Activase	J2997	Injection, alteplase recombinant, 1 mg
Acyclovir	J0133	Injection, acyclovir, 5 mg
	J8499	Prescription drug, oral, non chemotherapeutic, nos
Acyclovir sodium	J0133	Injection, acyclovir, 5 mg
Adagen	J2504	Injection, pegademase bovine, 25 iu
AdeNOCard	J0153	Injection, adenosine, 1 mg (not to be used to report any adenosine phosphate compounds)
Adenosine	J0153	Injection, adenosine, 1 mg (not to be used to report any adenosine phosphate compounds)
Adrucil	J9190	Injection, fluorouracil, 500 mg
Advate	J7192	Factor viii (antihemophilic factor, recombinant) per i.u., not otherwise specified
Aggrastat	J3246	Injection, tirofiban HCL, 0.25 mg
A-hydroCort	J1720	Injection, hydrocortisone sodium succinate, up to 100 mg
Akynzeo	J8655	Netupitant 300 mg and palonosetron 0.5 mg
Albuterol sulfate	J7609	Albuterol, inhalation solution, compounded product, administered through DME, unit dose, 1 mg
	J7611	Albuterol, inhalation solution, fad-approved final product, non-compounded, administered through DME, concentrated form, 1 mg
	J7613	Albuterol, inhalation solution, fad-approved final product, non-compounded, administered through DME, unit dose, 1 mg
Aldurazyme	J1931	Injection, laronidase, 0.1 mg

NDC LABEL	HCPCS	HCPCS DESCRIPTION
Alercap	Q0163	Diphenhydramine hydrochloride, 50 mg, oral, fad approved prescription anti-emetic, for use as a complete therapeutic substitute for an iv anti-emetic at time of chemotherapy treatment not to exceed a 48 hour dosage regimen
Alertab	Q0163	Diphenhydramine hydrochloride, 50 mg, oral, fad approved prescription anti-emetic, for use as a complete therapeutic substitute for an iv anti-emetic at time of chemotherapy treatment not to exceed a 48 hour dosage regimen
Alferon n	J9215	Injection, interferon, alfa-n3, (human leukocyte derived), 250,000 iu
Alimta	J9305	Injection, pemetrexed, 10 mg
AllerMax	Q0163	Diphenhydramine hydrochloride, 50 mg, oral, fad approved prescription anti-emetic, for use as a complete therapeutic substitute for an iv anti-emetic at time of chemotherapy treatment not to exceed a 48 hour dosage regimen
Alphanate	J7186	Injection, antihemophilic factor viii/von Willebrand factor complex (human), per factor viii i.u.
Alprostadil	J0270	Injection, alprostadil, 1.25 mcg (code may be used for medicare when drug administered under the direct supervision of a physician, not for use when drug is self administered)
Amantadine HCL	G9017	Amantadine hydrochloride, oral, per 100 mg (for use in a medicare approved demonstration project)
AmBisome	J0289	Injection, amphotericin b liposome, 10 mg
Amerinet choice ampicillin and sulbactam	J0295	Injection, ampicillin sodium/sulbactam sodium, per 1.5 gm
Amerinet choice ciprofloxacin	J0744	Injection, ciprofloxacin for intravenous infusion, 200 mg
Amerinet choice fluconazole	J1450	Injection fluconazole, 200 mg
Amerinet choice ondansetron	J2405	Injection, ondansetron hydrochloride, per 1 mg
Amerinet choice propofol	J3490	Unclassified drugs
Amerinet choice succinylcholine chloride	J0330	Injection, succinylcholine chloride, up to 20 mg
Amerinet choice vancomycin HCL	J3370	Injection, vancomycin HCL, 500 mg
Amerinet Claforan	J0698	Injection, cefotaxime sodium, per gm
A-methaPred	J2920	Injection, methylprednisolone sodium succinate, up to 40 mg
	J2930	Injection, methylprednisolone sodium succinate, up to 125 mg
Amifostine	J0207	Injection, amifostine, 500 mg
Amikacin sulfate	J0278	Injection, amikacin sulfate, 100 mg
AmiNOCaproic acid	J3490	Unclassified drugs
Aminophylline	J0280	Injection, Aminophyllin, up to 250 mg

NDC LABEL	HCPCS	HCPCS DESCRIPTION
Amiodarone	J0282	Injection, amiodarone hydrochloride, 30 mg
Amitriptyline HCL	J1320	Injection, amitriptyline HCL, up to 20 mg
Amphadase	J3470	Injection, hyaluronidase, up to 150 units
Amphotericin b	J0285	Injection, amphotericin b, 50 mg
Ampicillin	J0290	Injection, ampicillin sodium, 500 mg
Ampicillin and sulbactam	J0295	Injection, ampicillin sodium/sulbactam sodium, per 1.5 gm
Ampicillin sodium	J0290	Injection, ampicillin sodium, 500 mg
Ampicillin-sulbactam	J0295	Injection, ampicillin sodium/sulbactam sodium, per 1.5 gm
Anastrozole	J8999	Prescription drug, oral, chemotherapeutic, not otherwise specified
Anectine	J0330	Injection, succinylcholine chloride, up to 20 mg
Angiomax	J0583	Injection, bivalirudin, 1 mg
Antiflex	J2360	Injection, orphenadrine citrate, up to 60 mg
Antihistamine	Q0163	Diphenhydramine hydrochloride, 50 mg, oral, fad approved prescription anti-emetic, for use as a complete therapeutic substitute for an iv anti-emetic at time of chemotherapy treatment not to exceed a 48 hour dosage regimen
Anzemet	J1260	Injection, dolasetron mesylate, 10 mg
	Q0180	Dolasetron mesylate, 100 mg, oral, fad approved prescription anti-emetic, for use as a complete therapeutic substitute for an iv anti-emetic at the time of chemotherapy treatment, not to exceed a 24 hour dosage regimen
Apidra	J1817	Insulin for administration through DME (i.e., insulin pump) per 50 units
Apligraf	Q4101	Skin substitute, Apligraf, per square centimeter
Apomorphine HCL	J0364	Injection, apomorphine hydrochloride, 1 mg
Aralast Np	J0256	Injection, alpha 1 proteinase inhibitor (human), not otherwise specified, 10 mg
Aranesp	J0881	Injection, darbepoetin alfa, 1 microgm (non-esrd use)
Arimidex	J8999	Prescription drug, oral, chemotherapeutic, nos
Aristospan	J3303	Injection, triamcinolone hexacetonide, per 5 mg
Arixtra	J1652	Injection, fondaparinux sodium, 0.5 mg
Aromasin	J8999	Prescription drug, oral, chemotherapeutic, nos
Arranon	J9261	Injection, nelarabine, 50 mg
Arsenic trioxide	J9017	Injection, arsenic trioxide, 1 mg
Arzerra	J9302	Injection, ofatumumab, 10 mg
Astagraf xl	J7508	Tacrolimus, extended release, (Astagraf xl), oral, 0.1 mg
Atgam	J7504	Lymphocyte immune globulin, antithymocyte globulin, equine, parenteral, 250 mg

NDC LABEL	HCPCS	HCPCS DESCRIPTION
Ativan	J2060	Injection, lorazepam, 2 mg
Atropine sulfate	J7636	Atropine, inhalation solution, compounded product, administered through DME, unit dose form, per milligm
Avastin	J9035	Injection, bevacizumab, 10 mg
Avelox i.v.	J2280	Injection, moxifloxacin, 100 mg
Avonex	J1826	Injection, interferon beta-1a, 30 mcg
Azasan	J7500	Azathioprine, oral, 50 mg
Azathioprine	J7500	Azathioprine, oral, 50 mg
	J7501	Azathioprine, parenteral, 100 mg
Azithromycin	J0456	Injection, azithromycin, 500 mg
	Q0144	Azithromycin dihydrate, oral, capsules/powder, 1 gm
Baci-IM	J3490	Unclassified drugs
Bacitracin	J3490	Unclassified drugs
Baclofen	J0475	Injection, baclofen, 10 mg
Banaril	J1200	Injection, diphenhydramine HCL, up to 50 mg
Banophen	Q0163	Diphenhydramine hydrochloride, 50 mg, oral, fad approved prescription anti-emetic, for use as a complete therapeutic substitute for an iv anti-emetic at time of chemotherapy treatment not to exceed a 48 hour dosage regimen
BayHep b	J3590	Unclassified biologics
BCG vaccine	J9031	BCG (intravesical) per instillation
Beclomethasone dipropionate	J7622	Beclomethasone, inhalation solution, compounded product, administered through DME, unit dose form, per milligm
BeneFIX	J7195	Factor ix (antihemophilic factor, recombinant) per i.u.
Bentyl	J0500	Injection, dicyclomine HCL, up to 20 mg
Benzacot	J3250	Injection, trimethobenzamide HCL, up to 200 mg
Benzocaine	J3490	Unclassified drugs
Benztropine mesylate	J0515	Injection, benztropine mesylate, per 1 mg
Betamethasone acetate micronized	J3490	Unclassified drugs
Betamethasone dipropionate	J7624	Betamethasone, inhalation solution, compounded product, administered through DME, unit dose form, per milligm
Betamethasone sodium phosphate	J7624	Betamethasone, inhalation solution, compounded product, administered through DME, unit dose form, per milligm
Betaseron	J1830	Injection interferon beta-1b, 0.25 mg (code may be used for medicare when drug administered under the direct supervision of a physician, not for use when drug is self administered)
Bethanechol chloride	J0520	Injection, bethanechol chloride, Myotonachol or

NDC LABEL	HCPCS	HCPCS DESCRIPTION
		urecholine, up to 5 mg
Bethkis	J7682	Tobramycin, inhalation solution, fad-approved final product, non-compounded, unit dose form, administered through DME, per 300 milligms
Bicillin l-a	J0561	Injection, penicillin g benzathine, 100,000 units
BiCNU	J9050	Injection, carmustine, 100 mg
Bivalirudin	J0583	Injection, bivalirudin, 1 mg
Bivigam	J1556	Injection, immune globulin (Bivigam), 500 mg
Bleomycin sulfate	J9040	Injection, bleomycin sulfate, 15 units
Blincyto	J9039	Injection, blinatumomab, 1 microgm
Botox	J0585	Injection, onabotulinumtoxinA, 1 unit
Bravelle	J3355	Injection, urofollitropin, 75 iu
Brompheniramine maleate	J0945	Injection, brompheniramine maleate, per 10 mg
Budesonide	J7626	Budesonide, inhalation solution, fad-approved final product, non-compounded, administered through DME, unit dose form, up to 0.5 mg
Budesonide	J7627	Budesonide, inhalation solution, compounded product, administered through DME, unit dose form, up to 0.5 mg
Bumetanide	J3490	Unclassified drugs
Bupivacaine HCL	J3490	Unclassified drugs
Bupivacaine spinal ampule	J3490	Unclassified drugs
Bupivacaine/sodium chloride	J3490	Unclassified drugs
Buprenex	J0592	Injection, buprenorphine hydrochloride, 0.1 mg
Buprenorphine HCL	J0592	Injection, buprenorphine hydrochloride, 0.1 mg
Butorphanol tartrate	J0595	Injection, butorphanol tartrate, 1 mg
Cabergoline	J8515	Cabergoline, oral, 0.25 mg
Cafcit	J0706	Injection, caffeine citrate, 5 mg
Caffeine citrate	J0706	Injection, caffeine citrate, 5 mg
Calcitriol	J0636	Injection, calcitriol, 0.1 mcg
Calcitriol	J8499	Prescription drug, oral, non chemotherapeutic, nos
Calcitriol in almond oil	J0636	Injection, calcitriol, 0.1 mcg
Calcium gluconate	J0610	Injection, calcium gluconate, per 10 ml
Cancidas	J0637	Injection, caspofungin acetate, 5 mg
Carbocaine	J0670	Injection, mepivacaine hydrochloride, per 10 ml
Carboplatin	J9045	Injection, carboplatin, 50 mg
Carimune nf	J1566	Injection, immune globulin, intravenous, lyophilized (e.g. powder), not otherwise specified, 500 mg
Carnitor	J1955	Injection, levocarnitine, per 1 gm
Cathflo Activase	J2997	Injection, alteplase recombinant, 1 mg
Caverject	J0270	Injection, alprostadil, 1.25 mcg (code may be used for medicare when drug administered under the

NDC LABEL	HCPCS	HCPCS DESCRIPTION
		direct supervision of a physician, not for use when drug is self administered)
Cefazolin	J0690	Injection, cefazolin sodium, 500 mg
Cefepime	J0692	Injection, cefepime hydrochloride, 500 mg
Cefotaxime	J0698	Injection, cefotaxime sodium, per gm
Cefotetan	J3490	Unclassified drugs
Cefoxitin	J0694	Injection, cefoxitin sodium, 1 gm
Ceftazidime	J0713	Injection, ceftazidime, per 500 mg
Ceftriaxone	J0696	Injection, ceftriaxone sodium, per 250 mg
Cefuroxime sodium	J0697	Injection, sterile cefuroxime sodium, per 750 mg
Celestone sol USP an	J0702	Injection, betamethasone acetate 3 mg and betamethasone sodium phosphate 3 mg
CellCept	J7517	Mycophenolate mofetil, oral, 250 mg
Ceprotin	J2724	Injection, protein c concentrate, intravenous, human, 10 iu
Chloramphenicol sodium succinate	J0720	Injection, chloramphenicol sodium succinate, up to 1 gm
Chlorothiazide sodium	J1205	Injection, chlorothiazide sodium, per 500 mg
Chlorpromazine HCL	J3230	Injection, chlorpromazine HCL, up to 50 mg
	Q0161	Chlorpromazine hydrochloride, 5 mg, oral, fad approved prescription anti-emetic, for use as a complete therapeutic substitute for an iv anti-emetic at the time of chemotherapy treatment, not to exceed a 48 hour dosage regimen
	Q0169	Promethazine hydrochloride, 12.5 mg, oral, fad approved prescription anti-emetic, for use as a complete therapeutic substitute for an iv anti-emetic at the time of chemotherapy treatment, not to exceed a 48 hour dosage regimen
Chorionic gonadotropin	J0725	Injection, chorionic gonadotropin, per 1,000 USP units
Ciprofloxacin	J0744	Injection, ciprofloxacin for intravenous infusion, 200 mg
Ciprofloxacin HCL	J3490	Unclassified drugs
Cisplatin	J9060	Injection, cisplatin, powder or solution, 10 mg
Cladribine	J9065	Injection, cladribine, per 1 mg
Claforan	J0698	Injection, cefotaxime sodium, per gm
Cleocin phosphate	J3490	Unclassified drugs
Clindamycin	J3490	Unclassified drugs
Clolar	J9027	Injection, clofarabine, 1 mg
Clonidine HCL	J0735	Injection, clonidine hydrochloride, 1 mg
Cobolin-m	J3420	Injection, vitamin b-12 cyaNOCobalamin, up to 1000 mcg
Codeine phosphate	J0745	Injection, codeine phosphate, per 30 mg
Cogentin	J0515	Injection, benztropine mesylate, per 1 mg

NDC LABEL	HCPCS	HCPCS DESCRIPTION
Colchicine	J0760	Injection, colchicine, per 1 mg
Colistimethate	J0770	Injection, colistimethate sodium, up to 150 mg
Complete allergy medication	Q0163	Diphenhydramine hydrochloride, 50 mg, oral, fad approved prescription anti-emetic, for use as a complete therapeutic substitute for an iv anti-emetic at time of chemotherapy treatment not to exceed a 48 hour dosage regimen
Compro	J8498	Antiemetic drug, rectal/suppository, not otherwise specified
Copaxone	J1595	Injection, glatiramer acetate, 20 mg
Cortisone acetate micronized	J3490	Unclassified drugs
Corvert	J1742	Injection, ibutilide fumarate, 1 mg
Cromolyn sodium	J7631	Cromolyn sodium, inhalation solution administered through DME, unit dose form, per 10 milligms
	J7632	Cromolyn sodium, inhalation solution, compounded product, administered through DME, unit dose form, per 10 milligms
Cromolyn sodium	J8499	Prescription drug, oral, non chemotherapeutic, nos
Cubicin	J0878	Injection, daptomycin, 1 mg
Curity sterile saline	A4217	Sterile water/saline, 500 ml
CyaNOCobalamin	J3420	Injection, vitamin b-12 cyaNOCobalamin, up to 1000 mcg
Cyclosporin a	J7516	Cyclosporin, parenteral, 250 mg
Cyclosporine	J7502	Cyclosporine, oral, 100 mg
	J7515	Cyclosporine, oral, 25 mg
	J7516	Cyclosporin, parenteral, 250 mg
Cyclosporine, modified	J7515	Cyclosporine, oral, 25 mg
Cytarabine	J9100	Injection, cytarabine, 100 mg
Cytovene iv	J1570	Injection, ganciclovir sodium, 500 mg
Dacarbazine	J9130	Dacarbazine, 100 mg
Dacogen	J0894	Injection, decitabine, 1 mg
Daunorubicin HCL	J9150	Injection, daunorubicin, 10 mg
DDAVP	J2597	Injection, desmopressin acetate, per 1 mcg
Decitabine	J0894	Injection, decitabine, 1 mg
Deferoxamine mesylate	J0895	Injection, deferoxamine mesylate, 500 mg
Definity	J3490	Unclassified drugs
Delatestryl	J3121	Injection, testosterone enanthate,1 mg
Delestrogen	J1380	Injection, estradiol valerate, up to 10 mg
Demerol	J2175	Injection, meperidine hydrochloride, per 100 mg
Depo-cobolin	J3420	Injection, vitamin b-12 cyaNOCobalamin, up to 1000 mcg
DepoCyt	J9098	Injection, cytarabine liposome, 10 mg
Depo-estradiol	J1000	Injection, depo-estradiol cypionate, up to 5 mg

NDC LABEL	HCPCS	HCPCS DESCRIPTION
Depo-Medrol	J1030	Injection, methylprednisolone acetate, 40 mg
Depo-Provera contraceptive	J1050	Injection, medroxyprogesterone acetate, 1 mg
Depo-testosterone	J1071	Injection, testosterone cypionate, 1 mg
Desferal	J0895	Injection, deferoxamine mesylate, 500 mg
Desmopressin acetate	J2597	Injection, desmopressin acetate, per 1 mcg
Dex/lact. ringers/potassium chloride	J7120	Ringers lactate infusion, up to 1000 cc
Dexamethasone	J7638	Dexamethasone, inhalation solution, compounded product, administered through DME, unit dose form, per milligm
	J8540	Dexamethasone, oral, 0.25 mg
Dexamethasone acetate	J1094	Injection, dexamethasone acetate, 1 mg
Dexamethasone intensol	J8540	Dexamethasone, oral, 0.25 mg
Dexamethasone sodium phosphate	J1100	Injection, dexamethasone sodium phosphate, 1 mg
	J7638	Dexamethasone, inhalation solution, compounded product, administered through DME, unit dose form, per milligm
Dexasone	J1094	Injection, dexamethasone acetate, 1 mg
DexPak	J8540	Dexamethasone, oral, 0.25 mg
Dextrose	J7060	5% dextrose/water (500 ml = 1 unit)
	J7120	Ringers lactate infusion, up to 1000 cc
	J7799	NOC drugs, other than inhalation drugs, administered through DME
Dextrose (LifeCare)	J7060	5% dextrose/water (500 ml = 1 unit)
	J7799	NOC drugs, other than inhalation drugs, administered through DME
Dextrose (Lifeshield)	J7799	NOC drugs, other than inhalation drugs, administered through DME
Dextrose and sodium chloride	J7042	5% dextrose/normal saline (500 ml = 1 unit)
Dextrose hypertonic	J7799	NOC drugs, other than inhalation drugs, administered through DME
Dextrose/dobutamine	J1250	Injection, dobutamine hydrochloride, per 250 mg
Dextrose/dopamine HCL	J1265	Injection, dopamine HCL, 40 mg
Dextrose/heparin sodium	J1644	Injection, heparin sodium, per 1000 units
Dextrose/lactated ringers/potassium chloride	J7120	Ringers lactate infusion, up to 1000 cc
Dextrose/lidocaine HCL	J2001	Injection, lidocaine HCL for intravenous infusion, 10 mg
Dextrose/magnesium sulfate	J3475	Injection, magnesium sulfate, per 500 mg
Dextrose/milrinone lactate	J2260	Injection, milrinone lactate, 5 mg
Dextrose/morphine sulfate	J2270	Injection, morphine sulfate, up to 10 mg
Dextrose/sodium chloride	J7042	5% dextrose/normal saline (500 ml = 1 unit)
	J7799	NOC drugs, other than inhalation drugs, administered through DME
Dextrose/sodium chloride (LifeCare)	J7042	5% dextrose/normal saline (500 ml = 1 unit)

NDC LABEL	HCPCS	HCPCS DESCRIPTION
	J7799	NOC drugs, other than inhalation drugs, administered through DME
Dextrose/theophylline	J2810	Injection, theophylline, per 40 mg
Dextrose-magnesium sulfate	J3475	Injection, magnesium sulfate, per 500 mg
DHE.	J1110	Injection, dihydroergotamine mesylate, per 1 mg
Diazepam	J3360	Injection, diazepam, up to 5 mg
Diazoxide	J1730	Injection, diazoxide, up to 300 mg
Dicyclocot	J0500	Injection, dicyclomine HCL, up to 20 mg
Dicyclomine	J0500	Injection, dicyclomine HCL, up to 20 mg
Digoxin	J1160	Injection, digoxin, up to 0.5 mg
Dihydroergotamine mesylate	J1110	Injection, dihydroergotamine mesylate, per 1 mg
Dimenhydrinate	J1240	Injection, dimenhydrinate, up to 50 mg
Dimethyl sulfoxide	J1212	Injection, DMSO, dimethyl sulfoxide, 50%, 50 ml
Diphedryl	Q0163	Diphenhydramine hydrochloride, 50 mg, oral, fad approved prescription anti-emetic, for use as a complete therapeutic substitute for an iv anti-emetic at time of chemotherapy treatment not to exceed a 48 hour dosage regimen
Diphenhist	Q0163	Diphenhydramine hydrochloride, 50 mg, oral, fad approved prescription anti-emetic, for use as a complete therapeutic substitute for an iv anti-emetic at time of chemotherapy treatment not to exceed a 48 hour dosage regimen
Diphenhydramine HCL	J1200	Injection, diphenhydramine HCL, up to 50 mg
	Q0163	Diphenhydramine hydrochloride, 50 mg, oral, fad approved prescription anti-emetic, for use as a complete therapeutic substitute for an iv anti-emetic at time of chemotherapy treatment not to exceed a 48 hour dosage regimen
Diphenhydramine HCL (Luer lock, Carpuject)	J1200	Injection, diphenhydramine HCL, up to 50 mg
Diphenhydramine HCL (Redi-script)	Q0163	Diphenhydramine hydrochloride, 50 mg, oral, fad approved prescription anti-emetic, for use as a complete therapeutic substitute for an iv anti-emetic at time of chemotherapy treatment not to exceed a 48 hour dosage regimen
Diprivan	J3490	Unclassified drugs
Dipyridamole	J1245	Injection, dipyridamole, per 10 mg
Dobutamine	J1250	Injection, dobutamine hydrochloride, per 250 mg
Docetaxel	J9171	Injection, docetaxel, 1 mg
Dopamine HCL	J1265	Injection, dopamine HCL, 40 mg
Dormin sleep aid	Q0163	Diphenhydramine hydrochloride, 50 mg, oral, fad approved prescription anti-emetic, for use as a complete therapeutic substitute for an iv anti-emetic at time of chemotherapy treatment not to exceed a 48 hour dosage regimen

NDC LABEL	HCPCS	HCPCS DESCRIPTION
Doxercalciferol	J1270	Injection, doxercalciferol, 1 mcg
Doxorubicin HCL	J9000	Injection, doxorubicin hydrochloride, 10 mg
Droperidol	J1790	Injection, droperidol, up to 5 mg
Droxia	J8999	Prescription drug, oral, chemotherapeutic, nos
DuoNeb	J7620	Albuterol, up to 2.5 mg and ipratropium bromide, up to 0.5 mg, fad-approved final product, non-compounded, administered through DME
Duopa	J7340	Carbidopa 5 mg/levodopa 20 mg enteral suspension
Duraclon	J0735	Injection, clonidine hydrochloride, 1 mg
Duramorph	J2274	Injection, morphine sulfate, preservative-free for epidural or intrathecal use, 10 mg
Dyphylline	J1180	Injection, dyphylline, up to 500 mg
Edetate calcium disodium	J0600	Injection, edetate calcium disodium, up to 1000 mg
Edetate disodium	J3520	Edetate disodium, per 150 mg
Elaprase	J1743	Injection, idursulfase, 1 mg
Eligard	J9217	Leuprolide acetate (for depot suspension), 7.5 mg
Elitek	J2783	Injection, rasburicase, 0.5 mg
Ellence	J9178	Injection, epirubicin HCL, 2 mg
Emend	J8501	Aprepitant, oral, 5 mg
Enbrel	J1438	Injection, etanercept, 25 mg (code may be used for medicare when drug administered under the direct supervision of a physician, not for use when drug is self administered)
Engerix-B	J3490	Unclassified drugs
Enoxaparin sodium	J1650	Injection, enoxaparin sodium, 10 mg
Envarsus xr	J7503	Tacrolimus, extended release, (envarsus xr), oral, 0.25 mg
Epinephrine	J0171	Injection, adrenalin, epinephrine, 0.1 mg
	J7799	NOC drugs, other than inhalation drugs, administered through DME
Epirubicin HCL	J9178	Injection, epirubicin HCL, 2 mg
Epogen	J0885	Injection, epoetin alfa, (for non-esrd use), 1000 units
Epoprostenol	J1325	Injection, epoprostenol, 0.5 mg
Eptifibatide	J1327	Injection, eptifibatide, 5 mg
Erbitux	J9055	Injection, cetuximab, 10 mg
Erivedge	J8999	Prescription drug, oral, chemotherapeutic, nos
Erythrocin lactobionate	J1364	Injection, erythromycin lactobionate, per 500 mg
Estradiol cypionate	J1000	Injection, depo-estradiol cypionate, up to 5 mg
Estradiol valerate	J1380	Injection, estradiol valerate, up to 10 mg
Estrone	J1435	Injection, estrone, per 1 mg
Ethamolin	J1430	Injection, ethanolamine oleate, 100 mg

NDC LABEL	HCPCS	HCPCS DESCRIPTION
Ethanolamine	J3490	Unclassified drugs
Etopophos	J9181	Injection, etoposide, 10 mg
Etoposide	J9181	Injection, etoposide, 10 mg
Euflexxa	J7323	Hyaluronan or derivative, Euflexxa, for intra-articular injection, per dose
Eylea	J0178	Injection, aflibercept, 1 mg
Fabrazyme	J0180	Injection, agalsidase beta, 1 mg
Famotidine	J3490	Unclassified drugs
Fentanyl citrate	J3010	Injection, fentanyl citrate, 0.1 mg
Flebogamma	J1572	Injection, immune globulin, (Flebogamma/Flebogamma dif), intravenous, non-lyophilized (e.g. liquid), 500 mg
Flolan	J1325	Injection, epoprostenol, 0.5 mg
Floxuridine	J9200	Injection, floxuridine, 500 mg
Fluconazole	J1450	Injection fluconazole, 200 mg
Fludarabine phosphate	J9185	Injection, fludarabine phosphate, 50 mg
Flunisolide anhydrous	J7641	Flunisolide, inhalation solution, compounded product, administered through DME, unit dose, per milligm
Fluorouracil	J9190	Injection, fluorouracil, 500 mg
Fluphenazine decanoate	J2680	Injection, fluphenazine decanoate, up to 25 mg
Flutamide	J8999	Prescription drug, oral, chemotherapeutic, nos
Fomepizole	J1451	Injection, fomepizole, 15 mg
Fondaparinux sodium	J1652	Injection, fondaparinux sodium, 0.5 mg
Formoterol fumarate	J7640	Formoterol, inhalation solution, compounded product, administered through DME, unit dose form, 12 microgms
Foscarnet sodium	J1455	Injection, foscarnet sodium, per 1000 mg
Fosphenytoin sodium	Q2009	Injection, fosphenytoin, 50 mg phenytoin equivalent
Fragmin	J1645	Injection, dalteparin sodium, per 2500 iu
Furosemide	J1940	Injection, furosemide, up to 20 mg
Fuzeon	J1324	Injection, enfuvirtide, 1 mg
GamaSTAN	J1460	Injection, gamma globulin, intramuscular, 1 cc
Gammagard	J1566	Injection, immune globulin, intravenous, lyophilized (e.g. powder), not otherwise specified, 500 mg
	J1569	Injection, immune globulin, (Gammagard liquid), non-lyophilized,(e.g. liquid), 500 mg
Gammaked	J1561	Injection, immune globulin, (Gamunex/Gamunex-c/gammaked), non-lyophilized (e.g. liquid), 500 mg
Gammaplex	J1557	Injection, immune globulin (Gammaplex), intravenous, non-lyophilized (e.g., liquid) 500 mg
Gamunex-c	J1561	Injection, immune globulin, (Gamunex-

NDC LABEL	HCPCS	HCPCS DESCRIPTION
		c/gammaked), non-lyophilized (e.g. liquid), 500 mg
Ganirelix acetate	J3490	Unclassified drugs
Gemcitabine	J9201	Injection, gemcitabine hydrochloride, 200 mg
Gemzar	J9201	Injection, gemcitabine hydrochloride, 200 mg
Genahist	Q0163	Diphenhydramine hydrochloride, 50 mg, oral, fad approved prescription anti-emetic, for use as a complete therapeutic substitute for an iv anti-emetic at time of chemotherapy treatment not to exceed a 48 hour dosage regimen
Gengraf	J7502	Cyclosporine, oral, 100 mg
Gengraf	J7515	Cyclosporine, oral, 25 mg
Genotropin	J2941	Injection, somatropin, 1 mg
Gentamicin sulfate	J1580	Injection, Garamycin, gentamicin, up to 80 mg
	J7699	NOC drugs, inhalation solution administered through DME
Geodon	J3486	Injection, ziprasidone mesylate, 10 mg
Geridryl	Q0163	Diphenhydramine hydrochloride, 50 mg, oral, fad approved prescription anti-emetic, for use as a complete therapeutic substitute for an iv anti-emetic at time of chemotherapy treatment not to exceed a 48 hour dosage regimen
Glassia	J0257	Injection, alpha 1 proteinase inhibitor (human), (glassia), 10 mg
Gleevec	J8999	Prescription drug, oral, chemotherapeutic, nos
GlucaGen	J1610	Injection, glucagon hydrochloride, per 1 mg
Glycopyrrolate	J7643	Glycopyrrolate, inhalation solution, compounded product, administered through DME, unit dose form, per milligm
Gold sodium thiomalate	J1600	Injection, gold sodium thiomalate, up to 50 mg
Gonal-f	J3490	Unclassified drugs
Good sense antihistamine allergy relief	Q0163	Diphenhydramine hydrochloride, 50 mg, oral, fad approved prescription anti-emetic, for use as a complete therapeutic substitute for an iv anti-emetic at time of chemotherapy treatment not to exceed a 48 hour dosage regimen
Good sense nighttime sleep aid	Q0163	Diphenhydramine hydrochloride, 50 mg, oral, fad approved prescription anti-emetic, for use as a complete therapeutic substitute for an iv anti-emetic at time of chemotherapy treatment not to exceed a 48 hour dosage regimen
Graftjacket	Q4107	Skin substitute, GraftJacket, per square centimeter
Granisetron HCL	J1626	Injection, granisetron hydrochloride, 100 mcg
	Q0166	Granisetron hydrochloride, 1 mg, oral, fad approved prescription anti-emetic, for use as a complete therapeutic substitute for an iv anti-

NDC LABEL	HCPCS	HCPCS DESCRIPTION
		emetic at the time of chemotherapy treatment, not to exceed a 24 hour dosage regimen
Haloperidol	J1630	Injection, haloperidol, up to 5 mg
Haloperidol Amerinet choice	J1631	Injection, haloperidol decanoate, per 50 mg
Haloperidol decanoate	J1631	Injection, haloperidol decanoate, per 50 mg
Haloperidol lactate	J1630	Injection, haloperidol, up to 5 mg
Hectorol	J1270	Injection, doxercalciferol, 1 mcg
HepaGam b	J1573	Injection, hepatitis b immune globulin (HepaGam b), intravenous, 0.5 ml
Heparin lock flush	J1642	Injection, heparin sodium, (heparin lock flush), per 10 units
Heparin sodium	J1644	Injection, heparin sodium, per 1000 units
Hepflush-10	J1642	Injection, heparin sodium, (heparin lock flush), per 10 units
Herceptin	J9355	Injection, trastuzumab, 10 mg
Hizentra	J1559	Injection, immune globulin (Hizentra), 100 mg
Humalog	J1815	Injection, insulin, per 5 units
Humalog	J1817	Insulin for administration through DME (i.e., insulin pump) per 50 units
Humatrope	J2941	Injection, somatropin, 1 mg
Humira	J0135	Injection, adalimumab, 20 mg
Humulin	J1815	Injection, insulin, per 5 units
Humulin r u-500	J1817	Insulin for administration through DME (i.e., insulin pump) per 50 units
Hyaluronic acid	J3490	Unclassified drugs
Hydralazine HCL	J0360	Injection, hydralazine HCL, up to 20 mg
Hydrea	J8999	Prescription drug, oral, chemotherapeutic, nos
Hydrocortisone acetate	J1700	Injection, hydrocortisone acetate, up to 25 mg
Hydromorphone HCL	J1170	Injection, hydromorphone, up to 4 mg
Hydroxocobalamin	J3420	Injection, vitamin b-12 cyaNOCobalamin, up to 1000 mcg
Hydroxyprogesterone caproate	J1725	Injection, hydroxyprogesterone caproate, 1 mg
Hydroxyurea	J8999	Prescription drug, oral, chemotherapeutic, nos
Hydroxyzine HCL	J3410	Injection, hydroxyzine HCL, up to 25 mg
Hydroxyzine pam	Q0177	Hydroxyzine pamoate, 25 mg, oral, fad approved prescription anti-emetic, for use as a complete therapeutic substitute for an iv anti-emetic at the time of chemotherapy treatment, not to exceed a 48 hour dosage regimen
Hydroxyzine pamoate	Q0169	Promethazine hydrochloride, 12.5 mg, oral, fad approved prescription anti-emetic, for use as a complete therapeutic substitute for an iv anti-emetic at the time of chemotherapy treatment, not to exceed a 48 hour dosage regimen
Hydroxyzine pamoate	Q0177	Hydroxyzine pamoate, 25 mg, oral, fad approved

NDC LABEL	HCPCS	HCPCS DESCRIPTION
		prescription anti-emetic, for use as a complete therapeutic substitute for an iv anti-emetic at the time of chemotherapy treatment, not to exceed a 48 hour dosage regimen
Hylenex	J3473	Injection, hyaluronidase, recombinant, 1 USP unit
Hyoscyamine sulfate	J1980	Injection, hyoscyamine sulfate, up to 0.25 mg
HyperHEP b	J3590	Unclassified biologics
HyperRHO	J2788	Injection, rho d immune globulin, human, minidose, 50 microgms (250 i.u.)
	J2790	Injection, rho d immune globulin, human, full dose, 300 microgms (1500 i.u.)
	J2792	Injection, rho d immune globulin, intravenous, human, solvent detergent, 100 iu
Hypertet	J1670	Injection, tetanus immune globulin, human, up to 250 units
Hyqvia	J1575	Injection, immune globulin/hyaluronidase, (hyqvia), 100 mg immune globulin
Ibandronate sodium	J1740	Injection, ibandronate sodium, 1 mg
Idamycin pfs	J9211	Injection, idarubicin hydrochloride, 5 mg
Idarubicin HCL	J9211	Injection, idarubicin hydrochloride, 5 mg
Ifosfamide	J9208	Injection, ifosfamide, 1 gm
Ifosfamide/mesna (combo-pack)	J9999	Not otherwise classified, antineoplastic drugs
Imitrex	J3030	Injection, sumatriptan succinate, 6 mg (code may be used for medicare when drug administered under the direct supervision of a physician, not for use when drug is self administered)
Imlygic	J9999	Not otherwise classified, antineoplastic drugs
Imuran	J7500	Azathioprine, oral, 50 mg
Increlex	J2170	Injection, mecasermin, 1 mg
INFeD	J1750	Injection, iron dextran, 50 mg
Infumorph	J2274	Injection, morphine sulfate, preservative-free for epidural or intrathecal use, 10 mg
Insulin-Humalog	J1817	Insulin for administration through DME (i.e., insulin pump) per 50 units
Integra bilayer matrix wound dressing	Q4104	Skin substitute, Integra bilayer matrix wound dressing (BMWD), per square centimeter
Integra dermal regeneration template	Q4105	Skin substitute, Integra dermal regeneration template (DRT), per square centimeter
Integra matrix wound dressing	Q4108	Skin substitute, Integra matrix, per square centimeter
Integrilin	J1327	Injection, eptifibatide, 5 mg
Intron a	J9214	Injection, interferon, alfa-2b, recombinant, 1 million units
Invanz	J1335	Injection, ertapenem sodium, 500 mg
Ipratropium bromide	J3535	Drug administered through a metered dose inhaler
	J7644	Ipratropium bromide, inhalation solution, fad-

NDC LABEL	HCPCS	HCPCS DESCRIPTION
		approved final product, non-compounded, administered through DME, unit dose form, per milligram
	J7645	Ipratropium bromide, inhalation solution, compounded product, administered through DME, unit dose form, per milligm
Ipratropium bromide and albuterol sulfate	J7620	Albuterol, up to 2.5 mg and ipratropium bromide, up to 0.5 mg, fad-approved final product, non-compounded, administered through DME
Iressa	J8565	Gefitinib, oral, 250 mg
Irinotecan HCL	J9206	Injection, irinotecan, 20 mg
Itraconazole	J1835	Injection, itraconazole, 50 mg
Ixempra	J9207	Injection, ixabepilone, 1 mg
Kenalog	J3301	Injection, triamcinolone acetonide, not otherwise specified, 10 mg
Ketorolac tromethamine	J1885	Injection, ketorolac tromethamine, per 15 mg
Kinevac	J2805	Injection, sincalide, 5 microgms
Kogenate fs	J7192	Factor viii (antihemophilic factor, recombinant) per i.u., not otherwise specified
Kyprolis	J9047	Injection, carfilzomib, 1 mg
Lactated ringer's	J7120	Ringers lactate infusion, up to 1000 cc
Lantus	J1815	Injection, insulin, per 5 units
L-carnitine free base	J1955	Injection, levocarnitine, per 1 gm
L-carnitine HCL	J1955	Injection, levocarnitine, per 1 gm
Leucovorin calcium	J0640	Injection, leucovorin calcium, per 50 mg
Leukeran	J8999	Prescription drug, oral, chemotherapeutic, nos
Leuprolide acetate	J9218	Leuprolide acetate, per 1 mg
Levalbuterol	J7612	Levalbuterol, inhalation solution, fad-approved final product, non-compounded, administered through DME, unit dose, 0.5 mg
	J7614	Levalbuterol, inhalation solution, fad-approved final product, non-compounded, administered through DME, unit dose, 0.5 mg
Levetiracetam	J1953	Injection, levetiracetam, 10 mg
Levocarnitine	J1955	Injection, levocarnitine, per 1 gm
Levofloxacin	J1956	Injection, levofloxacin, 250 mg
Levoleucovorin calcium	J0641	Injection, levoleucovorin calcium, 0.5 mg
Levorphanol tartrate	J1960	Injection, levorphanol tartrate, up to 2 mg
Levulan Kerastick	J7308	Aminolevulinic acid HCL for topical administration, 20%, single unit dosage form (354 mg)
Lidocaine	J2001	Injection, lidocaine HCL for intravenous infusion, 10 mg

NDC LABEL	HCPCS	HCPCS DESCRIPTION
Lincocin	J2010	Injection, lincomycin HCL, up to 300 mg
Lincomycin HCL	J2010	Injection, lincomycin HCL, up to 300 mg
Linezolid	J2020	Injection, linezolid, 200 mg
Lioresal intrathecal refill kit	J0475	Injection, baclofen, 10 mg
Lioresal intrathecal screening kit	J0476	Injection, baclofen, 50 mcg for intrathecal trial
LMD in dextrose	J7100	Infusion, dextran 40, 500 ml
Lorazepam	J2060	Injection, lorazepam, 2 mg
Lovenox	J1650	Injection, enoxaparin sodium, 10 mg
Lucentis	J2778	Injection, ranibizumab, 0.1 mg
Lupron depot	J1950	Injection, leuprolide acetate (for depot suspension), per 3.75 mg
Lupron depot	J9217	Leuprolide acetate (for depot suspension), 7.5 mg
Magnesium sulfate	J3475	Injection, magnesium sulfate, per 500 mg
Makena	J1725	Injection, hydroxyprogesterone caproate, 1 mg
Mannitol	J2150	Injection, mannitol, 25% in 50 ml
	J7799	NOC drugs, other than inhalation drugs, administered through DME
Marcaine	J3490	Unclassified drugs
Marinol	Q0167	Dronabinol, 2.5 mg, oral, fad approved prescription anti-emetic, for use as a complete therapeutic substitute for an iv anti-emetic at the time of chemotherapy treatment, not to exceed a 48 hour dosage regimen
Matulane	J8999	Prescription drug, oral, chemotherapeutic, nos
Mediphedryl	Q0163	Diphenhydramine hydrochloride, 50 mg, oral, fad approved prescription anti-emetic, for use as a complete therapeutic substitute for an iv anti-emetic at time of chemotherapy treatment not to exceed a 48 hour dosage regimen
Medrol	J7509	Methylprednisolone oral, per 4 mg
Medroxyprogesterone acetate	J1050	Injection, medroxyprogesterone acetate, 1 mg
Megace	J8999	Prescription drug, oral, chemotherapeutic, nos
Megestrol acetate	J8999	Prescription drug, oral, chemotherapeutic, nos
Menadione	J3430	Injection, phytonadione (vitamin k), per 1 mg
Meperidine HCL	J2175	Injection, meperidine hydrochloride, per 100 mg
Mepivacaine HCL	J0670	Injection, mepivacaine hydrochloride, per 10 ml
Mercaptopurine	J8999	Prescription drug, oral, chemotherapeutic, nos
Meropenem	J2185	Injection, meropenem, 100 mg
Merrem iv	J2185	Injection, meropenem, 100 mg
Mesna	J9209	Injection, mesna, 200 mg
Methadone HCL	J1230	Injection, methadone HCL, up to 10 mg
Methocarbamol	J2800	Injection, methocarbamol, up to 10 ml
Methotrexate	J8610	Methotrexate; oral, 2.5 mg

NDC LABEL	HCPCS	HCPCS DESCRIPTION
Methotrexate sodium	J9250	Methotrexate sodium, 5 mg
	J9260	Methotrexate sodium, 50 mg
Methyldopate HCL	J0210	Injection, methyldopate HCL, up to 250 mg
Methylprednisolone acetate	J1030	Injection, methylprednisolone acetate, 40 mg
Methylprednisolone acetate	J1040	Injection, methylprednisolone acetate, 80 mg
Methylprednisolone acetate	J7509	Methylprednisolone oral, per 4 mg
Methylprednisolone sodium succinate	J2920	Injection, methylprednisolone sodium succinate, up to 40 mg
	J2930	Injection, methylprednisolone sodium succinate, up to 125 mg
Metoclopramide HCL	J2765	Injection, metoclopramide HCL, up to 10 mg
Metrodin	J3355	Injection, urofollitropin, 75 iu
Metronidazole	J3490	Unclassified drugs
Miacalcin	J0630	Injection, calcitonin salmon, up to 400 units
MICRhoGAM ultra-filtered plus	J2788	Injection, rho d immune globulin, human, minidose, 50 microgms (250 i.u.)
Midazolam	J2250	Injection, midazolam hydrochloride, per 1 mg
Milrinone lactate	J2260	Injection, milrinone lactate, 5 mg
Mitoxantrone	J9293	Injection, mitoxantrone hydrochloride, per 5 mg
Monoject prefill advanced	A4216	Sterile water, saline and/or dextrose, diluent/flush, 10 ml
Monoject prefill heparin lock flush	J1642	Injection, heparin sodium, (heparin lock flush), per 10 units
Morphine sulfate	J2270	Injection, morphine sulfate, up to 10 mg
	J2274	Injection, morphine sulfate, preservative-free for epidural or intrathecal use, 10 mg
Moxifloxacin HCL	J2280	Injection, moxifloxacin, 100 mg
Mycamine	J2248	Injection, micafungin sodium, 1 mg
Mycophenolate mofetil	J7517	Mycophenolate mofetil, oral, 250 mg
Mycophenolic acid	J7518	Mycophenolic acid, oral, 180 mg
Myfortic	J7518	Mycophenolic acid, oral, 180 mg
Myobloc	J0587	Injection, rimabotulinumtoxinB, 100 units
Nabi-HB	J3590	Unclassified biologics
Nafcillin	J3490	Unclassified drugs
Naglazyme	J1458	Injection, galsulfase, 1 mg
Nalbuphine HCL	J2300	Injection, nalbuphine hydrochloride, per 10 mg
Naloxone HCL	J2310	Injection, naloxone hydrochloride, per 1 mg
Naltrexone HCL	J3490	Unclassified drugs
Naropin	J2795	Injection, ropivacaine hydrochloride, 1 mg
Natrecor	J2325	Injection, nesiritide, 0.1 mg
Navelbine	J9390	Injection, vinorelbine tartrate, 10 mg
NebuPent	J2545	Pentamidine isethionate, inhalation solution, compounded product, administered through DME,

NDC LABEL	HCPCS	HCPCS DESCRIPTION
		unit dose form, per 300 mg
Neoral	J7502	Cyclosporine, oral, 100 mg
	J7515	Cyclosporine, oral, 25 mg
Neostigmine methylsulfate	J2710	Injection, neostigmine methylsulfate, up to 0.5 mg
Neo-synephrine HCL	J2370	Injection, phenylephrine HCL, up to 1 ml
Neulasta	J2505	Injection, pegfilgrastim, 6 mg
Neupogen	J1442	Injection, filgrastim (g-csf), excludes biosimilars, 1 microgm
Night time sleep aid	Q0163	Diphenhydramine hydrochloride, 50 mg, oral, fad approved prescription anti-emetic, for use as a complete therapeutic substitute for an iv anti-emetic at time of chemotherapy treatment not to exceed a 48 hour dosage regimen
Nipent	J9268	Injection, pentostatin, 10 mg
Nolvadex	J8999	Prescription drug, oral, chemotherapeutic, nos
Norditropin flexpro (prefilled purple pen)	J2941	Injection, somatropin, 1 mg
Normal saline flush	A4216	Sterile water, saline and/or dextrose, diluent/flush, 10 ml
Novaplus ampicillin	J0290	Injection, ampicillin sodium, 500 mg
Novaplus ampicillin and sulbactam	J0295	Injection, ampicillin sodium/sulbactam sodium, per 1.5 gm
Novaplus azithromycin	J0456	Injection, azithromycin, 500 mg
Novaplus butorphanol tartrate	J0595	Injection, butorphanol tartrate, 1 mg
Novaplus carboplatin	J9045	Injection, carboplatin, 50 mg
Novaplus cefazolin	J0690	Injection, cefazolin sodium, 500 mg
Novaplus cefoxitin	J0694	Injection, cefoxitin sodium, 1 gm
Novaplus Claforan	J0698	Injection, cefotaxime sodium, per gm
Novaplus Diprivan	J3490	Unclassified drugs
Novaplus epirubicin HCL	J9178	Injection, epirubicin HCL, 2 mg
Novaplus haloperidol decanoate	J1631	Injection, haloperidol decanoate, per 50 mg
Novaplus HepaGam b	J1573	Injection, hepatitis b immune globulin (HepaGam b), intravenous, 0.5 ml
Novaplus hydralazine HCL	J0360	Injection, hydralazine HCL, up to 20 mg
Novaplus midazolam HCL	J2250	Injection, midazolam hydrochloride, per 1 mg
Novaplus nafcillin	J3490	Unclassified drugs
Novaplus oxacillin	J2700	Injection, oxacillin sodium, up to 250 mg
Novaplus oxytocin	J2590	Injection, oxytocin, up to 10 units
Novaplus protamine sulfate	J2720	Injection, protamine sulfate, per 10 mg
Novaplus Tazicef	J0713	Injection, ceftazidime, per 500 mg
Novarel	J0725	Injection, chorionic gonadotropin, per 1,000 USP units
Novolin	J1815	Injection, insulin, per 5 units
NovoLog	J1815	Injection, insulin, per 5 units

NDC LABEL	HCPCS	HCPCS DESCRIPTION
	J1817	Insulin for administration through DME (i.e., insulin pump) per 50 units
Nplate	J2796	Injection, romiplostim, 10 microgms
Nutropin aq pen cartridge	J2941	Injection, somatropin, 1 mg
Nytol QuickCaps	Q0163	Diphenhydramine hydrochloride, 50 mg, oral, fad approved prescription anti-emetic, for use as a complete therapeutic substitute for an iv anti-emetic at time of chemotherapy treatment not to exceed a 48 hour dosage regimen
Octagam	J1568	Injection, immune globulin, (Octagam), intravenous, non-lyophilized (e.g. liquid), 500 mg
Octreotide acetate	J2354	Injection, octreotide, non-depot form for subcutaneous or intravenous injection, 25 mcg
Ofev	J8499	Prescription drug, oral, non chemotherapeutic, nos
Omnitrope	J2941	Injection, somatropin, 1 mg
Oncaspar	J9266	Injection, pegaspargase, per single dose vial
Ondansetron HCL	J2405	Injection, ondansetron hydrochloride, per 1 mg
	Q0162	Ondansetron 1 mg, oral, fad approved prescription anti-emetic, for use as a complete therapeutic substitute for an iv anti-emetic at the time of chemotherapy treatment, not to exceed a 48 hour dosage regimen
Opana	J2410	Injection, oxymorphone HCL, up to 1 mg
Opdivo	J9299	Injection, nivolumab, 1 mg
Orapred	J7510	Prednisolone oral, per 5 mg
Orencia clickject	J0129	Injection, abatacept, 10 mg
Orphenadrine citrate	J2360	Injection, orphenadrine citrate, up to 60 mg
Orthovisc (prefilled syringe)	J7324	Hyaluronan or derivative, Orthovisc, for intra-articular injection, per dose
Osmitrol	J7799	NOC drugs, other than inhalation drugs, administered through DME
Ovidrel	J3490	Unclassified drugs
Oxacillin	J2700	Injection, oxacillin sodium, up to 250 mg
Oxaliplatin	J9263	Injection, oxaliplatin, 0.5 mg
Oxytetracycline HCL	J2460	Injection, oxytetracycline HCL, up to 50 mg
Oxytocin	J2590	Injection, oxytocin, up to 10 units
Paclitaxel	J9267	Injection, paclitaxel, 1 mg
Pamidronate disodium	J2430	Injection, pamidronate disodium, per 30 mg
Papaverine HCL	J2440	Injection, papaverine HCL, up to 60 mg
Paricalcitol	J2501	Injection, paricalcitol, 1 mcg
Pediapred	J7510	Prednisolone oral, per 5 mg
Pegasys	J3490	Unclassified drugs
Peg-intron	J3490	Unclassified drugs
Penicillin g potassium	J2540	Injection, penicillin g potassium, up to 600,000

NDC LABEL	HCPCS	HCPCS DESCRIPTION
		units
Penicillin g procaine	J2510	Injection, penicillin g procaine, aqueous, up to 600,000 units
Penicillin g sodium	J3490	Unclassified drugs
Pentam	J7676	Pentamidine isethionate, inhalation solution, compounded product, administered through DME, unit dose form, per 300 mg
Pentobarbital sodium	J2515	Injection, pentobarbital sodium, per 50 mg
Perforomist	J7606	Formoterol fumarate, inhalation solution, fad approved final product, non-compounded, administered through DME, unit dose form, 20 microgms
Perphenazine	Q0169	Perphenazine, 4 mg, oral, fad approved prescription anti-emetic, for use as a complete therapeutic substitute for an iv anti-emetic at the time of chemotherapy treatment, not to exceed a 48 hour dosage regimen
	Q0175	Perphenazine, 4 mg, oral, fad approved prescription anti-emetic, for use as a complete therapeutic substitute for an iv anti-emetic at the time of chemotherapy treatment, not to exceed a 48 hour dosage regimen
Pfizerpen	J2540	Injection, penicillin g potassium, up to 600,000 units
Phenadoz	J8498	Antiemetic drug, rectal/suppository, not otherwise specified
Phenergan	J2550	Injection, promethazine HCL, up to 50 mg
Phenobarbital sodium	J2560	Injection, phenobarbital sodium, up to 120 mg
Phentolamine mesylate	J2760	Injection, phentolamine mesylate, up to 5 mg
Phenylephrine HCL	J2370	Injection, phenylephrine HCL, up to 1 ml
	J7799	NOC drugs, other than inhalation drugs, administered through DME
Phenytoin sodium	J1165	Injection, phenytoin sodium, per 50 mg
Phytonadione	J3430	Injection, phytonadione (vitamin k), per 1 mg
Piperacillin and tazobactam	J2543	Injection, piperacillin sodium/tazobactam sodium, 1 gm/0.125 gms (1.125 gms)
Pitocin	J2590	Injection, oxytocin, up to 10 units
Polocaine-mpf	J0670	Injection, mepivacaine hydrochloride, per 10 ml
Polygam	J1566	Injection, immune globulin, intravenous, lyophilized (e.g. powder), not otherwise specified, 500 mg
Potassium chloride	J3480	Injection, potassium chloride, per 2 mEq
Potassium chloride solution	J7120	Ringers lactate infusion, up to 1000 cc
Pralidoxime chloride	J2730	Injection, pralidoxime chloride, up to 1 gm
Prednicot	J7512	Prednisone, immediate release or delayed release, oral, 1 mg

NDC LABEL	HCPCS	HCPCS DESCRIPTION
Prednisolone	J7510	Prednisolone oral, per 5 mg
Prednisolone acetate micronized	J2650	Injection, prednisolone acetate, up to 1 ml
Prednisone	J7512	Prednisone, immediate release or delayed release, oral, 1 mg
Pregnyl	J0725	Injection, chorionic gonadotropin, per 1,000 USP units
Premarin intravenous	J1410	Injection, estrogen conjugated, per 25 mg
Premierpro rx ampicillin	J0290	Injection, ampicillin sodium, 500 mg
Premierpro rx furosemide	J1940	Injection, furosemide, up to 20 mg
Prialt	J2278	Injection, ziconotide, 1 microgm
Primatrix dermal repair scaffold	Q4110	Skin substitute, Primatrix, per square centimeter
Primaxin iv	J0743	Injection, cilastatin sodium; imipenem, per 250 mg
Privigen	J1459	Injection, immune globulin (Privigen), intravenous, non-lyophilized (e.g. liquid), 500 mg
Procainamide HCL	J2690	Injection, procainamide HCL, up to 1 gm
Prochlorperazine	J8498	Antiemetic drug, rectal/suppository, not otherwise specified
Prochlorperazine	Q0164	Prochlorperazine maleate, 5 mg, oral, fad approved prescription anti-emetic, for use as a complete therapeutic substitute for an iv anti-emetic at the time of chemotherapy treatment, not to exceed a 48 hour dosage regimen
Prochlorperazine edisylate	J0780	Injection, prochlorperazine, up to 10 mg
Prochlorperazine maleate	Q0164	Prochlorperazine maleate, 5 mg, oral, fad approved prescription anti-emetic, for use as a complete therapeutic substitute for an iv anti-emetic at the time of chemotherapy treatment, not to exceed a 48 hour dosage regimen
Procrit	J0885	Injection, epoetin alfa, (for non-esrd use), 1000 units
Progesterone	J2675	Injection, progesterone, per 50 mg
Progesterone in sesame oil	J2675	Injection, progesterone, per 50 mg
Progesterone micronized	J2675	Injection, progesterone, per 50 mg
Prograf	J7507	Tacrolimus, immediate release, oral, 1 mg
	J7525	Tacrolimus, parenteral, 5 mg
Prolastin-c	J0256	Injection, alpha 1 proteinase inhibitor (human), not otherwise specified, 10 mg
Prolia	J0897	Injection, denosumab, 1 mg
Promethazine	J8498	Antiemetic drug, rectal/suppository, not otherwise specified
	Q0169	Promethazine hydrochloride, 12.5 mg, oral, fad approved prescription anti-emetic, for use as a complete therapeutic substitute for an iv anti-emetic at the time of chemotherapy treatment, not to exceed a 48 hour dosage regimen

NDC LABEL	HCPCS	HCPCS DESCRIPTION
Promethazine HCL	J2550	Injection, promethazine HCL, up to 50 mg
	J8498	Antiemetic drug, rectal/suppository, not otherwise specified
	Q0169	Promethazine hydrochloride, 12.5 mg, oral, fad approved prescription anti-emetic, for use as a complete therapeutic substitute for an iv anti-emetic at the time of chemotherapy treatment, not to exceed a 48 hour dosage regimen
Promethazine HCL (Luer lock, Carpuject)	J2550	Injection, promethazine HCL, up to 50 mg
Promethazine HCL (Redi-script)	Q0169	Promethazine hydrochloride, 12.5 mg, oral, fad approved prescription anti-emetic, for use as a complete therapeutic substitute for an iv anti-emetic at the time of chemotherapy treatment, not to exceed a 48 hour dosage regimen
Promethegan	J8498	Antiemetic drug, rectal/suppository, not otherwise specified
Propofol	J3490	Unclassified drugs
Propranolol	J1800	Injection, propranolol HCL, up to 1 mg
Prostaglandin e1	J0270	Injection, alprostadil, 1.25 mcg (code may be used for medicare when drug administered under the direct supervision of a physician, not for use when drug is self administered)
Prostin vr pediatric	J0270	Injection, alprostadil, 1.25 mcg (code may be used for medicare when drug administered under the direct supervision of a physician, not for use when drug is self administered)
Protamine sulfate	J2720	Injection, protamine sulfate, per 10 mg
Protirelin	J2725	Injection, protirelin, per 250 mcg
Protonix	J3490	Unclassified drugs
Protopam chloride	J2730	Injection, pralidoxime chloride, up to 1 gm
Provocholine	J7674	Methacholine chloride administered as inhalation solution through a nebulizer, per 1 mg
Pulmicort Respules	J7626	Budesonide, inhalation solution, fad-approved final product, non-compounded, administered through DME, unit dose form, up to 0.5 mg
Pulmozyme	J7639	Dornase alpha, inhalation solution administered through DME, unit dose form, per milligm
Pyridoxine	J3415	Injection, pyridoxine HCL, 100 mg
Q-dryl	Q0163	Diphenhydramine hydrochloride, 50 mg, oral, fad approved prescription anti-emetic, for use as a complete therapeutic substitute for an iv anti-emetic at time of chemotherapy treatment not to exceed a 48 hour dosage regimen
Quality choice sleep aid	Q0163	Diphenhydramine hydrochloride, 50 mg, oral, fad approved prescription anti-emetic, for use as a complete therapeutic substitute for an iv anti-emetic at time of chemotherapy treatment not to

NDC LABEL	HCPCS	HCPCS DESCRIPTION
		exceed a 48 hour dosage regimen
Quelicin	J0330	Injection, succinylcholine chloride, up to 20 mg
Quenalin	Q0163	Diphenhydramine hydrochloride, 50 mg, oral, fad approved prescription anti-emetic, for use as a complete therapeutic substitute for an iv anti-emetic at time of chemotherapy treatment not to exceed a 48 hour dosage regimen
Ranitidine HCL	J2780	Injection, ranitidine hydrochloride, 25 mg
Rapamune	J7520	Sirolimus, oral, 1 mg
Rapidpaq dicopanol	Q0163	Diphenhydramine hydrochloride, 50 mg, oral, fad approved prescription anti-emetic, for use as a complete therapeutic substitute for an iv anti-emetic at time of chemotherapy treatment not to exceed a 48 hour dosage regimen
Recombivax hb	J3490	Unclassified drugs
Remicade	J1745	Injection infliximab, 10 mg
Remodulin	J3285	Injection, treprostinil, 1 mg
ReoPro	J0130	Injection abciximab, 10 mg
Resectisol	J7799	NOC drugs, other than inhalation drugs, administered through DME
Retisert	J7311	Fluocinolone acetonide, intravitreal implant
RhoGAM ultra-filtered plus	J2790	Injection, rho d immune globulin, human, full dose, 300 microgms (1500 i.u.)
Rhophylac	J2791	Injection, rho(d) immune globulin (human), (Rhophylac), intramuscular or intravenous, 100 iu
Rifadin iv	J3490	Unclassified drugs
Rifampin	J3490	Unclassified drugs
Rimso-50	J1212	Injection, DMSO, dimethyl sulfoxide, 50%, 50 ml
Risperdal consta	J2794	Injection, risperidone, long acting, 0.5 mg
Rite aid allergy	Q0163	Diphenhydramine hydrochloride, 50 mg, oral, fad approved prescription anti-emetic, for use as a complete therapeutic substitute for an iv anti-emetic at time of chemotherapy treatment not to exceed a 48 hour dosage regimen
Rituxan	J9310	Injection, rituximab, 100 mg
Robaxin	J2800	Injection, methocarbamol, up to 10 ml
Ropivacaine HCL	J2795	Injection, ropivacaine hydrochloride, 1 mg
Ropivacaine HCL-sodium chloride	J3490	Unclassified drugs
Saizen	J2941	Injection, somatropin, 1 mg
Saline solution	A4216	Sterile water, saline and/or dextrose, diluent/flush, 10 ml
Sandimmune	J7502	Cyclosporine, oral, 100 mg
	J7515	Cyclosporine, oral, 25 mg
	J7516	Cyclosporin, parenteral, 250 mg
Sandostatin	J2354	Injection, octreotide, non-depot form for

NDC LABEL	HCPCS	HCPCS DESCRIPTION
		subcutaneous or intravenous injection, 25 mcg
Sandostatin lar depot	J2353	Injection, octreotide, depot form for intramuscular injection, 1 mg
Sensorcaine-mpf	J3490	Unclassified drugs
Serabrina la France	Q0163	Diphenhydramine hydrochloride, 50 mg, oral, fad approved prescription anti-emetic, for use as a complete therapeutic substitute for an iv anti-emetic at time of chemotherapy treatment not to exceed a 48 hour dosage regimen
Serostim	J2941	Injection, somatropin, 1 mg
Signifor lar	J2502	Injection, Pasireotide long acting, 1 mg
Siladryl allergy	Q0163	Diphenhydramine hydrochloride, 50 mg, oral, fad approved prescription anti-emetic, for use as a complete therapeutic substitute for an iv anti-emetic at time of chemotherapy treatment not to exceed a 48 hour dosage regimen
Silphen	Q0163	Diphenhydramine hydrochloride, 50 mg, oral, fad approved prescription anti-emetic, for use as a complete therapeutic substitute for an iv anti-emetic at time of chemotherapy treatment not to exceed a 48 hour dosage regimen
Simply sleep	Q0163	Diphenhydramine hydrochloride, 50 mg, oral, fad approved prescription anti-emetic, for use as a complete therapeutic substitute for an iv anti-emetic at time of chemotherapy treatment not to exceed a 48 hour dosage regimen
Simulect	J0480	Injection, basiliximab, 20 mg
Sirolimus	J7520	Sirolimus, oral, 1 mg
Sleep tabs	Q0163	Diphenhydramine hydrochloride, 50 mg, oral, fad approved prescription anti-emetic, for use as a complete therapeutic substitute for an iv anti-emetic at time of chemotherapy treatment not to exceed a 48 hour dosage regimen
Sleepinal	Q0163	Diphenhydramine hydrochloride, 50 mg, oral, fad approved prescription anti-emetic, for use as a complete therapeutic substitute for an iv anti-emetic at time of chemotherapy treatment not to exceed a 48 hour dosage regimen
Sleep-tabs	Q0163	Diphenhydramine hydrochloride, 50 mg, oral, fad approved prescription anti-emetic, for use as a complete therapeutic substitute for an iv anti-emetic at time of chemotherapy treatment not to exceed a 48 hour dosage regimen
Smz-tmp	J3490	Unclassified drugs
Sodium chloride	A4216	Sterile water, saline and/or dextrose, diluent/flush, 10 ml
	A4217	Sterile water/saline, 500 ml
	A4218	Sterile saline or water, metered dose dispenser,

NDC LABEL	HCPCS	HCPCS DESCRIPTION
		10 ml
	J7030	Infusion, normal saline solution , 1000 cc
	J7040	Infusion, normal saline solution, sterile (500 ml=1 unit)
	J7050	Infusion, normal saline solution , 250 cc
	J7799	NOC drugs, other than inhalation drugs, administered through DME
Sodium chloride (LifeCare)	A4216	Sterile water, saline and/or dextrose, diluent/flush, 10 ml
	J7030	Infusion, normal saline solution , 1000 cc
	J7040	Infusion, normal saline solution, sterile (500 ml=1 unit)
	J7050	Infusion, normal saline solution , 250 cc
	J7799	NOC drugs, other than inhalation drugs, administered through DME
Sodium chloride (Luer lock)	A4216	Sterile water, saline and/or dextrose, diluent/flush, 10 ml
Sodium chloride concentrate	J7799	NOC drugs, other than inhalation drugs, administered through DME
Sodium chloride/respiratory therapy	A4216	Sterile water, saline and/or dextrose, diluent/flush, 10 ml
Sodium chloride/tobramycin sulfate (premix)	J3260	Injection, tobramycin sulfate, up to 80 mg
Sodium ferric gluconate complex in sucrose	J2916	Injection, sodium ferric gluconate complex in sucrose injection, 12.5 mg
Soliris	J1300	Injection, eculizumab, 10 mg
Solu-Cortef	J1720	Injection, hydrocortisone sodium succinate, up to 100 mg
Solu-Medrol	J2930	Injection, methylprednisolone sodium succinate, up to 125 mg
Somatuline depot	J1930	Injection, lanreotide, 1 mg
Sominex	Q0163	Diphenhydramine hydrochloride, 50 mg, oral, fad approved prescription anti-emetic, for use as a complete therapeutic substitute for an iv anti-emetic at time of chemotherapy treatment not to exceed a 48 hour dosage regimen
Sterile water bacteriostatic	A4216	Sterile water, saline and/or dextrose, diluent/flush, 10 ml
Streptomycin sulfate	J3000	Injection, streptomycin, up to 1 gm
Sufentanil citrate	J3490	Unclassified drugs
Sumatriptan succinate	J3030	Injection, sumatriptan succinate, 6 mg (code may be used for medicare when drug administered under the direct supervision of a physician, not for use when drug is self administered)
Sumavel DosePro	J3030	Injection, sumatriptan succinate, 6 mg (code may be used for medicare when drug administered under the direct supervision of a physician, not for

NDC LABEL	HCPCS	HCPCS DESCRIPTION
		use when drug is self administered)
Supprelin la	J9226	Histrelin implant (Supprelin la), 50 mg
Surgimend collagen matrix	Q4100	Skin substitute, not otherwise specified
Synercid	J2770	Injection, quinupristin/dalfopristin, 500 mg (150/350)
Synribo	J9262	Injection, omacetaxine mepesuccinate, 0.01 mg
Syrex	A4216	Sterile water, saline and/or dextrose, diluent/flush, 10 ml
Tacrolimus	J7507	Tacrolimus, immediate release, oral, 1 mg
Talwin lactate	J3070	Injection, pentazocine, 30 mg
Tamoxifen citrate	J8999	Prescription drug, oral, chemotherapeutic, nos
Tazicef	J0713	Injection, ceftazidime, per 500 mg
Terbutaline sulfate	J3105	Injection, terbutaline sulfate, up to 1 mg
	J7681	Terbutaline sulfate, inhalation solution, compounded product, administered through DME, unit dose form, per milligm
Testopel pellets	J3490	Unclassified drugs
Testosterone cypionate	J1071	Injection, testosterone cypionate, 1 mg
Testosterone enanthate	J3121	Injection, testosterone enanthate,1 mg
Testosterone propionate	J3490	Unclassified drugs
Theophylline	J2810	Injection, theophylline, per 40 mg
Thiamine HCL	J3411	Injection, thiamine HCL, 100 mg
Thiotepa	J9340	Injection, thiotepa, 15 mg
Thrombate iii	J7197	Antithrombin iii (human), per i.u.
Thymoglobulin	J7511	Lymphocyte immune globulin, antithymocyte globulin, rabbit, parenteral, 25 mg
Thyrogen	J3240	Injection, thyrotropin alpha, 0.9 mg, provided in 1.1 mg vial
Tice BCG	J9031	BCG (intravesical) per instillation
Tigan	J3250	Injection, trimethobenzamide HCL, up to 200 mg
Tigan	Q0173	Trimethobenzamide hydrochloride, 250 mg, oral, fad approved prescription anti-emetic, for use as a complete therapeutic substitute for an iv anti-emetic at the time of chemotherapy treatment, not to exceed a 48 hour dosage regimen
TissueMend	Q4109	Skin substitute, TissueMend, per square centimeter
TOBI	J7682	Tobramycin, inhalation solution, fad-approved final product, non-compounded, unit dose form, administered through DME, per 300 milligms
Tobramycin	J7682	Tobramycin, inhalation solution, fad-approved final product, non-compounded, unit dose form, administered through DME, per 300 milligms
	J7685	Tobramycin, inhalation solution, compounded product, administered through DME, unit dose

NDC LABEL	HCPCS	HCPCS DESCRIPTION
		form, per 300 milligms
Tobramycin sulfate	J3260	Injection, tobramycin sulfate, up to 80 mg
Tobramycin sulfate	J7685	Tobramycin, inhalation solution, compounded product, administered through DME, unit dose form, per 300 milligms
Topotecan HCL	J9351	Injection, topotecan, 0.1 mg
Treanda	J3490	Unclassified drugs
Trelstar depot	J3315	Injection, triptorelin pamoate, 3.75 mg
Trelstar la	J3315	Injection, triptorelin pamoate, 3.75 mg
Triamcinolone	J7684	Triamcinolone, inhalation solution, compounded product, administered through DME, unit dose form, per milligm
Triamcinolone diacetate	J3302	Injection, triamcinolone diacetate, per 5 mg
Triesence	J3301	Injection, triamcinolone acetonide, not otherwise specified, 10 mg
Triethylenethiophosphoramide	J9340	Injection, thiotepa, 15 mg
Trimethobenzamide HCL	J3250	Injection, trimethobenzamide HCL, up to 200 mg
	Q0173	Trimethobenzamide hydrochloride, 250 mg, oral, fad approved prescription anti-emetic, for use as a complete therapeutic substitute for an iv anti-emetic at the time of chemotherapy treatment, not to exceed a 48 hour dosage regimen
Trisenox	J9017	Injection, arsenic trioxide, 1 mg
Twilite	Q0163	Diphenhydramine hydrochloride, 50 mg, oral, fad approved prescription anti-emetic, for use as a complete therapeutic substitute for an iv anti-emetic at time of chemotherapy treatment not to exceed a 48 hour dosage regimen
Twinrix	J3490	Unclassified drugs
Tygacil	J3243	Injection, tigecycline, 1 mg
Tyvaso	J7686	NOC drugs, inhalation solution administered through DME
Unasyn	J0295	Injection, ampicillin sodium/sulbactam sodium, per 1.5 gm
Urea	J3350	Injection, urea, up to 40 gm
Valcyte	J3490	Immunosuppressive drug, not otherwise classified
Valganciclovir HCL	J8499	Prescription drug, oral, non chemotherapeutic, nos
Valstar	J9357	Injection, valrubicin, intravesical, 200 mg
Valu-dryl allergy	Q0163	Diphenhydramine hydrochloride, 50 mg, oral, fad approved prescription anti-emetic, for use as a complete therapeutic substitute for an iv anti-emetic at time of chemotherapy treatment not to exceed a 48 hour dosage regimen
Vancocin HCL	J3370	Injection, vancomycin HCL, 500 mg
Vancomycin HCL	J3370	Injection, vancomycin HCL, 500 mg

NDC LABEL	HCPCS	HCPCS DESCRIPTION
Vantas	J9226	Histrelin implant (Supprelin la), 50 mg
Varubi	Q9981	Rolapitant, oral, 1 mg
Vasceze heparin lock flush (Luer slip nozzle)	J1642	Injection, heparin sodium, (heparin lock flush), per 10 units
Vasceze sodium chloride (Luer slip nozzle)	A4216	Sterile water, saline and/or dextrose, diluent/flush, 10 ml
Vectibix	J9303	Injection, panitumumab, 10 mg
Velcade	J9041	Injection, bortezomib, 0.1 mg
Veletri	J1325	Injection, epoprostenol, 0.5 mg
Venofer	J1756	Injection, iron sucrose, 1 mg
Veritas collagen matrix	J3490	Unclassified drugs
Vfend	J3465	Injection, voriconazole, 10 mg
Vibativ	J3095	Injection, telavancin, 10 mg
Vinblastine sulfate	J9360	Injection, vinblastine sulfate, 1 mg
Vincristine sulfate	J9370	Vincristine sulfate, 1 mg
Vinorelbine	J9390	Injection, vinorelbine tartrate, 10 mg
Vistaril	Q0177	Hydroxyzine pamoate, 25 mg, oral, fad approved prescription anti-emetic, for use as a complete therapeutic substitute for an iv anti-emetic at the time of chemotherapy treatment, not to exceed a 48 hour dosage regimen
Vistide	J0740	Injection, cidofovir, 375 mg
Vitamin b12	J3420	Injection, vitamin b-12 cyaNOCobalamin, up to 1000 mcg
Vitrase	J3471	Injection, hyaluronidase, ovine, preservative free, per 1 USP unit (up to 999 USP units)
Water for injection	A4216	Sterile water, saline and/or dextrose, diluent/flush, 10 ml
	A4217	Sterile water/saline, 500 ml
WinRho sdf	J2792	Injection, rho d immune globulin, intravenous, human, solvent detergent, 100 iu
Xeomin	J0588	Injection, incobotulinumtoxin a, 1 unit
Xgeva	J0897	Injection, denosumab, 1 mg
Xolair	J2357	Injection, omalizumab, 5 mg
Xopenex	J7612	Levalbuterol, inhalation solution, fad-approved final product, non-compounded, administered through DME, concentrated form, 0.5 mg
Xopenex	J7614	Levalbuterol, inhalation solution, fad-approved final product, non-compounded, administered through DME, unit dose, 0.5 mg
Xylocaine	J2001	Injection, lidocaine HCL for intravenous infusion, 10 mg
Yondelis	J9999	Not otherwise classified, antineoplastic drugs
Zanosar	J9320	Injection, streptozocin, 1 gm
Zantac	J2780	Injection, ranitidine hydrochloride, 25 mg

NDC LABEL	HCPCS	HCPCS DESCRIPTION
Zembrace symtouch	J3030	Injection, sumatriptan succinate, 6 mg (code may be used for medicare when drug administered under the direct supervision of a physician, not for use when drug is self administered)
Zemplar	J2501	Injection, paricalcitol, 1 mcg
Zithromax	J0456	Injection, azithromycin, 500 mg
	Q0144	Azithromycin dihydrate, oral, capsules/powder, 1 gm
Zmax	Q0144	Azithromycin dihydrate, oral, capsules/powder, 1 gm
Zofran	J2405	Injection, ondansetron hydrochloride, per 1 mg
Zofran	Q0162	Ondansetron 1 mg, oral, fad approved prescription anti-emetic, for use as a complete therapeutic substitute for an iv anti-emetic at the time of chemotherapy treatment, not to exceed a 48 hour dosage regimen
Zofran odt	Q0162	Ondansetron 1 mg, oral, fad approved prescription anti-emetic, for use as a complete therapeutic substitute for an iv anti-emetic at the time of chemotherapy treatment, not to exceed a 48 hour dosage regimen
Zoladex	J9202	Goserelin acetate implant, per 3.6 mg
Zomacton	J2941	Injection, somatropin, 1 mg
Zorbtive	J2941	Injection, somatropin, 1 mg
Zortress	J7527	Everolimus, oral, 0.25 mg
Zosyn	J2543	Injection, piperacillin sodium/tazobactam sodium, 1 gm/0.125 gms (1.125 gms)
Zovirax	J8499	Prescription drug, oral, non chemotherapeutic, nos
Zyvox	J2020	Injection, linezolid, 200 mg